Examination of Musculoskeletal Injuries

Second Edition

Athletic Training Education Series

Sandra J. Shultz, PhD, ATC, CSCS
University of North Carolina at Greensboro
Peggy A. Houglum, PhD, ATC, PT
Duquesne University
David H. Perrin, PhD, ATC
University of North Carolina at Greensboro

David H. Perrin, PhD, ATC
Series Editor

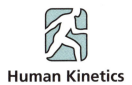

Human Kinetics

Library of Congress Cataloging-in-Publication Data

Shultz, Sandra J., 1961-
    Examination of musculoskeletal injuries / Sandra J. Shultz,
Peggy A. Houglum, David H. Perrin.-- 2nd ed.
        p. ; cm. -- (Athletic training education series)
    Rev. ed of: Assessment of athletic injuries. c2000.
    Includes bibliographical references and index.
    ISBN 0-7360-5138-4 (hard cover)
    1.   Sports injuries--Diagnosis--Examinations, questions, etc. 2.
Sports medicine--Examinations, questions, etc.
    [DNLM: 1.   Athletic Injuries--diagnosis--Examination Questions.
2.   Musculoskeletal System--injuries--Examination Questions. 3.
Physical Education and Training--methods--Examination Questions.
4.   Sports Medicine--methods--Examination Questions. QT 18.2
S562a 2005] I. Houglum, Peggy A., 1948- II. Perrin, David H.,
1954- III. Shultz, Sandra J., 1961- . Assessment of athletic
injuries. IV. Title. V. Series.
    RD97.S5383 2005
    617.1'027'076--dc22

                            2004022788

ISBN: 0-7360-5138-4

This book is a revised edition of *Assessment of Athletic Injuries,* published in 2000 by Human Kinetics.

The Web addresses cited in this text were current as of January 17, 2005, unless otherwise noted.

Acquisitions Editor: Loarn D. Robertson, PhD; **Developmental Editor:** Elaine H. Mustain; **Assistant Editor:** Sandra Merz Bott; **Copyeditor:** Jocelyn Engman; **Proofreader:** Red, Inc.; **Indexer:** Robert Swanson; **Permission Manager:** Dalene Reeder; **Graphic Designer:** Fred Starbird; **Graphic Artist:** Dawn Sills; **Photo Manager:** Kareema McLendon; **Cover Designer:** Keith Blomberg; **Photographer (cover):** Tom Roberts; **Photographers (interior):** Kelly J. Huff and Tom Roberts; **Art Manager:** Kelly Hendren; **Illustrators:** Argosy; **Printer:** Edwards Brothers

Printed in the United States of America   10 9 8 7 6 5 4 3 2 1

Human Kinetics
Web site: www.HumanKinetics.com

United States: Human Kinetics
P.O. Box 5076
Champaign, IL 61825-5076
800-747-4457
e-mail: humank@hkusa.com

Canada: Human Kinetics
475 Devonshire Road Unit 100
Windsor, ON N8Y 2L5
800-465-7301 (in Canada only)
e-mail: orders@hkcanada.com

Europe: Human Kinetics
107 Bradford Road
Stanningley
Leeds LS28 6AT, United Kingdom
+44 (0) 113 255 5665
e-mail: hk@hkeurope.com

Australia: Human Kinetics
57A Price Avenue
Lower Mitcham, South Australia 5062
08 8277 1555
e-mail: liaw@hkaustralia.com

New Zealand: Human Kinetics
Division of Sports Distributors NZ Ltd.
P.O. Box 300 226 Albany
North Shore City
Auckland
0064 9 448 1207
e-mail: blairc@hknewz.com

To my graduate students
Thanks for keeping me sharp!

As iron sharpens iron, so one person sharpens another....
Proverbs 27:17

Sandra J. Shultz

To my students whose daily inquiries toward
understanding and desire for knowledge provide
me with continual challenges, inspirations, and
stimulation. You are *my* teachers.

Peggy A. Houglum

Contents

Chapter 23   Musculoskeletal, Nervous, and Integumentary Conditions

Introduction to the Athletic Training Education Series

The five textbooks of the Athletic Training Education Series—*Introduction to Athletic Training*, *Examination of Musculoskeletal Injuries* (formerly *Assessment of Athletic Injuries*), *Therapeutic Exercise for Musculoskeletal Injuries* (formerly *Therapeutic Exercise for Athletic Injuries*), *Therapeutic Modalities for Musculoskeletal Injuries* (formerly *Therapeutic Modalities for Athletic Injuries*), and *Management Strategies in Athletic Training*—were written for athletic training students and as a reference for practicing certified athletic trainers. Other allied health care professionals, such as physical therapists, physician's assistants, and occupational therapists, will also find these texts to be an invaluable resource in the prevention, examination, treatment, and rehabilitation of injuries to physically active people.

The rapidly evolving profession of athletic training necessitates a continual updating of the educational resources available to educators, students, and practitioners. The authors of the five new editions in the series have made key improvements and have added important information. *Introduction to Athletic Training* includes a revised and simplified chapter on pharmacology. A new part I in *Examination of Musculoskeletal Injuries* makes this text one of the most comprehensive presentations of the foundational techniques for each assessment tool used in injury examination. Updated information on proprioceptive neuromuscular facilitation and sacroiliac joint evaluation and treatment is included in *Therapeutic Exercise for Musculoskeletal Injuries*, and a section on Pilates has been added. In *Therapeutic Modalities for Musculoskeletal Injuries*, a new chapter on evidence-based practice has been added, and the FDA's approval of laser treatment for selected injuries has led to a new chapter on this topic. Finally, the impact of the Health Insurance Portability and Accountability Act and the appropriate medical coverage model of the National Athletic Trainers' Association (NATA) are now addressed in *Management Strategies in Athletic Training*.

The Athletic Training Education Series offers a coordinated approach to the process of preparing students for the Board of Certification examination. If you are a student of athletic training, you must master the material in each of the content areas delineated in the NATA publication *Competencies in Athletic Training*. The Athletic Training Education Series addresses these competencies comprehensively and sequentially while avoiding unnecessary duplication.

The series covers the educational content areas developed by the Education Council of the National Athletic Trainers' Association for accredited curriculum development. These content areas and the texts that address each content area are as follows:

- Risk management and injury prevention (*Introduction* and *Management Strategies*)
- Pathology of injury and illnesses (*Introduction, Examination, Therapeutic Exercise*, and *Therapeutic Modalities*)
- Assessment and evaluation (*Examination* and *Therapeutic Exercise*)
- Acute care of injury and illness (*Introduction, Examination*, and *Management Strategies*)
- Pharmacology (*Introduction* and *Therapeutic Modalities*)
- Therapeutic exercise (*Therapeutic Exercise*)
- General medical conditions and disabilities (*Introduction* and *Examination*)
- Nutritional aspects of injury and illness (*Introduction*)
- Psychosocial intervention and referral (*Introduction, Therapeutic Modalities*, and *Therapeutic Exercise*)
- Health care administration (*Management Strategies*)
- Professional development and responsibilities (*Introduction* and *Management Strategies*)

The authors for this series—Craig Denegar, Susan Hillman, Peggy Houglum, Richard Ray, Ethan Saliba, Susan Saliba, Sandra Shultz, and I—are eight certified athletic trainers with well over a century of collective experience as clinicians, educators, and leaders in the athletic training profession. The clinical experience of the authors spans virtually every setting in which athletic trainers practice, including the high school, sports medicine clinic, college, professional sport, hospital, and industrial settings. The professional positions of the authors include undergraduate and graduate curriculum director, head athletic trainer, professor, clinic director, and researcher. The authors have chaired or served on the NATA's most important committees, including the Professional Education Committee, the Education Task Force, Education Council, Research Committee of the Research and Education Foundation, Journal Committee, Appropriate Medical Coverage for Intercollegiate Athletics Task Force, and Continuing Education Committee.

This series is the most progressive collection of texts and related instructional materials currently available to athletic training students and educators. Several elements are present in all the books in the series:

- Chapter objectives and summaries are tied to one another so that students will know and achieve their learning goals.
- Chapter-opening scenarios illustrate the importance and relevance of the chapter content.
- Cross-referencing among texts offers a complete education on the subject.
- Thorough reference lists allow for further reading and research.

To enhance instruction, each text includes an instructor guide and test bank. *Therapeutic Exercise for Musculoskeletal Injuries, Therapeutic Modalities for Musculoskeletal Injuries*, and *Examination of Musculoskeletal Injuries* each includes a presentation package. Presentation packages (formerly known as graphics packages) are usually in Microsoft PowerPoint format and delivered via CD-ROM. They contain selected illustrations, photos, and tables from the text. Instructors can use these to enhance lectures and demonstration sessions. Other features vary from book to book, depending on the subject matter; but all include various aids for assimilation and review of information, extensive illustrations, and material to help students apply the facts in the text to real-world situations.

Beyond the introductory text by Hillman, the order in which the books should be used is determined by the philosophy of each curriculum director. In any case, each book can stand alone so that a curriculum director does not need to revamp an entire curriculum in order to use one or more parts of the series.

When I entered the profession of athletic training over 25 years ago, one text—*Prevention and Care of Athletic Injuries* by Klafs and Arnheim—covered nearly all the subject matter required for passing the Board of Certification examination and practice as an entry-level athletic trainer. Since that time we have witnessed an amazing expansion of the information and skills one must master in order to practice athletic training, along with an equally impressive growth of practice settings in which athletic trainers work. You will find these updated editions of the Athletic Training Education Series textbooks to be invaluable resources as you prepare for a career as a certified athletic trainer, and you will find them to be useful references in your professional practice.

David H. Perrin, PhD, ATC
Series Editor

Preface

Examination of Musculoskeletal Injuries, formerly known as *Assessment of Athletic Injuries*, is one of five texts in the Athletic Training Education Series. *Examination of Musculoskeletal Injuries* addresses several areas of clinical practice you must master in order to pass the Board of Certification (BOC) examination, including pathology of injury and illnesses, assessment and evaluation, and general medical conditions and disabilities. According to the 2004 Role Delineation Study conducted by Columbia Assessment Services for the National Athletic Trainers' Association (NATA), certified athletic trainers devote approximately 23% of their time to clinical evaluation and diagnosis. Indeed, you will need to master the material in this book in order to properly manage, treat, and rehabilitate athletic injuries.

Each day of your career as a certified athletic trainer will present new challenges, and your ability to recognize, evaluate, and assess athletic injuries will prove essential to properly managing the broad spectrum of injuries you will encounter. These injuries will range from acute to chronic, obvious to subtle, and minor to life threatening. The essential components of the injury examination include obtaining an accurate injury history, inspecting the injured area and related structures, testing active and passive motion, conducting strength and neurological examinations, palpating bony landmarks and soft tissues, and examining function to determine an athlete's readiness to return to unrestricted physical activity. In addition, you will use special tests to isolate relevant structures and identify specific pathologies, including ligament stress testing and fracture examination. The order and extent to which you address these examination components will be determined in part by the injury acuity, the injury setting, and your initial history and observation. *Examination of Musculoskeletal Injuries, Second Edition*, uniquely presents injury examination strategies, dividing them into on-site, acute, and clinical protocols. These protocols allow you to focus your evaluation skills on emergent, nonemergent, and postacute conditions. Checklists provide the framework for developing a systematic approach to injury examination in each setting.

Examination of Musculoskeletal Injuries, Second Edition, is divided into three parts. Part I presents the general principles and foundational skills for each component of the injury examination. Chapters 1 and 2 review injury terminology and classifications and overview the general concepts and rationale for each of the essential components of the examination procedure. Chapters 3 through 9 delve into the specifics of each of these components (history, observation, palpation, range of motion, strength assessment, neurological examination, cardiovascular examination), presenting the goals, purposes, and general principles and techniques that you will need in order to perform the region-specific tests presented in part II. Because special tests are unique to each joint and typically incorporate the principles of several examination techniques, they are addressed in part II as they apply to specific body regions. Chapter 10 concludes part I by incorporating these individual examination components into systematic examination strategies tailored to injury acuity and environment.

Part II of *Examination of Musculoskeletal Injuries, Second Edition*, applies the general principles presented in part I to the recognition and examination of injuries and conditions specific to each body region. Chapters 11 through 20 address each body region and consist of four primary sections. Each chapter opens with functional anatomy, providing a brief overview of the primary anatomical characteristics of the region. Acute and chronic injuries specific to the region are presented next, with the focus on the etiology and signs and symptoms that will help you recognize and differentiate injuries commonly incurred by the physically active. Specific objective tests used to examine each region then follow, including tests for palpation, range of motion, strength, neurovascular status, special tests, and joint mobility. The chapter concludes by incorporating these tests into specific injury examination strategies for on-site injuries, immediate postinjuries, and injuries seen in the treatment facility. One or two scenarios precede the discussion of each examination strategy to orient you to the types of situations you can expect to encounter.

Completing the text, part III addresses the general medical conditions you are most likely to encounter in the physically active. The topics are presented here according to body system as presented in the Athletic Training Educational Competencies (National Athletic Trainers' Association 1999). Chapter 21 covers conditions of the eyes, ears, nose, and throat (EENT), respiratory and cardiovascular systems, and other viral conditions. Chapter 22 covers conditions affecting the digestive, endocrine, reproductive, and urinary systems. Disordered eating and sexually transmitted diseases are also discussed. Chapter 23 closes out part III with the general medical conditions affecting the musculoskeletal, nervous, and integumentary systems, as well as discussing other systemic diseases.

We have designed each chapter of *Examination of Musculoskeletal Injuries, Second Edition,* to optimize your understanding and mastery of the material. All chapters open with objectives that highlight key learning points and follow with a real-life scenario that illustrates the complexity and exciting challenge of athletic injury examination. Each chapter closes with a summary and a list of review and critical thinking questions to help ensure that you have adequately mastered the material. Throughout each chapter, you will find learning aids in the margins: definitions of terms that, while they are not defined in the text, may be unfamiliar to some readers; warnings marked by exclamation points to alert you to procedures you should not omit, as they may make the difference between complete recovery and permanent disability or even death; and facts designated by a lightbulb to remind you of statements made earlier in the text that are important to now recall.

NEW FOR THE SECOND EDITION

Substantial content has been added or revised in the second edition to make it more complete. One of the first things you will notice about the second edition is the global changes in terminology throughout the text, including the title. We have chosen to adopt the term *examination* rather than *assessment* or *evaluation* as we believe this term more purely and accurately defines the process used to identify an injury or illness. This rationale is addressed in detail in chapter 2. Taking the lead from the National Athletic Trainers' Association Board of Directors and the Pew Health Professions Commission, we have revised other terminology to include more of the athletic trainers' scope of practice and the various practice settings in which examination procedures are performed. To that end, you will often see the term *patient* used rather than *athlete*, and we have renamed the examination strategies *on-site, acute,* and *clinical* (formerly *on-field, sideline,* and *off-field*).

Part I presents primarily new content, including more detailed information on the fundamental components of injury examination. These principles are typically taught first in injury examination courses, and we have received consistent feedback that including more detailed information on these topics would be helpful to both instructors and students. Hence, these chapters focus more on the general how-to of each examination technique and provide a common reference point for many of the region-specific chapters in part II. Part I also presents in detail the examination procedures that are common to multiple joints (e.g., neurological and vascular examinations) for following chapters to refer back to. Also new to part I are detailed examination procedures for goniometric measurement, manual muscle testing, upper- and lower-quarter neurological screens, and posture and gait examinations.

Part II has been revised and reorganized to be more complete and streamlined. New to each chapter is a review of functional anatomy that is essential to injury examination for that region. The presentation of injuries specific to each body region is relatively unchanged, except where the discussions of some injuries have been clarified or new injuries have been added. While we have retained the unique presentation of injury examination strategies for various injury situations (on-site, acute, and clinical), we have addressed feedback that the presentation of objective tests in accordance with these examination strategies was confusing in the first edition. To streamline the chapters and give instructors greater flexibility in presenting the material, we have made a number of changes to the objective test section. All pertinent objective tests now appear together in one section preceding the discussion of specific examination strategies. Joint mobility examination has been moved to the end of the objective test section to allow instructors the flexibility to include or not include this advanced examination technique.

New to objective test sections are photos and technique charts for the specific motions tested with manual muscle testing and goniometry. Following the objective tests, situation-specific injury examination strategies focus less on the actual tests and more on the different approaches used for acute versus chronic injuries, as well as more on the general components of the subjective and objective examinations. Scenarios have been added to this section to provide an operational framework for the types of examinations to stimulate class discussion and help students use their clinical reasoning skills to decide which tests are most appropriate for certain situations. For each chapter, checklists have been revised to allow easy reproduction, aiding students by providing a study guide and also helping instructors evaluate student mastery of examination procedures.

The content in part III has also been revised and reorganized to be more complete yet streamlined. Content has been expanded to include more of the medical conditions listed in the educational competencies. New sections have been added for conditions of the musculoskeletal and reproductive systems, and significant content has been added to systemic disease, genitourinary, and cardiovascular sections. With the expanded content, this material now spans three chapters.

Also revised and available for instructors are an instructor guide and graphics package. The instructor guide includes case studies, course projects, chapter worksheets, sample test questions, and a sample course syllabus to assist with lecture and examination preparation. The Microsoft® PowerPoint graphics package is heavily weighted toward presenting the objective tests so that it is easily adaptable to each instructor's lecture content and style.

An exciting new addition to the second edition is a Web-based student resource. At this site, students will find copies of all checklists and pertinent tables that they can print and bring to class or review sessions to facilitate learning. To complement the black and white photos included in chapter 23, color slides for all the dermatological conditions are also available on the Web site for easy viewing. The Web site will remain available to anyone with the correct URL until a subsequent edition becomes available.

We trust you will find this new edition of *Examination of Musculoskeletal Injuries* an indispensable resource for developing your confidence in examining and differentiating the various pathologies that you will encounter over your career as a certified athletic trainer. This book can stand alone. It should be noted, however, that using the entire Athletic Training Education Series will be especially effective in preparing you for the challenging Board of Certification examination and for a gratifying career in athletic training and sports medicine.

Sandra J. Shultz, PhD, ATC, CSCS
Peggy A. Houglum, PhD, ATC, PT
David H. Perrin, PhD, ATC

Acknowledgments

A number of people have contributed to the development of this text whom we wish to recognize. We wish to extend our thanks to Scott T. Doberstein, MS, ATC, and John Cottone, EdD, ATC, for their critique of the first edition and excellent suggestions that were instrumental in significantly revising the second edition. Their efforts were followed by those of Mary Allen Watson, EdD, ATC, and Anthony S. Kulas, MEd, ATC, who reviewed and provided feedback on the newly developed content in part I. Special thanks also goes to Yohei Shimokochi and Elizabeth Spitz, who served as models for the more than 180 new photographs that have been added. We also wish to again acknowledge Dr. Kenneth E. Greer, professor and chairman of the department of dermatology, Dr. Theodore E. Keats, professor of medicine-radiology, the film library staff in the department of radiology, and Dr. Brian C. Hoard, associate professor of medicine-dentistry, all from the University of Virginia Health Sciences, for their assistance in obtaining photographs of dermatological conditions, radiographs of skeletal pathologies, Salter-Harris illustrations, and dental injuries that continue to be significant features in the second edition. This text has been greatly enhanced by the collective contributions of these outstanding individuals.

Finally, we would like to thank our publisher, Rainer Martens, at Human Kinetics, as well as acquisitions editor Loarn Robertson, developmental editor Elaine Mustain, assistant editor Sandra Merz Bott, and photographer Kelly Huff for their support and invaluable contributions to this effort.

Sandra J. Shultz, PhD, ATC, CSCS
Peggy A. Houglum, PhD, ATC, PT
David H. Perrin, PhD, ATC

Credits

Figures 3.1, 11.2, 11.3, 15.2, 16.2, 16.3, 19.1, and 19.2: Reprinted, by permission, from J. Watkins, 1999, *Structure and function of the musculoskeletal system* (Champaign, IL: Human Kinetics), 20, 63, 142, 142, 208, 210, 57, 59.

Figure 4.1 Reprinted, by permission, from B. Abernethy, S.J. Hanrahan, V. Kippers, L.T. Mackinnon, and M.G. Pandy, 2005, *The biophysical foundations of human movement* (Champaign, IL: Human Kinetics), 38.

Figures 5.2, 8.12, 9.5, 11.4, 12.5b, and 18.3: Reprinted, by permission, from R.S. Behnke, 2001, *Kinetic anatomy* (Champaign, IL: Human Kinetics), 13, 254, 260, 130, 42, 137, 186.

Figure 6.8, Chapter 7 Opening Photo, and 7.10: Reprinted, by permission, from P.A. Houglum, 2001, *Therapeutic exercise for athletic injuries* (Champaign, IL: Human Kinetics), 719, 681, 229.

Figure 7.1: Reprinted, by permission, from A.J. McComas, 1996, *Skeletal muscle* (Champaign, IL: Human Kinetics), 5.

Figure 7.9: Reprinted, by permission, from D.H. Perrin, 2005, *Athletic taping and bracing*, 2nd ed. (Champaign, IL: Human Kinetics), 55.

Figure 9.1: Reprinted, by permission, from B.J. Sharkey, 2002, *Fitness & health*, 5th ed. (Champaign, IL: Human Kinetics), 90.

Figure 9.2: Reprinted, by permission, from National Strength and Conditioning Association, 2000, *Essentials of strength training and conditioning*, 2nd ed. eds. T.R. Baechle and R.W. Earle. (Champaign, IL: Human Kinetics), 116.

Figures 11.10 and 14.14: Courtesy of Theodore E. Keats, MD.

Figures 12.1, 12.2, 12.5a, 13.3, and 13.4: Reprinted, by permission, from J. Loudon, S. Bell, and J. Johnston, 1998, *The clinical orthopedic assessment guide* (Champaign, IL: Human Kinetics), 86, 87, 72, 127, 125.

Figures 13.1 and 17.1: Reprinted, by permission, from W.C. Whiting and R.R. Zernicke, 1998, *Biomechanics of musculoskeletal injury* (Champaign, IL: Human Kinetics), 109, 150.

Figures 15.1 and 15.4: Reprinted, by permission, from C.M. Norris, 2000, *Back stability* (Champaign, IL: Human Kinetics), 28, 57.

I
Principles of Examination

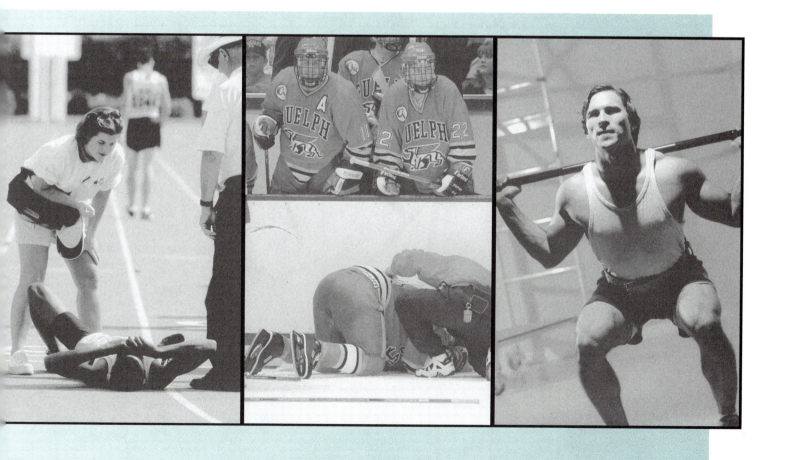

An examination is a systematic procedure through which the athletic trainer determines the severity, irritability, nature, and stage of an injury or illness. Part I of this text presents the principles of athletic injury examination, including the nine primary components of injury examination:

- History
- Observation
- Palpation
- Range of motion
- Strength
- Special tests
- Neurological status
- Circulatory status
- Functional capacity

The extent to which you will use each of these examination techniques and the order that you follow will depend on the specific injury scenario.

Chapter 1 helps you learn the basic injury terminology and classification criteria that are used throughout the text. Chapter 2 introduces the examination process by providing an overview of the goals and essential components of the subjective and objective portions of the examination. Chapters 3 through 9 describe the general terminology, principles, and techniques of the primary examination components, with the exception of special tests and functional tests. Because functional and special tests are unique to each joint and include principles of the other examination techniques (palpation, joint motion, strength, neurological, and circulatory testing), they are addressed as they apply to specific body regions in chapters 11 through 21. Chapter 10 closes part I by incorporating the individual examination components into systematic procedures tailored to injury acuity and environment.

Anatomical Nomenclature and Injury Classifications

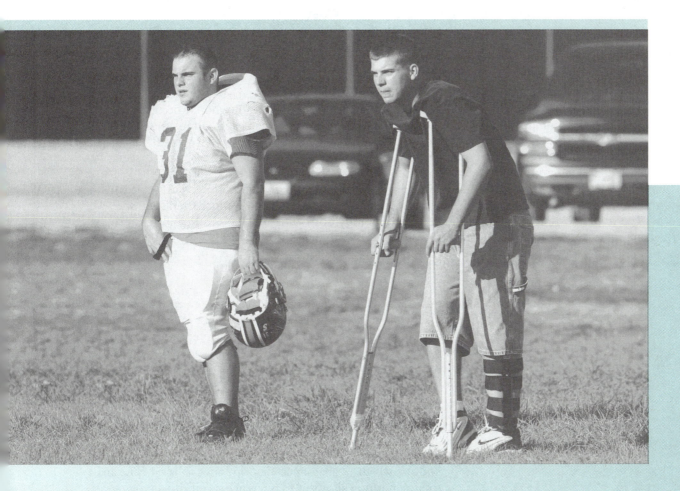

Objectives

After completing this chapter, the reader will be able to do the following:

1. Describe the anatomical reference position
2. Use appropriate terminology to describe the anatomical location and position of a structure relative to the rest of the body
3. Differentiate between a sign and a symptom
4. Classify injuries as either acute or chronic based on the onset and duration of symptoms
5. Define the common chronic inflammatory conditions, including signs and symptoms

6. Define the various classifications of closed soft tissue wounds, including degrees of severity
7. Define and classify closed and open wounds of the bone and joint articulations
8. Classify nerve injuries according to mechanism, severity, and signs and symptoms
9. Identify the classifications of open soft tissue wounds

Diane was looking forward to her new position as the first full-time head athletic trainer at Blue Ridge High School. Before hiring Diane, the school had no certified athletic trainer; a coach (who had taken a couple of athletic training courses in college) and the school nurse worked together to take care of the athletes when injury occurred. It wasn't long after the start of spring football that the athletic training room was packed with injured athletes.

"Steve, what can I help you with?" Diane asked the senior starting quarterback.

"Oh, my knee is acting up again. It seems to do this every year since I first injured it as a freshman. It hurts right here in the front below my kneecap. Coach said I strained it, but the nurse said I had tendinitis . . . so I don't really know what it is," Steve said. "What's the difference, anyway?"

"Well," Diane began to explain, "a strain is typically an acute injury caused by stretching or pulling a muscle or tendon. Tendinitis, on the other hand, is more of a chronic inflammation or irritation of the tendon."

"Chronic? Acute?" Steve asked.

"Sorry," Diane said. "Those are terms we use to describe how your symptoms began or how long you've had them. An acute injury is one that you usually know you have right when it occurs, and symptoms start almost immediately. With a chronic injury, the symptoms usually last longer and often appear gradually over time, and the person can't identify exactly when the injury occurred."

"Well, from what you're saying, tendinitis sounds more like it," Steve answered. "Boy, it sure would be nice, and less confusing, if everyone used the same words to describe my injury!"

Diane couldn't help but agree. She could recall a number of times when it had been difficult to determine an athlete's previous injury based on what the coach called it. Now, more than ever, she appreciated the importance of using consistent terminology both when documenting injuries and when communicating with parents, coaches, and other health professionals.

Clear communication is fundamental to your clinical practice. Proper anatomical reference and injury terminology are essential for communicating effectively with other health professionals and accurately documenting the findings of your examinations. This chapter reviews common anatomical terminology and injury classification systems that will help you both understand this text and clearly articulate the findings of your examinations. With few exceptions, these terms and systems will consistently apply to the different joints and body regions.

ANATOMICAL REFERENCE TERMINOLOGY

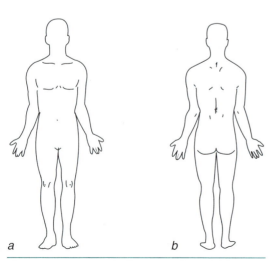

The **anatomical position** is the standardized position of the body on which all anatomical descriptions are based. The anatomical position allows us to reference specific body regions as related to the body as a whole (Moore 1992). It also allows us to describe the relationship of one anatomical landmark to another. For example, we can clearly describe the location of the tibial tubercle by indicating that it is anterior on the proximal tibia, just inferior to the patella. Whenever you refer to a body region or anatomical structure, you will always describe it relative to an anatomical reference position. Doing so will help you avoid confusion and misinterpretation of your findings.

Anatomical position can be described with the body either standing erect or lying **supine** (lying on the back), but it is probably easiest to visualize it as standing (figure 1.1). When the body is standing or lying supine, the head, eyes, and toes point directly forward. This is an anterior (front, or forward) position. The arms are positioned at the patient's side, with the

Figure 1.1 Anatomical position from (a) front and (b) back.

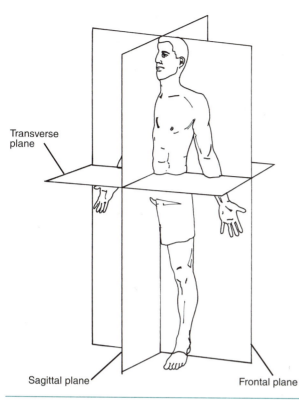

Transverse plane

Sagittal plane

Frontal plane

Figure 1.2 Anatomical planes.

Reprinted, by permission, from L. Cartwright and W.A. Pitney, 1999, *Athletic training for student assistants* (Champaign, IL: Human Kinetics), 4.

palms facing forward, and the lower limbs are straight and together with the feet pointing anteriorly.

From the anatomical reference position, we can define three anatomical planes (figure 1.2). Anatomical planes are imaginary planes that separate the body into left and right (**sagittal**), top and bottom (**transverse**), and front and back (**frontal**). At times, the sagittal plane is referred to as the **anterior–posterior plane**, and the frontal plane is referred to as the **coronal plane**. These planes of reference are useful when describing postural positions (chapter 4) and common movement patterns (chapter 6).

Table 1.1 lists terms that describe the position of body parts in reference to other parts of the body and the body itself in the anatomical reference position. The table also includes synonyms that are usually reserved for particular body regions. For example, **anterior** describes structures on or near the front of the body, while **posterior** describes structures on or near the back. The anterior surface of the hands is also commonly referred to as the palmar or ventral surface, while the posterior surface is also referred to as the dorsal aspect, or dorsum, of the hand.

Table 1.1
Chart of Anatomical Terms

Term	Synonyms	Term defined
Anterior	Ventral Palmar	Toward the front of the body
Posterior	Dorsal	Toward the back side of the body
Superior	Cranial Cephalic	Toward the head
Inferior	Caudal	Moving away from the head toward the feet
Medial		Toward the midline of the body
Lateral		Away from the midline of the body
Proximal		A position or attachment on the body that is in closer proximity to the trunk or origin of reference
Distal		A position or attachment on the body that is farther away from the trunk or origin of reference
Superficial		Nearer to the surface of the skin
Deep		Farther from the surface of the skin
Central		Nearer or closer to the center of a structure or system
Peripheral		Farther away from the center of a structure or system
Visceral		The covering of an internal organ
Parietal		The external wall of a body cavity

Adapted from K.L. Moore, 1992, *Clinically oriented anatomy,* 3rd ed. (Baltimore: Williams & Wilkins).

PHYSICAL MATURITY CLASSIFICATIONS

Physical maturity classifications allow us to define stages of physical growth. This standard classification system describes normal anatomic and physiologic development from infancy to older adulthood. These classifications are particularly relevant to this text in understanding the maturity and strength of the musculoskeletal system, but they are also used for differentiating physiological findings where appropriate (e.g., normal vital signs for child versus adult in chapter 9). Physical maturity is defined by the following classifications:

- **Infant** (0-12 months).
- **Childhood** (1-11 years) spans infancy to the onset of puberty and is characterized by steady growth and development. The skeleton is immature with epiphyseal (growth) plates open to allow bones to elongate. The age range of 1 to 5 years is considered young childhood and 6 to 11 years, middle childhood.
- **Adolescence** (11-13 through 18-20 years) spans the onset of puberty through full skeletal maturity. The onset of puberty is marked by the development of secondary sexual characteristics (pubic hair, menarche, and increased breast development in females; deepening voice and axillary pigmentation and facial hair in males) and peak height growth and weight gain (growth spurt). Skeletal maturity is marked by full closure (ossification, the formation of bone) of the epiphyseal plates and cessation of further growth in height. The age at which different bones complete ossification differs widely, ranging from early teens to early 20s. Because growth and development vary among individuals, it's difficult to name exact age limits. Adolescence begins approximately 2 years earlier in females than in males.
- **Adulthood** (18-40 years) indicates full physical maturity and development. Young adults are those aged 18 to 40 years. In this stage, bone and muscle mass increase through 25 to 30 years of age, after which mass levels off and then slowly declines.
- **Middle adulthood** (40-60 years) is marked by a gradual decline in strength, coordination, and balance.
- **Older adulthood** (greater than 60 years) spans the rest of the human being's life. This stage is marked by accelerating decline in strength, coordination, and balance. However, this decline can be highly individual depending on lifestyle, activity, nutrition, and disease.

INJURY CLASSIFICATIONS

Injuries are classified by the structure involved and the length of time experienced symptoms are present. In some cases subclassifications describe the severity of injury. This section defines the common injury classifications and subclassifications and cardinal signs and symptoms.

Sign Versus Symptom

A cardinal sign or symptom is classic and highly indicative of that condition.

Crepitus is a crackling, grating, or grinding sensation caused by abnormal movement between two structures.

The terms signs and symptoms are two separate injury descriptors rather than synonyms. A **sign** refers to a finding that is observable or that can be objectively measured, such as swelling, discoloration, deformity, **crepitus**, or redness. A **symptom**, on the other hand, denotes a subjective complaint or an abnormal sensation the patient describes that cannot be directly observed. Complaints or perceptions of pain, nausea, altered sensation, and fatigue are symptoms that patients commonly report.

Acute Versus Chronic

Injuries are classified as either acute or chronic. **Acute** injuries are conditions that have a sudden onset and are of short duration. They typically result from a single traumatic event or mechanism. Usually, the athlete clearly knows and recalls the mechanism of injury, as the signs and symptoms associated with the injury typically begin to surface immediately.

Snowball crepitus is a form of crepitus that sounds and feels as if you are compressing or rubbing the surface of a snowball with your fingers.

Chronic injuries, on the other hand, usually have a gradual onset and are of prolonged duration. Many times the exact mechanism or time of injury is not known. Chronic injury usually results from an accumulation of minor insults or repetitive stresses that would not be sufficient to cause injury if the same stress or insult were applied in an isolated event. Consequently, chronic injuries are primarily inflammatory conditions in which the demands on the tissue exceed its ability to heal and recover before additional stress is applied. Common inflammatory conditions are listed in table 1.2. Chronic injury often occurs following periods of inadequate rest or recovery, overuse of a muscle or body part, repetitive overloading of a structure, or repetitive friction between two structures. As such, these injuries may also be referred to as **overuse injuries**. Chronic injuries are often more difficult to treat than acute injuries, as the longer the pathologic state continues, the longer it takes for healing to occur and symptoms to subside.

Table 1.2
Common Chronic Inflammatory Conditions

Condition	Description	Signs and symptoms
Apophysitis	Inflammation of a bony projection or outgrowth that serves as a muscle attachment	Pain, tenderness, swelling, increased bony prominence, pain with muscle tension
Bursitis	Inflammation or swelling of a bursa (synovial-filled membrane that lies between adjacent structures to limit friction and ease movement)	Pain, redness, heat, palpable fluid accumulation, crepitus and/or fluid thickening
Capsulitis	Inflammation of a joint capsule	Pain, localized joint inflammation and swelling, decreased range of motion
Myositis	Inflammatory response in a muscle or its surrounding connective tissue; can lead to ossification	Pain, inflammation, tenderness, decreased range of motion; possible calcium deposit
Neuritis	Inflammation or irritation of a nerve or nerve sheath	Local and referred pain, pain with percussion, tenderness, impaired sensation and motor function
Periostitis	Inflammation of the membranous lining of a bone	Pain, palpable swelling or "bumpiness" and tenderness along the bone; pain with attaching muscle action
Tendinitis	Inflammation of a tendon attaching muscle to bone	Pain, swelling, palpable tenderness and crepitus; pain with active and resistive muscle action
Tendinosis	Microscopic tearing and degeneration of tendinous tissue from repetitive trauma	Chronic pain, palpable tenderness, decreased ROM, pain with passive stretch, pain and weakness with active and resistive muscle action
Tenosynovitis	Inflammation of the synovial sheath covering a tendon	Pain with palpation and movement of the tendon within the sheath; swelling or thickening, snowball crepitus, and decreased range of motion

CLOSED (UNEXPOSED) WOUNDS

Closed wounds include any injury that does not disrupt the surface of the skin. Although closed wounds are not always visually obvious, most result in noticeable signs (e.g., swelling, discoloration, and deformity) that aid in injury examination. Common examples of closed wounds include contusions, ligament sprains, muscle and tendon strains, inflammatory conditions, some bony fractures, joint dislocations, and neurovascular injuries.

Closed Soft Tissue Injuries

Closed injuries to soft tissue can occur as contusions, sprains, or strains. These types of soft tissue injuries are further classified according to the degree of severity or the extent of injury.

Contusion

A contusion, or bruise, refers to the compression of soft tissue by a direct blow or impact sufficient to cause disruption or damage to the small capillaries in the tissue. This trauma will cause local bleeding or hemorrhage, resulting in ecchymosis, or discoloration of the tissue. There will also be localized pain and tenderness. Ecchymosis and swelling may occur immediately or may be delayed, depending on the severity of injury. The severity of a contusion can be described as first degree, second degree, or third degree, usually according to the extent of tissue damage and functional impairment.

- **First degree.** A first-degree contusion involves only superficial tissue damage, causing minimal swelling and localized tenderness and no limitations in strength or range of motion.
- **Second degree.** A second-degree contusion is characterized by increased pain and hemorrhage caused by increased area and depth of tissue damage, resulting in mild to moderate limitations in range of motion, muscle function, or both.

A hematoma is a localized mass or "blood [hema] tumor [toma]" caused by an accumulation of blood in a confined area of a tissue or space.

- **Third degree.** A third-degree contusion is a severe tissue compression, resulting in severe pain, significant hemorrhage, and hematoma formation, as well as severe limitations in range of motion and muscle function. With third-degree contusions, you should suspect strongly that deeper structures (e.g., bone, muscle) may also have been damaged, but that such damage may be masked by the signs and symptoms associated with superficial soft tissue damage.

Sprain

A sprain is an injury to a ligament or capsular structure. Because ligaments attach one bone to another, sprains are associated with joint injury. Sprains result from forces that cause two or more connecting bones to separate or go beyond their normal range of motion, subsequently stretching and tearing the attaching ligament(s) or capsule. To describe the severity or extent of injury, a sprain is further classified as first degree, second degree, or third degree.

End feel is the quality of the feel or sensation felt by the examiner when applying pressure to the joint at the end of the range of motion.

Laxity denotes hypermobility or increased joint movement.

- **First degree.** A first-degree sprain is characterized by mild overstretching and does not cause any visual disruption in the tissue. Signs and symptoms include mild pain and tenderness over the involved ligament and little or no disability. Active and passive range of motions usually are not limited, but the athlete will typically experience pain at the end of the range as the ligament becomes taut. When the joint is stressed, the athlete will complain of pain, but you will notice a firm or definite end feel, without any joint laxity.

With first-degree sprains, inflammation and discoloration are usually minor and may be delayed until the next day. However, in some body regions, such as the lateral ankle, a relatively minor sprain can cause considerable and rapid swelling if a major capillary running adjacent to the ligament is disrupted. In other words, the degree of swelling and discoloration is not always a good indication of injury severity.

Stress testing *is a method of applying tension to a joint to evaluate the integrity of a ligament.*

Instability *is an abnormal joint movement caused by disruption of ligament or capsular integrity.*

- **Second degree.** With a second-degree injury, further stretching and partial disruption or macrotearing of the ligament occur. Second-degree injuries represent the broadest range of injury; therefore the severity of signs and symptoms and disability vary considerably. Signs and symptoms range from moderate to severe pain, point tenderness, ecchymosis, and swelling. Range of motion and normal function are usually limited secondary to pain and swelling. **Stress testing** will show varying degrees of joint instability (laxity), but the ligament will still be sufficiently intact to feel an end point where joint motion ceases.

- **Third degree.** A third-degree sprain is characterized by complete disruption (rupture) or loss of ligament integrity. The athlete may have felt or heard a "pop" at the time of injury. Signs and symptoms include immediate pain and disability, rapid swelling, ecchymosis, and loss of function. Stress testing of the ligament will reveal moderate to severe joint instability, and there will be no firm end feel or end point to joint motion. Third-degree injuries can be initially deceiving in that range of motion and stress testing are typically less painful than with second-degree injuries, since no tension is placed on the injured structure if it is completely torn.

Strains

Dyssynchrony *is a misfiring or mistiming of a muscle contraction.*

Whereas sprains involve stretching or tearing of a ligament, **strains** involve stretching or tearing of a muscle or tendon. Muscle and tendon strains occur most often as a result of a violent, forceful contraction or overstretching of the myotendon unit. Fatigue, lack of proper warm-up, and muscle imbalance or dyssynchrony are common predisposing factors. Similar to sprains, strains are classified by severity as first-degree, second-degree, and third-degree injuries.

- **First degree.** A first-degree strain is characterized by overstretching and microtearing of the muscle or tendon, but there is no gross fiber disruption. The athlete will complain of mild pain and tenderness but will typically have a full active and passive range of motion and little or no disability. Pain will usually accompany resisted muscle contraction. Following a first-degree strain, it is not uncommon for an athlete to continue to practice or compete, as pain and tenderness are often delayed until the next day.

- **Second degree.** Second-degree strains involve further stretching and partial tearing of muscle or tendon fibers. As with sprains, second-degree strains represent the broadest range of injury, and signs and symptoms can vary considerably. These include immediate pain, localized tenderness, and disability. Varying degrees of swelling, ecchymosis, decreased range of motion, and decreased strength will also be noted. The athlete will complain of pain with active muscle contraction and passive muscle stretch. Depending on injury severity, there may or may not be a palpable defect.

Palpable *means detectable by touching or feeling.*

- **Third degree.** In third-degree strains, a muscle or tendon is completely ruptured. Signs and symptoms include an audible pop, immediate pain, and loss of function of the myotendon unit. There will be a palpable defect in superficial muscles. Muscle hemorrhage and diffuse swelling will be present. Depending on the function or contribution of the injured muscle or tendon for a given movement, range of motion and strength may or may not be affected and may or may not be painful.

Bone and Joint Articulations

Articulation *refers to a union (joint) between two bones.*

The general classifications of closed wounds involving disruptions in a bone, joint surface, or joint articulation include fractures, dislocations, and subluxations.

Closed Fractures

Simple, or closed, fractures involve disruption in the continuity of a bone without disruption of the skin surface. Traumatic fractures are caused by direct impact or by an indirect force that exceeds the tensile strength of the bone. The direction of force or impact often dictates the type of fracture that results. Repetitive forces or impact at lower applied loads can also

Table 1.3
Classifications of Closed Fractures

Classification	Illustration	Description
Comminuted		Fracture resulting in multiple fragments or shattering of the bone at the site of injury.
Compression		Failure of the bone and subsequent compression or impaction of the fracture ends due to axial compression forces.
Greenstick		Incomplete fracture through the bone, most often occurring in young bones. Resembles the breaking of a "green stick."
Oblique		The fracture line extends obliquely or diagonally in relation to the long axis of the bone.
Spiral		An S-shaped fracture line that twists around and through the bone due to rotation or torsional forces.
Transverse		The fracture line runs transverse or horizontal to the long axis of the bone. Usually caused by direct lateral impact or stress failure.
Avulsion		The pulling away of a piece of bone secondary to tensioning of an attaching ligament, tendon, or muscle.
Osteochondral		A fracture that extends through the articular cartilage (i.e., joint surface) and into the underlying bone.
Stress of "fatigue"		Complete or incomplete failure of a bone due to repetitive stress or loading. Weakening and failure occur when bone breakdown/absorption exceeds bone production.

cause chronic weakening or failure of bone tissue resulting in a **stress fracture**. Table 1.3 presents the common classifications of closed fractures.

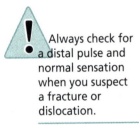

Always check for a distal pulse and normal sensation when you suspect a fracture or dislocation.

• **Traumatic (acute) fractures.** Signs and symptoms of a traumatic fracture include immediate pain, rapid swelling, bony tenderness, crepitus with movement of the bony fragments, and possible deformity if the fracture is displaced. False joint movement may also occur when the fracture is near a movable joint. With displaced fractures (misalignment of the bony fragments), there is always a danger of secondary injury (compression or tearing) to the surrounding soft tissue and neurovascular structures. Therefore, the examination process should always include determination of neurovascular status distal to the suspected fracture site.

For details on immediate care and immobilization of suspected fractures, refer to *Introduction to Athletic Training, Second Edition,* (Hillman 2005), chapter 8.

• **Stress fractures.** Signs and symptoms of stress fractures are not usually quite so obvious, and often the athlete initially dismisses them. The onset of pain is often gradual, but may appear suddenly once bone failure occurs. Pain or a deep ache may at first be noticeable only during activity and may subside with rest, progressing to more constant pain if the offending activity continues. Swelling will be minimal, and there will be localized tenderness over the fracture site.

Epiphyseal Injury

Epiphyseal injury or fracture involves the disruption or separation of the **epiphysis** or epiphyseal plate (growth plate). Epiphyseal injury is a concern in children and in adolescents before the cessation of growth, as disruption can cause premature closing and growth abnormalities in the involved bone. The most widely accepted classification system is the **Salter-Harris** classification system (Harris 1983) (see table 1.4). Signs and symptoms are consistent with those previously mentioned for closed fractures.

Dislocation

Joint **dislocation**, or **luxation**, is a complete disassociation of two joint surfaces. Joint dislocation most commonly results from forces that cause the joint to exceed its normal range of motion, forcing the bony articulation to separate. Consequently, joint dislocation usually involves severe stretching or complete disruption of the capsule and one or more of the supporting ligaments (third-degree sprain). Signs and symptoms include immediate pain, rapid swelling, deformity, and loss of function. As with displaced fractures, signs and symptoms associated with neurovascular impairment (impingement or tearing) may also be present and should be monitored. In some instances, joint dislocation may not be obvious if the joint spontaneously reduces immediately following the injury. In the case of a spontaneous reduction, the athlete may complain of a feeling of the joint slipping or "giving out," or a sensation of the joint "going out and coming back in." Chronic joint instability often follows an acute dislocation, precipitating recurrent episodes of dislocation or subluxation (see the next section) at lower forces and applied loads. This is particularly true of the patellofemoral, glenohumeral, and phalangeal joints.

Table 1.4
Salter-Harris Classifications of Epiphyseal Fractures

Classification	Illustration	Description
Type I		Complete separation of the epiphyseal plate (epiphysis from the metaphysis). No associated fracture.
Type II		Separation of the epiphysis with associated fracture of the metaphysis.
Type III		Fracture of the epiphysis extending from the ephiphyseal plate through the articular surface.
Type IV		Fracture extending through the ephiphysis, epiphyseal plate, and metaphysis
Type V		Crushing or compression of the epiphyseal plate. This injury has a high incidence of premature closure.

Descriptions adapted from R.B. Salter, 1999, *Textbook of disorders and injuries of the musculoskeletal system,* 3rd ed. (Philadelphia, PA: Lippincott, Wilkins & Wilkins).

Subluxation

Subluxation of a joint is an incomplete disassociation of two joint surfaces. Depending on the degree of subluxation, these injuries widely vary in signs and symptoms of pain, disability, swelling, and joint instability. Often, subluxations are difficult to identify, as deformity may be minimal and they often spontaneously reduce. History becomes important when identifying these injuries, and the athlete may complain of a sensation of the joint's slipping or momentarily giving out at the time of injury.

Nerve Injuries

Ischemia is tissue anemia caused by lack of blood flow to an area.

Nerve injury can result from compression or tensioning of the neural structure. Nervous tissue is very sensitive to compression and ischemia, and injury may occur secondary to a direct blow, acute swelling of tissue within an enclosed space, or any pathology that compromises the space through which the nerve courses. Laceration of the nerve can occur secondary to fracture, dislocation, penetrating trauma, or excessive tensioning or stretch. Signs and symptoms of pain, sensation, and motor function can vary considerably depending on the extent of nerve injury. Sensory impairment can range from **anesthesia** (no sensation) to **paresthesia** (tingling, burning, or numbness) to **hyperesthesia** (hypersensitivity), and motor function can range from no loss in muscle strength or function to weakness to complete loss of muscle function (paralysis).

Classifications for the extent of nerve disruption include neuropraxia, axonotmesis, and neurotmesis.

• The least severe nerve disruption is a **neuropraxia**, a transient and reversible loss in nerve function secondary to trauma or irritation. Neuropraxia entails mechanical deformation of the nerve but no disruption of the nerve fibers. Signs and symptoms of sensory and motor deficits are short-lived, ranging from a few seconds to two weeks depending on the extent of nerve trauma. A direct blow over the peroneal nerve at the proximal fibular head or the ulnar nerve at the medial elbow is a common mechanism for a neuropraxia.

• **Axonotmesis** denotes a partial disruption in the nerve. With an axonotmesis, sufficient nervous tissue is intact to allow eventual regeneration. However, signs and symptoms of sensory and motor deficits will be prolonged, lasting anywhere from two weeks to up to one year, so that considerable atrophy and weakness may result.

• **Neurotmesis**, the most severe nerve injury, is characterized by complete severance of the nerve, resulting in permanent loss of function of the innervated structures distal to the point of injury. With a neurotmesis, no regeneration is evident one year after the injury.

Other terms used to describe nerve pathology include neuralgia and neuroma.

• **Neuralgia** is an achiness or pain along the distribution of a nerve secondary to chronic irritation or inflammation. Neuralgia is a common symptom in nerve compression syndromes such as tarsal tunnel syndrome, ulnar nerve compression, carpal tunnel syndrome, and disc herniation. These syndromes will be discussed later in this text.

• A **neuroma** is a thickening of a nerve, or "nerve tumor," secondary to chronic irritation or inflammation.

OPEN (EXPOSED) WOUNDS

Open, or exposed, **wounds** are injuries that involve a disruption in the continuity of the skin, caused by friction or by blunt or sharp trauma. The classifications for open wounds are listed in table 1.5.

• An **abrasion**, or "strawberry," is particularly painful because of the large surface area that is exposed. Abrasions most commonly occur in soccer, baseball, and softball as a result of sliding. Floor burns are also abrasions, a consequence of sliding or of friction against a wooden floor as commonly occurs in basketball and volleyball. The use of knee pads in such

Table 1.5
Classification of Open (Exposed) Wounds

Classification	Description
Abrasion	Broad scraping or shearing off of the superficial skin layers with sliding of the skin against a rough or high-friction surface.
Blister	Separation and accumulation of fluid or blood between superficial skin layers secondary to repetitive friction or shearing movements.
Incision	A cut through all layers of the skin by a sharp object or instrument (e.g., knife), resulting in smooth, even wound edges.
Laceration	A tearing of the skin by blunt trauma to the skin over a bony prominence, resulting in jagged, uneven wound edges.
Puncture	A small disruption in the skin, caused by a sharp, penetrating object. Puncture wounds should be carefully examined for possible injury to underlying structures.
Avulsion	A tearing off or complete disassociation of a portion of skin.
Compound fracture/dislocation	Disruption in the skin surface secondary to penetration by a displaced fracture fragment or joint dislocation.

sports is effective in preventing these minor but painful superficial skin wounds. Signs and symptoms include a burning or stinging pain and minimal bleeding. It is important to cleanse these wounds thoroughly, making sure to remove all the dirt and debris to avoid infection.

• A blister—common in nonathletes as well as athletes—is an area of skin that is exposed to excessive friction or rubbing. Friction from new or ill-fitting shoes in the heel or toe region is a common cause of blisters in physically active people. Gymnasts and baseball and softball players commonly get blisters on the hands as a consequence of repetitive friction and rubbing between the hands and the bar or bat. Signs and symptoms include pain, redness, and accumulation of fluid (may be clear, serous, or blood-filled) between the superficial skin layers. Although the injury the blister creates is usually minor, the pain can be extremely limiting. It is important to avoid puncturing or removing the superficial skin layer, as pain and chance of infection are often significantly increased with exposure of the deeper tissue layers. Early examination and recognition of "hot spots" on the skin showing areas of friction, as well as the use of proper padding, can help prevent a blister from forming.

• An incision is usually caused by a knife or sharp object that makes a clean cut through the full thickness of the skin. Signs and symptoms include an observable disruption in the skin, possible separation or gapping of the wound edges if the skin is under tension, immediate bleeding, and minimal pain. Even small incisions in areas that are highly vascularized, such as the face, can cause considerable bleeding initially, although such bleeding can be quickly controlled with direct pressure.

• A laceration differs from an incision in that the cause is a blunt, rather than a sharp, trauma. With a laceration, the skin basically ruptures when a blunt force is exerted against a bony prominence. An elbow hitting an opponent's cheek during a rebound, a ball striking the eyebrow region, and a blocker making contact with an opponent's chin are common mechanisms for lacerations. Signs and symptoms are consistent with those of an incision, except that because the tissue is torn rather than cut, the wound edges are more jagged, and the blunt force may result in greater pain.

• A puncture wound can result when a pointed, sharp object penetrates the skin. These injuries can be deceiving in that there seems to be little observable tissue damage, and bleeding is often minimal. Evaluating and caring for puncture wounds should involve two primary concerns. If the depth of penetration is beyond the thickness of the skin layers, deeper structures that are not visible may be injured or damaged. In addition, puncture wounds are particularly susceptible to infection because they are difficult to clean given the limited exposure of the involved tissue.

- An **avulsion** is characterized by the complete tearing away of a portion of skin. The range of severity and signs and symptoms can be great, depending on the structures involved and the amount of tissue damage. A simple skin avulsion, the most common type, typically results when the skin is either caught on an unyielding object or pinched between two objects. Depending on the mechanism and the offending trauma, underlying tissues such as muscle, tendon, bone, and even an entire limb (amputation) can be torn away along with the skin, but these severe injuries rarely result from trauma incurred during physical activity.

Open wounds may be associated with an underlying (unexposed) injury. Paying careful attention to the mechanism by which the injury occurred, as well as to signs and symptoms that may be in addition to or out of proportion with what you would expect of the open wound, is important when evaluating these injuries. An obvious example is a **compound fracture** or **compound dislocation**. This injury occurs when a displaced fracture or joint penetrates the surface of the skin so that the bone or joint is exposed. Compound fractures and dislocations are most common in the fingers, but can occur with any joint dislocation or displaced long bone fracture. Crushing injuries that compress the soft tissue against the underlying bone and deeper tissue are another example of an open wound with an associated unexposed tissue injury.

Also of importance in evaluating and caring for open wounds is the use of proper precautions in the presence of blood or seeping wounds. Open, or exposed, wounds are also susceptible to infection and should be monitored for signs and symptoms of pus, increased pain, redness, swelling, heat, and red streaks running from the wound toward the trunk. If signs or symptoms of infection are present, the athlete should be referred for medical treatment and possible antibiotic therapy.

For further discussion of precautions in caring for open wounds, refer to *Introduction to Athletic Training, Second Edition,* (Hillman 2005), chapter 8.

SUMMARY

1. Describe the anatomical reference position.

   The anatomical reference position refers to the body standing erect or lying supine, with the head, eyes, and trunk facing forward; the arms at the side and palms facing forward; and the legs straight and together with the feet pointing forward.

2. Use appropriate anatomical terminology to describe the location and position of a structure relative to the rest of the body.

   A variety of terms describe the position and location of a body part. To define the position of a body part in relation to the body, positional terms such as anterior, posterior, superior, and inferior are used. To compare the position of one body part to another, terms such as lateral, medial, proximal, and distal are used. The use of these universally acceptable terms will help you communicate the findings of your examination to other health care professionals.

3. Classify injuries as either acute or chronic based on the onset and duration of symptoms.

   Injuries are classified as either acute or chronic. Acute injuries have a known mechanism and sudden onset; signs and symptoms usually surface immediately or shortly after the injury. Chronic injuries have a gradual onset and long duration. Often the person does not recall a specific mechanism of injury, and injury results from a repetitive stress over time.

4. Define the common chronic inflammatory conditions, including signs and symptoms.

Chronic inflammatory conditions can result from repetitive overuse, mechanical loading, and friction. A variety of tissues are susceptible to chronic inflammation, including bone, bursa, capsule, muscle, and tendon. Terms used to describe inflammatory conditions of various structures contain the suffix *itis*—for example, bursitis (inflammation of the bursa) and tendinitis (inflammation of the tendon).

5. Define the various classifications of closed soft tissue wounds, including degrees of severity.

Closed soft tissue wounds are generally classified as contusions (soft tissue compression), strains (stretching or tearing of muscle or tendon), and sprains (stretching or tearing of ligament). They are further classified by severity as first, second, or third degree. First-degree injuries, the least severe, are characterized by minimal pain and tissue disruption, and no loss of function. Second-degree injuries are injuries with moderate or partial tissue disruption. The signs, symptoms, and functional impairment associated with second-degree injuries can vary considerably, depending on the extent of tissue disruption. Third-degree injuries are the most severe; these are characterized by complete tissue disruption and severe functional impairment.

6. Define and classify closed and open wounds of the bone and joint articulations.

Injuries involving the bone or joint articulation include fractures and dislocations. A fracture occurs when the continuity of a bone is disrupted. Fractures are typically classified by the type, location, and extent of bony disruption, which is often dictated by the impact mechanism. When disassociation of two articular surfaces of a joint occurs, the injury is classified as either a dislocation (complete disassociation) or subluxation (partial disassociation), and is often accompanied by varying degrees of disruption in the supporting ligaments. Fractures or dislocations can be classified as open (compound) or closed wounds, depending on whether the displaced bone or joint segment penetrates the surface of the skin.

7. Classify nerve injuries according to mechanism, severity, and signs and symptoms.

Nerve injury can result from either compressive or tensioning forces placed on nerve tissues. Classifications for the extent of nerve disruption include neuropraxia, axonotmesis, and neurotmesis. Other terms used to describe more chronic nerve pathologies include neuralgia and neuroma. When an injury involves the nerve, there will be transient or permanent alterations in sensation and motor function, with signs and symptoms varying widely, depending on the extent of injury.

8. Identify the classifications of open (exposed) wounds.

Open wounds, or injuries that disrupt the continuity of the skin, are classified by the type of tissue disruption. Because the wound is exposed, you must use proper precautions when examining and treating these injuries and you should always closely monitor the wound for signs of infection.

REVIEW QUESTIONS

1. Compare and contrast the following injury terms, giving three or four examples of each:
   - Proximal versus distal
   - Lateral versus medial
   - Sign versus symptom
   - Closed (unexposed) versus open (exposed) wounds
   - Acute versus chronic

2. What is the difference between a strain and a sprain? Include in your discussion the common mechanisms and the ways in which the severity of these injuries is defined.

3. In the young athlete, what type of fractures might you expect that you wouldn't see in an adult?

4. How are joint dislocations and subluxations related to joint sprains?

5. Describe the grades of nerve injuries and the signs and symptoms associated with each.

6. List and describe the classifications of open wounds. What are some of the precautions and complications that you should be concerned about when dealing with open wounds?

7. For each of the following injuries, classify each as either acute or chronic and open or closed. Using proper classification terminology, describe what you believe the injury is.

   • A cut over the cheekbone caused by impact with another player's head.
   • Pain, tenderness, and crepitus in the Achilles tendon that has been present for more than 8 weeks.
   • Immediate localized swelling and discoloration over the shinbone after being struck by a baseball.
   • Enlargement of the bony prominence where the patellar tendon attaches to the tibia.
   • A turned ankle that causes pain, swelling, and discoloration. There is some joint laxity, but there is a definite end feel when applying pressure at the end of the motion.

CRITICAL THINKING QUESTIONS

1. Describe the position of the following structures using anatomical reference terms:
   • The hand relative to the elbow (1) with the arm at the side and (2) with the arm extended out in front.
   • The sole of the foot relative to anatomical reference position.
   • The top of the shoulder.
   • The scapula (1) on the trunk and (2) relative to the shoulder joint.
   • The patella relative to (1) the knee joint and (2) femur bone.
   • The left lung relative to the heart.

2. An athlete comes to you complaining of chronic pain in the anterior aspect of the knee. Given the anatomical structures in this area, what types of chronic inflammatory conditions might you suspect? Do you think you might be able to differentiate which structure is involved based on the signs and symptoms? Why or why not?

3. A worker comes into the industrial clinic complaining of pain, paresthesia, and muscle weakness in the lower leg. What types of nerve injuries might be associated with these signs and symptoms? Can you give examples of acute and chronic injury mechanisms that may cause these symptoms?

4. Over the phone, you are asked by a physician to describe an ankle injury. What are some of the important terms you would use to classify the type and severity of the injury in order to provide the physician with as much information as possible?

5. You are called onto the track where a sprinter is lying on the ground complaining of pain in the posterior thigh. She tells you that she was doing 60 m time trials and felt a pop and immediate pain in the muscle. In your examination, you note immediate swelling and a palpable defect on the medial side of the midposterior thigh. The athlete

is able to flex the knee with minimal discomfort, but she says it feels very weak. How would you classify this muscle injury? How would you rate the severity of injury based on these symptoms? Give reasons.

CITED REFERENCES

Harris, R.B. 1983. *Textbook of disorders and injuries of the musculoskeletal system.* 2nd ed. Baltimore: Williams & Wilkins.

Moore, K.L. 1992. *Clinically oriented anatomy.* 3rd ed. Baltimore: Williams & Wilkins.

ADDITIONAL RESOURCES

Hall, S.J. 1999. *Basic biomechanics.* 3rd ed. Boston: McGraw-Hill.

Hillman, S.K. 2004. *Introduction to athletic training.* 2nd ed. Champaign, IL: Human Kinetics.

Mosby's medical, nursing, and allied health dictionary. 2002. 6th ed. St. Louis: Mosby, Harcourt Health Sciences.

Thomas, C.L., ed. 1997. *Taber's cyclopedic medical dictionary.* 18th ed. Philadelphia: Davis.

Wilmore, J.H., and D.L. Costill. 2004. *Physiology of sport and exercise.* 3rd ed. Champaign, IL: Human Kinetics.

CHAPTER 2

Principles of Examination: An Overview

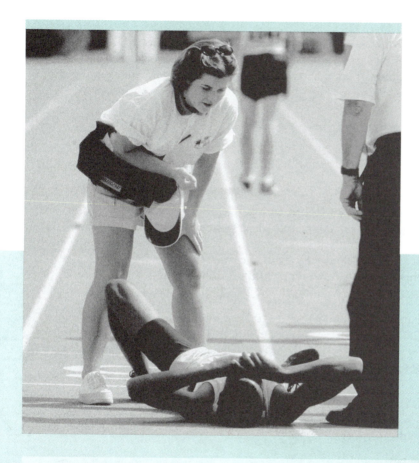

Objectives

After completing this chapter, the reader will be able to do the following:

1. Identify the two main segments that make up an examination
2. Explain the purpose and the components of the subjective segment
3. Identify the SINS of injury examination
4. Identify the general examination procedures of the objective segment
5. Explain the SOAP notes procedure for injury documentation

Throughout the initial week of Patrick's first semester in the professional phase of his athletic training program, he was enthralled with the way Mary Ann, his approved clinical instructor (ACI), examines patients. Patrick noticed that she follows the same procedure whether she is evaluating a knee sprain, a shoulder strain, or a case of Achilles tendinitis. Patrick also noticed that the tests Mary Ann uses during her examinations vary. So he asked her why she follows the same procedure each time and why she sometimes uses different tests for different injuries.

Patrick did well to observe Mary Ann's procedure for injury examinations. This chapter takes a bird's-eye view of each section of the examination process, and the remainder of part I delves into the specifics of each section. This chapter also details how to record your findings from each examination using SOAP notes.

PROPER USE OF TERMINOLOGY

Terminology, as discussed in chapter 1, must be defined so that all parties can communicate accurately and confidently.

An **assessment** is a procedure through which the clinician determines the severity, irritability, nature, and stage (SINS) of an injury. An **evaluation** is the systematic process that allows the clinician to make a clinical judgment. The assessment techniques and the evaluation processes that are used for identifying the injury and determining its care are so closely aligned that allied health professionals use the terms *assessment* and *evaluation* interchangeably. Furthermore, they use these terms in a manner that differs from common usage. For example, *Merriam-Webster's Collegiate Dictionary, Eleventh Edition,* (2003) defines *assess* as follows:

> **1 :** to determine the rate or amount of (as a tax) **2 a :** to impose (as a tax) according to an established rate **b :** to subject to a tax, charge, or levy **3 :** to make an official valuation of (property) for the purposes of taxation **4 :** to determine the importance, size, or value of (~ a problem) **5 :** to charge (a player or team) with a foul or penalty.

According to the same source, *evaluate* is defined as follows:

> **1 :** to determine or fix the value of **2 :** to determine the significance, worth, or condition of usu. by careful appraisal and study.

Examine is defined as follows:

> **1 a :** to inspect closely **b :** to test the condition of **c :** to inquire into carefully : INVESTIGATE **2 a :** to interrogate closely (~ a prisoner) carefully **b:** to test by questioning in order to determine progress, fitness, or knowledge ~ *vi.* : to make or give an examination.

Given these definitions, it seems most appropriate to use "examination" rather than "evaluation" or "assessment."

As often happens, daily practice affixes terminology so that it becomes part of the common language over time. Allied health professionals commonly refer to the examination process as "evaluating" or "assessing" the patient, but in the strictest sense of these words, this usage is incorrect. A patient is *examined*, not evaluated or assessed. It is only after health care professionals complete an examination that they assess or evaluate the results in order to determine a physical diagnosis and provide the most appropriate care or referral for the injury.

Another term that warrants discussion is *diagnosis*. When can you appropriately use this term? Taber's *Cyclopedic Medical Dictionary* (1993) defines **diagnosis** as follows:

1. The term denoting name of the disease or syndrome a person has or is believed to have. **2.** The use of scientific and skillful methods to establish the cause and nature of a person's illness. This is done by obtaining the history of the disease process; the signs and symptoms present; laboratory data; special tests such as X ray pictures and electrocardiograms. The value of establishing a diagnosis is to provide a logical basis for treatment and prognosis.

Taber's defines *physical diagnosis* as "diagnosis by external examination only," and *medical diagnosis* as "the entire process of determining the cause of the patient's illness or discomfort." A physician is the only one who has the authority to perform or order all necessary diagnostic tests required for the medical diagnosis, so this definition does not apply to athletic trainers and other allied health professionals.

Athletic trainers are within their standard of practice when they provide a diagnosis, physical diagnosis, athletic training diagnosis, or diagnostic label to an injury. Other allied health professions such as occupational therapy and physical therapy teach students to diagnose within their own practice parameters. Athletic trainers should not hesitate to use the term *diagnosis* when discussing examination conclusions. All allied health professionals, however, should refrain from using the term *medical diagnosis*, since it is exclusively identified with physicians.

Thus, although *examination* is a more accurate term, the terms *evaluation* and *assessment* have become part of common terminology and are easily recognized and accepted by all allied health professionals. *Diagnosis* and *physical diagnosis* are terms allied health professionals use to identify the results of their patient examination, while *medical diagnosis* is reserved for the diagnosis made by physicians. This text predominately uses *examination*, but it occasionally uses *assessment* and *evaluation*, not because they are correct but because they are familiar. Ultimately, allied health professionals should consider changing the way they converse to more accurately reflect what they do, and consistently use the terms *examination* and *diagnosis*.

EXAMINATION COMPONENTS

Before clinicians can make a diagnosis, they must thoroughly examine the injury by sequentially performing specific examination components. Some situations require more components than others. An introduction to all examination components follows, and chapter 10 presents their appropriate use.

Injury Survey

When an injury occurs, you must first eliminate any critical or life-threatening concerns before evaluating the injury itself. This initial process is called the injury survey. The injury survey is divided into primary and secondary surveys.

Primary Survey

A **primary survey** determines the status of life-threatening or limb-threatening conditions using the **ABCs** of emergency medical care: **a**irway, **b**reathing, and **c**irculation. Limb-threatening conditions include loss of pulse, severe bleeding, and neural compromise. Depending on the results of this primary survey you will either tend to these emergency conditions or move on to the secondary survey.

Secondary Survey

If the injured athlete is breathing and you have any bleeding under control, move on to a secondary examination to determine the presence of other injuries. The term *secondary* indicates that the primary survey has either been concluded or deemed unnecessary. A **secondary survey** is a rapid examination of the seriousness of the injury before the athlete is moved. The conclusions you draw from a secondary survey determine how you should remove a patient from the injury site. Both the primary and secondary surveys are outlined in more detail in chapter 10.

The remainder of this chapter introduces the elements of the injury examination that begins when you have completed your immediate surveys. Every examination includes a subjective and an objective segment, each of which is divided into other elements. Both segments focus on investigating the **SINS**—**s**everity, **i**rritability, **n**ature, and **s**tage—of an injury.

SINS

The subjective and objective segments of an examination create the total picture of an injury, identifying the SINS brings that picture into focus. Here is a look at each of the SINS elements.

Severity

The severity of the injury determines whether or not you refer the patient to a physician or other medical specialist. Most injuries involve soft tissue: ligament, capsule, fascia, tendon, and muscle. These soft tissue injuries are more often overuse injuries or acute first- or second-degree injuries and are less often third-degree injuries. While obviously you will refer the more severe injuries to a physician, you should never hesitate to refer injuries if you are unsure of their severity or what their proper disposition should be.

The severity of an injury is categorized as mild, moderate, or severe. You identify severity by the magnitude of the signs and symptoms: The more intense the signs and symptoms, the more severe the injury. A first-degree ankle sprain with little edema and pain is classified as mild, but a third-degree ankle sprain with laxity, intense pain, and significant edema is severe and requires referral.

Refer to chapter 1 for the full definitions of *mild, moderate,* and *severe* used for classifying first-, second-, and third-degree sprains and strains.

Irritability

The irritability of an injury relates to its stage, its extent, the structures injured, and the patient's level of pain tolerance. If you have not witnessed the injury but initially see the patient in your treatment facility (clinical examination), the injury history provides you with the irritability of the injury. Irritability is classified as mild, moderate, or severe based on the intensity of pain, the amount of time the pain has been present, and how much the pain interferes with activity and sleep. For example, if the person reports frequent episodes of severe pain (7-10 on a 10-point scale) with little relief, is unable to sleep through the night because of pain, and is often uncomfortable even without activity, the injury is very irritable. On the other hand, if the reports of pain are mild to moderate (0-3 or 4-6 on a 10-point scale, respectively) and the patient is able to perform his sport, although perhaps not optimally, the injury is minimally or moderately irritable.

You should identify the irritability of an injury before performing any tests. If the injury is very irritable, you will be unable to complete your examination because the patient will be unable to tolerate it. In this case, use an abbreviated examination that provides only the key information you need to begin treatment, deferring other tests until the irritability lessens. As a general rule, the less irritable the injury is, the more complete the examination can be.

Nature

The nature of the injury is classified according to the type of injury and the structure involved. A sprain or dislocation is an injury of a ligament or capsule, a strain is an injury of a muscle or tendon, a fracture is an injury of a bone, and an open wound is an injury of the skin and possibly other structures. Injury to inert tissue such as ligament, capsule, and bone causes pain with active and passive movement, whereas injury to muscle and tendon usually causes pain with active but not passive movement. Although the history helps you determine the nature of an injury, you must confirm your suspicions through special tests. These special tests are presented later in the chapters in part II.

Refer to chapter 1 for more information on injury classifications.

Stage

With an on-site or immediate examination at the time the injury occurs, the stage of the injury is obvious—it is new and therefore acute. By contrast, when the patient presents to you some time after the injury occurs, the injury could be at any one of three stages. Each stage presents different symptoms and signs. You should determine the injury's stage because the treatment approach differs for each stage. Injuries fall into one of three stages or classifications: acute, subacute, and chronic. Although these classifications are based on the healing process, there is no clear-cut delineation between the end of one stage and the beginning of another. There is also some disagreement as to how long each stage lasts and when each stage begins.

- An **acute** injury results from a sudden onset of macrotrauma and has a wide range of recovery depending on its severity. Although recovery from an acute injury may take some time, the primary initial symptoms that classify it as acute occur over the first 7 to 10 days after its onset. An injury can be considered acute up to 4 weeks. After this time, it is considered a subacute injury.

- A **subacute** injury classification is between the acute and chronic stages, 4 to 6 weeks after the onset of trauma (American Academy of Orthopaedic Surgeons 1991).

- A **chronic** injury does not resolve in a normal amount of time. Symptoms continue to interfere with activity. Conditions are classified as chronic 6 to 8 weeks after their onset, and they may last for several months. A chronic injury is different from a repetitive trauma injury. Repetitive trauma occurs when a tissue receives recurring stress at a level beyond its ability to cope. For example, an overuse syndrome is a repetitive trauma injury, but a low back sprain that continues to cause pain is a chronic problem. Without intervention for either chronic or repetitive trauma injuries, symptoms continue to aggravate the patient and interfere with activity.

These terms—*acute*, *subacute*, and *chronic*—are not always applied in a hard-and-fast manner. The purpose of the classification system is to help you appreciate the healing process and determine the appropriate treatment course.

Refer to *Therapeutic Exercise for Musculoskeletal Injuries, Second Edition*, (Houglum 2005) and *Therapeutic Modalities for Musculoskeletal Injuries, Second Edition*, (Denegar, Saliba, and Saliba 2005) for a more in-depth discussion of the healing process.

Subjective and Objective Segments

The SINS of any injury are identified through a thorough and accurate injury examination. You should identify the SINS during both the acute and clinical examinations. Use the subjective examination segment to create an image of the injury's SINS and the objective segment to then confirm or disprove your suspicions.

Subjective Segment

The **subjective** segment involves taking the history of the injury. The data you receive should provide you with an idea of the severity, irritability, and nature of the injury. Remember, the data you receive are only as good as the questions you ask. Your questioning should be as complete as possible so that you can gain information to guide your objective examination. Details of taking a history are presented in chapter 3.

Objective Segment

As the name implies, this part of the examination focuses on impartial evidence provided by the various tests you perform. The information you gathered in the subjective examination determines which tests you choose to perform.

During the **objective** segment, you perform tests to help you establish the severity and nature of the injury. If the objective tests do not confirm the hypotheses you formulated during the subjective segment, you must reexamine the patient for other possible injuries and then retest or refer her to another medical professional for further examination and diagnosis. It is crucial that you use common sense and let the subjective report dictate how aggressively you perform the objective examination. If the patient is in severe pain, do not perform a complete examination, but rather only 1 to 2 tests that can establish appropriate immediate treatment or referral. You may defer complete examination until there is less pain and the injury is less irritable. If the patient is able to tolerate a more extensive examination, proceed—but only as necessity and the level of pain dictate. Otherwise you may aggravate the injury and lose the patient's confidence in your ability to help him.

Testing During the Objective Segment

The objective segment of an examination is a routine process, requiring specific tests and the identification of responses to confirm your suspicions regarding the patient's diagnosis. The examination process presented here is recommended since it follows a logical sequence of events. Whether you implement this system or develop your own, you should use a consistent, sequential system each time you perform an examination. Such a system will make you less likely to forget a test and more likely to perform a thorough examination.

Objective Examination Comparisons

Since a goal of the objective examination is to define the injury, you must know what reproduces the patient's symptoms and what is normal for that patient. You can learn these factors by producing a comparable sign and by comparing the injured segment to the contralateral extremity.

Comparable Sign

With each test you perform, you are seeking a response. All objective tests should elicit a negative response if the tissue or structure is not injured and a positive response if it is. A positive response results from either a reproduction or alteration of the patient's symptoms. The reproduction of the patient's complaint of pain through testing is called a **comparable sign** (Maitland 1991). It is desirable to produce a comparable sign since the test that produced the sign will reveal the problem. A negative response, on the other hand, is seen when the test provides a normal result.

Components of the objective examination include observation, palpation, range of motion (ROM) tests, strength tests, special tests, neurovascular tests, and functional tests. One or more of these tests will produce a comparable sign. The information you obtain from these examination procedures and the procedures of the subjective segment provide a total picture of the injury: a diagnosis or clinical impression.

Bilateral Comparison

You should perform all of the objective tests bilaterally (**bilateral comparison**). To obtain reliable information from the tests, you need to understand the purpose of each test, compare the injured side with the uninjured side, and know the normal response for each test. You must also realize how changes in the patient's position can affect results. For example, the results of strength testing of shoulder flexion may depend on whether the patient is sitting or supine. It is important to examine the patient efficiently. If you do not understand the purpose of each test, you will use more tests than necessary, prolonging the examination and perhaps aggravating the condition.

Observation

Observation is a valuable skill that is used throughout all phases and types of examinations and treatments. Observing how the patient responds provides useful information about the patient's perception of the injury as well as clues about its nature and severity. Observation begins as soon as you see the patient and continues throughout the subjective and objective segments of an examination. Facial expressions and the eyes are windows into a patient's true response, and thus you should carefully watch them not only at the time of injury but also during the objective tests. You also should observe the patient's general posture, the way in which she holds or protects the injured part, and her willingness to move the injured segment. Observe for contour, alignment, and discoloration, and compare the right and left sides—they should be symmetrical. Observation is discussed in detail in chapter 4.

Palpation

Your sense of touch is critical to the objective portion of the examination. With concentration and practice, your sense of touch will develop just as your other clinical skills do. In addition to palpating for swelling, pain, and temperature, you will palpate for spasm, deformity, moisture, pulse, and general contour of soft tissue and bony prominences. Palpation is more thoroughly presented in chapter 5.

Range of Motion

Range of motion (ROM) testing includes active and passive motions. Some professionals also include resistive motion, or strength, in this category; however, strength is presented under its own category in this text. Active motion testing, which you will perform first, determines the integrity of the active or contractile tissue of the musculotendinous unit. Passive motion testing examines inert structures around the joint. Until you are familiar with the ROM tests, you may prefer to perform all the active motion tests first and then follow with all the passive motion tests. Once you are comfortable with the tests, however, it is recommended that you perform the active and passive motion tests by muscle or muscle group to limit patient movement from one position to another.

During ROM testing, you examine both the quality and quantity of physiological and accessory motion as well as test for pain. You may also test how the joint feels at the end of the range of motion (the joint's end feel). The various elements of ROM testing are presented in chapter 6.

Strength

Strength examination follows the active and passive ROM tests. Strength tests examine the musculotendinous resistive ability, the neuromuscular integrity of the contractile tissue, and the pain level of the contractile elements. The method you use to examine strength depends on the type of injury, available equipment, time, and place of examination. Isometric tests are typically performed first, followed by more specific manual muscle tests as warranted. Isometric tests, or **break tests**, are efficient and are usually performed with the joint in a neutral midrange position for multiple-joint muscles and in an end-range position for single-joint muscles. These positions limit the amount of stress applied to a joint and assure that you test for strength without interference from inert joint structures. If you discover a strength deficit with a break test, you may need to examine the muscle's strength throughout its entire range of motion. An extensive presentation of strength examination is found in chapter 7. If the patient has significant pain, it may not be possible to perform a strength test, and you will have to defer strength examination to a later date.

Special Tests

Special tests are unique to specific joints, body segments, or structures. For example, special tests for the knee differ from special tests for the ankle or shoulder. Some special tests for the knee examine the integrity of the menisci, while a special test for the ankle examines interosseus membrane integrity, and special tests for the shoulder investigate glenoid labrum stability. Each body segment requires unique tests for examining the degree of injury to unique soft tissue structures and bones of its area.

By the time you are ready to use special tests, history, palpation, ROM, and strength tests have narrowed the range of injury possibilities. Use special tests to eliminate or confirm a suspected condition as well as to quantify the integrity of a structure or the extent of an injury. Special tests should stress the structure adequately enough to allow you to either grade an abnormal response or reproduce the patient's symptoms. The stress must be great enough to elicit an accurate response but not so great that it aggravates the injury. In the beginning, finding this balance can be difficult.

Special tests do not provide a complete profile of the injury. Throughout the examination process you progressively focus the picture and narrow the possibilities of what the injury is. You must be careful not to rush the investigative process by making assumptions or focusing too quickly on one or two special tests. Remember to keep an open mind until your understanding of the injury, or the injury image, becomes certain.

Since the special tests are numerous and many are unique to each body segment, they are discussed in the chapters dealing with the various segments in part II. However, this chapter underlines general principles guiding the use of special tests.

Selecting the Tests

As noted earlier, deciding on the degree of stress or which special test to use requires good judgment. It is sometimes neither necessary nor appropriate to use a special test to stress an injury—for example, in the case of an elbow dislocation. A patient may simply be in too much pain to undergo a stress test; in this case it is better to defer the special test than to cause additional pain. Special tests confirm the severity and nature of the injury. The special tests presented throughout this text are those that clinicians most commonly use because of the tests' accuracy and demonstrated reliability. You must remember, however, that some of these tests may not have demonstrated reliability or may not be appropriate for some clinicians because of individual circumstances. For example, if you have a small hand and are evaluating a large patient, a McMurray test for the knee may not provide you with accurate or appropriate information. You will need to determine the most suitable tests for your examination based on the specific situation of the injury and your knowledge and skills.

Testing Technique

You should perform special tests only after you have explained to the patient what will occur. The special tests are performed on the uninvolved extremity first for two reasons, as already noted: (1) to familiarize the patient with the procedure so she is less apprehensive, encouraging relaxation that will achieve better test results, and (2) to learn what response to the test is normal for that patient. Since many special tests produce different results from one patient to another, you must establish a baseline for each person to determine whether the test is positive or negative. Depending on the test, the result is considered positive if it produces abnormal results compared to the uninvolved side in terms of laxity or stiffness, stability or instability, presence or absence of sounds, restriction or ease of movement, strength or weakness, normal or abnormal function, and presence or absence of pain.

Accuracy of Test Results

Always remember that negative or positive results of a single special test do not necessarily indicate the absence or presence of a specific injury. This is why all the factors of your examination are used in combination: to provide a full and consistent profile of the injury. Sometimes a positive result may falsely occur and complicate your examination results so that other tests are necessary for providing accurate results. Your skills and ability to perform the tests reliably can make a big difference in the test results, and thus experience plays an important role in the accuracy of the special tests. Another factor to consider is the accuracy of the specific special tests themselves, as some are more sensitive than others. However, though for some injuries there are several tests, it is not necessary to use all that are available. Remember, a special test intends to reproduce the patient's symptoms or create a comparable sign, so unless you require additional confirmation, one or two tests per structure are usually adequate for your examination and are better tolerated by the patient.

Neurological Status

You should perform a neurological examination if you suspect a nerve injury and the patient's symptoms include radiation of numbness, tingling, shooting pain, deep pain, burning pain, or weakness. Radiating neurological symptoms or referred symptoms (pain in a location other than the injury source) can result from pathology in the spinal cord, nerve roots,

See also Chapter 6, pages 90-91, for more information on general technique for ligament and capsular stress tests.

peripheral nerves, or soft tissue, and they occur secondary to disc herniations, fractures or dislocations, impingement or compression syndromes, nerve tensioning or stretching, and other traumas.

Neurological symptoms vary with the level of nerve injury. While unilateral symptoms often indicate a nerve root or peripheral nerve lesion, bilateral symptoms often indicate central cord pathology. The symptoms also differ for a nerve root versus a peripheral nerve injury. Because it is important to understand these differential systems and the innervation zones for each nerve root and peripheral nerve, a neurological examination is detailed in chapter 8.

Although there are specific neurological tests for specific body areas, the three primary neurological tests involve examination of sensory, motor, and reflex responses. These tests are designed for spinal cord and nerve root exams, but sensory and motor examination results can also produce peripheral nerve conclusions. Specific neurological tests and their implications are explained in chapter 8.

Vascular Status

Circulatory tests examine the integrity of the vascular system. You will often palpate pulses to determine the presence of blood flow. If the pulse weakens or disappears following an injury, the situation is a medical emergency, and you must provide for immediate and emergency medical referral to prevent loss of a limb or worse. You will note pallor or lack of capillary refill in areas of decreased blood flow or ischemia. Shock may also cause some of these pathological signs. Circulatory status along with tests and methods for recognizing vascular conditions are presented in chapter 9.

Functional Capacity

Functional tests are used only when the athlete is ready to return to former participation levels. These final tests determine not so much the nature or severity of an injury but rather the patient's ability to safely and fully resume all activities. Most commonly, you will perform these tests after a course of treatment following an injury rather than at the time of injury. Only in cases of minor injuries—if symptoms have subsided and all previous tests have demonstrated that the patient is able to return to participation—is functional testing a part of the immediate examination process. In these cases, you must perform functional tests before permitting the patient to return to full participation.

Functional testing helps you determine the patient's confidence and physical readiness to return to participation beyond what you can learn from standard strength and ROM testing. Functional testing requires specific tasks and controlled skill movements that mimic the physical demands and joint stresses inherent to the patient's sport or work activity. By having the patient perform these functional movements, you can also determine the quality of her performance in a more controlled environment and identify whether there is any apprehension or compensation with other movements in an effort to protect an area or avoid pain.

Specific functional tests are wide and varied. They will be unique to the specific demands of each case. Therefore, you should have a working understanding of the physical demands and stresses that a patient will experience so you can provide an appropriate functional examination.

Lower-Extremity Functional Tests

You can use the same generic functional tests for the lower extremity for nearly every activity that requires running. Examples of these tests include a progression of standing to walking to climbing stairs to jogging to running to sprinting. Once generalized running activities are completed, sport-specific activities should be included for a complete test series. Additional progressions can include performing activities forward, then backward, then in lateral and sudden change-of-direction motions, first in predetermined paths and then in sudden, unanticipated paths. Following this section is a progression of generic running activities for functional testing of the lower extremity. If the athlete's sport involves jumping, then the progression should also include activities such as jumps, bounding jumps, lateral jumps, and combinations of jumps and runs. The height of the jumps can progress from small and single to larger and multiple, depending on the sport's demands.

Generic Lower-Extremity Tests

1. Balance in standing such as the stork stand or tandem stand
2. Walking forward
3. Walking up and down stairs
4. Jogging forward
5. Running forward
6. Sprinting forward
7. Hopping forward
8. Jogging backward
9. Running backward
10. Sprinting backward
11. Jogging side to side
12. Running side to side
13. Sprinting side to side
14. Hopping forward
15. Hopping side to side
16. Hopping alternate feet
17. Hopping involved leg only
18. Skipping forward
19. Skipping backward
20. Skipping side to side
21. Jumping forward
22. Jumping backward
23. Sport-specific activities

The specific requirements of the patient's sport and position primarily determine the lower-extremity tests. For example, you should test a volleyball hitter with activities such as rapid side-to-side motions, sprinting with sudden stops and jumps, and repeated blocking jumps. You should test a hockey goalie with sudden abduction movements, sudden changes in direction, and sudden changes from skating forward to sideways to backward. You should test a hockey forward using forward and backward skating sprints, sudden changes of direction, and sudden stops, all in a progressive manner from long and slow to short and quick.

Upper-Extremity Functional Tests

Functional testing for the upper extremity also depends upon the specific sport and position demands. Generic upper-extremity tests include activities such as tossing and throwing, pushing and pulling, hitting and batting, and catching and receiving. These activities begin at a simple level, such as throwing over a short distance and at a low speed, and progress as the athlete's performance indicates, reaching a competitive level equivalent to the demands the patient will encounter when he returns to full participation. Some of these functional tests are listed in the box Upper-Extremity Functional Tests.

Upper-Extremity Functional Tests

1. Tossing
2. Throwing
3. Pitching
4. Hitting
5. Batting
6. Catching
7. Receiving
8. Standing on hands
9. Supporting body weight on arms
10. Sport-specific activities

Specific upper-extremity activities mimic the sport's participation demands. For example, you must test a male gymnast's ability to perform an iron cross on the rings before he returns to competition. A baseball pitcher's functional tests greatly differ from the gymnast's, and a baseball shortstop's tests vary from the pitcher's. You may evaluate a pitcher for consistency, form, speed, and the quality of his pitching. On the other hand, you may evaluate the shortstop for the accuracy and speed of his sidearm throw to different bases and his ability to field balls.

Each sport has specific functional activities. On some occasions, the athlete may participate in a sport that involves both upper- and lower-extremity activities. If the athlete has been out of participation for an extended time, you may need to functionally test both her upper and lower extremities. You must know the skills and demands of the sport to provide appropriate functional tests. If necessary, you should discuss the sport requirements with someone who is familiar with them. Table 2.1 presents some suggestions for functional tests.

Diagnostic Tests

Diagnostic tests, usually ordered by a physician, may be indicated to either confirm or eliminate any suspected diagnosis. A variety of diagnostic tests are available, and their use is determined in part by availability, physician preference, and the tissue involved. Laboratory tests such as blood and urine tests identify illness or organ injury; ultrasound scans rule out some organ and soft tissue injuries; and radiographic tests identify bone, ligament, or other soft tissue injury. Common radiographic tests for evaluating orthopedic injuries

Table 2.1

Examples of Functional Tests for Different Sports and Positions

Sport/position	Examples of functional tests
Football quarterback	Throwing short and long distances; scrambling via sudden cuts, lateral runs, sprints
Football lineman	Thrust from set stance; lateral runs; sprints forward; blocking maneuvers
Football receiver	Sprints forward, laterally, and backward; sudden changes in direction; catching while running; running and jumping
Soccer goalie	Sudden lateral moves; jumping; diving
Soccer forward	Sprints forward, laterally, and backward; dribbling and passing; overhead throws; tackling
Female gymnast	Handstands; jumping; sprinting forward; back and forward walkovers; handsprings; dismounts from bars and beam
Male gymnast	Handstands; jumping; sprinting forward; iron cross on rings; dismounts from bars, rings, and pommel horse
Basketball forward	Sprinting forward; lateral cuts; backward sprints; lay-ups; free throws
Basketball guard	Sprinting forward; lateral cuts; backward sprints; dribbling while running and cutting; 3-point shots
Baseball/softball outfielder	Sprinting 50 to 100 feet; base sliding; running and catching; hitting
Baseball/softball catcher	Squatting; sudden squat to stand; throw to second base; catching; sprinting 20 feet
Volleyball frontline player	Jumping up; jumping laterally; jump and hit the ball; approach the net for a hit or a block and jump
Volleyball setter	Sprint forward and laterally 15 feet; dive; set and pass

include X ray for fracture identification; magnetic resonance imaging (MRI) and computed tomography (CT) scans for soft tissue, meniscal, and ligamentous injuries; and bone scans for elusive bone injuries such as stress fractures. Although diagnostic examination techniques are not comprehensively covered in this text, appropriate tests will be noted where relevant in individual chapters of part II.

DOCUMENTING THE EXAMINATION

A final ingredient of utmost importance in your examination procedures is accurate and thorough documentation of your findings. Injury documentation is essential for a number of reasons. From a legal standpoint, you may need to reproduce records for a legal dispute or for verifying an insurance claim. From a more practical standpoint, other colleagues may care for your patient when you are not available, and accurate examination, injury, and treatment records assure continuity of care. Injury documentation also proves useful for reexamining injuries, allowing you to compare your findings from one examination to the next. It is never wise to rely on your memory, as you may forget critical findings.

Your documentation should be thorough but concise. It is likely that you will perform multiple examinations or treatments in a single day, so efficient documentation is essential if you wish to avoid getting bogged down in paperwork. Many computerized systems for tracking injuries are now available. Whether in written or computerized form, the same information is recorded.

All examination and treatment notes are legal documents. As such, you are required to manage them as legal documents. This means that you should make your notes in ink. The documents should be seen only by those treating the patient and be kept in a secured place. If an error is made in the document, it should be crossed out with a single line so it is still readable, with the initials of the person correcting the error written next to it.

See *Management Strategies in Athletic Training, Second Edition,* (Ray 2005) for details on record keeping, storage requirements, and HIPAA regulations.

SOAP Notes

The simplest and most common documentation procedure is called SOAP notes. **SOAP notes** include documentation of your **s**ubjective findings, **o**bjective findings, overall conclusions or **a**ssessment, and subsequent **p**lan for treatment or follow-up based on your examination and diagnosis. The record should contain all the information that may need to be recalled later. The sample examination form in this chapter provides an idea of the kinds of information that may be included. Clinicians devise examination forms to suit their own preferences and needs: some use an open-ended form like the one on page 32; others use a detailed fill-in-the-blank form that lists specific objective tests for each body region.

The subjective portion of the form includes the essential information from the history portion of the subjective examination, such as chief complaint, mechanism of injury, and reported signs and symptoms. Your subjective documentation should also provide a clear picture of the injury's SINS (see page 22).

The following is an example of documentation of the subjective examination:

> The patient reported to the athletic training clinic complaining of pain in her right anterior knee. She stated that the pain had appeared gradually over the last 3 to 4 days and denied any mechanism of injury. The patient is a freshman basketball player who in the last 2 weeks has begun intensive conditioning activities 2 hours a day in preparation for the season. Prior to this increase in activity, she had been on vacation and physically inactive for the previous month. She described the pain as an "ache" just below the patella while pointing to the infrapatellar tendon. Patient stated pain is worse at start of activity but improves with warm-up. Pain is worse during activities of jumping, squatting, and during rest after long-term sitting. Patient denies any previous injury to either knee.

From this written history, you can determine the location and nature of the injury and also get a sense of what may have caused the injury, the degree of irritability, the stage or duration of the injury, and the level of severity.

The objective portion of your documentation should present all the findings of your objective examination. It also includes information you obtained from any notes, chart information, or diagnostic tests performed. This includes your observations as well as the results of pertinent objective tests such as ROM, strength, neurovascular, and special tests.

The following is a continuation of the example just presented:

> Slight limp observed as she walked into the AT clinic. Upon inspection, mild swelling noted just inferior to patella in infrapatellar tendon region. No obvious deformity or discoloration noted. Able to complete a full active ROM into flexion and extension, some discomfort with active extension. No pain with passive ROM, except in full passive flexion. Strength = 5/5 on manual muscle testing for both knee flexion and extension with pain noted on resisted extension. Neurological examination and special tests for patellofemoral laxity were negative. Palpable tenderness and inflammation noted over infrapatellar tendon.

Soap Notes Form

Athlete's Name: _____   **Record/ID#** _____

Injury Date: _____   **Record Date:** _____

Sport: _____

Subjective (history):

_____

_____

_____

_____

Objective (observation, palpation, ROM, strength, neurological tests, special tests):

_____

_____

_____

_____

_____

_____

_____

_____

_____

_____

_____

_____

_____

_____

_____

_____

Assessment (impression):

_____

_____

Plan (treatment and disposition)

_____

_____

From *Assessment of Athletic Injuries* by S.J. Shultz, P.A. Houglum, and D.H. Perrin, 2000. Champaign IL: Human Kinetics

Notice that not every test within the objective examination is included in this account. Primarily, you want to report the important findings that clearly describe the injury. Although it is not necessary to document every negative finding, you may include the negative findings indicating that you ruled out other injuries or structures that would produce similar signs or symptoms. With practice, you will become more efficient in your written report and better able to discern what should be included. There is no need to write full sentences with SOAP notes.

The assessment portion of your documentation should include your impression of the injury. On the basis of the findings from your subjective and objective examination, you should now have a good sense of the diagnosis. Here is where you condense the results of your entire examination and draw conclusions. Unless it is clearly definitive, you may qualify your impression using wording such as "possible," "probable," or "rule out."

To continue with our example:

Assessment (or impression): R patellar tendinitis.

It is important to write down your impression or diagnosis, as it may change upon reexamination or as symptoms change.

Finally, documentation of the plan provides a written account of your immediate treatment and referral plans for the patient. Your short-term and long-term goals are also included here. If you referred the patient for further medical examination or if EMS was called, this should be documented in the plan. If the patient was removed from activity, allowed to return to activity, or advised to rest, this should be noted as well.

To finish our example:

Remove from activity. Pt to apply ice for 20 minutes daily over weekend. Patient will rest over the weekend and be reexamined on Monday.

Other essential information to include on your form are the patient's name and identification number, date of initial injury, date of documentation, and sport. Physical characteristics such as age, height, and weight may be important in some instances. It is also helpful if the form includes a full-body diagram to mark the location of the patient's pain and any referral pain patterns. Often, it is easier to draw these pain patterns than to describe them verbally. Write your documentation as soon after the injury examination as possible, while the information is fresh in your mind. You can often document your findings as you proceed through a clinical examination. With on-site and acute examinations this is more difficult, as you will probably be unable to write the report during the examination. For this reason it is a good idea to have a notepad among your field supplies where you can jot down important findings that may be difficult to recall later.

When providing treatment at the initial examination, record new SOAP notes for the treatment after completing the examination. The *S* portion can be brief, using a statement such as, "See initial examination." The *O* portion is the treatment provided. For example, ice × 15 minutes, immobilization, or wound cleansing with whatever is used to clean and dress the wound should be reported as part of the objective statements. The *A* portion includes your impression of the condition of the injury or patient after treatment. For example, "Edema around R knee ↓ by 2 cm at joint margin after Px." The *P* portion includes what your next procedure or treatment will be. You may state, "Begin ES to ↓ pain and edema next Rx. Cont. with immobilization × 5 days."

SUMMARY

1. Identify the main segments that make up an examination.

   The two main segments are the subjective segment and the objective segment.

2. Explain the purpose and the components of the subjective segment.

   The subjective examination includes the history from the patient and others who may provide additional information. The goal of the subjective examination is to obtain sufficient information on which to proceed to the objective examination.

3. Identify the SINS of injury examination.

   The combined subjective and objective portions of the injury examination provide critical information on the injury's SINS: severity, irritability, nature, and stage. You identify the severity to reveal the extent of the injury, establish whether referral is needed, and determine what care is appropriate. You determine the injury's irritability to provide information on the stage of the injury and the degree of exacerbation of the symptoms. The irritability also determines how aggressive you can be in the objective examination. The nature of the injury includes the type of injury and the tissues or structures involved. Stage of the injury is determined according to whether the complaint is acute or chronic. Together, the SINS allow you to form an accurate impression of the injury. After completing an examination and on the basis of the SINS, you should be able to make appropriate decisions regarding referral to another medical authority, the appropriateness of return to full or partial participation, and the proper course of treatment.

4. Identify the general examination procedures of the objective segment.

   During the objective examination it is desirable to produce a comparable sign and compare the injured segment to the contralateral side. Doing so provides a more accurate conclusion of all information obtained throughout the examination. The sequence of examination techniques is observation followed by palpation, active and passive ROM tests, strength tests, special tests, neurological and vascular examinations, and finally, functional tests.

5. Explain the SOAP notes procedure for injury documentation.

   The purpose of injury documentation is to provide a record of the injury examination—essential because such documentation may be needed for legal verification and protection, communication of findings with other health professionals, and comparison of findings upon reexamination. A SOAP note form is commonly used to document the Subjective findings, the Objective findings, your Assessment or diagnosis of the injury, and the immediate Plan of action. When documentation is not possible at the time of injury, it is important to have a pad of paper handy on the field so you can jot down the essential findings you will need to complete proper documentation later.

REVIEW QUESTIONS

1. You have not yet learned specific details about the subjective segment of an examination, but can you imagine some of the questions you should ask a soccer player about his ankle injury?

2. Why is it necessary to examine both active and passive ROM of a volleyball player with a shoulder injury?

3. What is a comparable sign and how is it determined? Why might a bilateral comparison be important in determining a comparable sign?

4. What is the purpose of palpation? What would you palpate for if a football player complained of subluxating his patella?

5. Describe break tests.

6. Under what conditions and for what presenting symptoms would a neurological examination be performed?

7. What kinds of tests would you use as functional tests for a basketball player to decide if she can return to the game after you've taped her sprained ankle?

8. Returning to the scenario at the beginning of the chapter, what do you think Mary Ann would say in answer to Patrick's questions?

CRITICAL THINKING QUESTIONS

1. An industrial worker comes into the clinic complaining of shoulder pain for the past 5 to 7 days. What is the order of the objective tests you would perform on him?

2. You are called out to the track because an athlete has collapsed on the track. You know nothing else about the injury at this point. What are the first things you will do when you get to the downed athlete?

3. A patient comes to you complaining of a knee injury. In the history you find that he had a second-degree sprain on the opposite knee just 6 months ago. How might this affect your examination and why?

CITED REFERENCES

American Academy of Orthopaedic Surgeons (AAOS). 1991. *Athletic training and sports medicine.* Rosemont, IL: American Academy of Orthopaedic Surgeons.

Maitland, D.G. 1991. *Peripheral manipulation.* Boston: Butterworth-Heinemann.

Merriam-Webster's Collegiate Dictionary. 11th ed. 2003. Boston: Houghton Mifflin.

Thomas, C.L. 1993. *Taber's cyclopedic medical dictionary.* Philadelphia: F.A. Davis.

ADDITIONAL RESOURCES

Caroline, N. 1995. *Emergency care in the streets.* Boston: Little, Brown.

Denegar, S., E. Saliba, and S. Saliba. 2005. *Therapeutic modalities for musculoskeletal injuries.* 2nd ed. Champaign, IL: Human Kinetics.

Hillman, S.K. 2005. *Introduction to athletic training.* 2nd ed. Champaign, IL: Human Kinetics.

Houglum, P.A. 2005. *Therapeutic exercise for musculoskeletal injuries.* 2nd ed. Champaign, IL: Human Kinetics.

Ray, R. 2005. *Management strategies in athletic training.* 3rd ed. Champaign, IL: Human Kinetics.

Taking a History

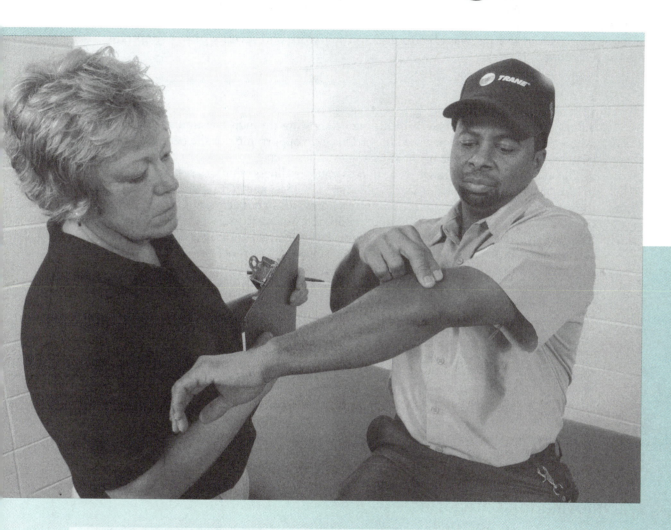

Objectives

After completing this chapter, the reader will be able to do the following:

1. Identify the main goals and features of taking a history

2. Ask pertinent, nonleading questions to determine the nature and severity of the injury

3. Differentiate the types of information that should be learned for emergent, acute non-emergent, and chronic examinations

4. Obtain a thorough history from any ill or injured athlete

At the end of Dr. Miller's athletic injury examination class, he challenged his students: "If you were unable to use your eyes to see or hands to touch, do you think you could figure out what injury or illness an athlete might have?" After considering this, Justin realized that without the benefit of sight or touch, he would not be able to use most of the injury examination techniques he had learned. Dr. Miller's challenge took on real meaning later that night, when one of the women's basketball players called him complaining of abdominal pain. It was only through asking a series of questions that he was able to discern the nature and severity of her symptoms and make the appropriate referral.

Taking a **history** is the process of learning or knowing through questioning the facts and events associated with an injury or illness. This is an opportunity for the patient to describe what happened and what he or she is feeling or experiencing.

Obtaining an accurate record of an athlete's injury or illness requires a systematic approach to learning about the events leading to the injury or illness and getting a clear description of the associated signs and symptoms. This history provides an initial impression of the severity, irritability, nature, and stage (SINS) of the condition. You can learn a tremendous amount of information about an athlete's condition simply by listening to the athlete describe the injury. When you carefully select your questions, you gain a useful picture of the athlete's complaint and a sense of the direction your objective examination should take. This chapter covers the general principles of taking a history as well as the specific information you should seek when evaluating emergent, acute, or chronic conditions.

INFORMATION TO SEEK

The first step in an injury examination is obtaining a history. This is the athlete's (or bystanders' if the athlete is unable to communicate) opportunity to describe the injury or illness, the athlete's response to the injury or illness, and previous events that may affect the current situation. Your questioning should be efficient and thorough—pertinent to the moment, but complete enough to allow you to formulate a plan for the remaining examination. Following in the next section are the primary categories of information you should seek when taking a history.

Information Categories

- **Chief complaint.** To quickly focus your historical examination, first determine the athlete's chief complaint. Ask questions like "What's wrong?" or "Where do you hurt?" to quickly determine the primary problem. You should always investigate the chief complaint first, even if it seems obvious. For example, you may note that a soccer player's leg is bleeding after a collision with the goalpost, but when you ask her, "Where do you hurt?" she may answer, "My head hurts." If an athlete has multiple complaints, ask him which complaint is bothering him most and begin your examination there.

- **Mechanism of injury.** The mechanism of injury is how the injury occurred. Injury occurs as a result of some force acting on the body that exceeds the tolerance of the tissues. With traumatic injuries, you should ascertain the direction, location, and velocity (speed) of the force. Certain injuries occur with certain types of forces, so learning the type of force imposed on the body also alerts you to the potential for tissue damage and the possible tissues involved (figure 3.1).

    - A **compressive force** usually results in crush injuries, which can range in severity from a simple contusion to a compression fracture of the cervical spine.

    - A **tensioning force** commonly results in muscle strains and joint sprains, which occur when the force exceeds the length and tensile strength of a tissue.

- A twisting force commonly causes joint injuries, such as when the anterior cruciate ligament of the knee tears when an athlete plants her foot and then rotates her body to change direction.

- A shearing force occurs when there is transverse displacement between two structures. The secondary result of a shearing force is possible compression or tensioning of the displaced structures. Brain tissue is particularly vulnerable to shearing forces (see chapter 19 for more information).

In addition to the type of force applied, the surface area the force impacts also affects the injury. Given the same velocity, a localized force can result in substantially greater tissue damage than the same force applied over a broader surface area. Whether the body is stationary or moving when the force is applied also dictates the amount of tissue damage.

Establishing the mechanism of injury helps you determine the nature and extent of the injury and may also alert you to areas you might not otherwise investigate based on the chief complaint alone. Ask "What happened?" or "How did it happen?" or "How did you get hurt?" to establish the mechanism of injury.

- **Nature of illness or injury.** The nature of an illness or injury describes its associated conditions. When an athlete suffers an acute injury, he typically can tell you the events surrounding the injury. On the other hand, an athlete with a chronic injury or a chief complaint of acute abdominal pain may not be able to answer questions such as "How did you get sick?" or "What caused it?" In these cases, you may need to inquire further about the signs and symptoms associated with their chief complaint and ask about the events leading up to their illness or injury before you can determine its nature.

Signs and Symptoms

Investigating the signs and symptoms the athlete is experiencing provides detailed information about the nature, severity, irritability, and stage of the injury or illness. Asking questions such as "How are you feeling?" or "What are you feeling?" or "Are you experiencing any pain?" helps you discern the athlete's symptoms. Asking them to grade the intensity of their symptom on a scale of 1 to 10 helps you determine the severity of their condition. You should also ask the athlete if she observed any unusual signs, such as hearing a "pop" when twisting a knee, feeling an unusual lump or defect in a tissue, or noting increased swelling and discoloration

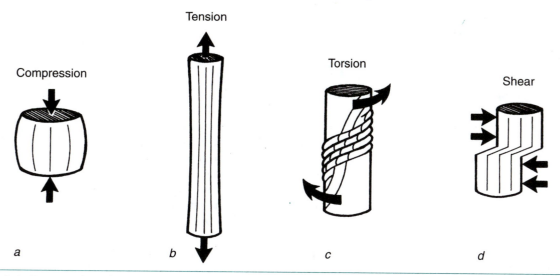

Figure 3.1 Types and mechanisms of injury forces: *(a)* compression, *(b)* tension, *(c)* torsional/twisting, and *(d)* shearing.

the day following an injury. Likewise, a bystander may note the athlete appeared disoriented and had an unusual breath odor before falling unconscious.

> A **sign** is a finding that can be observed or objectively measured, whereas a **symptom** is a subjective complaint or an abnormal sensation the patient describes.

- **Current signs and symptoms.** When asking questions about signs and symptoms, be careful not to lead the athlete. For example, it would be leading to ask, "Did you hear a pop when you twisted your knee?" A better question that allows the athlete to answer more accurately is, "Did you hear or feel anything when you injured your knee?" Also, "How would you describe your pain?" is better than "Is your pain more of a deep ache?" If the athlete has difficulty describing his symptoms, offer him a variety of options from which to choose. Remember, the history you obtain is only as good as the questions you ask, and its accuracy determines the course of the remaining examination.

> A *syncopal episode,* or *syncope,* is a temporary loss of consciousness resulting from inadequate blood flow to the brain.

- **Previous history and contributing factors.** You should also inquire about possible complaints, signs and symptoms, and events the athlete may have experienced before the onset of the injury or illness, or, if the examination is delayed, in the interim since the injury or first appearance of signs and symptoms. Inquiries about the patient's previous history help you identify any preexisting conditions, symptoms, or events that might relate to the athlete's current complaint. For instance, asking an athlete about preexisting medical conditions or how they felt just before fainting may help you understand the cause of their syncopal episode. If an athlete complains of a rash, you may want to inquire about any known allergies and potential exposure to allergens. In the case of chronic complaints, obtaining a prior history is imperative to understanding the underlying cause and nature of the injury. For example, if an athlete comes to you complaining of persistent pain and tenderness in her Achilles tendon for the past few weeks, you will need to ask when the symptoms began, if she remembers doing anything unusual before the start of the symptoms, what types of stress are applied to the tendon during normal daily activity as well as sport or exercise activity, and what types of activities make the symptoms better or worse.

> Refer to chapter 21 for more information about syncopal episodes.

A history of signs and symptoms also helps you determine the stage of the injury. A complaint of sharp, unrelenting abdominal pain that began the night before and has gradually increased suggests an acute and potentially serious condition. An industrial worker who reports elbow pain after a full day on the assembly line and later reveals that he has noted the pain on and off over the past 3 months is likely suffering from a chronic overuse condition. You need to ask additional questions that better define the nature and extent of the symptoms, the activities that aggravate or relieve symptoms, and the events leading to the onset of symptoms.

SITUATION-SPECIFIC HISTORY AND DEPTH OF INQUIRY

The time you spend and the information you seek when obtaining a history depend on the situation and may differ dramatically. When called to examine an unconscious victim, you are only concerned with getting the most important facts to guide your primary survey and course for immediate care until you are able to rule out any life-threatening conditions. When an athlete injures his ankle on the field, you only need to learn sufficient information to determine the course of your immediate examination and whether it is safe to remove the athlete to the sideline, where you can obtain a more detailed history and examine the condition more thoroughly.

The level of inquiry also depends on your knowledge of the events surrounding the injury. Let's assume you are attending basketball practice and observe an athlete turn his ankle when coming down from a rebound. In this case, you already have a good sense of the nature and mechanism of the injury. On the other hand, when an athlete comes to you complaining of vague shoulder pain that has gradually increased over the past 3 weeks, you need to spend more time investigating the nature of her complaint, the associated signs and symptoms, and the possible contributing factors before beginning the objective portion of your examination.

Essential History (Emergent Examination)

When you are dealing with a potentially life-threatening injury or illness, your immediate concern is performing a primary survey to determine if the athlete is conscious or unconscious; to assess airway, breathing, and circulation; and to check for profuse bleeding. If you did not see the event leading to the injury or illness, as you approach the athlete quickly ask bystanders if they know what happened in order to determine any essential history that will influence your immediate examination and care. If your primary examination reveals no immediate threats to life, you should identify any factors that may affect your ongoing emergency care. For instance, if an athlete is having difficulty breathing and his coach tells you he has chronic asthma, you can more quickly assess the situation and assist him in using his inhaler. If the athlete is unconscious, a quick check for a medical ID bracelet or a brief consultation with bystanders may provide important information about her medical history (e.g., history of diabetes or epilepsy) that may help guide your secondary examination. Once you determine that the athlete is stable, you can ask questions to specifically determine the nature and severity of her condition and guide your ongoing examination.

Focused History (On-Site Examination)

When taking an on-site history, you conduct a focused history, in which you only investigate the athlete's major complaint and any problems that are readily apparent and in need of attention before transporting the athlete off the field. If you were an eyewitness to the event, you may already have vital information regarding the mechanism and the forces involved. Witnessing the athlete's initial response to the trauma can provide valuable information as well. If you did not see the injury and the athlete is unconscious, ask bystanders what happened and how long the person has been unconscious. Questioning an athlete may be challenging if he is in a great deal of pain, but it may also calm him and shift his focus away from his pain or fear, thus easing the remainder of your examination.

You may find that the athlete's perspective greatly differs from your own or other bystanders' perspective. For example, although observers on the sideline may not have heard anything, the athlete may have experienced a pop or snap. An athlete may also experience torque or rotational forces that are not readily observed. Questions regarding the location and intensity of the athlete's symptoms help you determine an injury's severity and decide how to transport the athlete off the field. Does the athlete have pain? If she complains of neck or back pain and you suspect a spinal injury, ask if she is experiencing any numbness or tingling. If these symptoms are present, your examination should proceed accordingly (see chapter 8 for more information on neurological examination). Does the athlete complain of being dizzy, lightheaded, or nauseated? This type of questioning helps you quickly focus on the area of injury or nature of the illness and allows you to direct your examination appropriately.

During the on-site examination you should gather the information necessary for determining the general nature and extent of the injury and the best course of immediate action. You can defer the rest of the history to the acute examination once you know that it is safe to remove the athlete from the playing field (see the following discussion of detailed history as well as chapter 10 for more information on the acute examination).

Detailed History

In cases where there is no life-threatening condition and you can take time for a thorough examination, you should obtain a detailed history. A detailed history comprehensively explores the athlete's chief complaint, the mechanism of injury or nature of illness, the associated signs and symptoms, and any preexisting factors that may contribute to the current

When dealing with life-threatening conditions, you should immediately assess the level of consciousness and then airway, breathing, and circulation. (See chapters 9 and 10 for more information on how to conduct a primary survey.)

Diabetes *is an autoimmune disorder that causes a deficiency in glucose metabolism (chapter 22).*

Epilepsy *is a chronic condition characterized by recurring seizures (chapter 23).*

complaint. Unlike the essential and focused histories typically conducted when dealing with acute injury or illness, a detailed history applies to both acute and chronic conditions.

Current History

Once you have removed an athlete from the field, ask her again about her chief complaint and injury mechanism. These complaints commonly change within minutes after injury, and you often get a clearer impression of an athlete's condition once she has had the opportunity to calm down. Likewise, if you are unaware of an injury until the athlete walks into the athletic training room after practice, you will want to get a detailed picture of her chief complaint, mechanism of injury, and current signs and symptoms. Ask questions that will help you develop a good picture of the injury so that you can pay attention to the correct body segment during the objective examination. How did the athlete land? How was the injured extremity positioned at the time of impact? Did the athlete hear any noise or feel any unusual sensations? Was the pain immediate? Did the pain shoot or stay localized? Has the pain changed since it first began? Can the athlete pinpoint the pain? How does the athlete describe the pain? What is its intensity on a scale of 0 to 10, with 0 indicating no pain and 10 indicating unbearable pain? Does the injury hurt only when the athlete moves it or while she's at rest as well? Obtaining a thorough pain profile helps you determine the athlete's pain tolerance and the severity and location of the injury. It also helps establish how aggressive you can be during the objective portion of the examination. Remember to ask nonleading questions in order to gain the most accurate information about the signs and symptoms.

Examples of Leading and Nonleading Questions

Leading	*Nonleading*
Does your shoulder hurt?	Where is your pain?
Is the pain burning or stinging?	Can you describe the pain?
Does it hurt when you walk?	What activities increase your pain?
Did you hear a pop?	Did you hear or feel any unusual sounds or sensations?

History of Previous Injury or Illness

Obtaining a history of previous injury or illness gives you an idea of any medical conditions that may affect the current injury. For example, if the athlete has a history of rotator cuff surgery and now suffers an elbow strain, soft tissue tightness of her shoulder may be related to the excess stress that could have precipitated this elbow injury. Or, if the athlete broke a leg two years ago and was in a cast for six weeks, resultant tightness in the calf that was never completely resolved may affect your examination of today's ankle sprain. Whether the second baseman's diabetes is controlled will influence your level of concern about the laceration he received on his forearm from an opponent's cleat. That a fireman has previously sprained the same knee may influence your findings during ligament stress testing. It is also important to ask about the opposite, or uninvolved, side. While the uninjured side is typically used as the benchmark for what is normal for a person, it may not provide an accurate comparison depending on previous injuries.

Ask, for example, "Have you previously injured the same area or the surrounding area?" If so, find out how long ago the injury occurred and how severe it was. Also ask, "Have you ever injured the other side?" In either case, ask, "What were the diagnosis and treatment?" "What was the outcome of the treatment?" "How long was the recovery?" "Have you had any problems with the injury since then?" Asking questions such as, "Are you taking any medications?" "Do you take, or have you taken, steroids or recreational drugs?" "Do you have any other medical conditions that may affect this injury?" will lend further clarification to precipitating factors.

Questions for Specific Injury Situations

The following checklists provide appropriate questions to ask when dealing with acute, non-acute, and chronic injuries. Note the open-ended nature of the questions.

General Questions for Acute Injuries

What happened and how did it happen?

What position were you in when the injury occurred? (How they landed, whether the foot was rotated in or out)

Did you hear or feel any unusual sounds or sensations at the time of injury? (Snap or pop)

Do you feel any unusual sensations now? (Numbness, tingling, burning)

Where is the pain? (Have them point to the location of pain to find the area that is most painful)

Can you describe the pain?

- Quality of pain (Sharp, dull, achy)
- Intensity (Have the athlete rate the pain on a scale of 0-10)
- Localized or diffuse
- Referral of pain to other segments
- Changes in pain from when it started (intensified or lessened)

When does it hurt? (All the time, only when moved, only when touched or stressed)

What is the previous history of the body region? (Nature, severity, duration of symptoms; treatment received)

What is the previous history for the opposite side?

Are there any other medical conditions to be aware of?

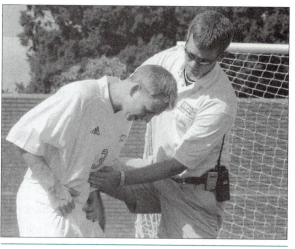

Figure 3.2 Know what questions to ask when. Asking detailed questions about previous unrelated injuries is clearly counterproductive in this situation.

General Questions for Nonacute Injuries

What happened and how did it happen? If the symptoms came on gradually, when did they first appear and what were you doing at the time?

What activities aggravate the injury now?

What makes it feel better?

When you work out, when do the symptoms come on and how long do they persist?

Do the symptoms interfere with daily activities, and if so, what activities?

Can you describe the pain?

- Quality of pain (sharp, dull, achy)
- Intensity (0-10 scale)
- Localized or diffuse
- Referral to other segments
- Changes in the pain from when it started (intensified or lessened over time)

Does the pain wake you up at night?

Is there any time during the day that the pain is worse or less, or is the pain activity related?

What treatment, if any, have you self-administered?

General Questions for Chronic Injuries

What hurts (what is the chief complaint)?

When did the injury occur?

Was it a sudden onset, or did the symptoms appear gradually over time?

If sudden, do you know how it happened or what caused it?

If gradual, when did the symptoms first appear and what were you doing at the time?

Can you describe the pain?

- Quality of pain (sharp, dull, achy)
- Intensity (scale of 0-10)
- Localized or diffuse
- Referral of pain to other segments
- Changes in pain from when it started (intensified or lessened over time)

When does it hurt?

Is the pain constant or intermittent?

Once the injury is irritated, how long does the pain last?

What activities make the pain worse?

How much do the pain or symptoms interfere with activity?

What activities make the pain better?

Have you made any abrupt or significant changes in training?

- Change in intensity, duration, training surface, type of activity
- Any change in training implements (tennis racket grip, bat weight, shoes)

What is the previous history for this body region (nature, severity, duration of symptoms; treatment received)?

What is the previous history for the opposite side?

Are there any other medical conditions to be aware of?

- Change in diet or weight?
- Recent illness?
- Other signs and symptoms?
- Existing medical conditions?
- Taking any medications or receiving any treatment?

Refer to the Web site http://www.HumanKinetics.com/ExaminationOfMusculoskeletalInjuries for printable versions of the checklists.

The history you obtain will guide you in your objective examination by profiling the SINS of the injury or illness. The SINS define the examination techniques you use and how aggressively you apply them.

Later chapters in part II include specific questions for particular regions of the body. If the athlete cannot recall a particular injury or illness that has caused the current symptoms, special medical questions may be required to rule out general medical problems, some of which could be serious. Such questions include, for example, if the athlete has recently experienced unexplained weight loss or recurring night sweats. These signs could indicate any one of several life-threatening conditions, such as cancer or acquired autoimmune deficiency syndrome, which should not be ignored. Fever could suggest an illness needing medical attention. You should ask a female athlete in her childbearing years if she is pregnant, as pregnancy may affect your treatment protocol. Other specific questions you should ask depend on the athlete's symptoms. Generally, complaints of symptoms that include dizziness, hearing or vision changes, coordination problems, unexplained weakness, and bowel or bladder dysfunction, can indicate neurological pathology. Chapters 21, 22, and 23 describe the signs and symptoms associated with a variety of common medical conditions that you should also be familiar with.

SUMMARY

1. Identify the main goals and features of taking a history.

   Obtaining a history serves as a fundamental first step in your athletic injury examination. The purpose of taking a history is to obtain, through a series of well-planned questions, an accurate record of an athlete's injury or illness. Asking questions that identify the athlete's chief complaint will help you determine the primary problem and focus your examination. Learning the mechanism of injury or nature of the illness informs you about how the injury occurred and events leading to the onset of the illness, which helps you better understand the nature of the condition. Asking about current and previous signs and symptoms details the nature of the condition and provides clues regarding the level of its severity, irritability, and stage. You can also learn important information from asking the athlete about previous injuries or events that may affect the current condition or your examination findings.

2. Ask pertinent, nonleading questions to determine the nature and severity of the injury.

   Careful questions sketch a picture of the athlete's complaint and symptoms and properly direct your objective examination. To gain an accurate picture of the athlete's injury or illness, your questioning should be efficient and thorough. Ask only pertinent questions, but ask enough questions to allow you to formulate a plan for the remaining examination. When asking questions about signs and symptoms, be careful not to lead the athlete, but instead allow him to answer as accurately as possible in his own words.

3. Differentiate the types of information that should be learned for emergent, acute nonemergent, and chronic conditions examinations.

   The extent of questioning depends on the injury scenario. When called to examine an unconscious athlete with a potentially life-threatening condition, concern yourself only with the essential facts that are necessary to guide your primary survey and immediate care until you stabilize the athlete. When an athlete is injured on the field, you will perform a more focused history to learn enough information to determine the course of your immediate examination and care and decide whether it is safe to remove the athlete to the sideline. Obtain a more detailed history in cases when there are no life-threatening conditions and you are in an environment conducive to a thorough examination. Unlike the essential and focused history that are typically only conducted when dealing with acute injury or illness, a detailed history applies to both acute and chronic conditions. For chronic conditions, you need to ask additional questions regarding events leading to the onset of symptoms, aggravating and relieving factors, and patterns of their signs and symptoms over time, including a detailed pain profile.

4. Obtain a thorough history from any ill or injured athlete.

   Obtaining a thorough current and previous history of an injury or illness guides your objective examination. When you complete the history portion of the examination, you should have an idea of the nature, stage, and irritability of the injury, which will define the examination techniques you use and how aggressively you apply them.

REVIEW QUESTIONS

1. When approaching an athlete on the field who has injured her ankle but otherwise appears to be in no acute distress, what are the primary questions you ask to determine or diagnose the nature of the injury?

2. How would the remaining questions in the history portion of the examination of this ankle injury differ when on the field and on the sideline?

3. Does witnessing an injury influence the questions you ask? Why or why not?

4. To establish the nature of an illness, what specific questions should you ask?

5. Is the question "Did you feel your knee shift when you twisted it?" a well-phrased question? Why or why not? If not, how would you phrase it differently?

6. Why is it important to understand the mechanism of injury? How does this information assist you in understanding the potential structures involved and the extent of tissue damage that may have occurred?

CRITICAL THINKING QUESTIONS

1. An industrial worker comes into the clinic complaining of shoulder pain for the past 5 to 7 days. What are some of the questions you might ask to determine the severity, irritability, nature, and stage of the injury?

2. Let's revisit the challenge that Justin faces in the opening scenario on page 38. If one of your athletes called you complaining of abdominal pain, what questions would you ask to determine the seriousness of the condition and whether the athlete needs to be examined?

3. You are in the athletic training facility treating one of your basketball athletes when Andrea, a soccer player, races in and tells you that her teammate, Brenda, is down on the field and not moving. What questions might you ask Andrea as you run out to the field to learn essential clues to the nature of Brenda's condition?

4. A tennis athlete comes into the athletic training facility complaining of right wrist pain. As you begin to ask the athlete questions about his injury, you notice that his right forearm is much smaller in circumference than his left forearm. What questions might you ask to learn the reason for this difference and whether it may be contributing to the current injury?

5. A basketball player goes down on the court after a rebound and grabs his right knee. As you evaluate this acute knee injury on the court, you notice that the athlete has a long, vertical scar on the uninjured (left) knee. When would it be appropriate to ask questions about this previous injury? What specific questions would you ask and how might this information affect your examination of the current injury?

ADDITIONAL RESOURCES

American Academy of Orthopaedic Surgeons (AAOS). 1999. *Emergency: Care and transportation of the sick and injured.* 7th ed. Sudbury, MA: Jones and Bartlett.

Caroline, N.L. 1995. *Emergency care in the streets.* 5th ed. Boston: Little, Brown.

Observation

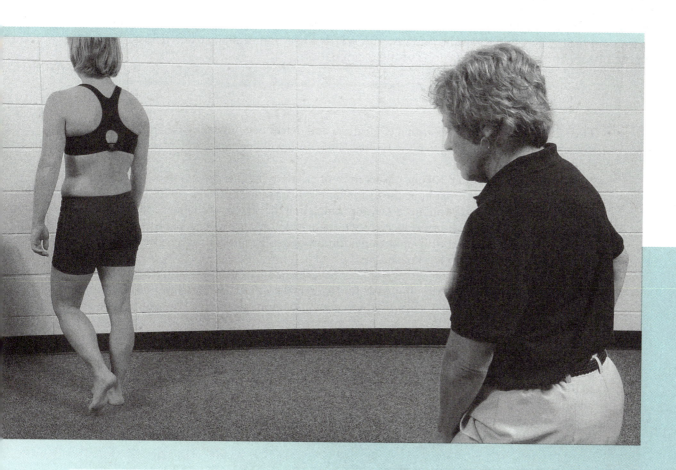

Objectives

After completing this chapter, the reader will be able to do the following:

1. Identify the main goals of the observation
2. Understand the elements of the global observation
3. Recognize the elements of the specific observation
4. Differentiate among the three somatotypes of body structure
5. Perform an examination of static posture
6. Be familiar with the parts of the stance and swing phases of gait
7. Describe the specific observations that should be routinely performed on the injured segment

Susan is doing well in her athletic training courses in the first semester of the professional phase of her curriculum. She has been working with Jonathan, her ACI, over the past month and has familiarized herself with the athletic training department of the local high school where Jonathan works. She mentioned to Jonathan that yesterday she learned the history, observation, and palpation sections of an examination, and that her class was rapidly moving into the other parts of a total examination. As she was explaining the details of what she learned, a volleyball player entered the athletic training facility and told them she had just injured her knee. Jonathan instructed Susan to perform the history and observation portions of the examination.

The athletic trainer observes with a clinical eye and delves beyond merely seeing, but looks to identify the abnormal, notice the unique, and continually compare the atypical with the typical.

As discussed in chapter 2, your observation of an injury begins the moment you see the patient and continues throughout the examination. It includes noticing details easily overlooked by the untrained eye but necessary for completing the picture of an injury. This chapter refines the definition of observation and presents suggestions that will make observations an automatic and critical part of your examination process. The goal of this chapter is to take your visual acuity to a new level of sensitivity.

Observation begins the objective portion of every examination and continues during the other tests you perform. Watching each test is crucial to understanding and interpreting the results. The sharper your skills of observation, the more accurately you will be able to diagnose the patient's injury.

A thorough observation provides information on the affected area, the degree to which the injury affects the athlete's function, and your probable role in healing the injury. The observation provides you with an initial impression of the injury and the athlete's response to the injury. As you examine the injury, your observation skills combined with tests provide additional clues to the severity and nature of the injury.

There is no universal agreement among clinicians about the meanings of *inspection* and *observation*. This text regards the terms as synonymous and uses them accordingly.

SYSTEM OF OBSERVATIONAL EXAMINATION

Observation must include global observations and specific observations. Global observations are your initial and overall impressions. Specific observations are performed after the history, during the posture and gait examination and the objective measures of the injured and noninjured segments.

Global Observation

General observation of the athlete without specific attention to the injury is involved in the global observation. The global observation includes initial and overall impressions.

- **Initial impressions on the field.** If you see the injury occur and must go onto the field, you will notice if the athlete is moving. If the athlete is not moving, you know immediately that the injury may be serious and requires urgent action. On the other hand, if the athlete is rolling on the ground, you know the injury is likely not life threatening. The athlete will instinctively protect the injured area, so the area she grasps influences your initial impression of the injury location.

- **Overall impressions on the field.** As you note your initial impressions, you begin to formulate an overall impression. The overall impression summarizes the immediate situation and provides you with direction for immediate care or a focus from which to begin your examination. Once you have observed the athlete's level of consciousness, your overall impression guides your actions as you arrive at the athlete's side. Your impression of the athlete's response to the injury determines if there is a need to calm the athlete before beginning the examination. Is the athlete calm or visibly upset? Is he in too much pain to converse? Is he hysterical? Once you begin physical examination of the injury, you continue to accumulate observations that direct your next actions. When the athlete is calm and stabilized, your observations determine the most appropriate means of transporting him off the field of play. Once the athlete is on the sidelines, your observations assist you in developing a final impression of the athlete's injury.

• **Initial impressions in the clinical setting.** If you see the patient's injury for the first time in your facility without witnessing the injury, you will still develop an initial impression. In this case, the initial impression includes observation of how the patient walks and stands. How does the patient hold the injured segment? Are there any gross deformities that can be readily observed? If the injured part involves the upper extremity, does it swing freely by the patient's side or is it held next to the body? Is the arm in a sling or splint? If the injury involves the lower extremity, is the patient using crutches or other assistive devices? Is the injury supported or splinted? Does the patient lurch or limp? If so, how much weight does the patient seem to put on the extremity? Is the patient walking with any gross differences from right to left such as a stiff knee or laterally rotated hip? Which joint does she seem to keep from moving through its normal motion? What facial expressions does she display as she walks? Does she grimace or is it otherwise obvious that she has discomfort walking?

• **Overall impressions in the clinical setting.** The patient's eyes reveal his true response to pain and should be carefully observed throughout the examination. As the patient reports his history, does he sit comfortably, or is he unable to find a comfortable position for very long? If the patient removes clothing to allow for examination, how well does he perform the task? Is he hesitant to move the injured segment? Is he able to perform the task independently, or does he require assistance?

Make global observations second nature because they are crucial during emergencies and nonemergencies alike.

Specific Observation

Once you complete the general observation, you will turn to a more **specific observation** to determine the precise injury and other areas of the body that may be affected by or aggravating to the injury site. These secondary areas are determined through observation of posture and gait. Later in this chapter we take an in-depth look at posture and gait analysis as well as observation of the injury.

• **Observation of Body Type.** Body types are divided into three categories, or **somatotypes: ectomorph, mesomorph,** and **endomorph.** Only 5% of the population possesses a pure body type; most people are a combination of the three types with a stronger tendency toward one (Nieman 2003). Somatotypes are strongly related to body weight rather than to the ratio of lean body mass to fat body mass. The ectomorphic body type has low to normal fat mass, has low muscle mass, and is underweight. The mesomorphic body type also has low to normal fat mass but has average to high muscle mass and may be average weight or overweight. The endomorphic body type has high fat and muscle mass and is overweight (see figure 4.1).

Because of their inaccuracies in describing an individual, somatotypes are not often presented clinically but are used to describe in general terms an individual's overall build. Somatotypes may be used when diagnosing eating disorders. However, without knowing the athlete's lean-to-fat body mass ratio and nutritional habits, looking only at somatotype may provide misleading results.

• **Observation of posture and gait.** Observation of overall posture is important because poor posture can contribute to an injury. For example, a forward head posture can worsen

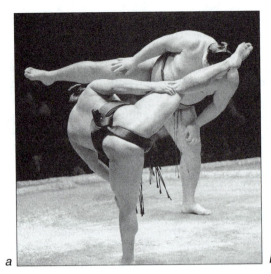
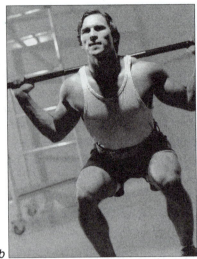
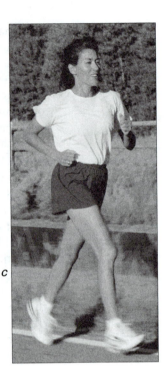

Figure 4.1 Somatotypes: *(a)* endomorph with high fat and muscle mass, *(b)* mesomorph with low to normal fat and average to high muscle mass, and *(c)* ectomorph with low to normal fat and low muscle mass.

a cervical sprain, and a round shoulder posture can negatively affect the shoulders' range of motion (ROM). Know what normal posture is in order to determine if the athlete has dysfunctional posture that may have aggravated or resulted from the injury. If the athlete has a lower-extremity injury, perform a gait analysis (discussed in "Examination of Gait" on page 54).

- **Observation of the injured segment.** Once you conclude your observation of body type and posture and gait, observe the injured segment in greater detail. Your overall impressions have been created from gross observation of how the patient holds or protects the injured segment. Now you continue with specific observations of the injured part as detailed in the Summary Observation Checklist.

Summary Observation Checklist

▷ *Global Observation On-Site*

☐ Is the athlete moving?

☐ Does the injury appear to be life threatening?

☐ Is the athlete protecting the injury?

☐ Is the athlete in need of urgent care?

☐ Are there gross deformities or is there severe bleeding?

☐ How is the athlete responding to the injury?

    ☐ What are the athlete's facial expressions?

    ☐ Is the athlete visibly upset?

    ☐ Is the athlete in too much pain to speak to you?

    ☐ Is the athlete's response appropriate for the injury?

☐ What is the best means of transporting the athlete off the field?

▷ *Global Observation in the Athletic Training Facility*

☐ How is the athlete standing?

☐ How is the athlete walking?

- ☐ Does the athlete use crutches?
- ☐ Does the athlete use a splint or sling?
- ☐ Is there an abnormal gait?
- ☐ Are there any other gross gait pathologies?
- ☐ How does the athlete move the injured segment?
- ☐ Are deformities apparent?
- ☐ What are the athlete's facial expressions?
- ☐ Does the athlete appear to be in discomfort?

▷ Specific Observation of Noninjury Segments

- ☐ What is the athlete's body type?
- ☐ What is the athlete's posture?
  - ☐ Anterior view
  - ☐ Lateral view
  - ☐ Posterior view
- ☐ Does the athlete have gait deviations?
  - ☐ Stride length
  - ☐ Gait rhythm
  - ☐ At heel strike
  - ☐ At foot flat
  - ☐ At midstance
  - ☐ At heel-off
  - ☐ At toe-off
  - ☐ During early, mid, and late swing
  - ☐ Each joint and segment from an anterior view
  - ☐ Each joint and segment from a lateral view
  - ☐ Each joint and segment from a posterior view

▷ Specific Observation of Injury Segment

- ☐ Gross deformity
- ☐ Bleeding
- ☐ Edema
  - ☐ Localized
  - ☐ Diffuse
- ☐ Ecchymosis
  - ☐ Proximal to the injury
  - ☐ Distal to the injury
- ☐ Skin redness
- ☐ Signs of infection
  - ☐ Pus
  - ☐ Swelling
  - ☐ Enlarged lymph nodes
  - ☐ Red streaks
- ☐ Lacerations
- ☐ Blisters or calluses
- ☐ Rash
- ☐ Muscle spasm
- ☐ Preexisting deformities

DETAILS OF SPECIFIC OBSERVATION

Conduct your specific observation systematically. A consistent routine reduces the chance of forgetting an item that may reveal crucial clues.

Examination of Posture

Examine posture with the patient in a static position and in as few clothes as possible to allow an unobstructed view of all postural elements. Correct posture minimizes stress on muscles, bones, and joints while incorrect posture places abnormal stress on these structures. The more posture deviates from the correct position, the greater the stress placed on the structures that work to maintain it.

Incorrect posture usually develops with gradual changes in muscle, tendon, or fascial support. Children under the age of four generally have good posture and mechanics. As early as elementary school, children develop poor sitting and standing habits, and abnormal posture becomes apparent. By the time an individual becomes a teenager or young adult, abnormal postural habits are entrenched. Poor posture becomes more exaggerated as people age and develop progressively greater tightness and weakness in already shortened or lengthened soft tissue structures, resulting in changes in bone alignment and stress distribution.

Incorrect posture can also occur rapidly following an acute injury if the athlete alters position to reduce pain, function with altered ability, or protect an injury. For example, a patient who experiences excessive swelling around the knee following an injury may not be able to stand with the knee fully extended, or a person suffering a cervical sprain may stand with the head thrust forward to relieve pain.

Sometimes an individual acquires an incorrect alignment because genetically determined joint or soft tissue characteristics cause the deformity over time, or the deformity present from birth becomes more apparent as the person ages.

You should include posture when examining any injury in the athletic training clinic. Posture can either result from injury or contribute to injury and should not be overlooked if you are to provide appropriate care. Examine posture by inspecting the anterior, lateral, and posterior views of the patient in the frontal and sagittal planes (figure 4.2).

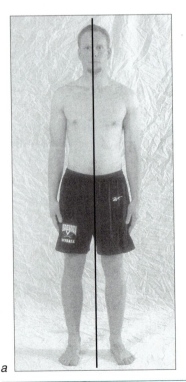 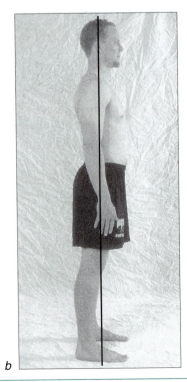 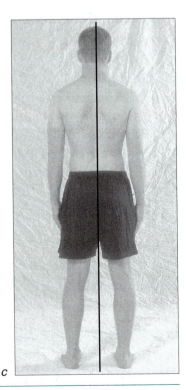

a   b   c

Figure 4.2 Correct standing alignment: *(a)* anterior, *(b)* lateral, and *(c)* posterior views.

Reprinted, by permission, from P.A. Houglum, 2001, *Therapeutic exercise for athletic injuries* (Champaign IL: Human Kinetics), 343-344.

Examination Procedure

A plumb line is often used as a reference of alignment for the body when examining posture. A **plumb line** is a string suspended overhead with a small weight, or plumb bob, attached at the end near the floor. Position the patient behind the line so you can see the body bisected by the plumb line.

- **Anterior view.** The patient faces you with the plumb line dividing his body into right and left halves. Use the checklist for the anterior view to identify any deviations from normal.
- **Lateral view.** Observe the lateral view from both the left and right sides so you can see any imbalances between the two. Use the checklist for the lateral view to identify any deviations from normal.
- **Posterior view.** This view includes some of the same items observed in the anterior view but should not be eliminated since it also reveals other factors such as foot arch positions, knee fossa alignment, scoliosis, and scapula height. The plumb line bisects the body as indicated in the posterior view checklist. Again, use the checklist to identify any deviations from normal.

Anterior, Lateral, and Posterior Posture Examination Checklists

▷ *Anterior Posture Examination Checklist*

- ☐ Plumb line bisects body in left and right halves
- ☐ Plumb line runs between the eyes and the center of the nose, mouth, chin, jugular notch, sternum, and navel; runs equidistant between the right and left foot
- ☐ Left and right halves of the body are mirror images of each other
- ☐ Arms rest at the sides of the body
- ☐ Hands are along the sides of the hips
- ☐ Patellae face anteriorly
- ☐ Knees straight and equidistant from the plumb line
- ☐ Toes pointed either forward or slightly laterally
- ☐ Ear lobes are level
- ☐ Acromion processes are even
- ☐ Axillary folds are even
- ☐ Lower rib margins are level
- ☐ Iliac crests are level
- ☐ Patellae are same height
- ☐ Tibial tuberosities are even
- ☐ Medial malleoli are level
- ☐ Muscle definition is symmetrical throughout

▷ *Lateral Posture Examination Checklist*

- ☐ Plumb line runs through the middle of the ear's auditory meatus, the bodies of the cervical spine, the acromion process, the midthoracic area, and the greater trochanter
- ☐ Plumb line runs slightly posterior to the patella and anterior to the lateral malleolus
- ☐ Anterior superior iliac spine (ASIS) and posterior superior iliac spine (PSIS) are close to level with each other
- ☐ Leg is perpendicular to the foot
- ☐ Hands are slightly forward of the elbow and beside the thigh
- ☐ Chin is parallel to the floor

(continued)

(continued)

▷ *Posterior Posture Examination Checklist*

☐ Plumb line bisects the head and all spinous processes from the cervical through the lumbar spine

☐ Left and right halves are mirror images of each other

☐ Ear lobes are level

☐ Shoulder heights are level (dominant may be slightly lower)

☐ Axillary folds are even

☐ Inferior angles of scapulae are level

☐ Vertebral scapular borders are equidistant and 5 cm (about 2 in.) from spine

☐ Scapulae rest on ribs between T2 and T7

☐ Iliac crests are level

☐ Popliteal fossa are same height

☐ Arms rest comfortably at sides with hands along sides of thighs

☐ Achilles tendons are perpendicular to floor

☐ Medial malleoli are level

☐ Two toes are visible laterally to each leg

☐ Muscle definition is symmetrical throughout

Postural Deviations

You should record postural deviations during the examination, ranking them as mild, moderate, or severe. Occasionally, a position may be considered normal, hyper-, or hypo-, while other postural deviations may be identified with names that define the abnormality but may not indicate severity. For example, genu recurvatum indicates hyperextension of the knee joint without relating the severity of the hyperextension. Placing a descriptor such as mild in front of these names can further qualify or quantify the deviation.

The examination process always includes comparison of left and right corresponding segments, because "normal" is often solely determined by comparison to the contralateral side. Normal for one person may not be normal for another person. For example, a gymnast will have much greater excursion in a straight leg raise than a baseball player, and a pitcher will have more glenohumeral lateral rotation than a first baseman. Each athlete must be compared only to herself and not to others.

Postural deviations cannot be recognized as abnormal unless normal posture is identified. You must know what is normal, or expected, in postural examination from all views. In part II, where the body regions and their associated injuries are discussed, postural deviations unique to those regions are presented. How to identify, treat, or modify the deviations, as well as the consequences of the deviations, are also discussed.

Examination of Gait

Gait examination is a dynamic examination. The way an athlete walks informs you of lower-extremity and trunk injuries. Gait is a complex activity that requires little or no thought when all segments function normally. However, when an injury interferes with normal function, gait becomes a chore at best and impossible at worst. Gait examination can reveal the severity, irritability, and nature of the injury.

Although gait varies greatly from one individual to another, there is a normal range. Individuals ambulate outside of this range because of an injury or habit; in either case, the risk of injury increases because abnormal gait applies additional stresses. For example, an athlete who walks or runs with exaggerated pronation is susceptible to injuries to the plantar fascia and Achilles tendon. An athlete who walks with excessive knee flexion due to tightness that limits extension places increased stress on the articular cartilage of the knee and magnifies the stresses on the lumbar spine since she is essentially walking with a shorter leg on one side.

As with posture, recognizing normal gait is the first step (no pun intended) to identifying abnormal gait. Since gait is so complex, let's simplify it by looking at its phases and components before identifying the key motions of each joint.

Gait Cycle

Gait, the person's manner of ambulation or locomotion, involves the total body. Gait speed determines the contribution of each body segment. Normal walking speed primarily involves the lower extremities, with the arms and trunk providing stability and balance. The faster the speed, the more the body depends on the upper extremities and trunk for propulsion as well as balance and stability. The legs continue to do the most work as the joints produce greater ranges of motion through greater muscle responses.

Gait encompasses a continuum from slow walking to fast running and has been described as a continual system of balance loss and recovery (Perry 1990). We propel the body from one leg to the other as muscles and momentum move the body forward. In the bipedal system, which human beings use, the three major joints of the lower body and pelvis work with each other to make walking efficient, using as little motion as necessary. The degree to which the body's center of gravity moves during forward translation defines efficiency. The body's center of gravity (CoG) moves both side to side and up and down during gait. In each direction CoG shifts less than 5 cm (2 in.). The foot clears the ground with just as much efficiency: a mere 1 cm (3/8 in.).

Gait is measured using a cycle. The point of heel contact of one extremity to the next point of heel contact of the same extremity completes one cycle. Walking involves two phases of gait: stance and swing-through (swing). Gait is a combination of open- and closed-chain activities. During the stance phase, the extremity bears the weight of the body (closed chain). The stance phase lasts the longest, comprising approximately 60% of the total gait cycle. During the first and last 10% of the stance phase, both feet contact the ground, and during the remainder of the stance phase only one lower limb supports the body's weight. During the swing phase (open chain), the limb does not bear weight.

Each gait phase is further divided into components, allowing clinicians to discuss gait patterns and deviations. There are two "languages," or systems, used to discuss gait phases. Since clinicians use both systems and you may encounter other health professionals who use one or the other, both are presented in figure 4.3.

Here are the gait phases, arranged sequentially:

1. **Heel strike or initial contact.** Heel strike (initial contact) is a very short period of time that begins the moment the foot contacts the ground and is the first instance of double support, or support from both lower limbs. At this time the foot is in about 5° of supination, hitting the ground on the lateral heel. The ankle is at neutral dorsiflexion–plantar flexion, the knee is at or near full extension, and the hip is in 30° of flexion.

2. **Foot flat or loading response.** Foot flat or loading response occurs during double support when the body absorbs the impact by rolling the foot into pronation, moving the ankle into 15° of plantar flexion, flexing the knee to 15°, and using the hip to maintain stabilization at 30° of flexion.

3. **Midstance.** As the name implies, midstance is the middle of the stance phase. During midstance the body is supported by a single leg. At the middle of midstance, the body's weight is directly over the supporting foot. The body begins to move from force absorption at impact to force propulsion forward. It does this by moving the body forward in front of the weight-bearing leg so the ankle now moves in to dorsiflexion as the knee and hip extend, and the foot supinates, converting it from a force-absorbing loose structure to a force-transmitting rigid lever.

4. **Heel-off or terminal stance.** This phase begins once the heel of the foot leaves the floor. The body is still in single-leg stance but the swing leg progresses ahead of the stance leg. The tibia of the swing leg is moving from perpendicular to the floor toward knee extension. The body's weight is over the metatarsal heads. The foot is supinated 5°, the ankle is plantar flexed, the knee is fully extended, and the hip is hyperextended 10°.

Closed chain refers to the proximal segment moving with the distal segment fixed (e.g., foot on the ground).

Open chain refers to the proximal segment (e.g., leg) being fixed with the distal segment (e.g., foot) allowed to freely move.

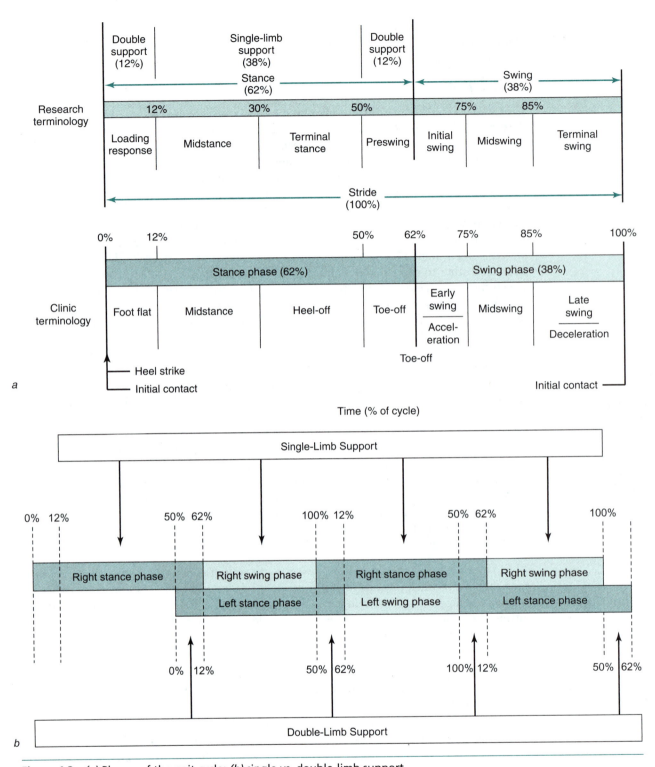

Figure 4.3 *(a)* Phases of the gait cycle; *(b)* single vs. double-limb support.

Reprinted, by permission, from P.A. Houglum, 2005, *Therapeutic exercise for musculoskeletal injuries,* 2nd ed. (Champaign, IL: Human Kinetics), 358.

5. Toe-off or preswing. Just before the heel of the swing leg hits the ground, toe-off of the weight-bearing leg begins its final phase. This is the second instance of double-limb support in the gait cycle. During preswing the weight-bearing lower limb prepares to transfer weight to the other limb. The great toe is dorsiflexed 60°, the ankle is plantar flexed 20°, the knee is flexed 35°, and the hip is neutral. The moment the toes come off the ground at the end of the preswing, the lower limb completes the stance phase and begins the swing phase.

6. Early swing or initial swing. Early swing is the first one-third of swing. The knee achieves maximum flexion at 60°, clearing the toe from the ground. The ankle assists by dorsiflexing to a neutral position. The hip assists by flexing 20° with some lateral rotation.

7. Midswing. Midswing occurs during the second one-third of the swing phase. It is marked by the tibia coming forward of the stance leg, perpendicular to the ground. The ankle remains neutral and the knee flexes approximately 30° while the hip continues into greater flexion.

8. Late swing or terminal swing. Late swing is the last one-third of swing. The swing leg prepares for weight acceptance by decelerating the rate of swing, maintaining the ankle in a neutral or slightly dorsiflexed position, continuing to extend the knee, and reaching for the ground by flexing the hip to 30°.

Gait continuously moves from one phase to another. The terms for identifying and discussing the topic are a means of communication. Within each component of each gait phase, ROM changes and muscle activity is modified. Figure 4.4 summarizes ROM activity in the hip, knee, and ankle during each of the gait phases.

Muscle Activity

During gait, muscles of the lower body act as accelerators, decelerators, or stabilizers. Accelerators propel the body forward while decelerators slow segmental movement to allow smooth, continuous motion, and stabilizers prevent needless motion. Muscles acting as accelerators work concentrically during the last half of stance and during swing to propel the extremity and body forward. The decelerators work eccentrically during the early part of stance to smooth forward motion by absorbing shock and slowing motion generated from the swing phase. Stabilizers work isometrically throughout the stance phase to keep the body upright and steady.

Stabilizer muscles include the trunk and hip extensors. Accelerators include the calf muscles and knee flexors during late stance and the hip flexors and ankle and toe extensors during swing. Decelerators and shock absorbers include the knee extensors, which control knee flexion, and the anterior toe and ankle muscles, which control plantar flexion of the ankle.

During gait, muscles cycle through periods of activity followed by periods of inactivity. This on-and-off system allows us to ambulate long distances without fatigue. Muscles that must work for unusually long periods because of abnormal posture or gait will experience early fatigue and excessive stress that they may not be able to tolerate, especially if sudden increases or changes in workouts occur.

Maximum Motion Requirements for Gait

Knowing the maximum ROM required by each joint during walking and running allows you to determine the patient's ability to walk or run without motion restriction. During walking, the greatest amount of ankle motion occurs at midstance and at toe-off. Midstance requires 10° of dorsiflexion, and toe-off needs 20° of plantar flexion. The knee moves from 0° of extension at heel strike to 60° of flexion at midswing. The hip ranges from 10° of hyperextension at heel-off to 30° of flexion during late swing and through foot flat.

Running Gait

Running gait differs from walking gait in that it has different phases, involves greater motions, and requires greater, quicker muscle activity. The stance phase during running is shorter, but the swing phase lasts longer. The faster an athlete runs, the greater the swing phase and the shorter the stance phase. During running, there is no time of double support, but there is a time when the body does not contact the ground. This phase is called the **double float** phase and occurs at the beginning of initial swing and the end of terminal swing. Running gait specifics vary with different running speeds. Generally, the faster the athlete's speed, the greater the athlete's stride, ranges of motion, and explosiveness of muscle activity. Ankle motion can increase to 75° and knee motion can be greater than 120°.

Normal Gait

	Stance 60%					Swing 40%		
	Heel strike	Foot flat	Midstance	Heel-off	Toe-off	Early swing	Midswing	Late swing
Trunk	Erect Neutral	Erect Neutral	Erect Neutral	Erect Neutral	Erect Neutral	Erect Neutral	Erect Neutral	Erect Neutral
Pelvis	Level Forward rotation	Level 5° forward rotation Upward lateral rotation	Level Neutral rotation	Level 5° posterior rotation Downward lateral rotation	Level Posterior rotation Downward lateral rotation	Level Posterior rotation moving forward Lateral position is down	Level Neutral lateral rotation moving up	Level 5° forward rotation
Hip	30° flexion Slight adduction Near-neutral rotation	30° flexion Slight adduction Slight rotation	Extends Slight adduction Slight medial rotation	10° hyper-extension Slight abduction	5° Neutral Extension Slight medial rotation 4° Abduction	20° flexion Slight lateral rotation 5° Abduction	Flexing Lateral rotation	30° flexion Mild lateral rotation going to medial rotation
Knee	Full extension Tibia in lateral rotation	15° flexion Tibia in medial rotation	Moves toward extension	Full extension	35° flexion	Cont. to 60° flexion Tibial lateral rotation	Begin to move to 30° flexion Tibial lateral rotation	Cont. to extend
Ankle	Neutral	15° plantar flexion Pronation	10° dorsi-flexion Starts to supinate	Moving into plantar flexion Supinating	20° plantar flexion	Moving to neutral	Neutral	Neutral
Toes	Neutral	Neutral	Neutral	MTP: 30° extension IP: Neutral	MTP: 60° extension IP: Neutral	Neutral	Neutral	Neutral

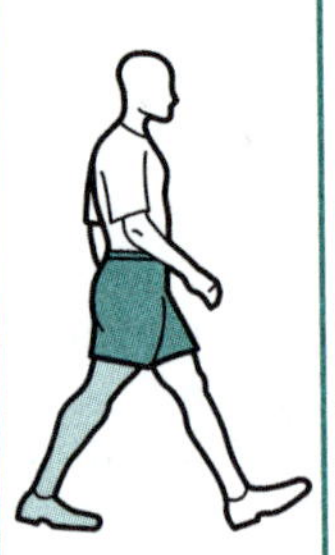

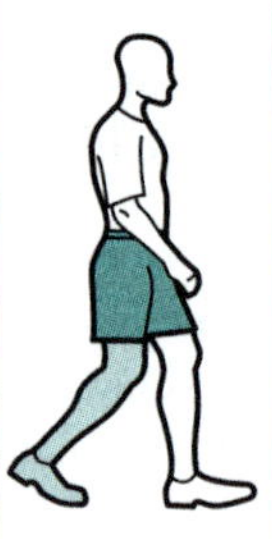

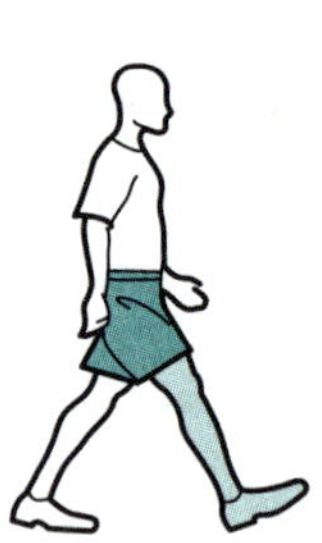

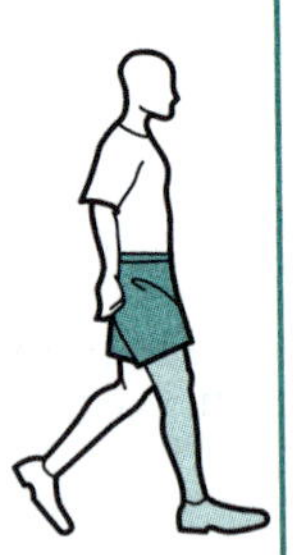

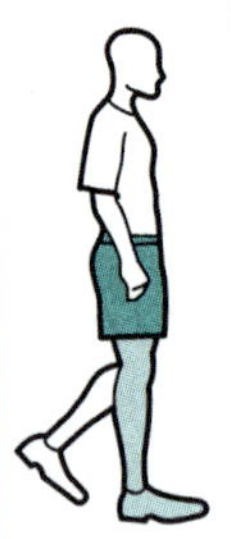

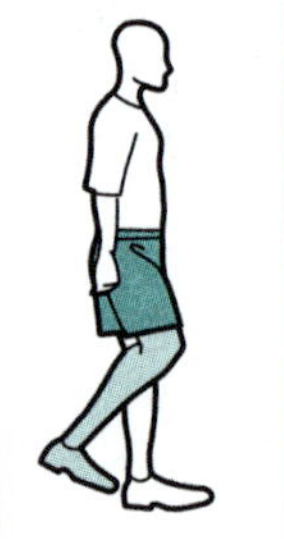

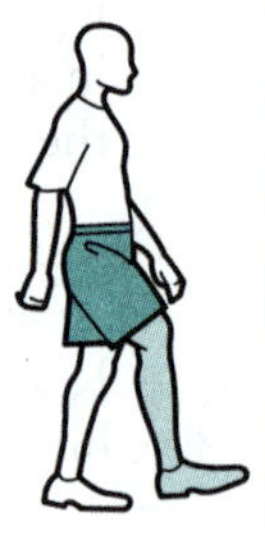

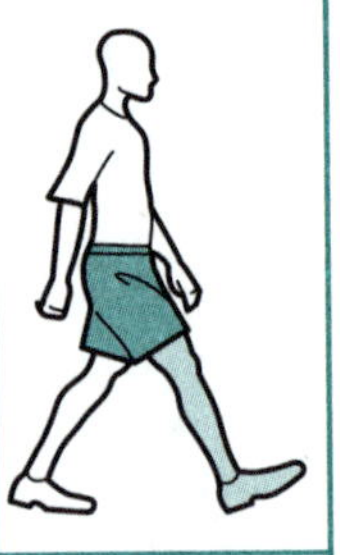

Figure 4.4 Normal gait kinetics of the hip, knee, and ankle.

Reprinted, by permission, from P.A. Houglum, 2001, *Therapeutic exercise for athletic inuries* (Champaign,IL: Human Kinetics), 385.

Procedure for Examining Gait

When you examine a patient's gait, watch how the patient walks during your global observation. Observe for symmetry and any obvious deviations from normal gait and use your sense of hearing as well as vision. Listen to the patient's feet hit the ground. Does each foot hit the ground with the same rhythm and intensity? Look at the patient's stride. Is the left stride the same length as the right stride? Next, look at each segment systematically. Observe the patient from anterior, lateral, and posterior views as she walks. The optimal way to examine gait is to record the patient on video and review it at a slow speed. If video is impossible, have the patient walk at a comfortable speed on a treadmill. If a treadmill is not available, have the patient walk in your facility as you make your observations. The Overall Gait Inspection checklist outlines the points you should examine.

Foot and Ankle Observation

Once you complete the overall observation, start the segmental examination, either beginning at the feet and moving up the chain or beginning at the head and moving to the feet. Be systematic. You should examine only one extremity's joint at a time before moving to the next joint or extremity. The Observation of the Foot and Ankle During Gait checklist provides a systematic process for observation of the foot and ankle.

Overall Gait Inspection

- ☐ Athlete has minimal clothing to allow good observation
- ☐ Athlete is relaxed
- ☐ Ask athlete to remove shoes
- ☐ Observe for symmetry in gait
- ☐ Listen for cadence
- ☐ Rhythm
- ☐ Symmetry
- ☐ Intensity
- ☐ Watch for stride length and stride width
- ☐ Look for smoothness of gait
- ☐ Observe from anterior, lateral, and posterior views
- ☐ Move to systematic segmental examination

Observation of Foot and Ankle During Gait

- ☐ Are you observing from anterior, posterior, and lateral views?
- ☐ Where does the foot hit the ground?
- ☐ Does the longitudinal arch change through weight bearing?
- ☐ Does the calcaneus change vertical alignment during stance?
- ☐ Does the calcaneus rotate quickly once it's non-weight bearing?
- ☐ Are the same number of toes evident laterally for each foot from behind the leg?
- ☐ Is muscle contraction evident?
- ☐ When does the heel come off the ground during stance?
- ☐ Does the ankle remain in neutral during swing?
- ☐ Is the gait smooth from foot flat to midstance?
- ☐ How does the left side compare to the right?

Knee Observation

As with the ankle, inspect the knee from anterior, posterior, and lateral views. The Observation of the Knee During Gait checklist provides a list of factors to examine during your observation.

Hip Observation

The hip is also observed throughout the stance and swing phases. The Observation of the Hip During Gait checklist guides you through observation of this joint.

Trunk and Upper-Extremity Observation

Do not forget to observe the position and movement of the head, trunk, and upper extremity during the patient's gait. These movements can provide important clues. The observations for these segments are outlined in the Observation of the Trunk and Upper Extremities During Gait checklist.

Observation of the Knee During Gait

- ☐ Are you observing from anterior, posterior, and lateral views?
- ☐ Is the knee in alignment with the ankle and hip from the anterior view?
- ☐ Does the patella remain forward during stance or does it rotate medically or laterally?
- ☐ Does the knee swing directly forward or circumduct during swing?
- ☐ Does the knee go from extension to partial flexion to extension during stance?
- ☐ Does the knee flex far enough during swing?
- ☐ How does the left knee compare to the right?

Observation of the Hip During Gait

- ☐ Are you observing from anterior, posterior, and lateral views?
- ☐ Is there slight lateral rotation at heel strike?
- ☐ Is adduction–abduction alignment good or does the hip adduct to cross toward the other leg during stance?
- ☐ Is the hip flexed with the trunk upright during heel strike?
- ☐ Does the hip move into hyperextension during heel-off?
- ☐ Is there sufficient hip flexion to clear the foot during swing?
- ☐ Is hip motion smooth throughout the gait cycle?
- ☐ Does the hip circumduct during swing?
- ☐ How does the left hip compare to the right?

Observation of the Trunk and Upper Extremities During Gait

- ☐ Are you observing from anterior, posterior, and lateral views?
- ☐ Does the trunk remain erect throughout the gait cycle?
- ☐ Does trunk rotation coincide with shoulder motion?
- ☐ Do the arms swing equally?
- ☐ Do the arms swing naturally from the shoulders?
- ☐ Do the shoulders appear relaxed?

Gait Deviations

When an injury occurs to the lower body, the patient usually is unable to ambulate normally, using instead an abnormal or pathological gait. Abnormal gaits occurring from acute injury are usually the result of pain. Pain is often associated or accompanied by edema, loss of function, or both. Any gait deviation resulting from pain is an **antalgic gait**. The hallmarks of an antalgic gait include spending less time on the injured extremity and more time on the healthy extremity, restricting motion of the injured segment, and using other techniques to apply less stress to the painful segment. For example, a patient with a lateral ankle sprain may walk with the extremity laterally rotated to limit ankle motion and places less stress on the lateral ankle. Or a patient with an injured knee may advance the extremity during the swing phase of gait by circumducting the hip, allowing the foot to clear the floor with minimal knee motion.

For a more detailed discussion on gait analysis, refer to *Therapeutic Exercise for Musculoskeletal Injuries, Second Edition,* (Houglum 2005), chapter 12.

Specific Observation of the Injury

Observation of the injury includes initial and continuous observations of the injured segment, the athlete's response to the injury, and the results of tests performed on the injured segment. You should always compare an injury site to its counterpart on the other side of the body to determine what is normal for the athlete. Is there any gross deformity? Gross deformity in a joint could indicate fracture or dislocation. Disruption of continuity in a long bone could indicate a fracture or muscle tear. These injuries indicate a need for medical referral and further examination on your part may not be necessary. Remember that along with observing the injury, you should also notice how the athlete responds to your requests to see the injury or move it. Watching the athlete's eyes for reactions is crucial.

If gross deformity is not present, continue observation of the injury site. Is any bleeding present? Is any edema present? Edema formation immediately following an injury can indicate a ligament or capsule injury. Diffuse edema occurs after the immediate injury response. If ecchymosis is also present, disruption of local blood vessels has accompanied the injury. If the injury is seen a day or more following the incident and swelling and ecchymosis are proximal to the injury site, the athlete has likely kept the injury elevated. However, if the swelling and ecchymosis are distal to the injury site, it is probable that the athlete has kept the injury in a primarily dependent position, allowing gravity to pull the fluid distally down the extremity.

You should also observe the skin. Redness may indicate an area of inflammation beneath the skin. If the injury site has redness along with swelling, pus, enlarged adjacent lymph nodes, extreme tenderness, and red streaks from the site running proximally, the site is probably infected. Are there any lacerations, scars, calluses, blisters, or rashes? If so, where are they, how large are they, and how do they appear in terms of color and discharge? Observation of other factors such as the presence of muscle spasm, ability or inability to use the injured segment, and preexisting congenital or structural deformities should be included in the visual examination of the injury before palpation.

In part II, you will see how the techniques of observation become part of the overall injury examination and how specific deviations and abnormal findings enable you to form a complete picture of an injury.

SUMMARY

1. Identify the main goals of the observation.

   The goals of a thorough observation are to fill in the total picture of the injury by determining the affected area, the degree to which the injury affects function, and the clinician's probable role in care. The observation provides an initial impression of the injury and the athlete's response to the injury. Combined with tests, it provides clues as to the severity and nature of the athlete's injury.

2. Understand the elements of the global observation.

Initial impressions begin as soon as you see the athlete. The athlete's response and movements help you form an impression of the severity and location of the injury. If you see the injury occur, notice whether the person is moving. A patient instinctively protects the injured area, so the injury location may be identified by the area the athlete grasps or immobilizes. As the initial impressions take shape, so does the overall impression. The overall impression is a summary of the immediate situation and directs immediate care, if necessary, or a focus from which to begin the examination.

3. Recognize the elements of the specific observation.

The specific observation determines both precise injury to the injured segment and possible involvement of noninjured segments. Observation of body type, overall posture, and gait are important because these elements can aggravate or contribute to an injury

4. Differentiate among the three somatotypes of body structure.

The ectomorphic body type has a low to normal fat mass, a low muscle mass, and is underweight. The mesomorphic body type also has a low to normal fat mass but has an average to high muscle mass and is average or overweight. The endomorphic body type has a high fat and muscle mass and is overweight.

5. Perform an examination of static posture.

Posture is inspected from anterior, lateral, and posterior views of the patient. From an anterior view, the plumb line bisects body into left and right halves, running between the eyes, the center of the nose, mouth, chin, jugular notch, sternum, and navel, and between the legs with equal distance between the right and left knees and feet. The left and right halves of the body should be symmetrical, a mirror image of each other. The arms should rest at the sides of the body with hands along the sides of the thighs. The patellae should face anteriorly with the knees straight, and the toes should point forward or slightly laterally. Left and right prominences should be parallel to each other (ear lobes, acromion processes, axillary folds, lower rib margins, iliac crests, patellae, tibial tuberosities, and medial malleoli). Muscle definition should be symmetrical in the chest, abdomen, hips, thighs, legs, shoulders, and arms.

From a lateral view, the plumb line in the sagittal plane runs through the middle of the ear's auditory meatus, the bodies of the cervical spine, the acromion process, the midthoracic area, and the greater trochanter. The plumb line continues down and runs slightly posterior to the patella and anterior to the lateral malleolus. The anterior (ASIS) and posterior (PSIS) iliac spines should be close to level with each other. The leg should be perpendicular to the foot. The hands should be slightly forward of the elbow but alongside the thigh. The chin should be parallel to the floor.

From the posterior view, the plumb line bisects the head and all spinous processes from the cervical through the lumbar spine. Left and right halves should be mirror images of each other. From this view the levels of the left and right segments are compared, including ear lobes, shoulder height (the dominant shoulder may be slightly lower than the nondominant shoulder), inferior angle of the scapulae, iliac crests, popliteal fossas, medial malleoli. The arms should rest comfortably at the sides with the hands next to the lateral thigh. The vertebral scapular borders should be equidistant from the plumb line (about 5 cm, 2 in., or 2 to 3 finger widths), as should be the knees and feet. The scapulae should rest against the posterior ribs between T2 and T7. The Achilles tendons should be vertical to the floor and you should be able to see the two lateral toes of each foot. Muscle definition of the back, hips, thighs, and legs should be symmetrical.

6. Be familiar with the parts of the stance and swing phases of gait.

One gait cycle lasts from the point of heel contact of one extremity to the next point of heel contact of the same extremity. Walking involves two separate phases of gait, stance and swing-through. The stance phase is the closed kinetic portion of gait and makes up approximately 60% of the total gait cycle. The swing phase is when the extremity is not bearing weight. During the first 10% and last 10% of the stance phase, both feet are in contact with the ground. During the middle portion of stance, only one lower extremity supports the body's weight. Stance phase is divided into heel strike (initial contact), foot flat (loading response), midstance, heel-off (terminal stance), and toe-off (preswing). Swing phase in divided into early swing (initial swing), midswing, and late swing (terminal swing).

7. Describe the specific observations that should be routinely performed on the injured segment.

Gross deformity of the injury site is observed first, followed by the presence of bleeding, edema, and ecchymosis. Other observations include signs present in the skin, such as redness, pus formation, adjacent enlarged lymph nodes, extreme tenderness, red streaks, lacerations, scars, calluses, blisters, rashes, and muscle spasms. The athlete's ability to use the injured segment and preexisting congenital or structural deformities should be included in the visual examination.

REVIEW QUESTIONS

1. How do global and specific observations differ?

2. Identify six items you would observe to create an overall impression of an athlete injured in a soccer game.

3. Why is it important to observe other parts of the body in addition to the injured part?

4. Explain how posture can influence an injury.

5. Why is it important to view posture from both anterior and posterior views?

6. How do gait characteristics change when an athlete switches from walking to running? What does this mean to the clinician working with an injured athlete?

7. How would you perform a gait analysis on an athlete who comes into the athletic training clinic complaining of a hip flexor strain?

8. What specific factors would you observe after making global observations of an injury to a player's forearm that has just occurred as she slid into home plate?

CRITICAL THINKING QUESTIONS

1. How would global observation of an injury differ between a football receiver you saw get injured on the field and a football receiver who came into the athletic training facility complaining of an injury he received in yesterday's practice?

2. If a right-handed baseball pitcher suffered a left knee sprain of his anterior cruciate ligament while sliding into second base, why would it be important to perform a posture and gait examination as part of your examination of the injury? Would you perform these examinations at the time of the injury or later in the athletic training facility? Why?

3. A volleyball player who underwent surgery 6 weeks ago to repair a dislocated ankle has been out of a post-op splint for 2 weeks. She still is not walking normally. What

do you think may be causing her abnormal gait? What substitutions would she use in her gait because of those problems?

4. A supervisor of aeronautical construction is in charge of two large, adjacent construction buildings. The floors of these buildings are concrete. Over the past 20 years he has walked at least 5 miles daily during the course of his work. In the past year he developed severe osteoarthritis of his talocrural joint. Rather than replace the joint, his surgeon fused the ankle. It is now 10 weeks since the surgery; he is bearing his full weight, but he does not walk normally. Can you describe what type of gait pattern he would have, given that his ankle is fused but he has no pain?

5. After suffering a medial collateral ligament sprain, a baseball outfielder had his right knee splinted for 6 weeks and was placed on crutches. Although he still has trouble walking normally, he is anxious to start running again now that he is off the crutches. What ranges of motion does he need in his hips, knees, ankles, and great toe before he can walk normally? What factors would you look for in his gait to determine when he could start running?

6. While serving as the athletic trainer for the women's basketball team during their invitational tournament, you see the team's center go up for a rebound and come down, landing on another player's foot. You hear a pop as she crumbles to the floor. What will you watch for as you go out onto the floor to examine her? What will you include in your global and specific observations?

7. You are working in an outpatient clinic. Your new 35-year-old patient suffered a patellar dislocation 7 days ago when she slipped on ice. Even though the knee remains painful and swollen, her physician wants her to begin treatment to restore motion and strength and relieve the pain and edema. Can you describe her gait and how it would vary from a normal gait?

8. Going back to the opening scenario at the beginning of this chapter, identify all the observations that Susan should make before Jonathan completes the examination of the volleyball player.

CITED REFERENCES

Nieman, D.C. 2003. *Exercise testing and prescription: A health-related approach.* 5th ed. New York: McGraw-Hill.

Perry, J. 1990. Gait analysis in sports medicine. *Instr Course Lect* 39:319-324.

ADDITIONAL RESOURCES

Houglum, P.A. 2005. *Therapeutic exercise for musculoskeletal injuries.* 2nd ed. Champaign, IL: Human Kinetics.

Sahrmann, S. 2002. *Diagnosis and treatment of movement impairment syndromes.* St. Louis: Mosby.

CHAPTER 5

Palpation

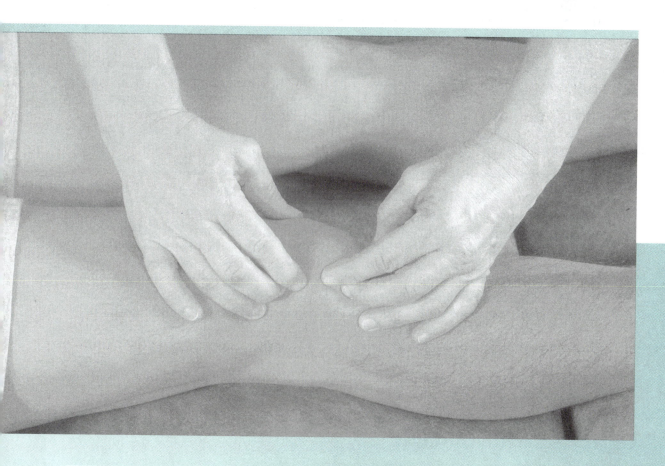

Objectives

After completing this chapter, the reader will be able to do the following:

1. Understand the role palpation plays in the objective examination
2. Describe the key personal and preparatory skills necessary for effective palpation
3. Acquire the proper technical skills for accurate examination
4. Identify various tissues based on known tissue characteristics
5. Develop a systematic approach for a palpation examination

Tom was in his first semester of an entry-level graduate athletic training program. During his clinical training, his approved clinical instructor (ACI) asked him to examine a basketball player's knee. After taking a history, he learned that the athlete's chief complaint was pain just below the patella immediately after an explosive jump. Tom's observation revealed mild swelling compared to the uninjured side. He then began his palpation, starting with direct, pinpoint palpation of the painful area. This caused the athlete considerable pain, and it seemed to Tom that everything else he tested also caused pain. In addition, he noticed that the athlete seemed apprehensive and had trouble relaxing.

Because of the pain and apprehension, Tom had a hard time determining the origin of the problem or specific tissue involved. When he sat down with his ACI to discuss his examination and findings, he was frustrated that he was not able to identify the problem. His ACI offered suggestions for improving his technical skills and approach to the palpation examination so that the next time, the athlete would be more at ease and Tom would better be able to distinguish between the potentially involved tissues.

Palpation is using the sense of touch to detect abnormalities and other critical details of an injury or illness. In this portion of the examination, you examine the surface of the body to detect tissue abnormalities, areas of asymmetry, changes in quality of movement or function, and other pathologies of the skin and underlying structures. Palpation consists of feeling with your hands for changes in tissue size, contour, organization, texture or consistency, tension or tone, and temperature or moisture, and checking for pain, swelling, muscle spasm, and tissue thickening. The goal of each palpation is to locate all pertinent structures, determine their characteristic feel, and examine them for the presence of pathology. In this chapter we describe the general principles and technical skills of a palpation examination, including palpation techniques and characteristic tissue qualities for the bony and soft tissue structures that you will commonly palpate.

GENERAL PRINCIPLES

Palpation is a valuable examination tool that we often take for granted, yet it requires specific skills to be effective. While some pathologies are easily identifiable, others may be missed due to inexperience or poor technique. The way you perform palpation also influences the athlete's comfort and confidence in your abilities. The following sections will help you hone your palpation skills to ensure patient comfort and confidence and to maximize your ability to discriminate between normal and abnormal tissue.

Foundational Skills

Before you can perform palpation examinations, you must master three related areas: anatomical knowledge, personal skills, and patient comfort.

1. **Anatomical knowledge.** For each region of the body you need to have a working knowledge of
   - the region's surface anatomy relative to the type, location, and depth of soft and bony tissues underlying the skin, and
   - the structural characteristics and general feel of each tissue to be palpated, so that you know what to feel for and can differentiate between healthy and pathological tissue.

A good test of your anatomical knowledge is to imagine the structures under the surface of the skin that you will be palpating. If you are unable to picture these structures, your knowledge of the area's anatomical landscape is lacking.

Even with a solid understanding of regional anatomy and tissue characteristics, effectiveness in distinguishing between various tissues also requires a number of personal and technical skills.

2. **Personal skills.** When applying your hands to an injured athlete, you must always convey confidence and professionalism. You should be relaxed and in a comfortable position, which conveys to the athlete that you are at ease and confident and allows you to better control the quality and sensitivity of your touch, ultimately improving the accuracy of your findings. It is always helpful to warm your hands by rubbing them or placing them inside your pockets before touching the athlete. Cold hands cause the athlete to tense and withdraw from your touch.

3. **Patient comfort.** Patient comfort is also important. Whenever possible, achieve optimal exposure of the area by removing sport equipment (e.g., shoulder pads) and excessive or heavy clothing that can impede your ability to adequately palpate specific structures. The athlete should then be comfortably positioned and draped, if needed, with a towel or sheet, so that he can relax. Always explain to the athlete what you plan to do before you begin your examination. When the athlete is comfortable and confident in your abilities, he will be less likely to tense up, which can impede your examination.

Palpation Technique

You must finely tune your palpation skills to discriminate between normal and abnormal tissue. Once you begin the examination, focus on what you are palpating as well as the athlete's response (e.g., is she wincing in pain from the pressure applied?). Avoid using your thumbs for the most part. The pads of your fingertips are the most sensitive part of the hand for identifying tissue texture, consistency, and size, while the back of the hand is best for sensing temperature and moisture. Use the pads of one or two fingers (usually index and middle fingers) for small areas, and use three or more finger pads over a large area. When performing palpation of a larger structure such as a major muscle belly, you may use the broader surface of your fingers or hand.

Maintain contact with the skin as you move from one structure to the next to stay aware of what structures are under your fingers. Every time you remove your fingers, you have to reorient yourself to these structures. Your touch should be deliberate and direct, but slow and gentle. While a deliberate, direct touch conveys confidence, pressing too firmly or abruptly can cause discomfort. Too much pressure also lessens tactile sensitivity. A touch that is too light may tickle the athlete, making it nearly impossible for him to relax. Your movement should be slow so that you can accurately distinguish between tissue structures. In some cases, you will want to keep your hands still while the tissues move beneath your hands. Biel (2001) describes the following palpation techniques:

- **Rolling and strumming.** Roll your fingers or thumb across the structure to identify ridges or lines in a bone as well as the direction of muscle fibers and general tone of a muscle.

- **Movement when palpating still structures.** When trying to determine the contour of a structure, move your hands slowly along its surface.

- **Stillness when palpating moving structures.** To feel the quality of a muscle contraction, keep your hands still while the muscle contracts beneath your hand.

- **Movement of a limb as a palpation tool.** The limb is moved in an active, passive, or resistive manner as you palpate the area or structure. For example, palpating the infrapatellar tendon while the knee flexes and extends allows you to feel for inflammation or abnormalities as the tendon loosens and tightens.

STRUCTURES TO PALPATE

The human body is made up of tissues that vary in structure and function. Thus, each tissue has its own characteristic feel, requiring certain palpation techniques and expected findings. Commonly palpated structures include skin, muscles, tendons, fasciae, ligaments, joint spaces, neurovascular structures, and bones. (Internal organs are also palpated for disease and injury, but these are covered in chapter 20 in the discussion of examination strategies for the thorax and abdomen.) The following sections will aid your understanding of common tissue structures that you will palpate and their normal characteristics with respect to temperature, orientation, thickness, mobility, and topography.

Skin

A *dermatome* is an area of the skin innervated by a specific nerve root.

Shock is a state of circulatory collapse in which the cardiovascular system does not circulate enough blood to the body.

⚠️ If an athlete's skin is cool and moist and she displays other signs and symptoms of shock, this is a medical emergency requiring immediate referral.

An *adhesion* is an undesirable attachment of two adjacent structures by fibrous connective tissue.

Palpation of the skin can detect inflammation and injury of underlying tissue, as well as the status of the body as a whole. Because the skin covers the entire surface of the body, it is always part of any palpation examination. The skin protects the internal structures and organs of the body and plays a crucial role in regulating body temperature. Most areas of the skin are also well innervated to communicate sensory stimuli (heat, pressure, touch, pain) from the external environment as well as receive stimuli referred from internal structures (e.g., dermatomes). The skin is typically warm and dry to the touch, and although relatively tough, it is quite supple and mobile, with some elasticity. Thickness and mobility vary depending on the body region, needed protection, and amount of joint movement. For example, the skin is thin and highly mobile over the back of the hand where the metacarpophalangeal joints flex, but it is much thicker and less mobile on the plantar surface of the foot where stability, protection, and padding are more important.

Use the back of the hand to palpate the skin for moisture and temperature. Warm, moist skin is common for the exercising athlete, and you need to be able to distinguish these findings from signs of serious illness. Cool, moist skin may indicate shock, while very hot, dry skin is characteristic of heat stroke. Under resting conditions, a localized increase in skin temperature may indicate an acute inflammatory condition or infection. Unusually cool skin may be a sign of impaired circulation or reduced blood flow, as can occur with a blood clot or vessel occlusion. Cool, clammy skin should always alert you to the risk of shock, especially when accompanied by other signs and symptoms of shock (see chapter 9).

Using the pads of the fingers, also palpate the skin for mobility, texture, and pain or change in sensory perception. The skin should be soft and pliable, gliding smoothly over bony prominences and underlying tissues. Because the skin attaches to the underlying superficial fascia, you will note some resistance to movement. Immobile skin may suggest excessive swelling that has already stretched the skin surface or adhesions between the skin and superficial fascia due to previous injury and scarring (e.g., surgical scar). Palpable tenderness may have several causes, including direct skin injuries (e.g., contusion) and damage to underlying structures. However, changes in skin sensitivity may also suggest pathologies in distant tissues that refer pain to the area (e.g., internal organs, nerve roots). These referred pain patterns are covered in part II.

Fascia

Fascia is dense connective tissue that enhances the form and function of the body. The superficial fascia lies just below the skin and, like the skin, covers the entire body (figure 5.1). The thickness and density of the superficial fascia vary. Fascia tends to be thinner where a high degree of mobility is required (e.g., back of the hand), and thicker in areas that are less mobile or need greater protection (e.g., plantar surface of the foot). It has a spongy, soft feel. When lightly moving the skin, the resistance you feel at the end of the range of the movement is due to the skin's attachment to the superficial fascia. Be aware that within the superficial fascia also course lymph vessels, blood vessels, and nerves.

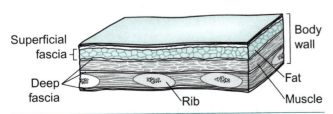

Figure 5.1 The superficial fascia lies just below the skin. The resistance felt when lightly moving the skin back and forth results from its attachment to the superficial fascia.

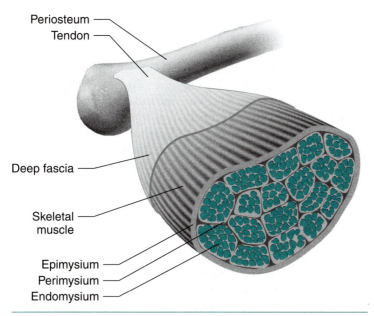

Periosteum
Tendon
Deep fascia
Skeletal muscle
Epimysium
Perimysium
Endomysium

Figure 5.2   The deep fascia is a thick, fibrous, continuous structure that envelops and separates muscles. It is smooth and firm to the touch.

Herniation is the protrusion or projection of a structure through the wall of the tissue that normally encases it.

The **deep fascia** is a thick, fibrous, continuous structure that envelops and separates muscles (figure 5.2). Because it is closely connected with the muscle that it envelops, it is difficult to clearly separate the two structures upon palpation. Deep fascia helps define the contours of each muscle, and it is smooth but firm to the touch. It is most notable when torn and the muscle herniates through the tear, in which case you feel smooth, firm fascia and then a raised, softer area where the muscle is emerging. Fascial herniations are commonly found over the anterior tibial compartment of the lower leg (see chapter 16).

When palpating the fascia, use both superficial and deep palpation. To examine the superficial fascia, gently move the skin horizontally and vertically, getting a sense of the degree to which the fascia restricts the mobility of the skin in each direction. Compare this mobility to the uninjured side or surrounding area. As previously noted, increased resistance may be a sign of swelling or adhesions. The skin should glide smoothly under your fingers. A bumpier feel may be a sign of inflammation. To examine the deep fascia, apply firmer pressure so that your palpation focuses on the deeper muscular level. In addition to fascial tears and herniations, you may note a very tender, distinct nodule, or myofascial **trigger point,** which is a focal, hypersensitive area within the myofascia (see chapter 11).

Myotendinous Unit

The **myotendinous unit** includes both contractile (muscle) and noncontractile (tendon and fascia) connective tissues that work together to move a body segment. The central nervous system controls muscle function to produce movement. The muscle belly has a soft, supple feeling, with a striated texture due to the parallel arrangement of the muscle fibers. You can follow the muscle fibers to determine the muscle's line of pull (or action) and to distinguish the muscle from adjacent muscles.

Muscle tension or tone depends on the contraction or relaxation of a muscle. You will note **hypertonia** (excessive tone) when the muscle is contracted or in spasm, while **hypotonia** (flaccid tone) suggests muscle atrophy or a loss of neural innervation. **Muscle fasciculations, tremors**, and **spasms** are involuntary muscle contractions that occur secondary to injury or pain. They can involve a few muscle fibers that are innervated by one motor unit (fasciculations), several motor units (tremors), and even the entire muscle (spasm); and they can involve either agonist or antagonist muscles. If present, these contractions are readily palpable in the injured and can be observed visually in superficial muscles.

Palpate muscle both parallel and perpendicular to the muscle fibers. You can easily recognize deformations in muscle contour through comparison with the uninvolved, contralateral side. Palpation of muscle tissue produces a soft, forgiving sensation. Depending on the contour and the area, an abnormal muscle palpation may indicate

- muscle strain,
- abnormal growth within the muscle (e.g., myositis ossificans),
- herniation of the fascia surrounding the muscle tissue,
- hypertonia, or
- hypotonia.

Edema is swelling resulting from fluid accumulation in the interstitial tissues.

When evaluating an injury with an open wound, you must wear gloves and observe universal precautions.

Increased thickening within the soft tissue can indicate edema caused by fluid accumulation in the tissue or space. Palpable defects in soft tissue may be associated with second- and third-degree strains.

As you proceed down the muscle belly, you will encounter the musculotendinous junction, where the muscle texture transitions from a striated feel to a smoother, firmer feel consistent with tendon tissue. Tendons are composed of dense connective tissue and are noncontractile. They have a smooth, rounded contour and are firm upon palpation when taut. Asking the athlete to move the limb or contract the muscle will help you distinguish between muscle and tendon. You should palpate the tendon for tenderness, inflammation, tissue thickening, and defects. If you palpate the tendon during movement, you may note some creptius, a grating or squeaky sensation that indicates inflammation. During active movement, the tendon should glide smoothly under your fingers.

Bone

Bone should be palpated for gross deformity, contour (e.g., surface irregularities), tenderness, and abnormal movement. Most healthy bones have irregular surfaces due to bony outgrowths (**prominences**), depressions, and attachments of ligaments and tendons. Because irregularities in surface and contour are common, you must have a good understanding of the bony anatomy for each region. You must also perform these palpations bilaterally, as bony surfaces can vary from person to person, and some areas may be naturally tender. Table 5.1 lists the common structural characteristics of bone and the types of bony surfaces you are likely to palpate.

As you palpate the bone surface, picture the position and normal contour of the bone as it lies under the surface of the skin. Identify any superficial bony prominences, depressions, grooves, and ridges along the bone's surface and feel for characteristic flares as you near the bone's proximal and distal ends. Palpation of bony structures should always produce a hard, unyielding sensation that distinguishes them from all other tissues.

Table 5.1
Palpable Bony Structures

Structure	Normal structural characteristics
Shaft	The body of a long bone, usually tubular in shape; the circumference of the bone often widens near its end to articulate with other bones
Head or condyle	The rounded end of a long bone that articulates with the joint
Epicondyle	The prominent aspect of the bone, just proximal to the condyle
Groove	A narrow, longitudinal depression in a bone, usually for passage of a tendon
Ridge or crest	A linear, raised elevation on the bone; very prominent ridges are called crests
Tubercle	A small and rounded projection or eminence
Tuberosity	A more prominent and large rounded projection or eminence
Apophysis	A small projection or outgrowth on a bone that serves as the attachment for a tendon
Epiphyseal plate	An area of growth between the shaft and the end of the bone that is present in the immature skeleton; the growth plate is often indistinguishable from the contour of the bone upon palpation and should not move upon palpation
Notch	An indentation in the end of a bone, usually to allow passage and protection of a ligament, nerve, artery, or tendon
Periosteum	The lining or covering of a bone that is normally indistinguishable from the bone's surface

Depending on the contour and area palpated, an abnormal bony palpation may indicate a fracture, a stress injury to the surface of the bone or attaching structures, or an abnormal bone growth. Displaced fractures are obvious, resulting in gross deformity in the bone contour. In the absence of gross deformity, abnormal movement accompanied by the sensation of crepitus or grinding when placing direct pressure on the bone indicates a nondisplaced fracture. If you note tenderness or swelling, determine the size of the area that is tender or swollen. Localized, pinpointed tenderness and swelling on the tibial shaft is more indicative of a bony defect or fracture, while diffuse tenderness and a bumpy texture along a broader surface of the bone (e.g., muscular attachments along the anterior medial shaft) usually indicate a stress injury resulting in periosteal irritation and swelling.

Abnormal growths or unusually large bony prominences may be sites of excessive friction or tensioning on the bone. In areas such as the back of the heel, excessive calcium formation may occur when repetitive pressure or friction from poorly fitting footwear is applied over an extended period of time. An enlarged apophysis, tubercle, or tuberosity accompanied by tenderness and a boggy feel may indicate excessive tensioning on the bone from the attached tendon. Each of these abnormalities is more easily recognized through comparison with the uninvolved, contralateral side.

Boggy refers to a soft, spongy feel, usually the result of localized inflammation.

Joint Structures

Effusion is when fluid (e.g., blood, synovial fluid) escapes and collects in the surrounding tissues.

Joint structures consist of a variety of dense connective tissues that stabilize articulating bones and provide lubrication between bones, as well as the muscles and tendons that cross the joint. You should palpate joint structures for tenderness, effusion, defect, and structural integrity. Common joint structures are listed in table 5.2.

Because it is often difficult to differentiate between joint structures, knowing the anatomy of a joint and the proximity of various joint structures is imperative. Capsular and bursa structures are not always readily palpable except when pathology is present. Swelling within a capsule or bursa produces tissue that feels soft and spongy to palpation. You may note thickening of capsular and bursa structures and the enclosed fluid over time with persistent, chronic, inflammatory conditions. When you note capsular swelling, consider the possibility of injury to the joint structures enclosed within the capsule, such as the osteochondral (bone–cartilage) surface, fibrocartilage, or ligament. Palpable swelling within the bursa most often indicates irritation or inflammation due to excessive pressure from a compressive force (e.g., direct blow) or frictional force (e.g., repetitive rubbing against adjacent structures). Defects such as a fold (e.g., **plica**) or pouch (e.g., **Baker's cyst**) in the capsular tissue may also be palpable. Pain and a sensation of pressure when palpating these structures also characterize inflammatory conditions.

Table 5.2
Palpable Joint Structures

Structure	Normal structural characteristics
Synovial capsule	A well-defined membranous connective tissue that surrounds and encloses the structures of a synovial joint
Articular cartilage	Smooth, hyaline cartilage that covers the articular surface of a bone
Bursa	A membranous connective tissue sac that contains synovium to reduce friction between adjacent structures
Joint line	A palpable separation between two articulating bones
Ligament	A taut, cordlike or bandlike fibrous connective tissue that connects bone to bone
Retinaculum	A band of membranous connective tissue that represents a thickening of the deep fascia at or near the joint and acts as a bowstring to hold tendons in place as they contract

Refer to chapter 17, page \bb\, for more information on plica syndrome and Baker's cyst.

Eversion is the outward movement of the sole of the foot away from the midline of the body.

Plantar flexion is the movement of the sole of the foot in an inferior direction, as occurs with pointing the toes.

Retinacula are thickened bands in the deep fascia that hold a tendon in place when a muscle contracts.

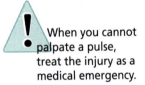
When you cannot palpate a pulse, treat the injury as a medical emergency.

Depending on joint position, a portion of the articular surface may be palpable. Check for tenderness and defects in the contour of the articular cartilage. Tenderness along the joint line may also indicate injury to the articular surface or the fibrocartilage discs that cushion the contour between some articulating bones. Palpate ligaments from insertion to origin, noting any tenderness or structural defects. Ligaments are most easily identified and palpated when they are slightly taut, so position the joint carefully to optimize ligament palpation. To determine retinaculum structural integrity and function, palpate retinacula while moving the tendons they stabilize. At the ankle, for example, palpate the extensor retinaculum for any bowstringing of the tendons with the toes extended, and palpate the lateral retinaculum behind the lateral malleolus when contracting the fibularis (peroneal) muscles during eversion and plantar flexion.

Neurovascular Tissue

Major arteries, veins, and nerves often run together in a thin fascial sheath as a **neurovascular bundle** where they cross the joint. These bundles are relatively mobile. They are protected by the musculoskeletal system, but they are palpable in various anatomical locations. While veins and arteries are hollow and easily collapsible upon palpation, nerves are more cordlike. Nerve tissue is also more sensitive to pressure than vessels. Palpate major arteries with the pads of your fingertips for the presence, strength, and rate of pulse. Do not use the thumbs, as they have a strong pulse of their own.

Periodically check peripheral pulses distal to an injury (and bilaterally for comparison) with any severe injury (e.g., fracture, dislocation, or crush), particularly severe injuries involving the part of the joint where main blood vessels traverse. These vessels can either be injured from the direct trauma or restricted due to secondary swelling immediately following an injury. Treat any loss of pulse as an emergency.

Gently palpate nerve roots, cords, and peripheral nerves for tenderness, mobility, and any thickening. Be careful not to "pluck" or overly compress the nerve, as this often produces pain and causes the athlete to withdraw.

Refer to chapter 9, page 156, for more information on examining peripheral pulses.

Lymphocytes are cells in the blood and lymphatic tissue that provide immunity from invading organisms.

Macrophages are the major phagocytic (destroyer) cells of the immune system.

Lymph Nodes

Lymph nodes are part of the immune system. They contain collections of lymphocytes and macrophages to filter and destroy microorganisms. A collection or chain of lymph nodes can be palpated in the groin, axilla, and anteriolateral and posteriolateral aspects of the neck (figure 5.3), where the nodes filter lymphatic flow from the pelvis, legs, arms, and head, respectively. On palpation lymph nodes are shaped like kidney beans, and they feel like firm nodules compared to the surrounding soft tissue. Palpable tenderness and enlargement of a node or chain of nodes indicate infection.

For more information on the role of lymphocytes and macrophages, refer to *Therapeutic Modalities for Musculoskeletal Injuries, Second Edition,* (Denegar, Saliba, and Saliba 2005).

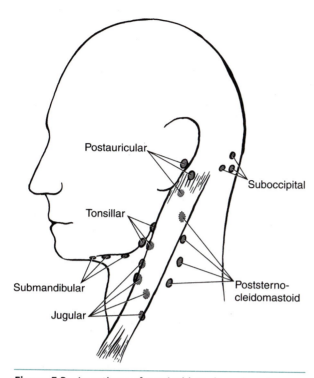

Figure 5.3   Locations of cervical lymph nodes.

Reprinted, by permission, from G.L. Landry and D.T. Bernhardt, 2003, *Essentials of primary care sports medicine* (Champaign, IL: Human Kinetics), 158.

PALPATION STRATEGIES

Palpate systematically so that you include all structures. If you establish a routine, following the same progression for each examination, you will avoid missing a structure. Noting landmarks that you can easily identify will help orient you to surrounding structures that are difficult to recognize.

For an accurate palpation examination, the athlete should be in a comfortable position and the injured segment should be supported. Before you begin, tell the athlete what you are going to do and ask her to report any pain during the palpation. Also observe facial expressions for signs of pain. The observed intensity and quality of the pain response are as important to identify as the athlete's subjective reports of pain. Remember to obtain a relative indication by asking the athlete to rate the pain on a scale of 0 to 10. You can sometimes perform palpation simultaneously on both the right and left sides. When this is impossible or inconvenient, palpate the uninvolved side first to determine the normal response for the athlete and to put the athlete at ease by showing him what to expect when you move to the injured side. You may need to recheck the uninvolved side to give the athlete a basis of comparison for the perceived level of pain or discomfort.

When performing the palpation examination, move from superficial to deeper structures and start away from the injury, palpating toward the injured site. For example, if the glenohumeral joint is injured, begin at the sternoclavicular joint and anterior structures and move laterally; then palpate the superomedial and posteromedial areas and move laterally before going on to the glenohumeral joint. This pattern gives the athlete the opportunity to alert you as you near the painful area.

Begin with light palpation of skin temperature and superficial soft tissue mobility before moving to deeper structures. Note how the skin moves against the underlying subcutaneous tissue and muscle. Does the skin move freely in all directions? Is the skin temperature normal compared to that on the other side? Follow palpation of the first layer of muscle by palpation of underlying muscle layers. Examine each layer for tissue mobility, swelling, texture, congruity, pain with pressure, and spasm. Finally, palpate the tendons, ligaments, and bony structures for tenderness, swelling, crepitus, and deformity. Biel (2001) suggests using the bones as a "trail guide" to help locate the tendon and ligament attachments.

You may encounter different types of fluid formation during your palpation examination, with each producing a characteristic response.

- Synovial swelling produces a boggy response that feels spongy to palpation.
- Fluid formation within soft tissue feels softer and moves when palpated.
- Edema caused by blood formation is usually warmer than other types of fluid formation and feels thicker or harder to palpation.
- Chronic swelling can feel leathery; in this condition, even cordlike fibrous band formations can be palpated. Recent soft tissue swelling that feels soft and gives or deforms with pressure is called **pitting edema**, whereas long-term leathery swelling is called **brawny edema**.

Following these guidelines, you can use the palpation examination to further solve the puzzle of the nature and severity of the injury.

SUMMARY

1. Understand the role palpation plays in the objective examination.

   Palpation uses the sense of touch to examine the surface of the body and detect tissue abnormalities, areas of asymmetry, changes in quality of movement or function, and other pathologies of the skin and underlying structures. The goal of each palpation examination is to locate all pertinent structures, determine their characteristic feel, and examine them for pathology.

2. Describe the key personal and preparatory skills necessary for effective palpation.

   Before you can properly perform your palpation examination for each region of the body, you need to have a good working knowledge of the region's surface anatomy, structural characteristics, and general feel of each tissue to be palpated. When applying your hands to an injured athlete, convey confidence and professionalism. Relax and maintain a comfortable position so you can better control the quality and sensitivity of your touch. Properly drape the athlete with a towel or sheet and warm your hands before palpating to help put the athlete at ease.

3. Acquire the proper technical skills for accurate examination.

   Palpation requires focus and fine-tuned skills for discriminating between normal and abnormal tissues. Use the pads of your fingertips to identify texture, consistency, and tissue size, and use the back of your hand to examine temperature and moisture. Maintain contact with the skin at all times as you move from one structure to the next. Your touch should be deliberate and direct to convey confidence, but slow and gentle to avoid causing discomfort or pain. Common palpation techniques include rolling and strumming, movement of the hands when palpating resting structures, stillness of the hands when palpating moving structures, and palpation during movement of a limb or body segment.

4. Identify various tissues based on known tissue characteristics.

   Different tissues varying in structure and function make up the human body. Each tissue has its own characteristic feel and requires certain palpation techniques and expected findings. Commonly palpated structures that you should distinguish by characteristic feel include the skin, muscles, tendons, fasciae, ligaments, joint spaces, neurovascular structures, lymph nodes, and bones.

5. Develop a systematic approach for a palpation examination.

   Perform palpation with a consistent routine, following the same progression for each examination to avoid inadvertently missing a structure. Always tell the athlete what you are going to do and ask him to report any pain during the palpation. Also observe facial expressions for signs of pain. Unless you can perform your palpation bilaterally, always palpate the uninvolved side first. Begin with light palpation of the skin temperature and general superficial soft tissue mobility and then move to deeper soft tissue structures. Examine each layer for tissue mobility, swelling, texture, congruity, pain with pressure, and spasm. Finally, palpate the tendons, ligaments, and bony structures for tenderness, swelling, crepitus, and deformity.

REVIEW QUESTIONS

1. Why is it important to develop a soft but direct touch in your palpation examination?

2. Describe the palpable characteristics that distinguish the following:
   - Ligament and tendon
   - Muscle and tendon
   - Skin and fascia

- Synovial and interstitial swelling
- Nerve and artery

3. What are some strategies for putting an athlete at ease before and during the palpation examination?

4. What are the challenges of palpating bony structures? How can accurate identification of bony structures aid palpation of specific soft tissue structures?

5. In addition to signs and symptoms associated with injuries to the skin tissue itself, what other information can you gain from palpating the skin surface?

6. What joint structures are typically not palpable unless swelling or inflammation is present?

CRITICAL THINKING QUESTIONS

1. After reading this chapter, reconsider the opening scenario. What suggestions do you think Tom's ACI gave and how would you have approached the examination differently?

2. Based on your knowledge of the pertinent anatomy, describe your strategy (order and approach) for palpating the structures around the elbow.

3. Describe what general techniques you would use to palpate the myotendinous unit.

4. Using the bony structures as a road map, identify the ligaments and tendons of the shoulder joint that can be palpated.

5. What palpable findings might suspected infection yield? Consider sites both local and distant to the injured area.

CITED REFERENCES

Biel, A. 2001. *Trail guide to the body: How to locate muscles, bones, and more.* 2nd ed. Boulder, CO: Books of Discovery.

ADDITIONAL RESOURCES

Kulas, A. Personal communication.

Moore, K.L. 1992. *Clinically oriented anatomy.* 3rd ed. Baltimore: Williams & Wilkins.

Mosby's medical, nursing, and allied health dictionary. 6th ed. 2002. St Louis: Mosby.

Thomas, C.L., ed. 1997. *Taber's cyclopedic medical dictionary.* 18th ed. Philadelphia: Davis.

CHAPTER 6

Examination of Motion

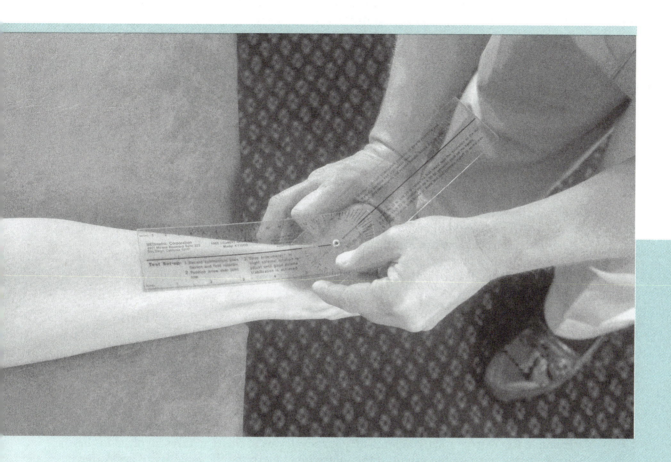

Objectives

After completing this chapter, the reader will be able to do the following:

1. Describe the differences between active and passive motion and between physiological and accessory motion

2. Identify the three normal end feels

3. Discuss the prerequisite knowledge and skills needed to examine range of motion (ROM)

4. Explain the technique used to measure range of motion (ROM)

5. Express the importance of recognizing a capsular pattern or motion

6. Explain the technique used to examine joint accessory motion

7. Present the procedure used to stress test a ligament

Once you have completed the history, observation, and palpation sections of the injury examination, you begin your range of motion (ROM) tests. As mentioned in chapter 2, range of motion includes active and passive motion and can also include resistive motion. Resistive motion, or strength, examination is presented in chapter 7. This chapter presents methods of examining active and passive ROM and their components, and discusses when to use each test and how to interpret the results. Although the specific measurements of each joint will be presented in detail in part II, general information regarding expectations of ROM are introduced here.

GOALS AND PURPOSES

The goal of examining range of motion is to objectively quantify the amount of active and passive motion available at and around the injury site. Observing the quality of movement is an important purpose of ROM measurement for it may tell you areas of pain or difficulty. If pain makes the injury very irritable, less active motion is possible. If little active motion but full passive motion is possible, the musculotendinous structure is the likely site of injury.

Examine ROM to confirm or eliminate your suspicions of the structures involved in the injury, help demonstrate the extent of the injury, and determine the integrity of active and passive elements that produce, support, and restrict joint movement. Recall that you should identify the injury's SINS (severity, irritability, nature, and stage) throughout your examination to make a diagnosis.

Normal range of motion is influenced by strength and active and passive tissue integrity. At the time an injury occurs, the injury's effect on the patient's ROM should not concern you as much as discerning any life-threatening injuries, the severity of the injury, and the best method of transport off the site. For this reason, you will rarely perform a full ROM examination on-site, but will examine ROM both on the sideline and in the athletic training clinic. You should be able to accurately examine ROM and all the components that contribute to normal motion. Normal ROM reduces risk of injury once the individual returns to full participation. This chapter identifies those components and provides information on how to interpret and record ROM examination results.

NORMAL RANGE OF MOTION

Osteokinematics refers to the movements of the long bones that produce motion. This motion occurs in an arc around a joint. Range of motion (ROM) describes the arc of motion through which a segment moves in a specific cardinal plane of motion. The three cardinal planes of movement are the sagittal, frontal, and transverse planes. Each cardinal plane of movement rotates around a corresponding axis. The sagittal plane divides the body into

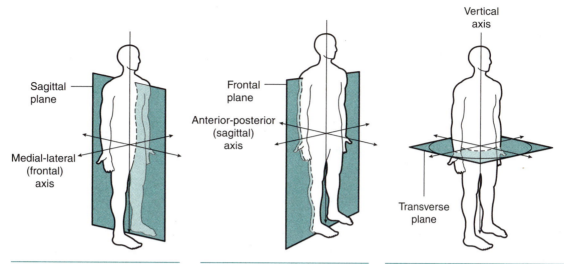

Figure 6.1 Sagittal plane.   **Figure 6.2** Frontal plane.   **Figure 6.3** Transverse plane.

Reprinted, by permission, from R.S. Behnke, 2001, *Kinetic anatomy (Champaign, IL: Human Kinetics), 27*

right and left segments and rotates around a medial–lateral axis; movements in the sagittal plane are flexion and extension (figure 6.1). The **frontal plane** divides the body into front and back segments and rotates around an anterior–posterior axis; motions in the frontal plane are abduction and adduction (figure 6.2). The **transverse plane** divides the body into upper and lower segments and rotates around a vertical axis; medial and lateral rotation and pronation and supination are movements produced in the transverse plane (figure 6.3). Some joints move in only one plane and others in more than one plane. For example, the elbow (humeroulnar) joint moves only in the sagittal plane around a medial–lateral axis to allow flexion and extension; such a joint is described as having one **degree of freedom**. The tibiofemoral joint has two degrees of freedom since it moves in two planes, the sagittal (flexion–extension) and the transverse (medial and lateral rotation) planes. The glenohumeral joint has three degrees of freedom because it moves in all three planes to produce flexion–extension, abduction–adduction, and medial–lateral rotation.

Range of motion is defined in degrees of motion. The two primary systems of measurement are the 180° system and the 360° system. Both systems are based on the **anatomical position** (see figure 1.1, page 4). The 360° system begins with extension and adduction positions at 180° and moves in arcs of motion toward 360°. This system is not used as frequently as the 180° system, in which the extension and adduction positions begin at 0° and move in arcs of motion toward 180°. For example, when using the 180° system the shoulder in the anatomical position starts at 0° and abducts to 180°, and the elbow begins at 0° and flexes to 145°.

Each joint has its own unique range of motion, but a "normal" ROM has been established for each joint. There is some dispute from one investigator to another as to the exact measures of these normal ranges, but for the most part, the disputes involve only a few joints and the disparity between them is a few degrees relative to the joint's full ROM.

You should know the expected ROM for each joint so that when examining the ROM of an injured joint, you will know whether the motion is normal or abnormal. In addition to standardized ranges of motion for each joint, normal may be defined differently for each individual. Examining the uninvolved extremity and knowing the patient's activities help you determine these individual differences. For example, normal ROM for shoulder lateral rotation is 90°, but a baseball pitcher's dominant shoulder commonly has a normal lateral rotation greater than 120°. If a warehouse worker suffers an ankle sprain, ROM on the contralateral extremity should be used to determine its normal range; if the uninvolved ankle has 15° of dorsiflexion, you can expect that the injured ankle should also have 15° of dorsiflexion.

You can view normal ranges of motion of the extremities in table 6.1. Variations in different authors' reports occur for some joint motions; these variations are indicated in the far right column of the table.

Table 6.1
Ranges of Joint Motion

Joint	Movement	Range of motion (start to end)	Variations in end ranges of motion
Shoulder	Extension–flexion	0-180°	150-180°
	Hyperextension	0-45°	40-60°
	Adduction–abduction	0-180°	150-180°
	Lateral rotation	0-90°	80-90°
	Medial rotation	0-90°	70-90°
	Horizontal abduction	30°	---
	Horizontal adduction	135°	---
Elbow	Extension–flexion	0-145°	120-160°
Forearm	Supination	0-90°	80-90°
	Pronation	0-80°	70-90°
Wrist	Extension	0-70°	65-70°
	Flexion	0-90°	75-90°
	Radial deviation	0-20°	15-25°
	Ulnar deviation	0-30°	25-40°
Thumb CMC	Abduction	0-70°	50-80°
	Flexion	0-45°	15-45°
	Extension	20°	0-20°
	Opposition	Tip of thumb to tip of #5	---
Thumb MCP	Extension–flexion	0-45°	40-90°
Thumb IP	Extension–flexion	0-90°	80-90°
#2-5 finger MCP	Flexion	0-90°	---
	Hyperextension	0-30°	30-45°
	Adduction–abduction	0-20°	---
#2-5 finger PIP	Extension–flexion	0-100°	100-120°
#2-5 finger DIP	Extension–flexion	0-90°	80-90°
Hip	Extension–flexion	0-120°	110-125°
	Hyperextension	0-15°	10-45°
	Abduction	0-45°	45-50°
	Adduction	0-20°	10-30°
	Lateral rotation	0-45°	36-60°
	Medial rotation	0-35°	33-45°
Knee	Extension–flexion	0-135°	125-145°

Joint	Movement	Range of motion (start to end)	Variations in end ranges of motion
Ankle	Dorsiflexion	0-15°	10-30°
	Plantar flexion	0-45°	45-65°
Subtalar joint	Inversion	0-30°	30-52°
	Eversion	0-15°	15-30°
MTP	Extension–flexion	0-40°	30-45°
	Hyperextension	0-80°	50-90°
IP	Extension–flexion	0-60°	50-80°

CMC = carpometacarpal; DIP = distal interphalangeal; IP = interphalangeal; MCP = metacarpophalangeal; MTP = metatarsophalangeal; PIP = proximal interphalangeal.

Based on information from Hoppenfeld 1976; Hislop and Montgomery 2002; AAOS 1965; Kendall, McCreary, and Provance 1993; Kapandji 1980; Esch and Lepley 1974; Gerhardt and Russe 1975.

PREREQUISITES FOR SUCCESSFUL ROM EXAMINATION

Two factors determine a joint's ROM: physiological motion and accessory motion. **Physiological motion** is the motion of the joint that occurs in the planes of motion. Physiological motion is divided into active motion and passive motion. **Active motion** is the motion the individual performs without assistance from an external source such as equipment or another individual. Another person or piece of equipment performs **passive motion** without assistance of the patient. A joint usually has slightly more passive motion than active motion because there is some joint motion at the end range of movement that is not under active control and is produced by passive stretching of soft tissue structures surrounding the joint (Norkin and White 2003).

Physiological Motion

Examine active and passive ranges of motion for the quantity of possible motion as well as the quality of the motion performed. You may see the term *active-assistive range of motion* (AAROM) in some readings and patient charts. **Active-assistive motion** refers to active motion combined with outside assistance required to complete the motion. This is a term used primarily in rehabilitation and is not presented in detail here. **Accessory motion** is the subtle, passive motion that occurs within and between the joint's inert structures, and it is necessary for full physiological motion. Physiological active and passive motion examination sometimes requires accessory motion examination to complete the ROM profile for the injured segment. Physiological motion examination is presented first and followed by accessory motion examination.

Active and passive ROM measurements provide different information, and you must examine both. You must also understand the specific structures stressed during each active and passive ROM and joint mobility test to narrow the possibilities of the nature of the injury. Here are the issues you must test and understand when investigating ROM:

- **Active range of motion.** Normal soft tissue and bony elements usually influence a joint's range of motion, but once injury occurs, pain, muscle spasm, and damaged tissue may also influence ROM. Measuring active motion informs you of the patient's ability and willingness to move the injured part and the quality and quantity of motion the individual can produce. Observation of the patient's motion and facial expressions can also reveal pain during active motion. Pain reduces active motion and makes the patient reluctant to move the segment. Weakness from injury to the musculotendinous element also reduces active motion. Pain, weakness, and injury to neural elements may also change coordination during motion. If the patient is unable to move the segment but feels no pain during the attempt, a nerve injury may be causing deficient active motion. Normal active range of motion measures for each joint are presented in the joint-related chapters in part II and summarized in table 6.1.

- **Passive range of motion.** Passive range of motion measures convey information about the inert structures surrounding the joint, eliminating muscle activity and its possible influences. Passive motion examination demonstrates the integrity of the joint capsule, ligaments, fascia, and articular surfaces of the joint. Passive motion can also provide information about the inert tissue surrounding muscle and tendons. Pain is possible during passive motion, so you must observe the patient's facial expressions during passive movement since some patients will not admit to pain that their expression reveals.

- **Normal end feel.** Passively moving a joint to the very end of its possible ROM provides additional information on the joint's end feel, or how the joint feels at the end of its motion. The barrier that prevents further motion at this point varies depending on the joint, and each joint has a unique end feel determined by that barrier. A normal end feel can be soft, firm, or hard. You will experience a soft end feel when the hamstrings muscles contacting the calf muscles block knee flexion, a firm end feel when the metacarpophalangeal (MCP) joint's capsule limits extension as the joint is pushed into hyperextension, and a hard end feel when the olecranon process encounters the olecranon fossa to prevent elbow extension (table 6.2).

- **Abnormal end feel.** Normal end feels become abnormal if they differ from the joint's usual end feel or if they occur sooner in the range of motion than is normal. For example, an elbow extension with a soft end feel is abnormal and a possible indication of edema. A firm end feel palpated prematurely in shoulder lateral rotation could indicate muscle spasm or a tight joint capsule. A hard end feel in knee extension at 30° of flexion could indicate a possible meniscal or bony fragment impeding joint motion. You may also encounter an empty end feel when the supporting structure tested is not intact. Additionally, if severe pain makes patients apprehensive, they may not allow you to go to an end feel by either objecting verbally or using muscle splinting to protect the joint.

Accessory Motion

If a joint lacks normal range of motion and the injury is not acute, you must perform additional motion tests to examine accessory joint motion. **Arthrokinematics** is the movement of joint surfaces relative to one another. These movements of joint surfaces are identified as rolls, slides (or glides), and spins. A **roll** occurs when a new point on one surface aligns with a new point on its opposing surface, much like a ball rolling on a table. A **slide** or **glide** occurs when one point on one surface contacts new points on the opposing surface like a braked car sliding on ice. Slides and rolls usually occur together. A **spin** occurs when one surface

Table 6.2
Normal End Feels

End feel	Description	Example
Soft	Two muscle bellies in contact with one another	Knee flexion, elbow flexion
Firm	Leathery or springy resistance from capsule or ligament	Ankle inversion, metacarpophalangeal hyperextension
Hard	Abrupt end feel from two bones meeting each other	Elbow extension

rotates on a stationary axis like a spinning top. In order for a joint to move, one or more of these movements must occur.

A joint may experience restricted ROM due to reduced arthrokinematics. Shortening of soft tissue surrounding joints, immobilization, weakness, and inflammation can cause a loss of joint mobility. If these conditions limit a joint's ROM, the joint capsule is affected, and characteristic patterns of motion develop. The unique pattern or motion restriction of a joint brought about by capsular changes is called a **capsular pattern** (Cyriax 1975). These capsular patterns are characteristic patterns of lost motion in the different plans of movement because of inert tissue tightness surrounding the joint (table 6.3). If you see a capsular pattern of motion, you should examine accessory motion after assessing ROM. Loss of motion that does not include a capsular pattern is likely the result of restricted tissue other than the capsule. Noncapsular patterns of motion can be caused by pain, muscle spasm, ligament restrictions, partial capsular restriction, muscle strains, and internal joint derangements.

Table 6.3
Capsular Patterns

Joints	Capsular pattern
Glenohumeral	Lateral rotation is more limited than abduction Abduction is more limited than flexion Flexion is more limited than medial rotation
Elbow	Flexion is more limited than extension Supination and pronation are equally limited
Wrist	Flexion and extension are equally limited Pronation and supination are mildly limited at the distal radioulnar joint
Finger	Abduction is more limited than adduction of the thumb CMC Flexion is more limited than extension of the MCPs and IPs
Hip	Medial rotation, abduction, and flexion are more limited than extension Generally, no limitation of lateral rotation
Knee	Flexion is more limited than extension

Ankle
    Talocrural
    Subtalar
	
	Plantar flexion is more limited than dorsiflexion
	Inversion is more limited than eversion

Foot and toes
    1st MTP
    2nd-5th MTP
    IP joint
	
	Extension is more limited than flexion
	Variable
	Extension is more limited than flexion

Lumbar spine	If a left facet is limited: Forward bending (FB) produces a deviation to the left Side bending right (SBR) is limited Side bending left (SBL) is unrestricted Rotation left (RL) is limited Rotation right (RR) is unrestricted
Cervical spine	If a left facet is limited: FB produces some deviation to the left SBR is unrestricted SBL is comparatively unrestricted RL is comparatively unrestricted RR is most limited

CMC = carpometacarpal; MCP = metacarpophalangeal; IP = interphalangeal; MTP = metatarsophalangeal.

MEASURING RANGE OF MOTION

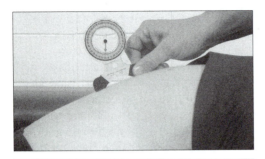

Figure 6.4 Goniometers similar to a carpenter level are called gravity-dependent goniometers, or inclinometers, and are used most often to measure motion in the spine.

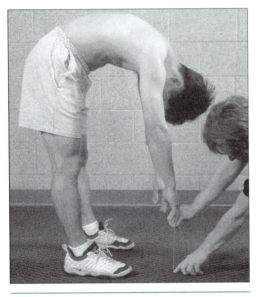

Figure 6.5 Use of a tape measure to examine ROM of the spine. See chapter 11 for details on measurement technique.

Reprinted, by permission, from P.A. Houglum, 2001, *Therapeutic exercise for athletic injuries* (Champaign, IL: Human Kinetics), 136.

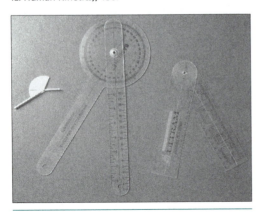

Figure 6.6 Different types of goniometers used to measure range of motion.

Reprinted, by permission, from P.A. Houglum, 2001, *Therapeutic exercise for athletic injuries* (Champaign, IL: Human Kinetics), 135.

Goniometry is the measurement of joint angles. The tool you will use to measure joints is a **goniometer**. There are many different types of goniometers on the market, but each has essentially the same structure: two arms (one stationary and one moveable) and an axis (fulcrum) that is surrounded by the body of the goniometer, which contains a measuring scale. The scale is usually similar to a protractor and calibrated in degrees. The scale can be either a 360° full-circle or a 180° half-circle. Goniometer arms range in length from 1 in. to 14 in. Use the long-armed goniometers to measure long bone joints such as the knee, and the short-arm goniometers to measure smaller joints such as the toe and finger interphalangeal joints. Goniometers similar to a carpenter level are called gravity-dependent goniometers, or inclinometers, and are used most often to measure motion in the spine (figure 6.4). Tape measures can also be used to identify lumbar range of motion if an inclinometer is not available (figure 6.5). Compare the measures found during the examination with previous measures or compare the left and right sides. Electric goniometers are also available but are usually reserved for research; they are more expensive and impractical for clinical use. Some of the more common goniometers are shown in figure 6.6. Calculate joint range of motion by measuring the angles between the beginning position and the ending position of available motion.

Measuring ROM accurately requires precision, and precision is achieved through practice and skillful observation. In addition to thoroughly mastering the material presented in this chapter, you must be able to position and stabilize the patient and segment to be measured, appropriately determine the end range of motion, identify and palpate the correct landmarks, apply the goniometer in the proper position, and read the goniometer correctly.

Positioning

Position involves four factors: the patient, the joint, the goniometer, and yourself. Incorrectly positioning any of these items can result in an inaccurate measurement of joint motion. You should position the patient so the joint to be measured can move through its ROM freely, without obstruction, and so you can easily observe the joint. The patient should be comfortable. If you need to measure several motions, you should plan the sequence of measurements so you will minimally change the patient's position. For example, you should measure all motions with the patient in prone before moving the patient to another position.

You must also carefully consider the position of the segment to be measured, particularly when measuring active motion. A segment that must lift against gravity may give a false active motion measurement if its muscles are not sufficiently strong enough to lift through the range of motion. When measuring passive ROM, performing too many activities at the same time such as stabilizing the part, holding the extremity against gravity, and aligning the goniometer may lead to a gross error of measurement. You should document the segment's position during ROM testing when recording the measurement.

Positioning the goniometer correctly is crucial; if the arms of the goniometer are not aligned properly, the measure will be inaccurate. Likewise, moving the axis of the goniometer off the joint line will yield

Prerequisite Knowledge for Measuring ROM

- Normal ranges of motion
- Proper stabilization
- Substitution patterns
- Normal end feels
- Landmarks
- Factors that can alter ROM
- Goniometric application
- Exact positioning of the goniometer axis, stationary arm, and moveable arm

Prerequisite Skills for Measuring ROM

- Position athlete and joint
- Stabilize athlete and joint
- Identify end ROM
- Palpate correct landmarks
- Apply goniometer correctly
- Check for proper alignment
- Read goniometer correctly

an incorrect measurement. The correct technique for goniometer alignment is discussed under Measurement Technique on page 86.

Finally, your position is just as important as the other factors in ROM measurements. Once you have placed the goniometer and assured proper alignment, you must read the goniometer at eye level for an accurate reading. For example, if you measure hip flexion and read the goniometer in an erect standing position, the results could differ by several degrees from the reading you would obtain if you knelt down to read the goniometer at eye level.

Patient Stabilization and Substitution

Stabilization is isolating the motion of the joint while eliminating unwanted motion from adjacent structures. You must stabilize the patient before measuring ROM or examining end feel to assure reliable results. Most often, you will stabilize the proximal joint segment and move the distal segment. You must isolate a joint motion to examine it accurately. If you allow both joint segments to move, true joint end feel may be inaccurate.

Moreover, if you do not stabilize the proximal segment, motion of other joints may contribute additional motion gains, exaggerating the joint's true motion and resulting in substitution. For example, if you measure shoulder flexion without appropriately stabilizing the shoulder, the patient can hyperextend the spine and falsely appear to have greater shoulder motion. Your knowledge of possible substitutions and an awareness of the patient's movement will assist in recognizing substitution patterns. Stabilization during ROM examination assures a truer execution of the test and a more accurate result.

Occasionally the patient's body weight may prevent unwanted motion. Most motions, however, require manual stabilization of the proximal segment to prevent unwanted motion. You must know how to stabilize the proximal segment while simultaneously using a goniometer to measure joint motion.

Measurement Technique

Goniometric measurement requires proper alignment of the stationary and moveable arms and the goniometer's axis (figure 6.7). Use bony landmarks to properly place these elements.

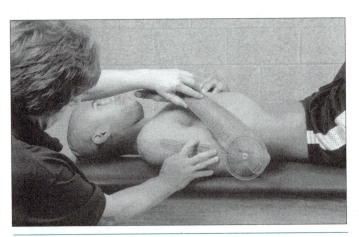

Figure 6.7 The axis is placed at the joint, the stationary arm is along the longitudinal aspect of the stabilized segment, and the moveable arm is placed in alignment with the moving segment.

Reprinted, by permission, from P.A. Houglum, 2001, *Therapeutic exercise for athletic injuries* (Champaign, IL: Human Kinetics), 137.

Place the stationary arm along the longitudinal axis of the stabilized joint segment and the moveable arm parallel to the longitudinal axis of the moving joint segment. When using a 180°-scale goniometer, you may need to reverse the stationary and moving arms before the moveable arm will register on the scale. Align the goniometer's axis with the joint's axis of motion. If the goniometer arms are accurately placed, the fulcrum will be positioned correctly.

To correctly align the goniometer arms, position yourself so your line of vision is at the same level as the goniometer. Checking both arms more than once before reading the scale also assures correct alignment. Oftentimes, you will align the stationary arm and then unwittingly move it again when adjusting the moveable arm; even highly experienced clinicians make a habit of checking and rechecking the goniometric arm and axis positions before reading the measurement.

Before measuring range of motion, you should explain to the patient what you will do. Take measurements at the start and end positions of the joint motion. If you are only interested in the end of the ROM, it is assumed that the start position is 0° and has been verified by visual determination. ROM examination is usually performed on the uninvolved extremity before the injured extremity. Performing the examination in this sequence provides you with an idea of what to expect when you examine ROM of the injured segment.

Range of Motion Measurement Technique

☐ Explain the technique to the patient

☐ Position the patient comfortably

☐ Position the segment to be measured at the beginning of its motion

☐ Stabilize the proximal portion of the segment

☐ Palpate bony landmarks

☐ Move to eye level

☐ Position the stationary arm

☐ Position the moveable arm

☐ Assure alignment of the fulcrum with the joint's axis

☐ Observe for substitution

☐ Recheck stationary and moveable arm positions

☐ Record measurement

☐ Stabilize proximal segment

☐ Move joint to end motion position

☐ Locate bony landmarks

☐ Realign stationary and moveable arms

☐ Observe for substitutions

☐ Recheck alignment of both arms and fulcrum

☐ Record measurement

The final factor in ROM measurement is recording the measure. Some facilities use forms listing normal ranges of motion and you can simply fill in the blanks with the patient's measurements. If such a form is not available, you should record the date, the patient's position (seated, prone), the type of motion (active or passive), and the side of the body and joint measured. Note any pain or other abnormal reactions that occur during the examination. If the patient lacks full motion, record the degrees as a range. For example, if a patient lacks 20° of knee extension and has full knee flexion motion, record ROM as 20-145°. If the patient has excessive motion, or hypermobility, use a minus to indicate excessive mobility. For example, if the patient has 15° of hyperextension of the knee and normal flexion motion, record –15-145°.

Avoid using a visual estimate to determine range of motion. The visual estimate may be off and can easily vary among clinicians, and it is not an objective measure. Especially avoid estimating if you use the measurement to identify a deficiency, record progress, or determine a patient's readiness to return to normal activity levels.

ACCESSORY MOVEMENT EXAMINATION

Joint restriction, as mentioned, is reflected in capsular patterns unique to each joint. If joint mobility is normal, the joint has a certain amount of **joint play**, the amount of motion within a joint that is not controlled by volitional movement but must be present for full ROM to occur. It is also called **accessory movement.** Capsular restriction reduces accessory motion. If accessory motion is reduced, physiological motion will also be diminished.

Joint Accessory Movement Rules

Immediate injuries do not display capsular patterns of movement. A joint loses its capsular mobility after several days or weeks of inflammation, immobilization, or restricted motion. If the joint's capsule does not move on a regular basis, it can adhere to adjacent structures and to itself, eventually losing its mobility and ability to achieve full range of motion. If a patient's history includes such a profile and a capsular pattern is evident during ROM examination, you should further examine the capsule.

When you see a capsular pattern of movement, you should examine the amount of joint accessory motion by using joint mobilization techniques. The joint mobilization techniques used for examination are similar to those used for treatment, with a few exceptions. Whether treating or examining, you must examine the uninjured contralateral joint to determine the value of "normal" for your patient since each person has a different amount of normal play within his joints. Joint play, or joint accessory motion, varies with age, with younger individuals generally having more joint play than older persons. Females also usually have more joint play than males.

The unique factor of joint mobilization that separates examination from treatments is that you will *always* perform an examination with the joint in its resting position. A **resting position** is the position where the capsule is loosest and the bone ends are the least congruent with one another. Each joint has its own unique resting position. Before you perform the examination you should know these resting positions. The resting positions are listed in table 6.4.

In the mobilization technique, one aspect of the joint is stabilized as the mobilization force is applied close to the joint at the other aspect. Perform joint mobility examination with the patient in a relaxed position, since muscle tension prevents accurate examination of joint play. Support the extremity and initially place the joint in a resting position so that the ligaments are at a resting length and the joint's surface contact is minimal. Examine one motion at a time. Apply the forces to the joint parallel to the plane of the joint surface; use enough force to produce accurate findings but not enough to cause excessive pain. As with other tests, examine the uninvolved side first.

Although joint mobilization techniques differ depending on the specific joint, most joints can be tested initially with a longitudinal force. A longitudinal force is applied as a **distraction,** or **traction,** technique by pulling the distal segment of the joint away from the proximal segment. This test determines general capsular mobility and overall mobility. If distraction

Table 6.4
Joint Resting Positions

Joint	Resting position
Finger MCPs and IPs	20° flexion
Wrist	0°
Elbow: humeroulnar	70° flexion, 10° supination
Elbow: humeroradial	Full extension and supination
Elbow: radioulnar	70° flexion, 35° supination
Glenohumeral	55° flexion, 20-30° horizontal abduction
Hip	30° flexion, 30° abduction, slight lateral rotation
Knee: tibiofemoral	20-25° flexion
Knee: patellofemoral	Full knee extension
Ankle and midfoot: talocrural	10° plantar flexion
Ankle and midfoot: subtalar and midtarsal	Midrange of inversion and eversion
Forefoot and toes: #1 MTP	20° dorsiflexion
Forefoot and toes: #2-5 MTP and IP	20° plantar flexion

MCP = metacarpophalangeal; IP = interphalangeal; MTP = metatarsophalangeal.

For information on applying joint mobilization for treatment refer to *Therapeutic Exercise for Musculoskeletal Injuries, Second Edition,* (Houglum 2005), chapter 6.

produces a restricted feel, additional tests will be necessary to further identify precise locations of restriction. You can examine most joints with anterior–posterior and posterior–anterior capsular mobilization techniques. These techniques are both glide maneuvers in which you move one end of the joint in a straight anterior–posterior (AP) or posterior–anterior (PA) direction on its opposing joint surface. These techniques examine the mobility of the anterior and posterior capsules in joints such as the shoulder, knee, and wrist.

Apply lateral glides using AP and PA movements laterally instead of anteriorly or posteriorly to examine lateral stability or restriction of a joint such as the shoulder, ankle, wrist, and the interphalangeal joints. Particular applications or other more specialized applications for each joint are discussed in later chapters.

Joint Accessory Examination Technique

As with physiological ROM examination techniques, joint accessory motion examination techniques require stabilizing one end of the joint while moving the other. The proximal end is usually stabilized while the distal end of the joint is moved. If you do not stabilize the joint properly, you will make an inaccurate determination of joint play. Occasionally the body can stabilize itself such as when the patient's weight lies on the scapula to stabilize it while you examine the glenohumeral joint of the shoulder. Other times, however, you will need to provide stabilization by securing the proximal segment. For example, when you examine the wrist joint, you must stabilize the distal forearm before moving the wrist.

Once you have determined that a capsular pattern exists, position the patient so he is comfortable and the involved extremity is supported. Before applying the joint mobilization

Accessory Joint Motion Examination Technique

- ☐ Explain the technique to the patient
- ☐ Position the patient comfortably
- ☐ Apply technique to contralateral joint
- ☐ Stabilize proximal segment
- ☐ Place hands as close as possible to joint
- ☐ Place the joint in its resting position and distract the joint
- ☐ Apply glide force parallel to joint surface
- ☐ Repeat technique on involved joint
- ☐ Compare to noninjured joint
- ☐ Record findings

examination technique, explain the procedure and its purpose to the patient. Begin on the uninvolved contralateral extremity, applying a distraction to the joint in its resting position. Keeping your hands as close to the joint as possible, apply AP and PA glide techniques to examine the patient's normal joint play. Apply the glide force parallel to the joint's surface. Next, perform the same technique on the involved joint and compare its results to those for the noninjured joint.

Remember that proper glide techniques are applied parallel to the joint surface and that you must go to the end of the available joint play motion in order to obtain an accurate examination. This means that once you feel the capsule's resistance, continue until joint motion becomes impossible. Use a firm but slow technique to identify when resistance occurs and any changes in intensity occur before you reach the end of movement. Applying the technique in such a manner will not damage the capsule, but it will provide valuable information useful for both examination and treatment. There are exceptions to this procedure if moving the joint to its end feel is not possible. For example, if the patient has too much pain to become comfortable for the examination or experiences muscle spasm, the technique will not produce a reliable result. Of course, neither joint mobilization examination nor treatment techniques should be used on a hypermobile joint.

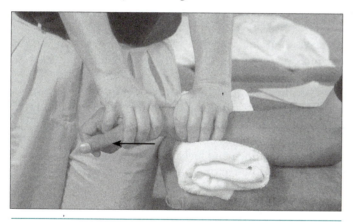

Figure 6.8 Notice that the stationary hand is on the distal forearm very near the wrist joint while the treatment hand is placed just distal to the joint line. The mobilization force is applied parallel to the joint surface.

Recording Results

Use your knowledge of what is normal for the patient to determine the amount and location of joint restriction. Grade the amount of restriction by comparing the motion loss to the contralateral side and what is normal for the patient's gender, age group, and functional requirements. This restriction can be categorized as slight, moderate, or severe, or a more precise examination can be made in percentages of normal. For example, when examining a 20-year-old baseball pitcher with glenohumeral loss of motion and a capsular pattern, you may find a "moderate loss of joint play in the anterior and inferior capsule of the right glenohumeral joint" or "40% loss of joint mobility in the anterior capsule and 60% loss of joint mobility in the inferior capsule of the right shoulder."

Recording the joint mobilization examination in the patient's medical record can be abbreviated to demonstrate the direction of joint accessory motion technique and the results.

Some examination forms devote space to joint play results, making recording results merely a matter of filling in the direction and percentage of joint play. If you use a narrative report instead, acceptable abbreviations still make the recording of joint play results simple. For example, you should indicate the joint, position tested, and direction of the force applied, and results of the test as follows: ⓡ G-H, resting position: PA = 40% N ant capsule, 60% N inf capsule; AP = WNL. The AP joint mobilization technique can also be abbreviated with a down arrow with a dot in the center to represent the joint (⬇), and PA can be abbreviated with an up arrow with a dot in the center (⬆).

SPECIAL TESTS: LIGAMENT AND CAPSULE STRESS TESTS

Some special tests used to examine injured joints include stress tests for the ligaments and capsule. These do not examine joint ROM or capsule tightness, but identify ligaments or capsules that have been damaged. These tests investigate the joint for signs of laxity rather than tightness or mobility. When laxity is present, the test is positive for a sprain.

Indications for Ligament Stress Tests

A sprain is an injury to a ligament or capsular structure. Because ligaments connect bones, sprains are associated with joint injury. Sprains result from forces that cause two or more connecting bones to separate or go beyond their normal range of motion, subsequently stretching and tearing the attaching ligaments or capsule.

Grading of Ligament Laxity

Apply ligament and capsule stress tests when you suspect a sprain. Sprains are classified as first, second, or third degree. For a quick review of the classifications of ligament injuries see pages 8-9. The injury is graded or classified according to the amount of motion the stress test produces. With a grade I or first-degree sprain, the stress test demonstrates pain and a leathery or firm end feel but no laxity. A stress test applied to a grade II or second-degree sprain shows some displacement, significant pain, and an end feel that is initially loose but becomes leathery or firm as the ligament slack is taken up. A grade III or third-degree injury is present when the stress test demonstrates an open end feel and severe pain. Although pain response is individually based and determined by factors other than severity of injury, as a rule, the greater the severity of injury, the greater the pain.

Stress Test Technique

By the time you use stress tests, the history and palpation have narrowed the range of injury possibilities. Special tests like ligament stress tests either eliminate or confirm a suspected condition as well as define the integrity of a structure or the extent of an injury. These tests stress the structure enough to either demonstrate an abnormal response or reproduce the patient's symptoms. The stress applied must be great enough to elicit an accurate response but not so great that it further aggravates the injury. For an inexperienced clinician, finding this balance can be difficult at times.

Perform ligament stress tests only after you have explained to the patient what will occur. As noted, you should test the uninvolved extremity first for two reasons:

- To familiarize the patient with the procedure to reduce his apprehension and help him relax so that the result may be more accurate
- To provide knowledge of what is normal for that individual. Since ligament laxity varies among individuals, you must establish a baseline for each patient to determine whether the test is positive or negative.

Ligament and Capsule Stress Test Technique

☐ Explain the technique to the patient
☐ Position the patient comfortably
☐ Stabilize proximal segment
☐ Grasp distal segment
☐ Position joint in correct position
☐ Apply stress in proper direction with sufficient force to stretch ligament or capsule

Depending on the test, a positive result produces different results between the involved and uninvolved sides in terms of laxity or stiffness, stability or instability, and the presence or absence of pain. The greater the positive result, the greater the degree of injury.

With the patient in a comfortable position, stabilize the proximal segment of the joint being tested. Position the joint appropriately for the ligament stress test, grasp its distal end with a firm, confident hand, and stress the ligament in the appropriate direction. This direction is usually perpendicular to the ligament and stretches the ligament. Apply the force smoothly and sufficiently to stress the ligament or capsule.

SUMMARY

1. Describe the differences between active and passive motion and between physiological and accessory motion.

   Active motion is performed by the patient without assistance from an external source such as equipment or another individual. Another person or piece of equipment performs passive motion on the patient without his assistance. Physiological motion occurs in the planes of motion of the joint and is divided into active and passive motion. Accessory motion in the joint is not controlled by volitional movement but must be present for full range of motion to occur.

2. Identify the three normal end feels.

   End feel describes how the joint feels when moved to the end of its motion. The barrier that prevents further motion varies depending on the joint, and each joint has a unique end feel that is determined by the barrier. A normal end feel can be soft, firm, or hard. A soft end feel example occurs when the hamstring muscles contacting the calf muscles block knee flexion, a firm end feel occurs when the MCP joint's capsule limits extension as the joint is pushed into hyperextension, and a hard end feel occurs when the olecranon process encounters the olecranon fossa to prevent elbow extension.

3. Discuss the prerequisite knowledge and skills needed to examine range of motion (ROM).

   The prerequisite knowledge for measuring ROM includes knowing and understanding normal ranges of motion, proper stabilization, possible substitution patterns, normal end feel for the joint being tested, correct landmarks, factors that can alter ROM, and the proper use of the goniometer, specifically, where to place the stationary and moveable arms. The prerequisite skills for measuring ROM include positioning the patient and joint comfortably, stabilizing the patient and the joint to be measured, identifying the end range of motion, palpating the correct landmarks, applying the goniometer correctly on the segment, and reading the goniometer correctly.

4. Explain the technique used to measure range of motion (ROM).

   Proper application of the ROM technique includes explaining the technique to the patient prior to performing it, positioning the patient and yourself comfortably, positioning the segment to be measured at the beginning of its motion, stabilizing the proximal portion of the joint, palpating bony landmarks, positioning yourself so you are at eye level to the joint, positioning the stationary arm of the goniometer to align with the proximal joint segment, positioning the moveable arm parallel to the moving joint segment, making sure alignment of the fulcrum with the joint's axis is correct, observing the patient for unwanted substitution, rechecking the stationary and moveable arm positions for correct alignment, and recording measurement.

5. Express the importance of recognizing a capsular pattern or motion.

If a capsular pattern or motion exists, the accessory movements of the joint are restricted. Joint accessory motion must be present for the joint to possess full ROM.

6. Explain the technique used to examine joint accessory motion.

Before applying the joint mobilization examination technique, explain the procedure to the patient. Begin within the uninvolved contralateral extremity and apply a distraction to the joint in its resting position. Keeping your hands as close to the joint as possible, apply AP and PA glide techniques to examine the patient's normal joint play. Apply the glide force parallel to the joint's surface. Next, perform the same technique on the involved joint. Compare the injured and noninjured joint and record the results.

7. Present the procedure used to stress test a ligament.

With the patient in a comfortable position, stabilize the proximal segment of the joint to be tested. Position the joint appropriately for the ligament stress test, grasp the joint's distal end with a firm, confident hand, and stress the ligament in the appropriate direction. This direction of stress is usually perpendicular to the ligament and stretches the ligament. Apply the force smoothly and sufficiently to stress the ligament or capsule.

REVIEW QUESTIONS

1. Why is there usually more passive range of motion in a joint than active range of motion?
2. Why is it important to include range of motion as part of an injury examination?
3. Give an example of an accessory motion in any joint.
4. What might cause a soft end feel during passive knee extension? What is the normal end feel?
5. Identify and explain the different arthrokinematic motions.
6. What are the normal ranges of motion for abduction and lateral rotation of a shoulder joint?
7. What is the resting position for the tibiofemoral joint?
8. When would you use a ligament stress test as a special test?
9. What would be the result of a stress test on a grade II ligament sprain?

CRITICAL THINKING QUESTIONS

1. When measuring range of motion of a patient's hip, knee, and ankle joints, how would you organize the measurement process to minimize changes in the patient's position?
2. Identify the possible substitutions a patient might use while performing active shoulder flexion, abduction, lateral rotation, and medial rotation motions. How would you proactively prevent those substitutions?

3. If a patient's extension–flexion range of motion in the knee is 15-90°, would you perform an accessory motion examination? Why? What motions would you perform?

4. Using appropriate abbreviations, write an examination note that included the following ROM findings: wrist flexion was at 75°, wrist extension was at 75°, ulnar deviation was at 10°, radial deviation was at 5°, supination was at 20°, and pronation was at 20°. Joint accessory motion found the capsule to have only one-quarter the normal joint mobility of the anterior and posterior capsules.

5. If a volleyball player landed on another player's foot and suffered what you suspected to be a sprain of the lateral ankle ligaments, how would you position the ankle to stress the lateral ankle ligaments?

6. If you were Linda in the opening scenario of this chapter, what would you tell Chris so that he stopped viewing each ROM measurement of each joint as different to help him remember ROM measurement techniques?

CITED REFERENCES

American Academy of Orthopaedic Surgeons (AAOS). 1965. *Joint motion: Method of measuring and recording.* Chicago: AAOS.

Cyriax, J.H. 1975. *Textbook of orthopaedic medicine. Vol 1: Diagnosis of soft tissue lesions.* Baltimore: Williams & Wilkins.

Esch, D., and M. Lepley. 1974. *Evaluation of joint motion: Methods of measurement and recording.* Minneapolis: University of Minnesota Press.

Gerhardt, J.J., and O.A. Russe. 1975. *International SFTR method of measuring and recording joint motion.* Bern: Huber.

Hislop, H.J., and J. Montgomery. 2002. *Daniels and Worthingham's muscle testing. Techniques of manual examination.* Philadelphia: WB Saunders.

Hoppenfeld, S. 1976. *Physical examination of the spine and extremities.* New York: Appleton-Century-Crofts.

Houglum, P.A. 2005. *Therapeutic exercise for musculoskeletal injuries.* 2nd ed. Champaign, IL: Human Kinetics.

Kapandji, I.A. 1980. *The physiology of the joints. Vol. 2. Lower limb.* New York: Churchill Livingstone.

Kendall, F.P., E.K. McCreary, and P.G. Provance. 1993. *Muscles: Testing and function.* 4th ed. Baltimore: Williams & Wilkins.

Norkin, C.C., and D.J. White. 2003. *Measurement of joint motion.* Philadelphia: FA Davis.

CHAPTER 7

Examination of Strength

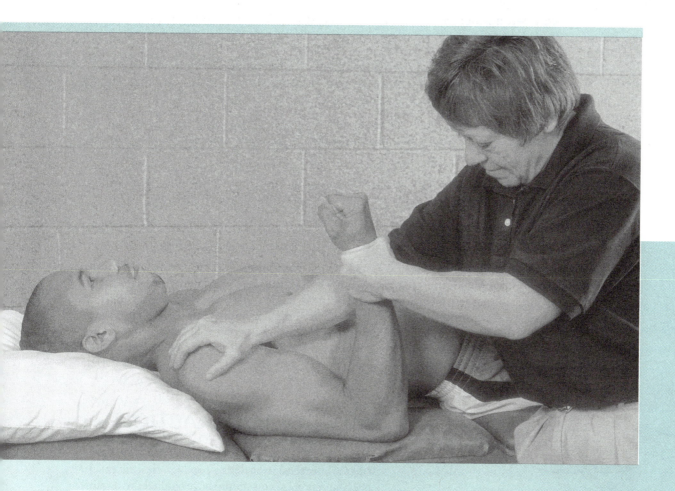

Objectives

After completing this chapter, the reader will be able to do the following:

1. Identify the main goals and features of the strength examination

2. Understand the effect of pain on the accuracy of the strength examination

3. Describe and demonstrate the types of manual muscle examination

4. Differentiate between isometric, isotonic, and isokinetic modes of instrumented strength examination

5. Become familiar with the instruments used for objective isometric strength examination

6. Perform an isotonic strength examination using a repetition maximum test

7. Describe the role of isokinetic testing in athletic injury examination and the type of measures computerized isokinetic dynamometry provides

95

One of the crucial skills needed to perform an accurate musculoskeletal injury examination is the ability to determine muscle performance. Examination of strength allows you to

- identify underlying deficits during prescreening evaluations to prevent injury, and
- quantify muscle weakness and dysfunction once injury occurs.

This chapter presents the general principles of strength examination and the common manual and instrumented strength examinations you may use in the examination of musculoskeletal injuries. Whether you are on the field or in the clinic and whether you are dealing with an acute injury or a chronic injury will largely dictate the method and detail of the strength examination. In this chapter we first review the functional neuroanatomy and mechanisms of muscle contraction. Then we focus on the general techniques of the strength examination, the type of data that can be derived from each test, and how to interpret the data. Part II addresses specific strength examinations for each joint.

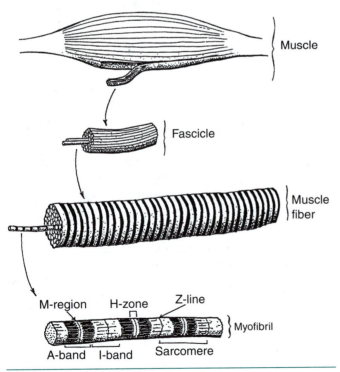

Figure 7.1 Structural components of muscle.

MUSCLE CONTRACTION

Muscles are complex biological structures that contract and extend in order to produce movement. In previous courses, you should have studied the organization of muscle tissue and the mechanisms of muscle contraction. Here is a brief review of both.

Functional Neuromuscular Anatomy

The gross functional contractile unit consists of a muscle and its connective tissue, tendon, and nerve supply. Bundles of muscle fibers called fascicles constitute the actual muscle (figure 7.1). Each muscle fiber within the fascicle consists of myofibrils that run the length of the fiber and are formed by a series of sarcomeres arranged end to end. The sarcomere is the smallest contractile unit of the muscle and contains the myofilaments actin and myosin.

These muscular components are linked together by layers of connective tissue that serve two functions. The first function is to attach the muscle to bone and allow it to exert force. Layers of connective tissue converge and extend beyond the contractile portions of the muscle and blend with the tendon before attaching to the bone. The second function is to separate and group muscle units in order to allow individual fibers and fasciculi to function independently as well as coordinate with other units.

The connective tissue layers include the epimysium, perimysium, and endomysium (see figure 5.2). The epimysium is the outermost layer and sheathes the entire muscle. The perimysium surrounds and gives shape to each fascicle. The deep layer of the perimysium, the endomysium, divides to surround each muscle fiber in the fascicle. Deep to the endomysium is a plasma membrane called the sarcolemma. Within the sarcolemma is sarcoplasmic fluid that contains fuel sources (e.g., ATP), organelles, and enzymes in addition to the bundle of myofibrils comprising the muscle fiber. Each myofibril is surrounded by an extensive network of sarcoplasmic reticulum and transverse tubules that communicate with the sarcolemma to control and provide for rapid contraction and relaxation of contractile units.

Muscle function requires communication with the central nervous system (spinal cord and higher cortical centers) via peripheral nerves. A single peripheral nerve consists of motor (efferent), sensory (afferent), and autonomic fibers. The motor neurons allow the central nervous system to communicate with the muscle and consist of a cell body located in the anterior horn of the spinal cord, an axon with a relatively large diameter, and terminal branches that innervate a group of muscles fibers (Basmajian and DeLuca 1985; Lamb and Hobart 1992). Sensory, or afferent, neurons transmit information from the muscle and other peripheral structures back to the central nervous system. This information is produced by proprioceptors that include the muscle spindle, Golgi tendon organ, and joint receptors. The proprioceptors' specific functions in initiating motor response and control are discussed in chapter 8. **Autonomic nerve fibers** act on structures such as smooth muscle glands and blood vessels to heighten and restore body functions (i.e., blood pressure, heart rate) in response to the environment. They are not involved in skeletal muscle function.

Autonomic nerve fibers act on structures such as smooth muscle, glands, and blood vessels to heighten and restore body functions (i.e., blood pressure, heart rate) in response to the environment.

Review of Excitation–Contraction Coupling

The physiological mechanisms responsible for muscular activation are well documented in the literature and are summarized here. The activation of an alpha motor (efferent) neuron via the central nervous system results in a nerve action potential that is transported along the motor nerve toward the muscle by saltatory conduction. When this excitatory stimulus reaches the motor end plate, the release of transmitter substances across the end plate to the postsynaptic cleft forms an end plate potential. This in turn creates a sodium ion (Na^+) influx at the muscle fiber membrane that results in charge separation and an end plate (synaptic) potential that triggers a sarcolemmal action potential (Enoka 2002). This action potential travels in both directions along the sarcolemma via the t-tubules. Then, by an unknown mechanism, this action potential causes calcium channels to open and release calcium ions (Ca^{++}) into the intracellular space. The Ca^{++} bind to troponin, allowing access to the actin molecule, which then binds with myosin. Finally, the splitting of adenosine triphosphate (ATP) provides energy for myosin to tightly bind and swivel on the actin, causing the actin and myosin to slide on one another and shorten the sarcomere. This process cycles repeatedly in each sarcomere in a muscle fiber. The sum total of the sarcomeres shortening in response to an action potential results in a muscle contraction.

A motor unit is the smallest functional unit of the neuromuscular system and consists of a single motor neuron and all the muscle fibers it innervates. Upon stimulation of the motor neuron, all the muscle fibers within the unit fire nearly simultaneously. Depending on the strength of contraction required, smaller motor units are recruited first followed by the larger motor units, allowing for a gradual increase in force.

GOALS AND PURPOSES

Strength testing determines the level of pain (by muscle inhibition), the resistive capabilities of the muscle being tested, and the neuromuscular integrity of the contractile (active) tissues surrounding the injured area. During an acute examination, you will usually perform isometric tests first, followed by more specific manual muscle tests (MMTs) through a part or full range of motion (ROM). During a nonacute injury examination in the clinic, you may also employ instrumented strength examinations that encompass isometric, isotonic, and isokinetic modes of strength testing in order to obtain a more objective measure of strength capacity.

Pain or apprehension can strongly influence the outcome of any strength test. Specifically, strength testing that produces pain causes a withdrawal response where the athlete demonstrates less strength than she would if she felt no pain. Athletes who fear that the test will cause pain, regardless of whether actual pain is experienced, may also demonstrate reduced strength. In these cases, strength output may be inaccurate. You should indicate on the evaluation that the test produced pain or apprehension and then retest at a later date when the athlete is more comfortable and able to produce a maximal effort.

A muscle's capacity to produce force can be examined through a static or dynamic contraction and through manual and instrumented methods. Manual break tests and instrumented isometric (static) examination reveal the amount of tension a muscle can generate against a resistance that does not permit observable joint movement. Manual muscle testing (MMT) and instrumented isotonic (dynamic) strength examination, or the application of force through all or part of a joint's ROM, are examined with concentric (shortening) or eccentric (lengthening) contractions. Isokinetic (dynamic) strength examination, however, allows athletes to exert as much force and angular joint movement as they can up to a set velocity. Each method of strength examination is covered in the following sections.

MANUAL STRENGTH EXAMINATION

You will frequently perform manual strength examinations to obtain an efficient, gross measure of a muscle's ability to produce force through either a static (fixed joint position) or dynamic (through a ROM) contraction. **Manual strength tests** include any strength evaluation where the examiner applies the resistance. Manual strength examination is most appropriate for on-site and acute evaluations, as it does not require equipment. Another advantage of manual strength testing is that you can carefully control and quickly adjust your resistance in response to the athlete's efforts, and you can alter the applied resistance through the ROM to allow the athlete to achieve maximal effort throughout the test (Kisner and Colby 2002). The primary disadvantage is that the findings rely on your subjective measurement of the patient's strength capabilities, and the measurement may vary between you and other clinicians depending on your strength compared to that of the athlete. A related disadvantage is that the examination can have limited value if you are relatively small in stature and are testing a large muscle group in a tall, strong athlete.

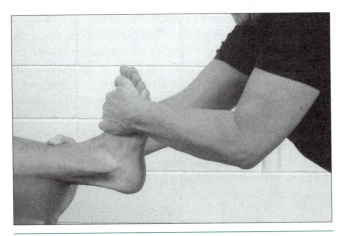

Figure 7.2 Break tests are a quick and efficient form of manual isometric strength examination. The tests are usually performed with the joint in a neutral, midrange position.

Break Tests

Break tests are a quick and efficient form of manual isometric strength examination. Perform break tests with the joint in a neutral, midrange position (figure 7.2) to limit the stress applied to the joint and eliminate interference from inert (noncontractile) joint structures. After positioning the joint, stabilize the proximal segment and instruct the athlete to hold the position as you attempt to move the joint or "break" the position by applying a matching resistance (equal and opposite to their effort) to the distal segment. Rather than applying a sudden, maximal force that overpowers and moves the joint, gradually build resistance to a maximum over 3 to 5 seconds as the athlete matches your resistance.

You can further confirm active tissue injury by stretching the muscle in the direction opposite its motion. For example, if a strength test has a positive result of pain and some weakness from the wrist extensors, you may also note pain while stretching the wrist extensors with passive wrist flexion and elbow extension.

Initial break test results will yield one of four results:

1. Strong and painless, indicating a normal response (the athlete's injury is not neuromuscular)

2. Strong and painful, indicating a lesion in the muscle or tendon

3. Weak and painless, indicating either a nerve injury or musculotendinous rupture

4. Weak and painful, indicating a serious injury that could range from a fracture to an unstable joint

The second category, strong and painful, is most commonly seen in acute injury evaluations and ranges from slight weakness with some pain for a mild muscle strain to moderate weakness with moderate pain for a second-degree strain to little loss of strength with more pain for tendinitis.

In the third category, weak and painless, contractile function can be lost without eliciting pain if the muscle tendon unit experienced a complete disruption so that when the muscle contracts, there are no fibers remaining intact that would be stressed upon contraction. Weakness without pain can also result from temporary or permanent injury to the motor nerve that stimulates the muscle to contract. A weak and painless result can range from slight weakness when only a minor contributing muscle of a functional muscle group is affected (e.g., rupture of the plantaris while the gastrocnemius remains intact), to moderate weakness when a primary contributor to a functional muscle group is affected (e.g., rupture of the long head of the biceps while the short head of the biceps, brachialis, and brachioradialis are still intact), to complete paralysis (e.g., loss of function of all primary and secondary movers due to a nerve root injury).

When documenting the results of a break test, grade the muscle according to the maximum resistance against which it holds. Table 7.1 contains an isometric grading scale you can use to document your findings. Note the presence or absence of pain along with the grade. To achieve consistent grading from test to test, always perform the break test in the same joint position, as strength varies depending on joint range. For this reason, you may also wish to perform break tests in different joint positions to get a more accurate picture of the athlete's strength.

Table 7.1
Break Test Grading Scale

Grade	Description
5	Maintains test position against gravity and maximal resistance
4	Maintains test position against gravity and moderate resistance
4–	Maintains test position against gravity and less than moderate resistance
3+	Maintains test position against gravity and minimal resistance
3	Maintains test position against gravity with no resistance

Adapted, by permission, from H.M. Clarkson, 2000, *Musculoskeletal examination: Joint range of motion and manual muscle strength*, 2nd ed. (Philadelphia: Lippincott, Williams & Wilkins, 24).

Manual Muscle Testing

Manual muscle testing (MMT) examines muscle strength using applied resistance against gravity through a full or partial ROM. In this case, allow the joint to move and match your resistance to the athlete's, providing the maximal resistance the athlete is capable of overcoming.

MMT provides more information than break tests since it examines muscle function throughout the ROM and better delineates individual muscle contributions. It is entirely possible that an athlete who has sustained a grade I muscle strain may achieve a strength grade of 5 when performing a break test at midrange. However, when the muscle test begins with the muscle in a more lengthened position, you may note a lesser grade. This discrepancy may be the result of more stress applied to the injured muscle fibers because the muscle is in a lengthened position, or because the contribution of other supporting muscles (**synergists**) changes in the extended position.

MMT can also better delineate the location and reason for weakness. For example, weak resisted elbow flexion can be caused by the biceps brachii, the brachialis, or the brachioradialis. Through proper joint positioning and applied resistance, MMT can isolate each muscle and identify the specific muscle or muscles causing the weakness. (See chapter 13 for specific MMTs that differentiate these muscles.)

> *Synergists* are muscles that work with the prime mover to assist joint motion. Their contribution to joint motion varies depending on joint orientation and position.

Manual Muscle Testing Technique

Perform MMT by stabilizing the proximal segment of the limb with one hand while applying resistance to the distal segment with the other. Generally, you will stabilize the body segment where the muscle originates and apply resistance to the body segment where the muscle inserts. To maximize your resistance, apply force at the distal end of the segment. This creates a longer lever arm, requiring greater muscle force to overcome the same resistance (figure 7.3), and it is mechanically advantageous because it allows you to use less force to resist the motion.

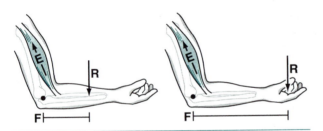

Figure 7.3   Maximize your resistance by applying force at the distal end of the moving segment.

Apply your resistance in a direct line with the orientation of the muscle to be tested. Position the athlete to best isolate the muscle or muscle group to be tested and to either maximize or eliminate the effects of gravity. For example, to test biceps strength against gravity, seat the athlete on the edge of a table to stabilize the trunk and allow free, unrestricted movement of the elbow through a full ROM. Use your dominant hand to apply resistance to the distal, anterior surface of the athlete's supinated forearm while stabilizing the humerus with your other hand (figure 7.4). This hand position best isolates the biceps brachii and maximizes the muscle's direct line of pull in achieving elbow flexion. Alternatively, to test strength of the brachialis, apply resistance to the posterior aspect of the pronated forearm while the trunk and humerus are stabilized as when testing biceps strength against gravity.

When performing MMT, watch for any evidence of muscle substitution or compensatory movements. Muscle substitution is the use of other muscles, usually synergists, to create motion. Compensatory movements refer to changes in body position that either reduce the stress placed on the muscle or maximize the use of synergists or other nearby muscles. Examples of compensatory movements include external rotation of the hip during hip flexor testing to minimize the effects of gravity and allow the hip adductors to aid movement; external rotation of the humerus to allow

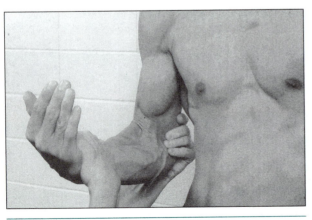

Figure 7.4   Hand positioning for MMT of the biceps brachii.

the long head of the biceps to assist a weakened deltoid in performing shoulder abduction; "hiking" or flexing of the hip joint during knee flexion to lengthen the hamstring muscles; and shrugging of the shoulder when testing lateral flexion of the cervical spine in an effort to bring the shoulder near the ear.

To help prevent compensatory movements and muscle substitution, carefully adhere to proper athlete positioning and segment stabilization. Other strategies include clearly instructing the athlete how to perform the movement and palpating the working muscle to ensure it maximally contracts (Clarkson 2000).

Grading Manual Muscle Tests

Grade manual muscle tests according to the amount of resistance you can apply with or without the muscle working against gravity. A gravity-dependent position is one in which the muscle works against the forces of gravity (e.g., knee extension in a seated position), while a gravity-eliminated position is a position in a plane of motion that absorbs or minimizes the effects of gravity (e.g., knee extension in side-lying).

Grading typically uses a scale of 0 to 5, with 5 representing normal strength (maximal resistance against gravity) and 0 representing no strength (no evidence of muscle contraction with gravity eliminated) (table 7.2). Grades 3, 4, and 5 are for tests where the muscle works against gravity, and grades 4 and 5 are for tests with manually applied resistance. Grades 1 and 2 are for tests where gravity is eliminated or minimized. You will not usually see grades 0, 1, or 2 in acute athletic injuries except with musculotendinous ruptures or nerve disruptions.

Table 7.2
Grading Criteria for Gravity-Resisted Muscle Strength

Medical Research Council	Daniels and Worthingham	Description
5	Normal	Patient completes ROM against gravity and against maximal resistance
4+		Patient completes ROM against gravity and against nearly maximal resistance
4	Good	Patient completes ROM against gravity and against moderate resistance
4–		Patient completes ROM against gravity and against minimal resistance >50% range
3+		Patient completes ROM against gravity, against minimal resistance <50% range
3	Fair	Patient completes ROM against gravity with no manual resistance
3–		Patient does not complete ROM against gravity but does complete more than half the range
2+		Patient initiates ROM against gravity or completes range with gravity minimized against slight resistance
2	Poor	Patient completes ROM with gravity minimized
2–		Patient unable to complete ROM with gravity minimized
1		Muscle contraction can be palpated but there is no joint motion
0	Zero	No palpable contraction or joint motion

Data from Medical Research Council, 1943, *Aids to the investigation of peripheral nerve injuries,* 2nd ed. rev. (London: H.M.S.O.); and L. Daniels and C.A. Worthingham, 1980, *Muscle testing,* 4th ed. (London: W.B. Saunders).

Summary of Manual Muscle Testing Technique

☐ Identify origin, insertion, and motion of muscle or muscle group to be tested.

☐ Consider possible compensation.

☐ Position athlete for maximal support and stabilization.

☐ Position self for best mechanical advantage and appropriate line of resistance.

☐ Stabilize proximal segment.

☐ Apply resistance to distal portion of the moving segment in direct line of pull with muscle function.

☐ Provide clear instructions for the athlete's movement.

☐ Complete the motion, watching for compensatory or substitution movements.

☐ Reposition the athlete to test with gravity minimized or eliminated if unable to complete the motion against gravity.

☐ Document appropriate grade.

The only way to obtain an accurate strength examination is to apply sufficient resistance. This requires that you properly position yourself to maximize your ability to apply manual resistance in line with the muscle action. It is also essential to apply MMT consistently each time to accurately determine changes in the athlete's status upon reevaluation and to compare limbs bilaterally. This includes consistently positioning the athlete, the examiner relative to the athlete, and the location of your stabilizing hand and applied resistance.

INSTRUMENTED STRENGTH EXAMINATION

Instrumented strength examination uses a variety of objective measurement devices and systems to quantify strength and other parameters of muscle function. Instrumented strength examination provides specific, numerical measures of muscle performance, allowing accurate documentation of the extent of dysfunction and reliable examination (quantifiable comparison) from one evaluation to the next. The primary disadvantages of instrumented strength examination are the devices' cost, lack of portability, and lack of practicality for on-site evaluations.

Depending on the capabilities of the device, instrumented strength examination allows the quantitative measurement of the following muscle functions:

- **Force,** or the measured amount of tension a muscle or muscle group produces at the location of the applied resistance

- **Torque,** or the measurement of the force exerted by a muscle about a joint's axis of rotation (torque is the product of the force applied at the location of the resistance and the distance of the applied resistance from the joint's axis of rotation, or force × distance)

- **Work,** or the total force applied over the length of a contraction and displayed as the area under the strength curve

- **Power,** or the time required to perform work (if you know the quantity of time required to produce work, you can determine the muscle's ability to generate power)

- **Endurance,** or the muscle's capacity to produce force over a series of consecutive contractions or its ability to maintain a sustained contraction over a period of time

Instrumented strength examination includes isometric, isotonic, and isokinetic modes. Each mode has advantages and disadvantages (see "Comparison of Isometric, Isotonic, and Isokinetic Examination Techniques") that will help you determine which is the most appropriate for a given injury situation.

Comparison of Isometric, Isotonic, and Isokinetic Examination Techniques

Isometric

Advantages

- Useful when joint motion is contraindicated.
- Requires minimal or no equipment.

Disadvantages

- Measures strength of a specific joint position.
- Lacks objective strength measurement.

Isotonic

Advantages

- Includes both concentric and eccentric strength components.
- Permits simultaneous examination of multiple joints or muscles.
- Allows examination in closed-chain, weight-bearing positions.
- Quantifies measurement of strength.

Disadvantages

- Limits maximal strength examination to the weakest point in the range.
- Cannot quantify other parameters of muscle performance (torque, work, or power).
- Allows stronger muscles to compensate or substitute for weaker muscles during multi-joint or muscle examinations.

Isokinetic

Advantages

- Isolates weak muscle groups.
- Provides maximal resistance throughout the examined ROM by using accommodating resistance.
- Provides inherent safety mechanism by using accommodating resistance.
- Quantifies torque, work, and power.

Disadvantages

- Requires expensive equipment not conducive to on-site examinations.
- Limits reliable examination to isolated muscle groups moving the limb through cardinal planes of motion.
- Examines primarily non-weight-bearing, open-kinetic chain positions.

Adapted from D.H. Perrin, 1993, *Isokinetic exercise and assessment* (Champaign, IL: Human Kinetics), chapter 9.

Isometric Strength Examination

Isometric strength examination measures a muscle's potential for producing static force against immovable resistance. Its primary advantage is that it can identify a muscle group around a joint that may be limited in motion because of pain, pathology, or equipment or bracing. Its primary disadvantage is that its findings are limited to the specific point of resistance application within the joint's ROM (similar to break tests). A number of instruments are available for measurable examination of isometric strength, including grip and pinch dynamometers, handheld dynamometers, and cable tensiometers. These devices are relatively inexpensive, though they vary considerably in sophistication and cost. While some are specific to body regions, others are capable of testing most major muscle groups. Accurate measurement depends on several factors, including body position, joint angle, hand position, and correct positioning of the instrument. These devices are typically used for clinical evaluations or for documenting quantifiable progress over time.

Grip and Pinch Dynamometers

Grip and pinch dynamometers measure the strength and endurance of an athlete's gross and fine motor grip. Grip dynamometers measure overall muscle function in the forearm and hand, while pinch dynamometers provide a more specific examination between muscles in the thumb and opposing fingers. In these devices, a strain gauge measures strength as force (in kilograms or pounds), usually at the location where resistance is applied. The measurement gauge often consists of a dial that shows real-time force and an indicator needle that remains at the peak force recorded until manually reset by the examiner. This system allows you to determine the maximum force that the athlete can achieve as well as the muscle's ability to sustain force over time. Both analog and electronic systems are available.

Accurate measurement of grip or pinch strength depends on body position, device position, grip or pinch size, and testing method. For example, you will obtain a different strength value when the strength test is performed with the elbow at the side and flexed to 90° versus when the elbow is fully extended. A grip or pinch that is too small or wide yields lower strength values than a midrange position.

Grip dynamometers are usually adjustable to accommodate different hand sizes. Perform grip measures in a standardized position to improve measurement reliability and ensure that strength changes upon reevaluation are due to changes in the muscle rather than testing technique. Always record instrument settings along with your findings for consistent instrument positioning.

To perform a grip strength test, adjust the grip size to a comfortable midrange grip. Position the upper arm vertically at the side, and either flex the elbow to 90° (figure 7.5) or fully extend it. The wrist and forearm should be in a neutral position. Have the athlete perform 2 or 3 submaximal contractions to get a comfortable grip and become familiar with the device. For testing, ask the athlete to perform three maximal grips lasting 3 to 5 seconds each and allow 30 to 60 seconds of rest between trials. Record the average or peak of the three trials. Test grip strength bilaterally to compare the injured and noninjured sides. To accurately interpret strength imbalances, know which hand is dominant and whether any other strength differences between hands may be expected due to sport-specific training demands.

Pinch strength can be used with various grips (figure 7.6) to more accurately examine fine motor skills and task-specific grasping functions. The **chuck grip,** also known as the digital prehension pinch, measures the force exerted between the thumb and 2nd and 3rd digit pads. The **tip grip** determines opposition strength by measuring the force exerted between the tip of the thumb and the tip of the other digits. The **lateral pinch grip** measures grasping strength by placing the dynamometer between the pad of the thumb and the medial aspect of the index finger. As with grip strength testing, consistent athlete and dynamometer positioning are essential for test repeatability and accuracy. Test protocol is similar to the grip strength test.

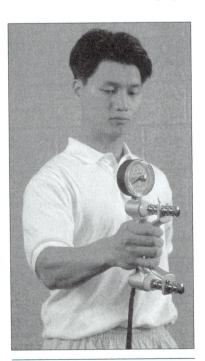

Figure 7.5 Examining hand and arm strength using a grip dynamometer.

For more information on fine motor skills of the hand, refer to *Therapeutic Exercise for Injured Athletes, Second Edition,* (Houglum 2005), chapter 19.

Handheld Dynamometers

Handheld dynamometers are equipped with a small, internal load cell capable of measuring muscular force during isometric contractions (figure 7.7). A handheld dynamometer enhances muscle strength quantification during manual isometric muscle testing (break tests). Perform the manual break test as before (see page 98), but with the dynamometer placed between your resistive hand and the position on the athlete's limb through which you apply resistance (figure 7.8). When the athlete generates muscle force in an attempt to keep you from moving the joint, the instrument records the maximal force encountered.

The accuracy and consistency of the handheld dynamometer have often been challenged when examining large muscle groups in healthy athletes, particularly because these dynamometers rely on adequate examiner strength and stabilization of the dynamometer. However, handheld dynamometer measures of knee extensor strength have been shown to be reliable between examiners of varied experience when tester strength is not a limitation (Bohannon and Wikholm 1992). The advantages of the handheld dynamometer compared to other instrumented methods are substantially lower costs and their practicality and efficiency in a variety of clinical settings.

Cable Tensiometers

Cable tensiometers were originally designed to measure the tension of aircraft control cables and then refined by Clark in 1948 for measuring the strength of muscle groups. Cable tensiometers are similar to handheld dynamometers in that they measure isometric strength. However, where handheld dynamometers measure the compressive or "push" force of the muscle through resistance applied between the examiner's hand and the athlete's limb via a load cell, cable tensiometers measure the applied tension or "pulling force" of the muscle via a strain gauge.

Secure one end of the cable tensiometer to a fixed object, with the athlete either gripping or attached (strapped) to the opposite

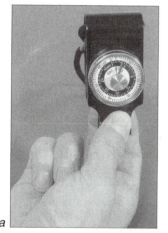
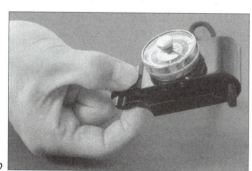
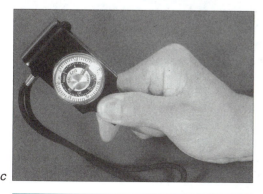

Figure 7.6 Examination of pinch strength using (a) chuck, (b) tip, and (c) lateral pinch grasping tasks.

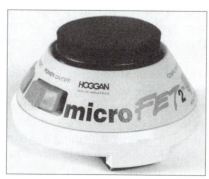

Figure 7.7 A handheld dynamometer.
Courtesy of Hoggan Health Industries

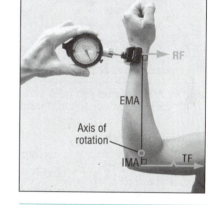

Figure 7.8 One example of the variety of handheld dynamometers available to objectively measure isometric strength for trunk and extremity muscles. The dynameter is placed on the extremity's distal surface and held in place by the clinician while the patient attempts to move the extremity. The maximum output is indicated on the dynamometer. RF = resistive force, EMA = external moment arm, IMA = internal moment arm, TF = triceps force.

Reprinted from *Kinesiology of the musculoskeletal system: Foundations for physical rehabilitation*, E.A. Neumann, Copyright 2002, with permission from Elsevier.

end. When the muscle contracts, a pulling resistance is applied in line with the strain gauge device. The gauge system is similar to the systems previously described, measuring isometric force in kilograms or pounds with a dial system that provides both real-time and maximal force readings.

The advantages of recording muscle strength using a cable tensiometer instead of more sophisticated devices are similar to those of most handheld dynamometers. While both types are relatively portable, the cable tensiometer has the added advantage of not being dependent on examiner strength and positioning. The trade-off, however, is that the unit must be secured to a stationary object in such a way that the athlete can be optimally positioned to create the correct line of pull for the desired muscle.

Isotonic Strength Examination

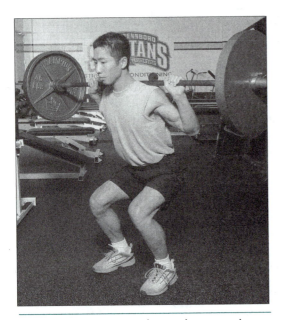

Figure 7.9 A squat can be used to assess isotonic strength of the hip and thigh.

Closed kinetic chain is movement of the body with the distal segment working against a fixed or immovable object.

Isotonic strength is examined as the patient lifts a fixed amount of weight through a ROM. It has also been called dynamic constant resistance (Fleck and Kraemer 2004). Isotonic strength can be measured objectively with dumbbells, barbells, and various commercial strength training devices. A distinct advantage of isotonic resistance is that it permits examination of functional strength by testing multiple joints simultaneously. For example, the bench press determines strength of the upper body while the leg press or squat identify strength of the lower body, simultaneously testing hip extension, knee extension, and plantar flexion (figure 7.9). Individual muscle groups can also be isolated. For example, you can isolate the biceps with dumbbell curls, the soleus with a bent-knee toe raise, and the quadriceps with a knee extension. Another advantage of isotonic examination is that it examines lower-extremity strength in a more functional, weight-bearing or closed-kinetic chain position.

Isotonic strength is commonly determined by testing the maximal weight that can be lifted through a joint's ROM for a set number of repetitions, usually either 1 (1RM) or 10 (10RM). Multiple test trials are usually required to identify the maximal weight the athlete can lift for the desired number of repetitions. The strategy is to begin with a weight lighter than the maximal amount and gradually approach the predicted maximum. When the athlete can exceed the set number of repetitions, she moves to an incrementally higher weight after an appropriate rest period. The athlete completes the test when she is able to lift the weight for the desired number of repetitions but not one repetition more. To obtain an accurate test, the athlete must warm up, maintain proper form throughout the test, take sufficient rest intervals between attempts, and be familiar with the task (Wathen 1994).

- **1-repetition maximum (1RM).** Identifying the maximal weight an athlete can lift for a single repetition is a true maximal strength test. Athletic trainers and strength and conditioning specialists typically use the 1RM to determine a healthy, mature athlete's muscular strength and then prescribe the appropriate intensity, usually expressed as a percentage of the athlete's 1RM, for subsequent training sessions. Because the 1RM is a maximal strength test, it is not used with an injured athlete, child, or adolescent. The 1RM is most appropriate for evaluation of healthy athletes, such as a preseason orthopedic evaluation of an athlete's conditioning or identification of any strength deficits from fully recovered injuries. To avoid injury with 1RM testing, start the athlete with a lighter weight so they can warm up or familiarize the muscle to the task before performing a maximal contraction. The National Strength and Conditioning Association (Semenick 1994) recommends beginning single repetition attempts at about 50% of the expected maximum, then increasing the weight to 75%, 90%, 100%, and higher until the 1RM is reached.

• **10-repetition maximum (10RM).** If an athlete is recovering from an injury, is untrained, or has no previous experience with a 1RM test, perform a 10-repetition maximum (10RM). The 10RM is similar to a 1RM and identifies the maximal weight an athlete can lift exactly 10 times. By consulting published tables, you can use the 10RM to predict maximal strength (NSCA 1994). Because 10RM tests can require multiple sets to identify the maximal weight, you must allow sufficient rest between sets to ensure that you examine strength rather than resistance to fatigue. A rest of 2 to 4 minutes is recommended. Starting with a weight that is too light can fatigue the athlete if he must perform too many sets before reaching his maximum, resulting in an artificially low maximum weight value. Ideally, you can identify an athlete's 10RM within five attempts (Wathen 1994).

*The **length–tension relationship** describes the force (tension) a muscle can generate at any given muscle length along its range.*

RM tests are limited by their inability to control test velocity or contribution from accessory muscle groups. Isotonic examination against a fixed resistance can also be limited in the sense that the amount an athlete can lift through her weakest part of the examined ROM determines the maximal force she can overcome. To address this limitation, some machines offer variable resistance that attempts to accommodate strength variations over a ROM by using an elliptical cam. The cam provides the least resistance where the ability to produce force is correspondingly lowest (end ranges of motion) and the greatest resistance where the muscle is at its optimal **length–tension relationship** and mechanical advantage (midrange). How well this variable resistance works depends on how well the person's size fits the machine.

Isokinetic Strength Examination

The concept of isokinetic resistance was introduced in 1967 by Hislop and Perrine (figure 7.10). As mentioned, isokinetic strength testing allows the athlete to exert as much force as possible against a resistance arm set to a fixed angular velocity. When the limb exceeds the preset velocity limit, the dynamometer counters the force to maintain a constant movement rate. In other words, no matter how hard and fast the muscle contracts to move the limb, the resistance arm will only move as fast as the selected speed allows.

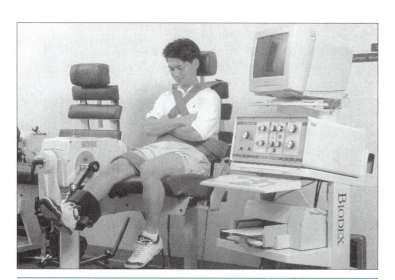

Figure 7.10 Strength test for knee extension using an isokinetic dynamometer.

The primary advantage of isokinetic strength testing is that it examines the muscle's maximal capabilities throughout the entire ROM. For example, at the midrange of joint motion, where muscles are at their optimal length–tension relationship for binding actin and myosin and greatest mechanical advantage, the isokinetic dynamometer maintains a preset velocity and the muscle produces more force. Conversely, at the extremes of the joint's ROM, where muscles are at a physiological and mechanical disadvantage, the dynamometer still maintains its velocity but the muscle produces less force.

Because isokinetic testing does not require a fixed resistance to move through the weakest point in a given arc of motion (as with isotonic strength testing), it records the maximal voluntary force a muscle generates at any given angle in the ROM. It may also be a safer alternative for examining injured athletes since the dynamometer's resistance immediately disengages when the athlete experiences any pain or discomfort during the test.

Isokinetic Torque Curve

Isokinetic testing devices can express muscle output throughout the ROM as a curve via an analog signal sent from the dynamometer. The normal concentric isokinetic curve is illustrated

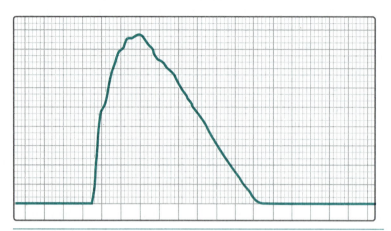

in figure 7.11. Isokinetic resistance adjusts to the amount of force generated by a given muscle group. The combined length–tension relationship and overall effectiveness of a muscle contraction are greatest at the middle of a joint's available ROM and lesser near the beginning and end of the range. The isokinetic curve reflects the muscle's variations in generated force as it contracts through a joint's ROM. You can determine several isokinetic measures of muscle performance from this torque or force curve (see next section "Measures of Muscle Performance").

Figure 7.11   Normal concentric isokinetic torque curve.

*An **artifact** is a change or alteration in the curve that is not consistent with expected results.*

Several factors contribute to a normal, smooth, and coordinated muscle contraction, producing the characteristic isokinetic torque curve. For example, the muscle group and joint must be free from pain or injury. An isokinetic dynamometer accommodates pain by disengaging when the patient produces less force. Pain originating from a musculotendinous unit or from an articulation crossed by a muscle group frequently results in **artifacts** within the torque curve.

Some clinicians suggest that certain pathologies produce characteristic artifacts in the isokinetic torque curve. For instance, some believe that isokinetic testing of a knee with a deficient anterior cruciate ligament (ACL) against a distally positioned resistance pad results in a bimodal (double-peak) torque curve. The purported mechanism for this characteristic curve suggests that as the quadriceps muscle group begins to contract in the absence of an intact ACL, producing the first peak, other soft tissue structures about the knee "catch" the anterior translation that occurs at the proximal tibia, causing the second peak. Figure 7.12 shows torque curves from a normal knee and an ACL-deficient knee that suggest using such curves to predict joint pathologies is questionable. While some clinicians claim to predict a variety of muscle and joint pathologies (e.g., chondromalacia patella, subluxing patella, knee plica syndrome) from torque curves, there is little to no scientific evidence to validate these claims. Interpretation of the torque curve should be limited to a muscle's capacity to produce torque, work, and power.

Measures of Muscle Performance

Computerized isokinetic dynamometers extract several measurement parameters from the isokinetic torque curve, including peak and average torque, peak and average force, work, and power. They can also obtain many of these values for a specific angle or ROM.

If a muscle's force or torque has been examined throughout the entire ROM, the measurement may be reported as either a peak or average value. **Peak torque** is the greatest torque produced at any point in the ROM. **Average torque** is calculated from the tension produced by the muscle throughout the entire ROM. Using average torque values to compare pretest, posttest, and bilateral muscle group performance necessitates careful standardization of the tested ROM. In contrast, peak torque is likely to occur within the midrange of motion and standardization may not be as essential as when studying average values. Peak and average torque are the most common isokinetic parameters for examining human muscle performance. More recently, clinicians have also used **angle specific torque,** the torque produced at any designated point throughout the ROM.

If known, the amount of force produced by a given muscle contraction over a certain distance (the area under the force/displacement curve) may be expressed as work. If the

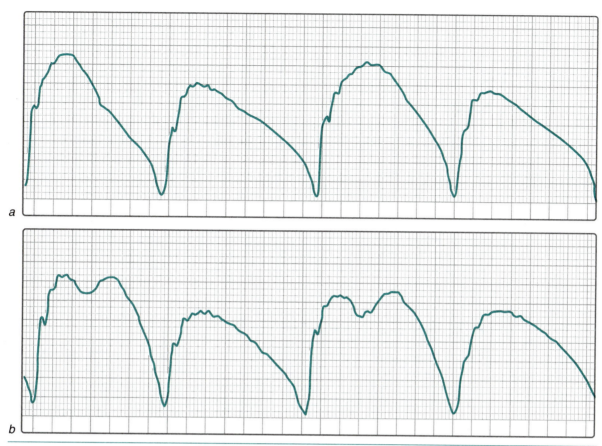

Figure 7.12 Torque curves from *(a)* an ACL-deficient knee and *(b)* a normal knee indicate that torque curve characteristics alone should not be used to predict pathologies.

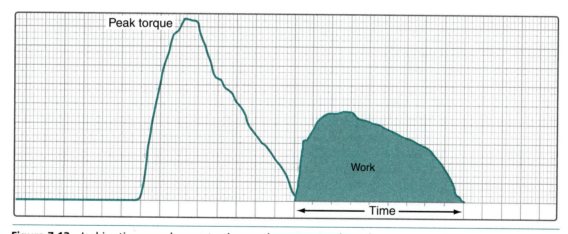

Figure 7.13 Isokinetic curve demonstrating peak torque, work, and power.

quantity of time required to achieve the measured work is known, the muscle's ability to generate power may be determined. Figure 7.13 illustrates peak torque, work, and power as indicated by a normal isokinetic torque curve. As can be seen in figure 7.14, return of peak torque following injury may not represent return to the muscle's average torque, work, or power capabilities.

The advent of active dynamometry in the mid-1980s allowed clinicians to quantify torque, work, and power in both concentric and eccentric modes of contractions and at slow, intermediate, and fast velocities. Today, most isokinetic dynamometers test velocities up to 300

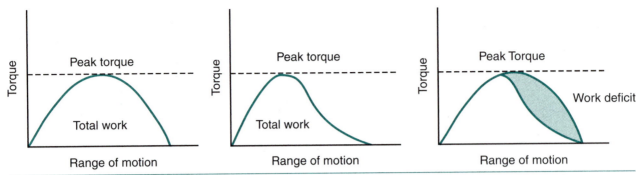

Figure 7.14   Two curves *(a-b)* showing equal peak torques *(c)* but very different average torque and work.

degrees per second (°/second) and some test as high as 500° per second. The ability to test at a wide range of velocities has fueled the misconceptions that slow isokinetic velocities reflect muscle strength and that torque produced at higher velocities represents power. These are misconceptions because, as previously defined, torque, work, and power are independent of test velocity.

Principles of Isokinetic Testing

Factors that interfere with accurate and reliable examination of human muscle performance deserve careful attention in the development of standard test protocols. A thorough musculoskeletal screen should precede any isokinetic evaluation. Athletes experiencing muscle spasm or joint restriction due to pain, inflammation, effusion, or muscle contracture should not be examined for isokinetic strength. Athletes should also be screened for any evidence of cardiovascular problems or disease to determine the appropriateness of maximal-effort strength testing.

For an isokinetic strength examination to yield accurate results, the following factors must be addressed:

- **Education, familiarization, and warm-up.** Isokinetic resistance is still a novel sensation for many patients. If an athlete does not understand that she will only encounter resistance if she exceeds the test velocity, she may not maximize her effort. Instruct the athlete by saying, "I want you to push and pull as hard as you can." Familiarize her with the test velocity and mode of contraction (eccentric versus concentric) using warm-up repetitions at each velocity. Three submaximal efforts followed by three maximal contractions are adequate to obtain reliable measurements of isokinetic peak torque, work, and power (Perrin 1986).

- **Body position, stabilization, and joint alignment.** Follow manufacturer guidelines for positioning and stabilizing the athlete to isolate the targeted muscle group and eliminate as much accessory muscle contribution as possible. Stabilize the athlete minimally at the waist and chest. To eliminate contribution from the upper extremities during a lower-extremity test, place the arms across the chest. Similarly, the knee should not bear weight during upper-extremity examination. Most manufacturers provide a manual that describes stabilization procedures and how to align with the dynamometer each joint the unit can test.

- **Gravity correction.** When a limb moves through a gravity-dependent position during isokinetic examination, use correction procedures to account for the weight of the dynamometer's lever arm and the limb being tested. When working against gravity, the limb must exert additional force to accelerate, usually reducing the recorded torque output. Conversely, acceleration of the limb with gravity erroneously increases torque values. The importance of gravity correction can be demonstrated with seated reciprocal knee extension and flexion. In this case, quadriceps strength (knee extension against gravity) is underestimated while hamstring strength (knee flexion with gravity) is overestimated. The effects of gravity not only reduce the accuracy of the test, but can also confound reciprocal muscle-group ratios. Determining the strength ratio from uncorrected values inflates the ratio so that the hamstrings appear stronger in relation to the quadriceps than they really are. A similar phenomenon can occur in seated shoulder internal and external rotation absolute values and reciprocal ratios when the shoulder is abducted to 90°. To avoid erroneous deficits between bilateral limbs or between tests, use the same gravity correction value from test to test and limb to limb. Gravity correction values should not vary greatly between limbs side to side unless significant muscle atrophy exists in the injured extremity.

- **Overshoot phenomenon.** Abruptly engaging an isokinetic dynamometer's resistance can result in a transient peak or spike in the isokinetic torque curve. A similar spike can occur when quickly decelerating at the end of a ROM. These artificial spikes are particularly troublesome at high velocities and can result in artificially high peak torque values. To guard against overshoot spikes and inaccurate test results, most isokinetic dyamometers have a ramping system that controls the rate of acceleration or a damping system that controls the rate of deceleration. Newer models have a preloading mechanism that requires a muscle to generate a considerable amount of tension before the dynamometer will begin to move at the set velocity. Because overshoot occurs mostly at the beginning and end ranges of motion, a filter may also be employed to ignore the first and last few degrees of the ROM. Although these methods guard against artifacts and overshoots in the torque curve, they may eliminate or alter some aspects of the torque curve itself, so you should understand the capabilities of your isokinetic equipment and employ these parameters across all tests for a given joint. You should also understand the implications of the procedures for reducing artifacts and erroneous torque values so that you can accurately interpret the test.

- **Appropriate test protocol.** A variety of test protocols are available for examining isokinetic torque, work, and power. Test protocols should define periods of warm-up and rest, test velocities, number of sets and repetitions to be performed, and provision of verbal encouragement or visual feedback. Several factors influence the ultimate selection of test protocols, including the muscle group to be tested, the stage of injury, the age and overall fitness of the athlete, and the sport activity the athlete engages in. Discussion of these factors is beyond the scope of this chapter; however, this chapter does provide a general protocol you may follow in the box below.

Recommended Protocol for Isokinetic Examination

1. Musculoskeletal screen
2. General body stretching and warm-up
3. Patient setup with optimal stabilization
4. Alignment of joint and dynamometer axes of rotation
5. Verbal introduction to the isokinetic concept
6. Gravity correction when appropriate
7. Warm-up (3 submaximal, 3 maximal repetitions)
8. Rest (3 seconds-1 minute)
9. Maximal test at slow velocity (4-6 repetitions)
10. Rest (3 seconds-1 minute)
11. Maximal test at fast velocity (4-6 repetitions)
12. Rest (3 seconds-1 minute)
13. Multiple repetition endurance test
14. Testing of contralateral extremity for bilateral comparison
15. Recording of test details and position settings to ensure replication on retest
16. Explanation of results to patient

Interpreting Isokinetic Test Results

An isokinetic evaluation produces a profile that you can use to predict susceptibility to injury in a healthy athlete, identify muscle performance deficits resulting from injury, monitor an injured athlete's rehabilitation, and examine an athlete's readiness to return to play. Depending on instrument capabilities, interpretation of the isokinetic evaluation usually involves careful analysis of the subject's ability to generate torque, work, or power.

- **Measuring peak torque, work, and power.** Peak torque may be identified as either the true peak or average. Because several isokinetic contractions are necessary to obtain a true peak value, the average of the peak values for several consecutive torque curves (average peak) may better indicate the muscle's maximal performance and may tend to be more stable over time. The advantage of true peak torque is that it can identify muscle performance for a restricted ROM. Average torque is measured across the entire torque tracing. The advantage of average torque is that it is less sensitive to artifacts. Because average torque is measured from the complete curve, the tested ROM must be consistent between bilateral and repeated tests. The work capacity of a single muscle group may be determined by calculating the total area under one or a series of consecutive torque curves. Power is determined by identifying the time required to perform work within a single or several repetitions. Most isokinetic instruments have computer software to perform these calculations.

- **Measuring endurance.** Endurance is determined by identifying the muscle's capacity to produce force over a series of consecutive isokinetic contractions. Isokinetic endurance can be quantified

  - as the number of repetitions required for the maximum torque value to fall below 50% of the maximum value recorded in the first few repetitions, or

  - as the percent decline over a certain number of repetitions or amount of time.

When using computer interfacing that calculates work, the total work performed over multiple contractions can also represent endurance capacity.

- **Peak torque relative to body weight.** Variations in body size and somatotype within the physically active population make it challenging to determine an adequate level of torque for all athletes. One useful technique for individualizing the interpretation of an isokinetic evaluation is to normalize torque to the person's body weight. Peak torque normalized to body weight (dividing peak torque by body weight) enables you to compare subjects despite varying body size and structure. When making comparisons you must also use consistent unit values. Torque can be expressed as newton meters (N·m) or foot-pounds (ft-lbs) and weight as kilograms (kg) or pounds (lbs). Different units can yield very different normalized values. We recommend expressing all data in accordance with SI units (N·m and kg).

SI units (Système International d'Unités) are the international standard for reporting measurements.

- **Bilateral muscle group comparisons.** Isokinetic examination accurately compares contralateral limbs so long as the test protocol for both sides is consistent in all respects. You should always test the uninjured side first so that the athlete learns what to expect and will be less apprehensive when you test the injured side. However, you should first determine if you need to adjust the test protocol for the injured side (e.g., adjust for restricted ROM), as you should use the same adjustments when testing the uninjured side in order to obtain an accurate comparison. Although the torque values of the uninjured extremity are often used to identify deficits on the injured side, limb dominance and the effects of neuromuscular specificity of various sports on bilateral strength relationships can confound this logic. While bilateral differences due to these factors are usually minimal in the lower extremity, athletes participating in bilaterally asymmetric upper-extremity activities (e.g., tennis, throwing) may differ in strength as much as 15% between dominant and nondominant sides (Perrin, Robertson, and Ray 1987).

SUMMARY

1. Identify the main goals and features of the strength examination.

   Strength testing examines the level of pain (via muscle inhibition), resistive capabilities, and neuromuscular integrity in the contractile (active) tissues surrounding the injured area. Strength examination allows you to identify underlying deficits during prescreening evaluations to help prevent injury, and to quantify muscle weakness and dysfunction once injury occurs.

2. Understand the effect of pain on the accuracy of the strength examination.

   Pain or apprehension can strongly influence any strength test. Pain causes an autonomic withdrawal of contraction strength so that the athlete demonstrates less strength than if there were no pain. Athletes who are apprehensive and simply fear the test will cause pain may also demonstrate reduced strength. When a strength test produces pain or apprehension, you should document these findings and retest the athlete at a later date when she is more comfortable and able to produce a maximal effort.

3. Describe and demonstrate the types of manual muscle examination.

   Manual muscle examination includes both static and dynamic contractions. The break test is an isometric muscle test that is performed with the joint in a neutral, midrange position. While stabilizing the proximal segment, instruct the athlete to hold the joint position as you attempt to move the joint or "break" the position by applying matching resistance to the distal segment. Gradually build your resistance to a maximum over 3 to 5 seconds as the athlete matches your force. Manual muscle testing (MMT) is a dynamic form of manual strength examination performed through a full ROM, allowing better isolation of individual muscles. MMTs are graded and interpreted on the amount of resistance the muscle applies. Grading is typically based on a 0- to 5-point scale, with 5 representing normal strength (maximal resistance against gravity) and 0 representing no strength (no evidence of muscle contraction with gravity eliminated). Grades 3, 4, and 5 are for tests with the muscle working against gravity, and grades 4 and 5 are for tests against manually applied resistance. Grades 1 and 2 are for tests with gravity eliminated or minimized.

4. Differentiate between isometric, isotonic, and isokinetic modes of instrumented strength examination.

   Instrumented strength examination uses a variety of objective measurement devices and systems to quantify strength and other parameters of muscle function. The primary benefit of instrumented strength examination is that it provides specific, numerical measures of muscle performance. Instrumented strength examination includes isometric, isotonic, and isokinetic tests. Isometric strength examination measures a muscle's maximal potential to produce a static force against an immovable resistance, isotonic strength examination measures potential to lift a fixed amount of weight through a ROM, and isokinetic strength examination measures capacity to accelerate the limb and generate torque at a fixed angular velocity. Each mode has advantages and disadvantages that determine which test is most appropriate for each injury.

5. Become familiar with the instruments used for objective isometric strength examination.

   Instruments include grip and pinch dynamometers, handheld dynamometers, and cable tensiometers. Grip and pinch dynamometers measure the strength and endurance of gross and fine motor grips. Handheld dynamometers are equipped with a small internal load cell capable of measuring compressive or pushing force during isometric contractions. Handheld dynamometers can be used to enhance the quantification of muscle strength during manual isometric muscle testing (e.g., break tests). Cable tensiometers use a strain gauge to measure the applied tension or pulling force of a muscle. The measurement gauge on these instruments often consists of a dial that provides real-time force and an indicator that remains at the peak force recorded until manually reset by the examiner.

6. Perform an isotonic strength examination using a repetition maximum test.

Isotonic strength is commonly determined by testing the maximum amount of weight a muscle can move through a joint's ROM for a set number of repetitions, usually either 1 (1RM) or 10 (10RM). Because the 1RM is a true maximal strength test, it is not used to examine injured athletes. You should perform a 10RM test on an athlete who is recovering from a previous injury, is untrained, or has no experience with a 1RM test. Begin with a weight lighter than the maximum the athlete can lift and gradually approach the predicted maximum. When an athlete exceeds the set number of repetitions on an attempt, have him lift an incrementally higher weight after resting the appropriate amount. The test is completed and maximum strength determined when the athlete lifts the weight exactly the desired number of repetitions. To obtain accurate results, the athlete must begin with a proper warm-up, maintain correct form, receive sufficient rest between attempts, and be familiar with the task.

7. Describe the role of isokinetic testing in athletic injury examination, and the type of measures computerized isokinetic dynamometry provides.

Isokinetic strength examination may be a safer alternative for testing an injured athlete in that the resistance of the dynamometer immediately disengages when the athlete experiences any pain or discomfort during the test. The primary advantage of isokinetic strength testing is that it examines the muscle's maximal capabilities throughout the entire ROM. Because there is no fixed resistance to move through the weakest point in an arc of motion (as with isotonic strength testing), isokinetic testing records the maximum voluntary force generated at any given angle in the ROM. The values that can be derived from the isokinetic torque curve include peak and average torque, peak and average force, work, power, endurance, torque to body weight normalization, and reciprocal muscle group ratios.

REVIEW QUESTIONS

1. What is the difference between torque and force?

2. On a manual break test, what would a strong and painful result likely indicate?

3. When performing a MMT for knee extension strength, the athlete is unable to lift the limb against your maximal resistance, but is able to complete most of the range with moderate resistance. How would you grade this test?

4. What are the key factors for obtaining an accurate grip strength test?

5. What are the advantages and disadvantages of isotonic strength examination for injured athletes?

6. Describe the features of a typical isokinetic torque curve. What factors (both human and instrumental) can alter the torque curve?

7. What is the difference between peak torque, average torque, and angle-specific torque?

8. What is the overshoot phenomenon in isokinetic testing? How can you control overshoot?

CRITICAL THINKING QUESTIONS

1. A pitcher comes to you complaining of weakness and fatigue during repetitive throwing. Your evaluation reveals no evidence of injury, and MMT does not reveal any gross deficits. You decide to perform an instrumented strength examination. What types of strength examination would you use, and what muscle groups would you test? Based on the athlete's sport, how would you interpret your findings when comparing his uninvolved side?

2. Consider the opening scenario. Let's assume Amy has access to the following strength testing equipment:

   a. Full line of isotonic strength equipment (free weights and machines) in the corporate gym

   b. Cable tensiometer

   c. Isokinetic dynamometer

   What strength examinations should Amy perform knowing she has to test 50 employees? How would she determine if an employee's strength profile is adequate for their job's demands?

3. You are the head athletic trainer at a local high school and a freshman arrives with a history of previous injury to the anterior cruciate ligament, which was reconstructed one year ago. She has provided a note from her physician indicating that she is fully recovered and cleared for participation. As part of your preseason testing, you feel it is important to do a full strength examination of her lower extremities. What instrumented tests would you use and why? What would be the benefits or disadvantages of a multijoint strength examination compared to isolated muscle group examination? What important comparisons would you make to determine the strength recovery on the injured side?

4. You are the new head athletic trainer at a university. The athletic director has informed you that the previous athletic trainer was pushing for the department to purchase an isokinetic strength testing system and asks for your opinion. You realize that isokinetic units are costly and you will need a strong justification for this purchase. Based on what you have learned about the advantages and disadvantages of isokinetic dynamometry, how would you justify its purchase to the athletic director?

CITED REFERENCES

Basmajian, J.V., and C.J. DeLuca. 1985. *Muscles alive: Their functions revealed by electromyography*. Baltimore: Williams & Wilkins.

Bohannon, R.W., and J.B. Wikholm. 1992. Measurements of knee extension force obtained by two examiners of substantially different experience with handheld dynamometer. *Isokinet Exerc Sci* 2(1): 5-8.

Clark, H.H. 1948. Objective strength tests of affected muscle groups involved with orthopedic disabilities. *Res Q* 19: 118-147.

Clarkson, H.M. 2000. *Musculoskeletal assessment: Joint range of motion and manual muscle strength*. 2nd ed. Philadelphia: Lippincott Williams & Wilkins.

Daniels, L., and C.A. Worthingham. 1980. *Muscle testing*. 4th ed. London: W.B. Saunders.

Enoka, R.M. 2002. *Neuromechanical basis of kinesiology*. 3rd ed. Champaign, IL: Human Kinetics.

Fleck, S.J., and W.J. Kraemer. 2004. *Designing resistance training programs*. 3rd ed. Champaign, IL: Human Kinetics.

Kisner, C., and L.A. Colby. 2002. *Therapeutic exercise: Foundation and techniques*. 4th ed. Philadephia: F.A. Davis.

Lamb, R., and D. Hobart. 1992. Anatomic and physiologic basis for surface electromyography. In *Selected topics in surface electromyography for use in the occupational setting: Expert perspectives*, ed. G.L. Soderberg.

Cincinnati: National Institute for Occupational Safety and Health. NIOSH Publication No. 91-100: 5-22.

Medical Research Council. 1943. *Aids to the investigation of peripheral nerve injuries.* 2nd ed. rev. London: H.M.S.O.

Perrin, D.H. 1986. Reliability of isokinetic measures. *J Athl Train* 10:319-321.

Perrin, D.H., R.J. Robertson, and R.L. Ray. 1987. Bilateral isokinetic peak torque, torque acceleration energy, power, and work relationships in athletes and nonathletes. *J Orthop Sports Phys Ther* 9: 184-189.

Semenick, D.M. 1994. Testing protocols and procedures. In *Essentials of strength and conditioning.* Eds. T.R. Baechle and R.W. Earle. Champaign, IL: Human Kinetics.

Wathen, D. 1994. Load assignment. In *Essentials of strength and conditioning.* Eds. T.R. Baechle and R.W. Earle. Champaign, IL: Human Kinetics.

ADDITIONAL RESOURCES

Portions of this chapter were adopted from Perrin, D.H. 1993. *Isokinetic exercise and assessment.* Champaign, IL: Human Kinetics.

Houglum, P.A. 2005. *Therapeutic exercise for injured athletes.* 2nd ed. Champaign, IL: Human Kinetics.

Kendall, F.P., E.K. McCreary, and P.G. Provance. 1993. *Muscles: Testing and function.* 4th ed. Philadelphia: Lippincott Williams & Wilkins.

National Strength and Conditioning Association (NSCA). 1994. *Essentials of strength and conditioning.* Eds. T.R. Baechle and R.W. Earle. Champaign, IL: Human Kinetics.

Examination of Neurological Status

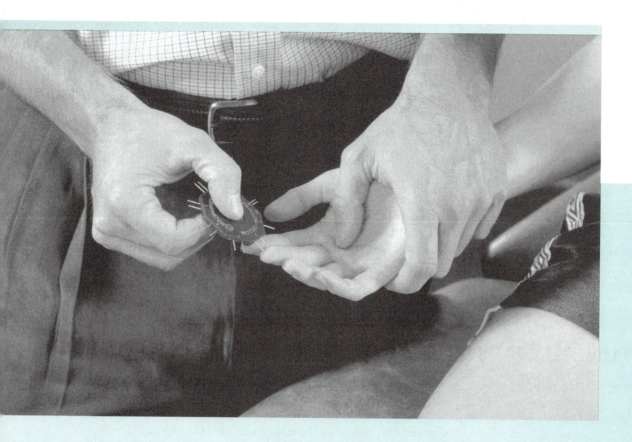

Objectives

After completing this chapter, the reader will be able to do the following:

1. Define the structures that comprise the central and peripheral nervous systems

2. Describe the function of a nerve plexus and its clinical implications for neurological examination

3. Identify the signs and symptoms for neurological testing and what differentiates an upper motor neuron lesion from a lower motor neuron lesion

4. Define sensory nerve function and how it is examined and interpreted

5. Define motor nerve function and how it is examined and interpreted

6. Differentiate among deep, superficial, and pathological reflexes and how each is examined

7. Identify the primary branches of the cervical and brachial plexuses and perform the appropriate sensory, motor, and reflex tests for each nerve root and peripheral nerve

8. Identify the primary branches of the lumbar and sacral plexuses and perform the appropriate sensory, motor, and reflex tests for each nerve root and peripheral nerve

9. Perform and interpret general neurological screening exams for suspected injuries to the head and upper and lower extremities

T akisha, a field hockey player, sought out Lance Smith, ATC, in the athletic training room to tell him about back and leg pain she experienced after a heavy lifting session. When Lance asked Takisha to describe the problem, she told him, "Lance, my back is killing me! It all started when I was completing my last set of squats. As I was lifting the weight, someone yelled at me from behind and it kind of startled me and I think I turned around part way to look. My back really hurt initially, then the pain eased up some, but then later in the evening and all day yesterday, I started having back spasms and my left leg and hip started hurting. Even when I lie down and try to take the weight off my legs, it still hurts."

"Can you pinpoint or describe the leg pain?" Lance asked.

Takisha thought for a moment before responding, "It's a little hard to describe. I can't really pinpoint the pain to any one location. It just seems to run down the inside of my leg. The pain is sort of dull and tingling and at times it burns a little bit. For some reason, I'm having a little trouble walking, too."

Lance recognized these signs and symptoms as neurological and was concerned that her back injury was irritating one or more of the spinal nerve roots. He decided to perform a full neurological examination.

Neurological tests examine the integrity of the central and peripheral nervous systems. Because neurological compromise can have serious and even life-threatening consequences, it is crucial to determine if the nerve structures are intact and functioning normally following an injury. This chapter addresses neuroanatomy; principles of neurological examination; and specific sensory, motor, and reflex tests for examining spinal and peripheral nerve integrity in the upper and lower extremities. This chapter also describes neurological tests that apply to multiple regions in the upper and lower extremities. However, specific neurological tests for the brain and thoracic spine are covered in chapters 19 (Head and Face) and 20 (Thorax and Abdomen).

FUNCTIONAL NEUROANATOMY

The nervous system enables the body to continuously adjust to its internal and external environments. The nervous system is divided into central and peripheral systems. The **central nervous system** includes the brain and spinal cord. The **peripheral nervous system** consists of all other neural structures, including the cranial nerves arising from the brain and the cervical, thoracic, and lumbosacral spinal nerve roots arising from the spinal cord via a ventral root containing motor (efferent) nerve fibers and a dorsal root containing sensory (afferent) nerve fibers (Moore 1992). These spinal nerves then split into two braches (rami): The dorsal rami run posteriorly and supply nerves to the skin and extensor muscles of the neck and trunk while the ventral rami supply nerves to the limbs and anteriolateral regions of the trunk (Kendall 1983; Moore 1992). Chapter 7 (page 97) reviews the functional anatomy of peripheral nerves.

Nerve Plexuses

The ventral rami branches at the neck, shoulder, lumbar, and sacral regions to form the cervical, brachial, lumbar, and sacral plexuses. A **nerve plexus** interconnects multiple spinal nerves through a series of uniting, dividing, reuniting, and intertwining offshoots that ultimately mixes peripheral nerves that emerge from the plexus as terminal branches (Kendall 1983). In some cases, this nerve network may result in a single peripheral nerve being supplied by as many as five spinal nerves. Table 8.1 identifies the spinal nerves that form the cervical, brachial, lumbar, and sacral plexuses and their primary peripheral branches. Consult an anatomy text to review the anatomical orientation and innervations for each

Table 8.1
Nerves of the Cervical, Brachial, Lumbar, and Sacral Plexus

Plexus	Spinal nerve root	Peripheral nerve branches
Cervical	C1	Lesser occipital (C2, sometimes C3)
	C2	Greater auricular (C2, C3)
	C3	Transverse cervical (C2, C3)
	C4	Supraclavicular (C3, C4)
		Phrenic (C3-C5)
Brachial	C5	Dorsal scapular (ventral rami of C5, sometimes C4)
	C6	Long thoracic (ventral rami C5-C7)
	C7	Subclavius (superior trunk, C5, sometimes C4, C6)
	C8	Suprascapular (superior trunk, C5, C6, sometimes C4)
	T1	Lateral pectoral (anterior division of C5-C7)
		Medial pectoral (medial cord, C8, T1)
		Medial brachial cutaneous (cutaneous nerve of the arm) (medial cord, C8, T1)
		Medial antebrachial cutaneous (cutaneous nerve of the forearm) (medial cord, C8, T1)
		Upper subscapular (posterior cord, C5, C6)
		Thoracodorsal (posterior cord, C6-C8)
		Lower subscapular (posterior cord, C5, C6)
		Musculocutaneous (terminal branch of lateral cord, C5-C7)
		Median (terminal branch of the lateral and medial cords, C5-C7, C8, T1)
		Ulnar (terminal branch of the medial cord, C8, T1, sometimes C7)
		Axillary (terminal branch of the posterior cord, C5, C6)
		Radial (terminal branch of the posterior cord, C5-C8, T1)
Lumbar	T12	Ilioinguinal and iliohypogastic (L1)
	L1	Femoral (L2-L4)
	L2	Obturator (L2-L4)
	L3	Genitofemoral (L1, L2)
	L4	Lateral femoral cutaneous (dorsal branches, ventral rami L2, L3)
Sacral	L4*	Common peroneal (posterior divisions, L4-S2)**
	L5*	Tibial (anterior divisions, L4-S3)**
	S1	Pudendal (S2-S4)
	S2	Superior gluteal (dorsal divisions, L4-S1)
	S3	

* Comprise the lumbosacral trunk (L4, L5; joins the lumbar and sacral plexus).
** Represent the anterior and posterior divisions of the *sciatic nerve* (L4-S3).

of these plexuses. This chapter discusses the functional anatomy, the sensory and motor innervations, as well as the neurological examination procedures for each spinal plexus and its peripheral branches.

GENERAL PRINCIPLES OF THE NEUROLOGICAL EXAM

You will perform a series of sensory, motor, and reflex tests to determine the integrity of the nerves you suspect may be injured. Before discussing specific neurological tests, the following sections describe the goals of the neurological exam; the principles of sensory, motor, and reflex testing; and how to interpret your findings.

Goal and Purpose

The goal of the neurological examination is to rule out any brain, spinal, or peripheral nerve pathology. Neurological conditions are typically divided into upper and lower motor neuron lesions. **Upper motor neuron lesions** are injury to the corticospinal or pyramidal tracks in the brain or spinal cord. Signs and symptoms associated with an upper motor neuron lesion include hemiplegia, paraplegia, and quadriplegia, depending on the location and extent of injury. Other signs and symptoms are spasticity, loss of voluntary control, sensory loss, and abnormal superficial and pathological reflexes. **Lower motor neuron lesions** are injury to nerve structures in the anterior horn of the spinal cord and in the spinal and peripheral nerves. Complete transection of the nerve results in total paralysis. Partial transection results in varying symptoms and levels of dysfunction, depending on the nerves involved. Signs and symptoms of lower motor neuron lesions include decreased muscle tone, sensory loss, progressive muscle atrophy, and diminished or absent spinal reflexes. Superficial and pathological reflexes are not affected.

Perform a neurological exam if you suspect a nerve injury and the athlete's symptoms include sensory changes (radiation of numbness, tingling, shooting pain, deep pain, or burning pain), weakness, or paralysis. Radiating, or referred, symptoms can result from pathology in the spinal cord, nerve roots, or peripheral nerves secondary to disc herniations, fractures, or dislocations; impingement or compression syndromes; nerve tensioning or stretch; or other nerve trauma. Neurological symptoms vary with the level of injury. Whereas unilateral symptoms indicate a nerve root or peripheral nerve lesion (lower motor neuron), bilateral symptoms often result from central cord or brain pathology (upper motor neuron).

Referred symptoms are experienced away from the site of injury.

The symptoms differ for nerve root and peripheral nerve injuries. Because nerve roots from the cervical and lumbar spine send branches to more than one peripheral nerve, the symptom profile is more diffuse with a nerve root lesion than with a peripheral nerve lesion. For example, the C7 nerve root has branches that innervate the ulnar, median, and radial nerves, so an injury to the C7 nerve root could cause symptoms affecting all three peripheral nerves. On the other hand, an injury to the radial nerve, a peripheral nerve, affects primarily the posterolateral hand.

Sensory Function Testing

Sensory nerves receive information from the peripheral environment and within the body and forward this information to the central nervous system in order to regulate the body's functions. The sensory modalities include vision, hearing, taste, smell, and touch. Sensory perceptions arise from a variety of afferent receptors located in the skin that relay information to the central nervous system (table 8.2). These receptors are specific to mechanical (light touch, pressure, vibration), thermal (temperature), chemical (chemical irritants), and noxious (pain) stimuli.

The patient's sense of touch is typically examined during neurological examination, because this sense reveals the integrity of specific nerves and is more easily stimulated without hurting the athlete. The sense of touch can be examined by direct touch over a specific nerve

Table 8.2
Sensory Receptor Types and Functions

Receptor	Function
Mechanoreceptors	Sense mechanical deformation of the skin surface (light touch, pressure, stretch, vibration)
Thermoreceptors	Sense heat or cold
Nociceptors	Sense pain from damaging chemical, mechanical, and thermal stimuli
Chemoreceptors	Sense chemical irritants that effect cellular metabolism

distribution (**primary sensation**), by asking the patient to identify a particular structure or texture by feeling the object with the eyes closed (**cortical sensation**), or by differentiating stimuli between two or more distinct points (**sensory discrimination**). This chapter focuses on primary sensation, or the perception of light touch, for examining the neurological integrity of specific nerves.

To perform the sensory test for light touch, run your fingertips lightly over the athlete's skin. Abnormal responses to light touch include the inability to feel anything (**anesthesia**), a different response compared to the response of the uninjured side (**paresthesia**), a hypersensitivity or irritability upon touch (**hyperesthesia**), and sensation in a different area (**referred**). Make bilateral comparisons whenever possible and ask the athlete to close her eyes or position her so she cannot see when or where you perform the test.

Sensory tests examine the integrity of afferent nerves and show when the sensory signal from the periphery is received and processed centrally. The sensory test serves as a scanning technique for quickly examining sensation. If the athlete reports any abnormal response (unusual sensation, different sensation when compared bilaterally to the uninjured side), perform a more detailed examination over a specific nerve root distribution. Ask the athlete if he feels anything and if so, what he feels and how it compares to the sensation he felt on the opposite side. If you are not sure the athlete has correctly perceived the light touch, you should ask him if he feels anything when in fact you are not touching him. If the athlete's response is unclear, repeat the test over the questionable area.

If the sensory test is positive, perform other sensory tests examining deep pressure or pain over the appropriate nerve distributions. Test superficial pain with a pinprick or pinwheel and then deep pressure pain by applying firm, noxious pressure over a larger area, such as squeezing the trapezius muscle, pinching the soft tissue in the webs between the hand's digits, or rubbing the sternum. Test temperature perception by placing hot and cold objects against the skin, and test vibration by touching a tuning fork to a bony prominence and questioning the athlete about her perception of vibration. Test proprioception by moving the athlete's joint and asking her to indicate the direction of movement or the new position of the limb. If tools for these examinations are not available on-site, wait until the athlete is removed to the athletic training facility. A positive sign on any sensory test indicates a possible neurological injury and you should refer the athlete to a physician for further examination.

Proprioception is the patient's awareness of the position or movement of her body or body segment.

Motor Function Testing

Because muscles communicate with the central nervous system through peripheral nerves, neurological motor tests are performed the same way as the manual muscle tests for strength examination described in chapter 7. As neurological motor tests, they are used to identify the injured peripheral nerve or nerve root instead of testing muscle and joint function. For example, if you suspect an athlete has a rotator cuff strain, you will use a manual muscle test to examine the strength of the rotator cuff muscles, but if she has suffered a cervical injury that has damaged the C6 and C7 nerve roots, you will use the manual muscle tests to identify which muscles have been affected. Sections later in this chapter discuss specific motor tests for the upper and lower extremities. When performing motor testing, it is good practice to first check if the athlete is able to actively move the injured segment before you apply manual resistance.

Reflex Testing

A **reflex** is an involuntary response to a stimulus that requires an intact pathway between the stimulation point and the responding organ (i.e., muscle). Testing a reflex examines the sensory and motor pathways of a nerve. Reflexes are specific to the stimulated area and are predictable. Observe for any abnormal response that could indicate neurological dysfunction. You may perform deep tendon, superficial, and pathological reflex tests to examine integrity of neural pathways.

Deep Tendon Reflexes

Muscle spindles are specialized muscle fibers arranged parallel to the contractile (extrafusal) muscle fibers. They sense changes in muscle tension and length and control muscle tone.

Deep tendon reflexes are caused by stimulation of an intact musculotendinous unit deep beneath the skin. Deep tendon reflexes are tested to examine lower motor neuron (distal to the spinal cord) lesions. In their simplest form, deep tendon reflexes are **monosynaptic reflex arcs**, meaning they are composed of one afferent neuron that is stimulated by its sensory receptor and directly synapses with an alpha motor neuron, resulting in muscular excitation or inhibition (Eccles 1981; Enoka 1994; Kandel, Schwartz, and Jessell 1995). This type of reflex, also called the M1 response, spinal reflex, or short loop reflex, originates at the spinal cord and is generated by a local stimulus (e.g., tendon tap), resulting in a gross, quick movement that requires no cortical input. Other reflexes receive input from higher brain centers and may involve one or more interneurons that mediate the reflex response. These reflexes have a longer latency and are called M2, intermediate, **long latency**, or long loop reflexes.

The knee-jerk reflex, or patellar tendon tap, is a well-known example of a monosynaptic, deep tendon reflex examination and is illustrated in figure 8.1. When the patellar tendon receives a brisk tap from a reflex hammer, the tendon and the quadriceps quickly stretch. As the quadriceps stretch, sensory receptors within the muscle spindle relay this information to the central nervous system via sensory (afferent) neurons. Once the spinal cord receives this sensory stimulus, within 20 to 30 milliseconds it directly synapses with the motor neurons that innervate the quadriceps, causing a brief but rapid contraction. The sensory neurons also synapse indirectly with motor neurons innervating the antagonist (opposing) muscles, in this case the hamstrings, to inhibit their contraction.

Deep tendon reflexes are graded on a scale of 0 to 4 (table 8.3). Use a reflex hammer to provide a brisk,

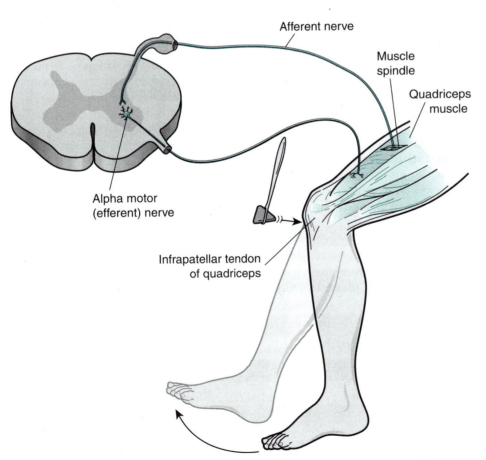

Figure 8.1 Neural pathway of the knee-jerk reflex.

light tap to a slightly stretched tendon. Perform 3 to 5 taps to examine the reflex for nerve root involvement. If you have difficulty eliciting a reflex response, have the athlete isometrically pull apart crossed ankles (when testing for an upper-extremity response) or clasped hands (when testing for a lower-extremity response) (figure 8.2). This technique, called Jendrassik's maneuver, increases the nervous system's sensitivity to improve deep tendon reflex response. Because this technique can mediate the strength of the reflex, you must use it consistently on comparative and repeat testing.

Because deep tendon reflexes primarily identify lower motor neuron lesions (spinal or peripheral nerve injury), diminished or absent reflex responses are most common. However, deep tendon reflexes may also produce evidence of upper motor neuron lesions. In the case of a central nerve injury (upper motor neuron lesion), the tendon tap will produce a clonus, an exaggerated reflex. Exaggerated reflexes should be further examined using superficial and pathological reflexes specific to upper motor neuron lesions. This issue is discussed in the sections on superficial and pathological reflexes (see page 125).

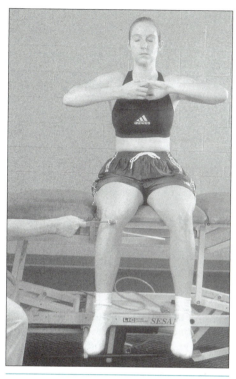

Figure 8.2 Jendrassik's manuever.

Test deep tendon reflexes to confirm suspected nerve injuries but do not use these tests alone for neurological examination because many variables influence their results. Although deep tendon reflexes are automatic involuntary responses, they can be influenced in either an inhibitory or excitatory fashion. For example, older and younger athletes may demonstrate less reflex activity, and reflexes may become hyperactive when a patient exercises. Some athletes simply have normally diminished or excessive reflexes.

Pain, previous or anticipated events, motivation, and central fatigue can also modulate the strength of the spinal stretch reflex (Kandel, Schwartz, and Jessell 1995; Taylor et al. 1996). An increase in muscle spindle discharge that increases excitatory input to the motor neuron pool can occur after a brief bout of intense activity as long as the muscle is not appreciably stretched (Enoka 1994; Nelson and Hutton 1985). Accumulation of chemical byproducts of anaerobic fatiguing exercise can also influence sensory feedback from the muscle, changing motor neuron excitation and force output (Duchateau and Hainaut 1993; Hakkinen 1994, Johansson, Djupsojobacka, and Sjolander 1993). Keep these factors in mind and test the patient's reflexes bilaterally, comparing the injured and uninjured sides.

Table 8.3
Reflex Grading Scale

Grade	Interpretation	Indication
0	Absent reflex	Complete loss of neuromuscular integrity (injury to a nerve root or peripheral nerve)
+1	Diminished reflex	Reduced neurological function (incomplete injury to a nerve root or peripheral nerve)
+2	Normal reflex	Normal neurological integrity and function
+3	Exaggerated reflex	Upper motor neuron lesion (brain or spinal cord injury); hypersensitivity may also occur following brief, intense bouts of activity
+4	Clonus	Upper motor neuron lesion

Technically, testing any tendon could elicit a deep tendon reflex, but only a few tendons are commonly used (see table 8.4).

Superficial Reflexes

Superficial reflexes are cutaneous reflexes elicited by stimulating the skin over areas where the central nervous system (spinal cord) mediates movement. Examine superficial reflexes to check for upper motor neuron lesions by lightly stroking the skin with a fairly pointed object, such as the sharp end of a reflex hammer. The absence of a superficial reflex indicates an upper motor neuron lesion and becomes more significant when hyperreflexia (exaggerated reflex) is noted with the corresponding deep tendon reflex.

Table 8.4 lists the commonly examined superficial reflexes. Although not often used to examine peripheral nerve injury, reflexes that produce a unilateral response may further confirm spinal cord pathology.

Pathological Reflexes

Pathological reflexes are abnormal reflexes specific to particular diseases. Because the central nervous system mediates pathological reflexes, they are similar to superficial reflexes. However, contrary to superficial reflexes, absence of a pathological reflex is normal while presence indicates disease or injury caused by an upper motor neuron lesion. For instance, a **clonus test** determines whether the central nervous system is functioning properly. To perform a clonus test, abruptly stretch a muscle and observe the response. A normal response is no reflex or a simple stretch reflex. A damaged central nervous system, however, produces a hyperactive stretch reflex characterized by rhythmic muscle contractions. The clonus test is usually performed at the ankle (sudden, forceful dorsiflexion stretch) (see figure 8.5), knee (sudden, forceful downward thrust on the patella), or the wrist (sudden, forceful extension of the wrist), depending on the location of the suspected lesion. Table 8.4 lists these and other pathological reflexes you should be familiar with. While a pathological reflex that occurs on only one side may also indicate a lower motor neuron lesion, these tests are typically performed bilaterally to determine the presence of brain injury.

REGION-SPECIFIC NEUROLOGICAL EXAMINATION

To effectively evaluate the neurological status of a particular body region, you must understand the sensory and motor innervations for each spinal nerve and peripheral nerve branch associated with a particular nerve plexus. This section focuses on dermatome, myotome, and reflex tests for each plexus and its peripheral nerves, providing an examination checklist for the upper and lower quarters (extremities). Later in this text you will learn neurological examinations for specific body regions, but if you master the general principles and tests for each plexus, you can easily apply the more specific tests. We will defer discussion of neurological examination procedures for the head and the abdominal area to the chapters that cover those regions (see chapters 19 and 20).

To evaluate afferent (sensory) nerve function, perform sensory testing with light touch over specific **dermatomes**, areas of the skin supplied by a particular spinal nerve. To evaluate efferent (motor) nerve function, perform manual muscle tests against **myotomes**, groups of muscles innervated by a single spinal segment. Knowing the sensory and motor distributions of the peripheral nerves will help you more accurately examine the integrity of nerves at a location distal to an upper- or lower-extremity injury. The following sections describe the specific sensory, motor, and reflex tests for each plexus and the primary peripheral nerve branches for the upper and lower extremities. The sensory and motor distributions of spinal and peripheral nerves can vary considerably from person to person, and at times the distributions of adjacent nerves may overlap. For this reason this chapter presents the locations considered to provide the most pure examination for each nerve, but these locations are not absolute.

Table 8.4

Deep Tendon, Superficial, and Pathological Reflexes

Reflex	Neural segment	Stimulus and response
Deep tendon		
Achilles	S1	Plantar flexion upon striking the tendon (normal)
Biceps	**C5**, C6	Elbow flexion upon striking the tendon (normal)
Brachioradialis	C5, **C6**	Radial deviation upon striking the tendon (normal)
Jaw	Cranial V	Mouth closes upon striking anterior chin (normal) Exaggerated (UMNL)
Medial hamstring	**L5**, S1	Knee flexion upon striking the semimembranosis tendon (normal)
Lateral hamstring	**S1**, S2	Knee flexion upon striking the biceps femoris tendon (normal)
Patellar	L2, L3, **L4**	Knee extension upon striking the infrapatellar tendon (normal)
Tibialis posterior	L4, **L5**	Plantar flexion and inversion upon striking the tibialis posterior just behind the medial malleolus (normal)
Triceps	C7	Elbow extension upon striking the triceps tendon (normal)
Superficial		
Abdominal Upper Lower	 T7-T10 T10-L1	Movement of the umbilicus toward the area being stroked (normal); if unilateral, pinpointing the involved quadrant indicates the approximate level of lesion
Anal	S2-S4	Anal sphincter contracts with touching or stroking the perianal skin (normal)
Cremasteric	T12, L1, L2	Scrotum contracts and testicle retracts with stroking the skin on the anterior, inner thigh (normal); unilateral absence indicates LMNL injury at L1, L2; bilateral absence indicates UMNL
Gluteal	L4, L5 S1-S3	Gluteal muscles contract with stroking the overlying skin (normal).
Lumbar	T12-L5	Back extensor muscles contract with stroking the skin overlying the erector spinae muscles (normal)
Plantar	S1, S2	Toes flex with lightly stroking the plantar surface of the foot (normal)
Pathological		
Clonus	UMNL	Antagonist and agonist muscle groups rapidly alternate involuntary contraction and relaxation with a sudden, forced stretch of a muscle (pathological); usually performed at the wrist (extension), ankle (dorsiflexion), or knee (downward force on the patella to stretch the quadriceps)
Babinski	UMNL (Pyramidal Tract)	Great toes extend and other toes splay (extend and abduct) with stroking the lateral plantar surface and across the sole foot (pathological)
Chaddock		Great toes extend and other toes splay with stroking the side of the foot distal to the lateral malleolus (pathological)
Gordon		Great toes extend and other toes splay with compressing or squeezing the calf muscle (pathological)
Oppenheim		Great toes extend and other toes splay with stroking downward on the anteriomedial tibial surface (pathological)

LMNL = lower motor neuron lesion, UMNL = upper motor neuron lesion.

Cervical Plexus

Table 8.5 shows dermatome, myotome, and reflex distributions for spinal and peripheral nerves arising from the **cervical plexus**, the primary sensory supply to the neck and scalp and the primary motor supply to the neck musculature and the diaphragm. Examine the cervical plexus whenever you suspect injury to the upper cervical spine region.

Functional Anatomy

The cervical plexus is formed by spinal nerves arising from the ventral rami of C1 through C4 as well as a few nerves from C5. Cutaneous branches arise from C2 to C4 to supply the skin of the neck and scalp. Motor branches supply the anterior and lateral muscles of the neck. The **phrenic nerve** that arises from C3 through C5 is crucial. Because it is the only motor nerve supplying the diaphragm, injury to the upper cervical region that causes paralysis also affects breathing.

Dermatomes

Test dermatomes by lightly touching the skin covering the top of the head (C1), the temporal and occipital regions (C2), the posterior cheek and lateral neck (C3), and the top of the shoulder (C4) (figure 8.3). Test each dermatome bilaterally for equal sensation and any abnormal sensation such as shooting pain, numbness, tingling, or hypersensitivity.

Myotomes

Check myotomes by performing active and resistive manual muscle tests of the neck musculature. Place the muscle at midlength and instruct the athlete to work against your resistance. The C1 and C2 nerve root innervates the neck flexor muscles (figure 8.4a), C3 innervates the lateral cervical flexors (figure 8.4b), and C4 innervates the muscles that shrug the shoulders (figure 8.4c).

Table 8.5
Sensory, Motor, and Reflex Distributions for the Cervical Plexus

Nerve root	Dermatome	Myotome	Reflex
C1	Top of head	(Cervical flexion)	None
C2	Temporal, occipital regions of the head	Cervical flexion (longus colli, sternocleido-mastoid, rectus capitus)	None
C3	Posterior cheek, neck	Lateral neck flexion (trapezius, splenus capitis)	None
C4	Superior shoulder, clavicle area	Shoulder shrug (trapezius, levator scapulae)	None

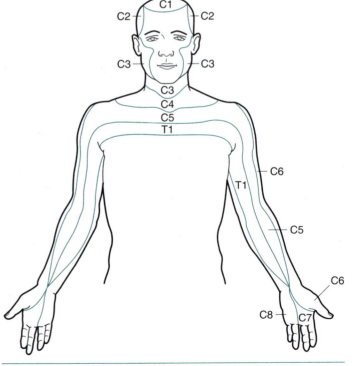

Figure 8.3 Sensory distribution for the cervical spine and the brachial plexus (C1-T1).

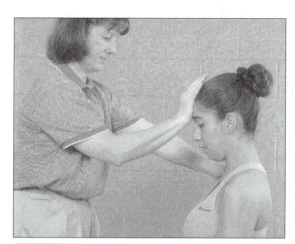
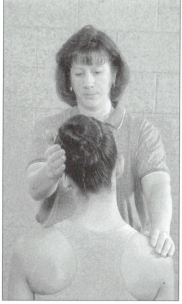
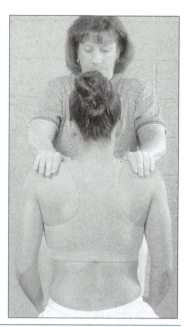

Figure 8.4 Myotome examination for *(a)* neck flexion, *(b)* lateral neck flexion, and *(c)* shoulder shrugging.

Reflexes

There are no deep tendon reflexes for the cervical plexus. To test for upper motor neuron lesions, perform a clonus test bilaterally (figure 8.5). This is done by applying a sudden stretch to a muscle and observing the reflex response. A normal response produces either no reflex, or at best, a simple stretch reflex. With damage to the central nervous system however, a hyperactive stretch reflex occurs, characterized by repetitive, rhythmic contractions of the muscle.

Brachial Plexus

Table 8.6 shows sensory, motor, and reflex distributions for spinal nerves and primary terminal branches of the **brachial plexus**, the primary neural supply to the upper extremities. You will need to know this distribution in order to select appropriate neurological tests when examining injuries to the lower cervical

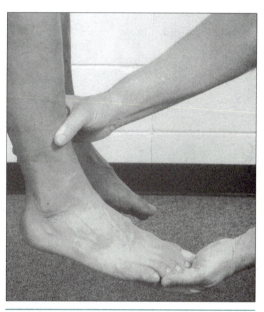

Figure 8.5 Clonus test for upper motor neuron lesion.

spine, shoulder girdle, and upper extremities. Depending on the level of injury, the appropriate tests will either focus on the spinal nerves or their terminal branches.

Functional Anatomy

The brachial plexus begins in the cervical region. It exits the spinal column just lateral to the anterior scalene muscle and courses through the axilla into the upper extremities. The brachial plexus is formed by a series of spinal rami (roots), trunks, divisions, cords, and terminal branches (figure 8.6). Cervical spinal nerves C5 and C6 form the upper (superior) trunk, C7 forms the middle trunk, and C8 and the thoracic spinal nerve T1 form the lower (inferior)

Table 8.6
Sensory, Motor, and Reflex Distributions for the Brachial Plexus

Nerve root/nerve	Dermatome	Myotome	Reflex
C5	Deltoid patch, lateral upper arm	Shoulder abduction (deltoid), elbow flexion (biceps)	Biceps (brachioradialis)
C6	Lateral forearm, radial side of hand, thumb, and index finger	Elbow flexion (biceps, supinator), wrist extension	Brachioradialis (biceps)
C7	Posterior lateral arm and forearm, middle finger	Elbow extension (triceps), wrist flexion	Triceps
C8	Medial forearm, ulnar border of hand, ring and little finger	Ulnar deviation, thumb extension, finger flexion and abduction	None
T1	Medial elbow, arm	Finger abduction (hand intrinsics)	None
Musculocutaneous (C5-C7)	Lateral forearm	Elbow flexion (biceps)	None
Median (C5-C7 and C8, T1)	Distal radial aspect, index finger	Thumb pinch, opposition, and abduction	None
Ulnar (C8, T1, some C7)	Distal ulnar side of 5th finger	Abduction, 5th finger (abductor digit minimi)	None
Axillary (C5, C6)	Lateral arm, deltoid patch	Shoulder abduction (deltoid)	None
Radial (C5-C8, T1)	Dorsal web space, between thumb and index fingers	Wrist extension, thumb extension	None

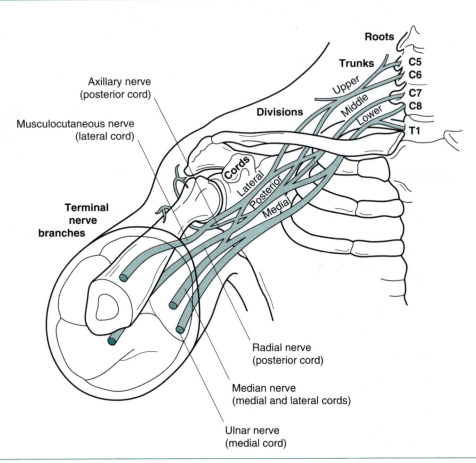

Figure 8.6   The brachial plexus nerve roots, trunks, divisions, cords, and terminal branches.

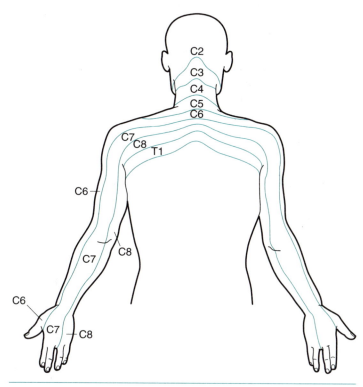

Figure 8.7   Dermatome distribution for the brachial plexus.

trunk. Each trunk divides into anterior and posterior divisions to form cords, which are named according to their relationship to the axillary artery. The anterior division of the upper and middle trunks (C5-C7) unite to form the lateral cord. The medial cord arises from the anterior division of the lower trunk (C8-T1), and the posterior cord is formed by the posterior divisions of the upper, middle, and lower trunks (C5-C8).

Two terminal branches arise from each of these cords. The lateral cord gives rise to the musculocutaneous nerve and the lateral contribution to the median nerve. The medial cord gives rise to the ulnar nerve and medial contribution to the median nerve. The posterior cord gives rise to the axillary and radial nerves. The brachial plexus also receives some communication from C4 and T2.

Dermatomes

Figures 8.7 and 8.8 map the typical sensory distribution for the upper extremity (see also figure 8.3). Note that the sensory distribution (dermatome) for a nerve root differs from that for a peripheral nerve. These sensory distribution zones may vary somewhat from one athlete to another.

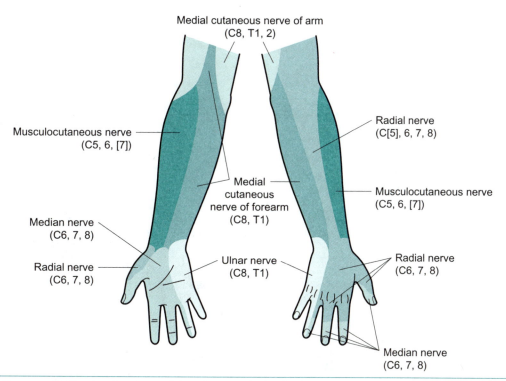

Figure 8.8   Sensory distribution for the peripheral nerves in the forearm and hand.

Perform sensory testing of spinal dermatomes for the brachial plexus with light touch over the mid-deltoid on the upper lateral (outer) arm (C5), the lateral forearm and radial side of the hand (C6), the middle finger (C7), the medial (inner) forearm and ulnar side of the hand (C8), and the medial side of the upper arm (T1). Sensory distributions for the terminal branches include the lateral forearm (musculocutaneous), dorsal web space and posterior forearm (radial), radial aspects of the second and third fingers (median), lateral border of the fifth finger (ulnar), medial forearm (medial cutaneous nerve of the forearm), medial upper arm (medial cutaneous nerve of the arm), and inferior portion of the deltoid and lateral arm (axillary).

Myotomes

Use muscle strength tests on muscles innervated by cervical spinal nerves C5 through T1 to examine myotomes. Use shoulder abduction to test C5 (figure 8.9a), elbow flexion and wrist extension to test C6 (figure 8.9b), elbow extension to test C7 (figure 8.9c), thumb extension to test C8 (figure 8.9d), and finger abduction to test T1 (figure 8.9e).

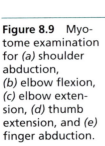

Figure 8.9 Myotome examination for *(a)* shoulder abduction, *(b)* elbow flexion, *(c)* elbow extension, *(d)* thumb extension, and *(e)* finger abduction.

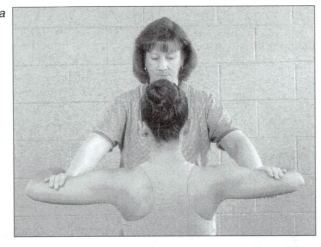

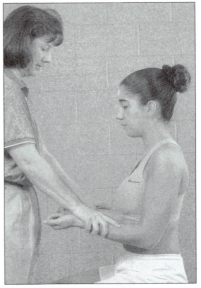

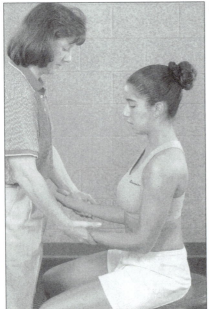

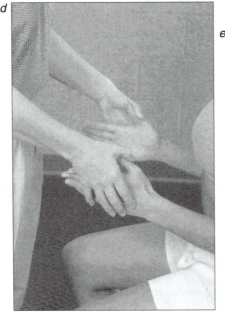

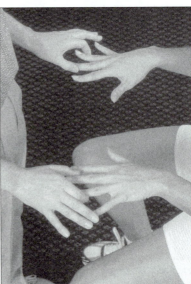

To examine motor function of the peripheral nerves, perform manual muscle testing for the median, ulnar, radial, and musculocutaneous nerves. Use thumb opposition and pinch strength to test the median nerve (figure 8.10a), abduction of the fifth finger to examine the ulnar nerve (figure 8.10b), and wrist or thumb extension to examine the radial nerve (figure 8.10c). The musculocutaneous nerve does not innervate muscle past the elbow, so use elbow flexion as the most distal examination for the integrity of this nerve.

Reflexes

Perform deep tendon reflexes over the biceps (figure 8.11a), brachioradialis (figure 8.11b), and triceps (figure 8.11c) tendons to examine spinal segments C5, C6, and C7, respectively. Apply a clonus test as described for the cervical plexus (see page 127) to the lower extremities to check for an upper motor neuron injury.

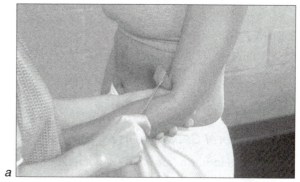

a

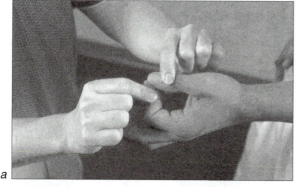

a

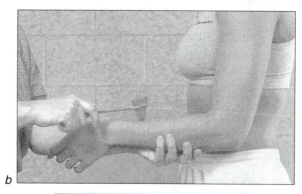

b

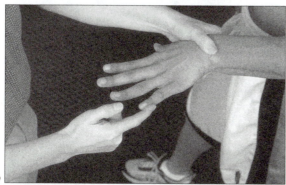

b

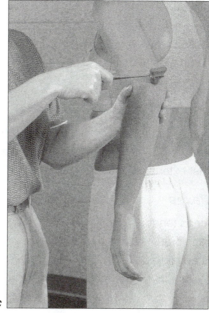

c

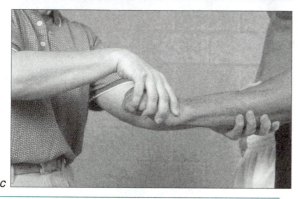

c

Figure 8.10 Motor testing of (a) thumb opposition (median nerve), (b) fifth finger abduction (ulnar nerve), and (c) wrist extension (radial nerve).

Figure 8.11 Deep tendon reflex examination of the (a) biceps, (b) brachioradialis, and (c) triceps tendons.

The following checklist is provided as a summary of the complete neurological screen for the cervical and brachial plexuses.

Checklist for Upper-Quarter Neurological Screen

▷ *Dermatomes*

- ☐ Top of head (C1)
- ☐ Temporal and occipital regions of scalp (C2)
- ☐ Posterior cheek (C3)
- ☐ Top of shoulder (C4)
- ☐ Mid-deltoid (C5)
- ☐ Lateral forearm and radial side of hand (C6)
- ☐ Middle finger (C7)
- ☐ Medial forearm and ulnar side of hand (C8)
- ☐ Medial side of arm (T1)

▷ *Peripheral Sensory Distributions*

- ☐ Lateral forearm (musculocutaneous)
- ☐ Dorsal web space of hand (radial)
- ☐ Radial aspect of 2nd and 3rd fingers (median)
- ☐ Lateral border of 5th finger (ulnar)
- ☐ Medial forearm (medial cutaneous nerve of the forearm)
- ☐ Medial arm (medial cutaneous nerve of the arm)
- ☐ Inferior deltoid and lateral arm (axillary)

▷ *Myotomes*

- ☐ Forward neck flexion (C1, C2)
- ☐ Lateral neck flexion (C3)
- ☐ Shoulder shrug (C4)
- ☐ Shoulder abduction (C5)
- ☐ Elbow flexion and wrist extension (C6)
- ☐ Elbow extension (C7)
- ☐ Thumb extension (C8)
- ☐ Finger abduction (T1)

▷ *Peripheral Motor Distributions*

- ☐ Thumb opposition and pinch strength (median nerve)
- ☐ Abduction of the 5th finger (ulnar nerve)
- ☐ Wrist extension and thumb extension (radial nerve)

▷ *Reflexes*

- ☐ Biceps tendon (C5)
- ☐ Brachioradialis tendon (C6)
- ☐ Triceps tendon (C7)
- ☐ Clonus test (upper motor neuron lesion)

Lumbar and Sacral Plexuses

Table 8.7 shows sensory, motor, and reflex distributions for spinal and peripheral nerves arising from the lumbar and sacral plexuses, the primary neural supplies to the pelvis, hip, and lower extremity. Subsequent chapters discussing the lumbar and lower extremity regions refer back to this table.

Table 8.7

Sensory, Motor, and Reflex Distributions for the Lumbar and Sacral Plexuses

Nerve root/nerve	Dermatome	Myotome	Reflex
L1	**Back, over greater trochanter and groin**	Hip flexion (psoas), iliacus, pectineus, sartorius	None
L2	Back, wrapping around to anterior superior thigh and **medial thigh above knee**	Hip flexion (psoas), hip adductors	(Patellar tendon)
L3	Back, upper gluteal, anterior thigh, **medial knee** and lower leg	Knee extension (quadriceps)	Patellar tendon
L4	Medial gluteals, lateral thigh and knee, **anterior medial lower leg,** dorsomedial aspect of foot and big toe	Ankle dorsiflexion and inversion (anterior tibialis)	Patellar tendon
L5	Lateral knee and upper **lateral lower leg, dorsum of foot**	Great toe extension (extensor hallucis)	Medial hamstring tendon
S1	Buttock, posterolateral thigh, **lateral side** and **plantar surface of the foot**	**Ankle plantar flexion** (gastrocnemius, soleus), **ankle eversion** (fibularis muscles), hip extension (gluteals), knee flexion (hamstrings)	Achilles tendon (lateral hamstring tendon)
S2	Buttock, posteriomedial thigh, posterior, medial heel	**Knee flexion** (hamstrings), great toe flexion (flexor hallucis longus)	(Lateral hamstring tendon)
Obturator (L2-L4)	None	Hip adduction (adductor brevis, magnus, longus, gracilis)	None
Femoral (L2-L4)	None	Knee extension (quadriceps, iliacus, pectineus, sartorius)	None
Superior gluteal (L4-S1)	None	Hip abduction (gluteus medius and minimus, tensor fascia)	None
Inferior gluteal (L5-S2)	None	Hip extension (gluteus maximus)	None

(continued)

Table 8.7
(continued)

Nerve root/nerve	Dermatome	Myotome	Reflex
Deep fibular (peroneal)	Dorsal web space, between 1st and 2nd digits	**Great toe extension** (extensor hallicus), toe extension (extensor digitorum longus and brevis) and dorsiflexion (tibialis anterior)	None
Superficial fibular (peroneal)	Lateral lower leg	Ankle eversion (fibularis longus and brevis)	None
Tibial (thigh)	None	Knee flexion (semintendinosis, semimembranosis, long head biceps femoris)	Hamstring
Tibial (lower leg)	Posterior heel, lateral aspect of ankle and foot (medial sural cutaneous nerve)	Ankle plantar flexion (gastroc, soleus)	Posterior tibialis
Medial plantar	Medial 3 digits	Great toe abduction (abductor hallicus), toe flexion with ankle plantar flexed (flexor hallicus and digitorum brevis)	None
Lateral plantar	5th digit and lateral side, 4th digit	Abduction, 5th digit (abductor digiti mini)	None

Bolded text indicates primary, purest test.

Functional Anatomy

The lumbar plexus is a network of nerves arising from the ventral rami of the first four levels of the lumbar spine, L1 through L4 (figure 8.12a). The most important branches of the lumbar plexus are the obturator and femoral nerves, which are supplied by L2 through L4. The obturator nerve supplies the adductor muscles of the thigh while the femoral nerve supplies the iliopsoas and knee extensors. A portion of L4 joins all of L5 to form the lumbosacral trunk, a large nerve that joins the sacral plexus and is considered separate from the lumbar plexus. The sacral plexus includes the lumbosacral trunk and the ventral rami of the S1 through S4 sacral spine nerves (figure 8.12b).

The two main nerves of the sacral plexus are the sciatic and pudendal nerves. The sciatic nerve is the main branch of the sacral plexus and is formed by spinal nerves L4 to S3, which converge at the anterior inferior border of the piriformis muscle. The sciatic nerve is actually two nerves, the tibial nerve and common fibular (peroneal) nerve, which run together in a single sheath until they separate into terminal branches midway down the thigh.

The tibial nerve represents the medial or anterior division of the sciatic nerve and innervates the posterior aspect of the thigh and leg and the plantar surface of the foot. Primary terminal branches of the tibial nerve include the genicular branches that supply the knee joint; the tibial branch that supplies the gastrocnemius, soleus, plantaris, and popliteus muscles; and the medial sural cutaneous nerve that supplies sensation to the lateral aspect of the ankle and foot. The tibial nerve then divides posterior to the medial malleolus to form the medial plantar nerve and lateral plantar nerve that supply the muscles of the foot.

The common fibular nerve represents the lateral or posterior division of the sciatic nerve, supplying the hip extensors, thigh abductors, and toe extensors and ankle evertors and dorsiflexors. Similar to the tibial nerve, the common fibular nerve has genicular branches to

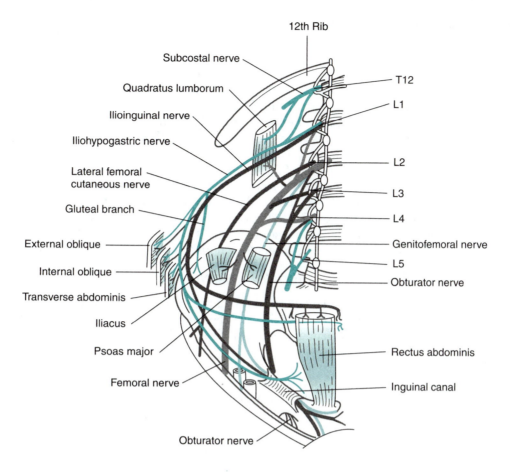

12th Rib

Subcostal nerve

Quadratus lumborum

Ilioinguinal nerve

Iliohypogastric nerve

Lateral femoral cutaneous nerve

Gluteal branch

External oblique

Internal oblique

Transverse abdominis

Iliacus

Psoas major

Femoral nerve

Obturator nerve

T12

L1

L2

L3

L4

Genitofemoral nerve

L5

Obturator nerve

Rectus abdominis

Inguinal canal

a   **Lumbar plexus**

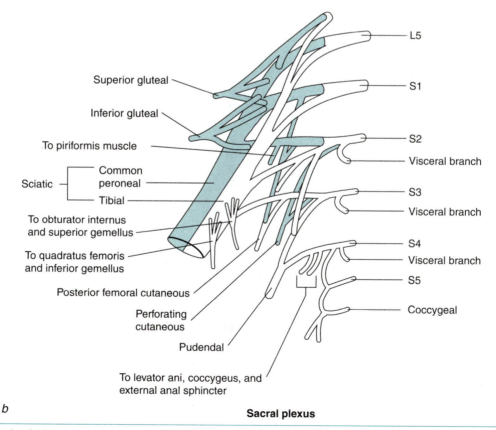

Superior gluteal

Inferior gluteal

To piriformis muscle

Sciatic — Common peroneal / Tibial

To obturator internus and superior gemellus

To quadratus femoris and inferior gemellus

Posterior femoral cutaneous

Perforating cutaneous

Pudendal

To levator ani, coccygeus, and external anal sphincter

L5

S1

S2

Visceral branch

S3

Visceral branch

S4

Visceral branch

S5

Coccygeal

b   **Sacral plexus**

Figure 8.12   The *(a)* lumbar and *(b)* sacral plexuses.

supply the knee joint and the lateral sural cutaneous nerve to provide sensation to the skin over the calf. The common fibular nerve then splits near the head of the fibula into its two terminal branches, the superficial and deep fibular (peroneal) nerves. The **deep fibular nerve** supplies the muscles in the anterior compartment of the leg and provides sensation for the skin between the first and second digits of the foot. The **superficial fibular nerve** supplies the fibular muscles in the lateral compartment of the leg and provides sensation for the skin over the distal anterior aspect of the leg and the dorsum and digits of the foot.

The **pudendal nerve** arises from separate branches of S2 through S4 to supply the muscles of the perineum and provide sensation to the external genitalia. The **superior gluteal nerve** also arises from the sacral plexus (L4-S1) to supply the gluteus medius and minimus and the tensor fascia latae. Other, smaller peripheral extensions of the sacral plexus innervate the piriformis (S1-S2), pelvic diaphragm (S3-S4), quadratus femoris (L4-S1), and obturator externus (L5-S2).

Lower-Quarter Neurological Screen

Following are directions and illustrations for the tests that make up a complete neurological screen of the lower quarter. Use the checklist on pages 140-141 to ensure that you do not miss any steps when screening the nerves of the lumbar and sacral plexus.

Dermatomes

Figure 8.13 shows the typical sensory distribution for both the lumbar and sacral plexuses. Perform sensory testing for the lumbar and sacral plexuses with the light touch or the pinprick

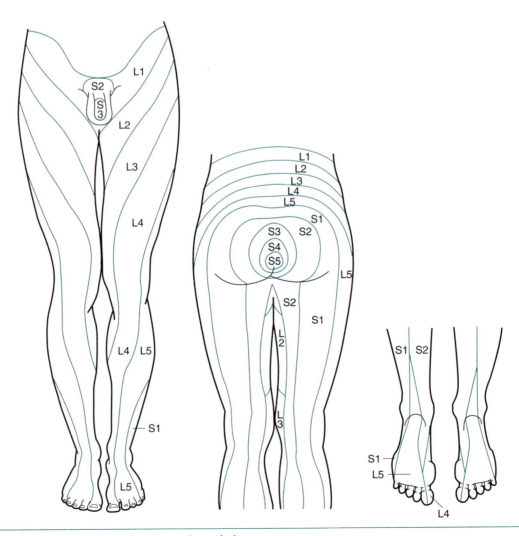

Figure 8.13   Dermatomes for the lumbar and sacral plexuses.

method over the lateral hip and groin (L1), anterior medial thigh (L2), medial aspect of the knee (L3), medial lower leg (L4), lateral lower leg and foot dorsum (L5), lateral plantar foot (S1), and posterior thigh (popliteal fossa) and posterior medial heel (S2).

Perform peripheral sensory examination when you suspect neurological injury in the lower extremity, such as femoral fracture, knee dislocation, or anterior compartment syndrome. Peripheral nerves for the lower extremity include the deep peroneal, superficial peroneal, tibial, and medial plantar nerves (table 8.7). The sensory distribution for each of these nerves is shown in figure 8.14. Test deep peroneal nerve sensation using light touch in the dorsal web space. Examine the superficial peroneal nerve over the dorsum of the foot and the lower

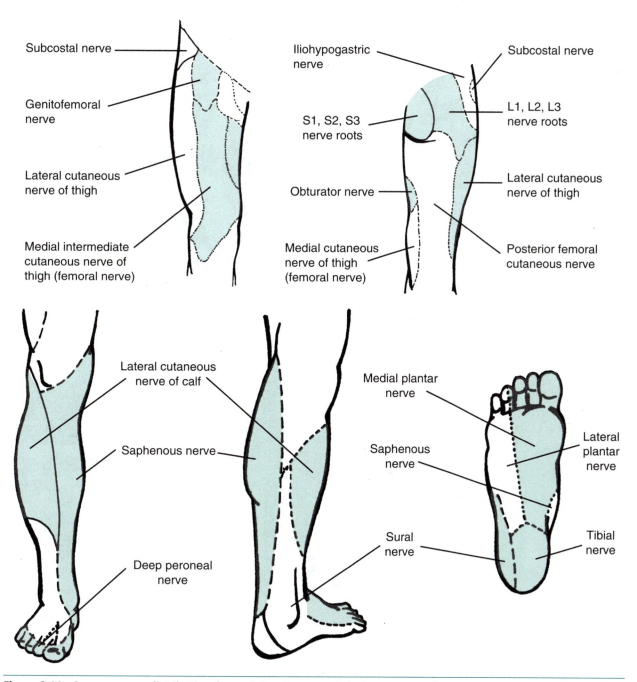

Figure 8.14   Sensory nerve distribution for peripheral nerves of the lower extremity.

Reprinted, by permission, from J. Loudon, S. Bell, and J. Johnston, 1998, *The clinical orthopedic assessment guide* (Champaign, IL: Human Kinetics), 152, 189.

lateral leg. Test the tibial nerve over the posteriomedial plantar heel, and examine the medial plantar nerve over the medial plantar surface of the foot.

Myotomes

Motor tests for the lumbar and sacral plexuses include manual resistance to hip flexion (L1-L2), knee extension (L3-L4), ankle dorsiflexion (L4), great toe extension (L5), ankle eversion or hip extension (S1), and knee flexion (S2) (figure 8.15a-f).

When you suspect nerve injury at the knee or below, also examine the peripheral nerves emanating from the lumbosacral plexus (figure 8.16a-e). Use plantar flexion and toe flexion to examine the posterior tibial nerve that innervates the muscles in the posterior compartment, use ankle eversion to examine the superficial peroneal nerve that innervates the lateral compartment muscles of the lower leg, and use dorsiflexion and great toe extension to

Figure 8.15 Motor tests for the lumbar and sacral plexuses include manual resistance to hip flexion (L1-L2), knee extension (L3-L4), ankle dorsiflexion (L4), great toe extension (L5), ankle eversion or hip extension (S1), and knee flexion (S2) (figure 8.15, a-f).

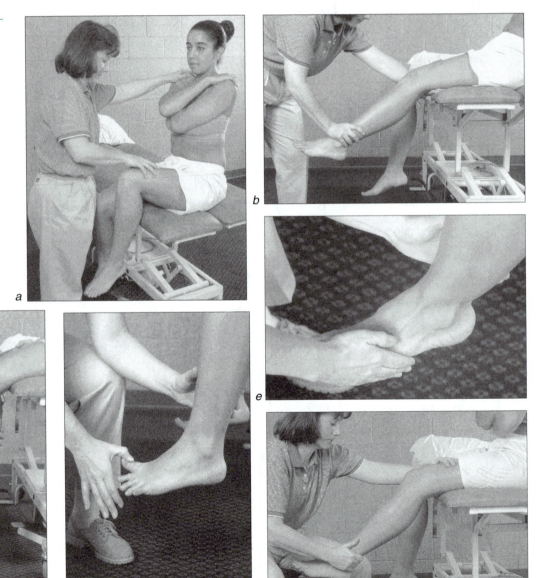

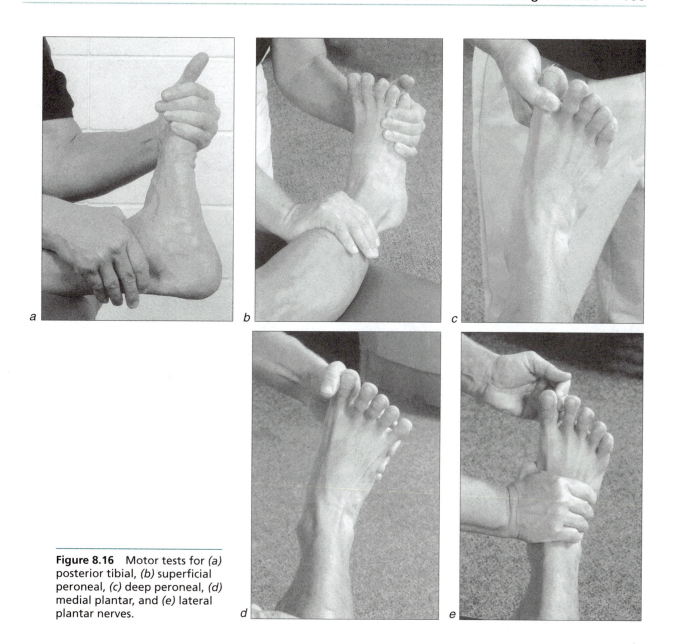

Figure 8.16 Motor tests for *(a)* posterior tibial, *(b)* superficial peroneal, *(c)* deep peroneal, *(d)* medial plantar, and *(e)* lateral plantar nerves.

examine the deep peroneal nerve that innervates the muscles in the anterior compartment of the lower leg. Use great toe abduction and adduction to examine the medial and lateral plantar nerves, respectively.

Reflexes

Superficial reflexes can be examined by stroking the skin along the inner thigh (cremasteric), the bottom of the foot (plantar), the buttocks (gluteal), and around the anus (anal) (see table 8.4). Deep tendon reflexes for the lumbar and sacral plexuses can be examined with a brisk tendon tap over any lower-extremity tendon, but typically the quadriceps (L3-L4) (figure 8.17a), Achilles (S1-S2) (figure 8.17b), and hamstring (L5-S1) (figure 8.17c) tendons are tested. Grade the response using the scale described on page 123.

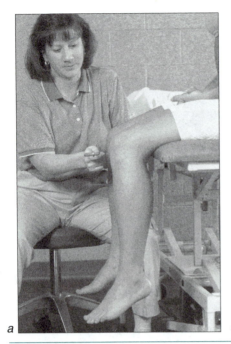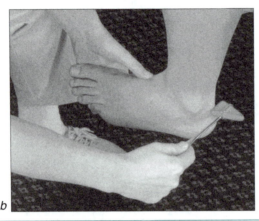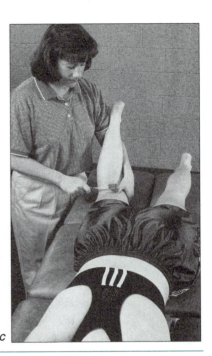

a   b   c

Figure 8.17   Reflex testing for the *(a)* patellar tendon, *(b)* Achilles tendon, and *(c)* medial hamstring tendon.

Use this checklist as a summary of the complete neurological screen for the lumbar and sacral plexus.

Checklist for Neurological Examination of the Lumbar and Sacral Plexuses

▷ Dermatomes

☐ Lateral hip and groin (L1)
☐ Anterior medial thigh (L2)
☐ Medial aspect of the knee (L3)
☐ Medial lower leg (L4)
☐ Lateral lower leg and dorsum of foot (L5)
☐ Lateral plantar foot (S1)
☐ Popliteal fossa and posterior medial heel (S2)

▷ Peripheral Sensory Distributions

☐ Dorsal web space (deep fibular)
☐ Dorsum of foot and lateral, lower leg (superficial fibular)
☐ Posterior medial plantar heel (tibial)
☐ Medial plantar surface of the foot (medial plantar)

▷ Myotomes

☐ Hip flexion (L1, L2)
☐ Knee extension (L3, L4)
☐ Ankle dorsiflexion (L4)
☐ Great toe extension (L5)
☐ Ankle eversion (S1)
☐ Knee flexion (S2)

▷ *Peripheral Motor Distributions*

- ☐ Plantar flexion and toe flexion (tibial)
- ☐ Ankle eversion (superficial peroneal)
- ☐ Great toe extension (deep peroneal)

▷ *Deep Tendon Reflexes*

- ☐ Patellar tendon (L3, L4)
- ☐ Tibialis posterior tendon (L4, L5)
- ☐ Achilles tendon (S1, S2)
- ☐ Medial hamstring tendon (L5, S1)
- ☐ Lateral hamstring tendon (S1, S2)

▷ *Superficial Reflexes*

- ☐ Cremasteric (T12, L1)
- ☐ Gluteal (L4, L5, S1-S3)
- ☐ Plantar (S1, S2)
- ☐ Anal (S2-S4)

SUMMARY

1. Define the structures that comprise the central and peripheral nervous systems.

   The central nervous system includes the brain and spinal cord, and the peripheral nervous system consists of all neural structures distal to the brain and spinal cord, including the cranial nerves arising from the brain and the cervical, thoracic, and lumbosacral spinal nerves arising from the ventral root (motor nerves) and dorsal root (sensory nerves) of the spinal cord. A single peripheral nerve consists of motor (efferent), sensory (afferent), and autonomic nerve fibers.

2. Describe the function of a nerve plexus and its clinical implications for neurological examination.

   A nerve plexus connects multiple spinal nerves, uniting, dividing, reuniting, and intertwining them. Ventral rami at the neck (C1-C4), shoulder (C5-T1), lumbar (T12-L3), and sacral (L4-S3) regions form the cervical, brachial, lumbar, and sacral plexuses, respectively. The terminal branches that arise from the plexus are often supplied by more than one spinal level.

3. Identify the signs and symptoms for neurological testing and what differentiates an upper motor neuron lesion from a lower motor neuron lesion.

   You should perform a neurological exam when you suspect nerve injury and the athlete's symptoms include sensory changes (i.e., radiation of numbness, tingling, shooting pain, deep pain, or burning pain), weakness, or paralysis. Neurological symptoms vary with the level of nerve injury.

   Upper motor neuron lesions result from injury to the corticospinal or pyramidal tracts in the brain or spinal cord. Signs and symptoms of an upper motor neuron lesion include hemiplegia, paraplegia, or quadriplegia, depending on the location and extent of injury, and may also include loss of voluntary control, spasticity, sensory loss, and abnormal superficial and pathological reflexes. Lower motor neuron lesions are conditions of the peripheral motor system caused by injury to the spinal and peripheral nerves and nerve structures in the anterior horn of the spinal cord. Complete transection of the nerve results in total paralysis of the innervated muscle(s). Unilateral symptoms indicate a nerve root or peripheral nerve (lower motor neuron) lesion, while bilateral symptoms indicate central cord or brain (upper motor neuron) pathology.

4. Define sensory nerve function and how it is examined and interpreted.

Sensory nerves receive information from the outside environment and from within the body through specialized end organs. The nerves forward this information to the central nervous system, which regulates the body's functions. Sensory information from the skin is the result of mechanical (light touch, pressure, vibration), thermal (temperature), chemical (chemical irritants), and noxious (pain) stimuli.

The ability to sense light touch is most often examined by directly touching a specific nerve distribution (primary sensory testing), by asking an athlete to identify a particular structure or texture by feeling the object with the eyes closed (cortical sensation testing), or by differentiating stimuli between two or more distinct points (sensory discrimination testing). Abnormal responses include an inability to feel anything (anesthesia), a different response compared to that of the uninjured side (paresthesia), a hypersensitivity or feeling of irritability upon touch (hyperesthesia), and sensation in an area other than the one touched (referred). Sensory examinations are performed bilaterally.

5. Define motor nerve function and how it is examined and interpreted.

Muscle function depends on communication with the central nervous system (spinal cord and higher cortical centers) via motor (efferent) nerve fibers in the peripheral nerves. Motor nerve function is examined using manual muscle tests that follow the course of the cervical, brachial, or lumbosacral nerve root plexuses. Neurological motor tests are performed and interpreted in the same way as manual muscle tests for orthopedic examination (see chapter 7). Manual muscle tests for motor nerve examination are performed over myotomes, groups of muscles innervated by a single spinal segment.

6. Differentiate among deep, superficial, and pathological reflexes and how each is examined.

A reflex is an involuntary response to a stimulus that requires an intact pathway between the stimulation point (sensory) and the responding organ (motor). To examine the integrity of neural pathways, perform deep, superficial, or pathological reflex tests.

Deep tendon reflexes are caused by stimulation of a structure deep beneath the skin, usually an intact musculotendinous unit, by striking the tendon with a hammer. Deep tendon reflexes are graded on a scale of 0 to 4, with 1 being a diminished reflex, 2 being a normal reflex, 3 being an excessive or exaggerated reflex, and 4 being a clonus or very brisk reflex response. Superficial reflexes are cutaneous reflexes that are elicited by lightly stroking the skin with a pointed object over areas where movement is mediated by the central nervous system. Movement toward the stimulation site is considered normal. Pathological reflexes are abnormal reflexes that are specific to a particular disease. They are similar to superficial reflexes because the response is mediated by the central nervous system.

Deep tendon reflexes are usually tested to determine the presence of a lower motor neuron lesion, characterized by diminished reflexes. Superficial and pathological reflexes are used to identify upper motor neuron lesions, indicated by the absence of a superficial reflex, presence of a pathological reflex, or an exaggerated deep tendon reflex.

7. Identify the primary branches of the cervical and brachial plexuses and perform the appropriate sensory, motor, and reflex tests for each nerve root and peripheral nerve.

The cervical plexus is formed by spinal nerves arising from the ventral rami of C1 through C4, with a few nerves coming from C5. Cutaneous branches arise from C2 through C4 to supply the skin of the neck and scalp. Motor branches supply the anterior and lateral muscles of the neck. The brachial plexus begins in the cervical region. It exits the spinal column just lateral to the anterior scalene muscle and then courses through the axilla into the upper extremity. It is formed by the ventral rami of cervical spinal nerves C5 through C8 and thoracic spinal nerve T1, and it provides sensation and motor function to the upper extremity.

Sensory testing is performed over the top of the head (C1), the temporal and occipital regions of the scalp (C2), the posterior cheek (C3), the top of the shoulder (C4), the mid-deltoid (C5), the lateral forearm and radial side of the hand (C6), the middle finger (C7), the medial forearm and ulnar side of the hand (C8), and the medial side of the arm (T1). Motor tests are performed for forward neck flexion (C1-C2), lateral neck flexion (C3), shoulder shrugging (C4), shoulder abduction (C5), elbow flexion and wrist extension (C6), elbow extension (C7), thumb extension (C8), and finger abduction (T1). Reflex testing includes deep tendon reflexes for the biceps (C5), brachioradialis (C6), and triceps (C7) tendons for lower motor neuron lesions and a clonus test for upper motor neuron lesions.

8. Identify the primary branches of the lumbar and sacral plexuses and perform the appropriate sensory, motor, and reflex tests for each nerve root and peripheral nerve.

The lumbar plexus arises from the ventral rami of the first four levels of the lumbar spine (L1-L4 spinal nerve). The most important branches of the lumbar plexus are the obturator and femoral nerves. The obturator nerve supplies the adductor muscles of the thigh while the femoral nerve supplies the iliopsoas and knee extensor muscles. The sacral plexus is composed of the lumbosacral trunk (L4-L5) and the ventral rami of S1 through S4 sacral spinal nerves.

The two main nerves of the sacral plexus are the sciatic and pudendal nerves. The sciatic nerve is composed of two divisions, the tibial nerve and common fibular (peroneal) nerve. The tibial nerve innervates the posterior aspect of the thigh and leg and the plantar surface of the foot, while the common fibular nerve supplies the hip extensors, abductors of the thigh, and extensor muscles of the foot and the evertor and dorsiflexor muscles of the ankle.

Sensory testing is performed over the lateral hip and groin (L1), anterior medial thigh (L2), medial knee (L3), medial lower leg (L4), lateral lower leg and dorsum of foot (L5), lateral plantar foot (S1), and popliteal fossa and posterior medial heel (S2). Motor testing is performed for hip flexion (L1-L2), knee extension (L3-L4), ankle dorsiflexion (L4), great toe extension (L5), ankle eversion (S1), and knee flexion (S2). Deep tendon reflexes include the infrapatellar (L3-L4), tibialis posterior (L4-L5), Achilles (S1-S2), medial hamstring (L5, S1), and lateral hamstring (S1, S2) tendon reflexes. Superficial reflexes for upper motor neuron lesions include the cremasteric (T12, L1), gluteal (L4, L5, S1-S3), plantar (S1-S2), and anal (S2-S4) reflexes.

9. Perform and interpret general neurological screening exams for suspected injuries to the head and upper and lower extremities.

To effectively evaluate the neurological status of a particular body region, you must understand the sensory and motor innervations for each spinal nerve and peripheral nerve branch associated with a particular neural plexus. To evaluate afferent nerve function, perform sensory testing with light touch over dermatomes, the area of the skin that is supplied by a particular spinal nerve.

To evaluate efferent (motor) function, manual muscle tests are performed against myotomes, or groups of muscles innervated by a single spinal segment. Peripheral nerves also have specific sensory and motor distributions, and knowing these will help you examine the integrity of nerves at a location distal to an upper- or lower-extremity injury. Since sensory and motor distributions of spinal and peripheral nerves can vary considerably from person to person, tests are performed bilaterally whenever possible, allowing comparison of the injured and uninjured sides. Reflex testing helps confirm suspected nerve injuries but should not be used as the sole tool for neurological examination, since many variables can influence their results.

REVIEW QUESTIONS

1. What terminal branches and contributing nerve roots supply the following sensations and movements?
   - Sensation over the tip of the middle finger
   - Sensation over the dorsal web space of the foot
   - Sensation over the dorsal web space of the hand
   - Sensation over the lateral border of the fifth finger
   - Grip strength
   - Toe raise

2. Of the various touch senses that can be examined, why is light touch most commonly used?

3. What sensory tests would you use to examine the following senses?
   - Superficial pain
   - Deep pressure pain
   - Temperature
   - Vibration
   - Two-point discrimination

4. What are the differences between manual muscle tests for neurological injury examination and orthopaedic injury examination?

5. By what mechanism does a tendon tap elicit a muscular response? What factors can alter the strength of the response?

6. What is Jendrassik's Maneuver and how is it used in neurological testing for the upper and lower extremity, respectively?

7. An exaggerated reflex indicates what type or types of neurological conditions?

8. Compare and contrast the following pathological reflexes: Chaddock, Babinski, Gordon, and Oppenheim.

9. What important motor nerve arising from the cervical plexus can threaten life if injured?

CRITICAL THINKING QUESTIONS

1. You are covering the state football championships when the team's star receiver comes off the field holding his arm. The player says he landed awkwardly on his right shoulder and side of his neck, causing a lateral stretch of his lower cervical and shoulder region. He complains of numbness, burning, and weakness in his right arm and is desperately trying to shake off the pain so he can go back into the game. Which nerve plexus is likely involved in the receiver's injury and what tests should you use to examine sensory and motor function before allowing the receiver to return to the game?

2. Consider the opening scenario, where Takisha complained of back pain with shooting pain in her left hip and anterior thigh after incorrectly lifting a heavy weight. When she walked in, Larry noticed she seemed to have a hard time lifting her foot, instead hiking her hip to swing her leg around so she could clear her foot from the ground. Larry's examination reveals reduced sensation over the medial and lateral lower leg and weakness (grade 3-5) with manual muscle testing for ankle dorsiflexion and extension of her great toe on the left side compared to the right side, which tested normal. Deep tendon and superficial reflexes were normal except for a slightly diminished patellar tendon reflex. What is the likely cause of Takisha's neurological symptoms and at what spinal level should Larry suspect injury? Is this an upper or lower motor neuron lesion? Justify your answer.

3. You are evaluating a gymnast who has fallen off the uneven parallel bars and has dislocated her elbow. What peripheral nerves may be affected by this injury and what neurological tests would you perform to rule out injury to these nerves? What neurological tests would you not perform, given the type of injury you are dealing with?

4. A baseball player takes a line drive to his anterior shin. You notice considerable swelling and tightness in his anterior compartment and are concerned that bleeding in the area may cause excessive pressure and possibly compress the nerves in the compartment. What nerves may be involved in injury to the anterior compartment of the lower leg, and what tests would you use to examine them? If you note reduced sensation and motor function, would you consider this a medical emergency? Why or why not?

CITED REFERENCES

Duchateau, J., and K. Hainaut. 1993. Behavior of short and long latency reflexes in fatigued human muscles. *J Physiol* 471:787-799.

Eccles, J.C. 1981. Physiology of motor control in man. *Appl Neurophysiol* 44: 5-15.

Enoka, R.M. 1994. *Neuromechanical basis of kinesiology*. 2nd ed. Champaign, IL: Human Kinetics.

Hakkinen, K. 1994. Neuromuscular fatigue in males and females during strenuous heavy resistance training. *Electromyogr Clin Neurophysiol* 34(4): 205-214.

Johansson, H., M. Djupsojobacka, and P. Sjolander. 1993. Influences on the gamma-muscle spindle system from muscle afferents stimulated by KCl and lactic acid. *Neurosci Res* 16(1): 49-57.

Kandel, E.R., J.H. Schwartz, and T.M. Jessell, eds. 1995. *Essentials of neural science and behavior*. Norwalk: Appleton and Lange.

Kendall, F.P., and E.K. McCreary. 1983. *Muscles: Testing and function*. 3rd ed. Baltimore: Williams & Wilkins.

Moore, K.L. 1992. *Clinically oriented anatomy*. 3rd ed. Baltimore: Williams & Wilkins.

Nelson, D.L., and R.S. Hutton. 1985. Dynamic and static stretch responses in muscle spindle receptors in fatigued muscle. *Med Sci Sports Exerc* 17(4): 445-450.

Taylor, J.L., J.E. Butler, G.M. Allen, and S.C. Gandevia. 1996. Changes in motor cortical excitability during human muscle fatigue. *J Physiol* 490(2): 519-528.

ADDITIONAL RESOURCES

Hoppenfeld, S. 1976. *Physical examination of the spine and extremities*. Norwalk: Appleton and Lange.

Magee, D.J. 1992. *Orthopedic physical examination*. 2nd ed. Philadelphia: W.B. Saunders.

Mosby's medical, nursing, and allied health dictionary. 6th ed. 2002. St. Louis: Mosby.

Thomas, C.L., ed. 1997. *Taber's cyclopedic medical dictionary*. 18th ed. Philadelphia: Davis.

Examination of Cardiovascular and Respiratory Status

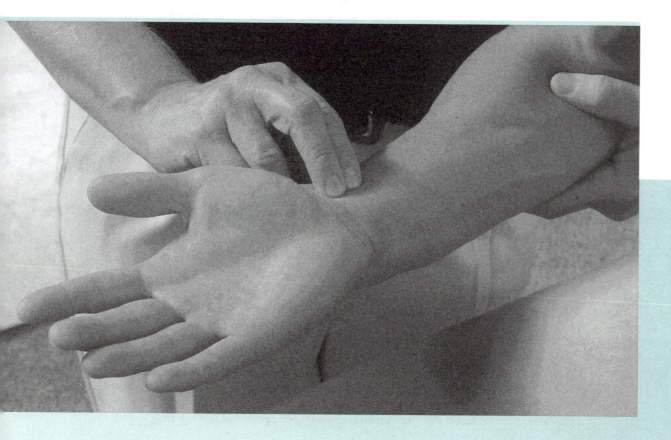

Objectives

After completing this chapter, the reader will be able to do the following:

1. Identify the functional components of the cardiorespiratory system necessary for adequate blood perfusion
2. Identify the components and functional importance of the peripheral vascular system
3. Identify the primary vessels and pulse points of the upper and lower limbs
4. Examine systemic cardiovascular and respiratory status by recording vital signs
5. Examine peripheral circulation and vascular status
6. Identify the etiology, stages, and signs and symptoms of shock

Body tissues need adequate circulation to meet their needs for oxygen (O_2), nutrients, and waste removal. Without sufficient O_2, cell death occurs within minutes. The brain and central nervous system tightly regulate heart rate, blood pressure, and respirations to maintain sufficient perfusion of blood and O_2 to the working tissue. While the body has an incredible ability to adjust cardiovascular parameters to meet altered demands on the system (e.g., exercise, injury, or disease), sometimes an injury or illness severely affects these systems, leading to cardiovascular compromise and a life- or limb-threatening situation. In this chapter, you will learn when to anticipate cardiovascular and respiratory compromise and how to quickly examine cardiorespiratory function. It is essential to identify the signs and symptoms of cardiovascular compromise both locally and systemically so that you can provide prompt and effective care.

FUNCTIONAL ANATOMY AND PHYSIOLOGY

The cardiorespiratory system includes the heart, lungs, arteries, veins, and capillaries that sustain life by delivering blood to the tissues to meet the cells' O_2, nutrient, and waste-removal needs. Cardiorespiratory function is controlled by the brain and peripheral receptors that sense changes in blood pressure and gases (primarily O_2, but also carbon dioxide [CO_2] and hydrogen ions [H^+]) to maintain respiration, heart rate, and blood pressure. While the intricate physiological mechanisms that control cardiorespiratory function are beyond the scope of this text, this chapter overviews the functional anatomy of the heart, lungs, and peripheral circulatory system to help you understand the examination of vital functions and the presence of cardiovascular or respiratory compromise, which are presented later in the chapter.

Lungs

The lungs receive air from the atmosphere through the mouth and nose, where it passes through the oropharynx and nasopharynx, past the larynx and vocal cords, and into the trachea. The trachea divides into two **bronchi** that each connect with a lung. Each bronchus divides into a number of **bronchiole** branches that eventually terminate into small, thin-walled membranous sacs called **alveoli.** Each of these air sacs is surrounded by a network of capillaries to allow O_2 from the inhaled air to cross the membrane and bind to hemoglobin in the blood so it can be transported to tissues throughout the body (figure 9.1). Conversely, CO_2 and other metabolic waste gases are transported from the blood into the alveoli, where they are exhaled into the environment.

The brain strictly regulates the amount of O_2 and CO_2 exchanged in the lungs and maintains arterial O_2, CO_2, and pH levels within a narrow limit. Inhalation is an active process, during which the diaphragm and intercostal muscles contract to expand the chest cavity, reducing intrathoracic pressure and thus drawing air into the lungs. In contrast, exhalation is a passive process, brought about by muscle relaxation that contracts the chest cavity and forces air out of the lungs. Under resting conditions, respiratory rate and depth remain relatively consistent. However, whenever metabolic demands increase (e.g., exercise, disease, fever),

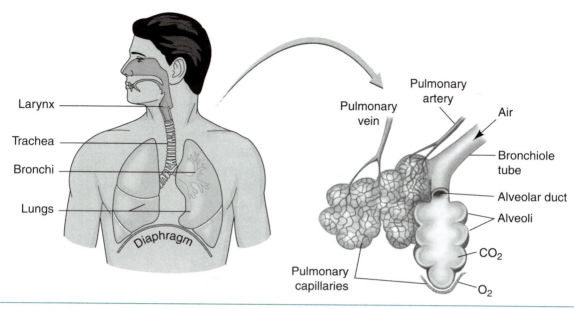

Larynx

Trachea

Bronchi

Lungs

Diaphragm

Pulmonary vein

Pulmonary artery

Air

Bronchiole tube

Alveolar duct

Alveoli

CO_2

O_2

Pulmonary capillaries

Figure 9.1 Capillary network surrounding the alveoli for gas exchange.

the body produces more CO_2, so breathing rate and depth increase to reduce CO_2 to normal levels. As we will discuss, a number of acute and chronic conditions can affect the mechanical or chemical processes of respiration, resulting in respiratory distress and compromise.

Heart

The **heart** pumps blood through the lungs and the peripheral circulatory system. It is located beneath the sternum and contains four chambers: two superior chambers, or **atria**, that receive blood from the peripheral circulatory system (right atrium) and the lungs (left atrium), and two inferior chambers, or **ventricles**, that pump blood into the lungs for oxygenation (right ventricle) or into the peripheral circulatory system to deliver the newly oxygenated blood to the body (left ventricle) (figure 9.2). The heart collects deoxygenated blood from the upper body through the **superior vena cava** and from the lower body through the **inferior vena cava**. The deoxygenated blood then enters the right atrium, where it passes through the **tricuspid (AV) valve** into the right ventricle to be pumped into the left and right **pulmonary arteries** for delivery to the lungs. In the lungs, gas exchange across the pulmonary capillaries and alveoli removes CO_2 and allows O_2 to bind to hemoglobin. The blood then passes into the left atrium and through the **bicuspid (mitral) valve** into the left ventricle where it is pumped back into the periphery through the aorta.

The blood exits each chamber of the heart through a one-way valve that prevents backflow and ensures consistent flow through each chamber. Blood is pumped through the chambers by smooth, coordinated contractions of the heart muscle. The contraction of heart muscle propagates from cell to cell, and the contraction rate is regulated by the autonomic nervous system. Under normal conditions, the electrical impulse begins at the sinoatrial (SA) node, also known as the heart's pacemaker, located in the superior area of the atria. It then travels to the antrioventricular (AV) node, moving through the **Purkinje fibers** in the ventricles. If this electrical network is disturbed due to injury or O_2 deficiency, the heart may stop or beat inefficiently. When the heart ceases to function properly, insufficient O_2 is delivered and cell death occurs in a matter of minutes.

Purkinje fibers extend from the bundle branches (originating from the AV node) to the myocardium in the ventricle to complete the cardiac conduction system.

Peripheral Circulation

The **peripheral circulatory system** includes arteries, arterioles, capillaries, venules, and veins that communicate with the various tissues of the body (figure 9.3). The peripheral circulation begins at the **aorta,** the sole vessel arising from the left ventricle, to supply blood to the

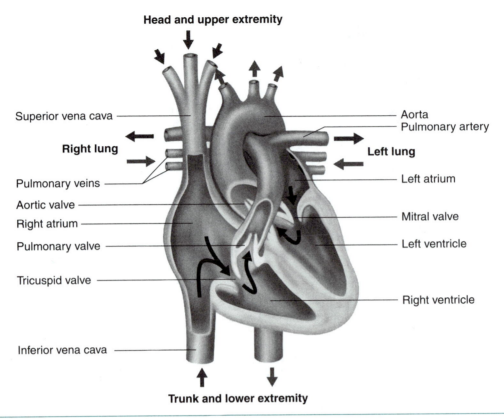

Figure 9.2 Chambers, valves, and primary vessels of the heart.

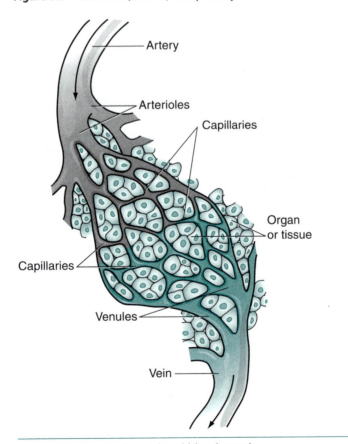

Figure 9.3 Levels of peripheral blood vessels.

primary arteries. The arterial branches serve as the primary blood conduits and give rise to smaller branches (arterioles) that terminate in a network of capillaries (capillary bed) where nutrients are exchanged with the surrounding tissues.

For the circulatory system to function appropriately, it must maintain consistent flow volume, meaning that the volume exiting the heart must match the volume that is returning to the heart at any given time. To accomplish this, the circulatory pathway is in series. Vessels that are in parallel (e.g., primary arteries) have similar pressure but different flow depending on their diameter, while vessels that are in series (e.g., from artery to arteriole to capillary) have different pressure but maintain consistent flow by varying their cross-sectional area. For example, pressure in the aorta and arteries is fairly constant, averaging 100 mmHg, but it drops considerably in the arterioles to 10 to 15 mmHg. With this pressure drop, there is less force pushing the blood through the smaller vessels, so one might expect flow to decrease. However, the total flow volume is held constant by a substantially greater total cross-sectional area of the arterioles and capillaries compared to the total cross-sectional area of the arteries. This system of progressively smaller but more numerous vessels slows blood flow sufficiently in the capillary beds to allow nutrient exchange with the target cells while maintaining consistent flow volume throughout the system and back to the heart.

Following nutrient exchange, the blood returns to the heart through a series of venules and veins. The venous system begins at the end of the capillary beds as venules that eventually converge to form larger and larger veins leading back to the heart via the superior and inferior vena cava. The deep veins typically have the same name as their accompanying artery. The venous system plays a critical role in cardiovascular function, controlling approximately 80% of the blood volume and acting as a blood reservoir. Smooth muscle within the walls of the venules expands and contracts, storing or mobilizing blood volume depending on the needs of the system. As discussed later in this chapter, shock can severely compromise the capabilities of this reservoir.

Primary Aortic Branches

The aorta is the largest blood vessel in the body. The first branch of the aorta is the ascending aorta, which becomes the left and right coronary arteries that supply the heart muscle. As the aorta continues, it gives rise to three primary arterial branches: the brachialcephalic artery that subsequently divides into the right common carotid and right subclavian arteries; the left common carotid artery; and the left subclavian artery. While the carotid arteries supply the head and neck, the subclavian arteries lead to a series of arterial branches that deliver oxygenated blood to the trunk and upper extremity. The aorta then continues on as the descending aorta, terminating in the lower abdomen and splitting into the two common iliac arteries that proceed to the lower extremities.

Severe orthopedic injuries (fractures, dislocations, and severe crush injuries) may compromise the circulatory system. These conditions are discussed in specific chapters. You should be aware of the primary vessels that pass through the upper and lower extremities and how to locate pulse points for palpation of cardiovascular function.

Primary Vessels of the Upper Limb

The primary vessels of the upper extremity are illustrated in figure 9.4. As the left and right subclavian arteries continue into the upper limbs, they become the axillary artery and repeatedly branch to supply the shoulder and axilla. The axillary artery then becomes the brachial artery as it passes through the axilla and courses into the upper arm along the medial aspect of the biceps brachii muscle and into the cubital fossa. In the cubital fossa, the brachial artery divides at the neck of the radius into the radial and ulnar arteries that supply the forearm. The radial artery and ulnar artery converge at the hand to form the deep and superficial palmar arches and digital arteries that supply the hand and fingers.

Two deep brachial veins accompany the radial, ulnar, and brachial arteries and return blood from the upper limbs to the axillary veins and ultimately to the superior vena cava. The medial cubital vein is a superficial vein located in the cubital fossa that is commonly used for venipuncture.

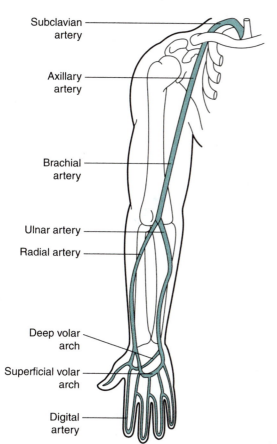

Figure 9.4 Primary arteries of the upper extremity.

Reprinted, by permission, from J.E. Donnelly, 1999, *Living anatomy* (Philadelphia: Lippincott, Williams & Wilkins), 93.

Venipuncture refers to puncturing a vein with a needle or similar device to draw blood, deliver fluids intravenously, and deliver medications.

Primary Vessels of the Lower Limb

Figure 9.5 is a schematic of the arterial supply to the lower limbs. Blood supply enters the lower limb from the femoral artery, which arises from the external iliac artery, a division of the common iliac artery. As the femoral artery courses along the anterior medial thigh,

Anterior   **Posterior**

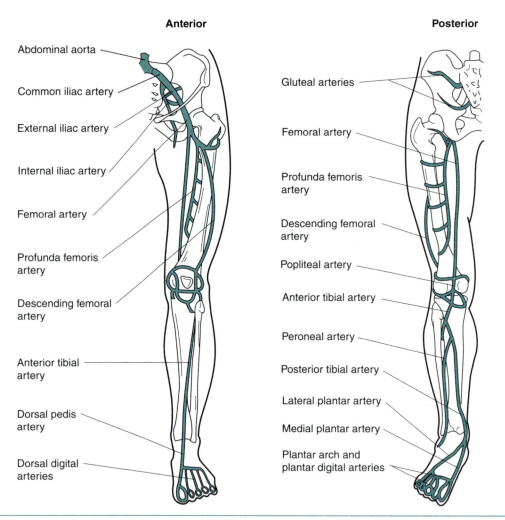

Abdominal aorta

Common iliac artery

External iliac artery

Internal iliac artery

Femoral artery

Profunda femoris
artery

Descending femoral
artery

Anterior tibial
artery

Dorsal pedis
artery

Dorsal digital
arteries

Gluteal arteries

Femoral artery

Profunda femoris
artery

Descending femoral
artery

Popliteal artery

Anterior tibial artery

Peroneal artery

Posterior tibial artery

Lateral plantar artery

Medial plantar artery

Plantar arch and
plantar digital arteries

Figure 9.5   Primary arteries of the lower extremity.

it branches to supply the thigh. The femoral artery then crosses the posterior knee, where it becomes the **popliteal artery** and branches to supply the knee joint. The popliteal artery divides into the anterior and posterior tibial arteries to supply the lower leg. The anterior tibial artery courses through the anterior compartment of the lower leg, supplying the anterior compartment and also sending contributory branches to the vascular network of the knee and ankle joints.

The **anterior tibial artery** exits the anterior compartment midway between the medial and lateral malleoli and becomes the **dorsalis pedis artery**, supplying the foot. The **posterior tibial artery** passes deep in the posterior compartment of the lower leg after giving rise to the peroneal artery near the distal border of the popliteus muscle. It then runs along the posterior medial surface of the tibia, just posterior to the tibialis posterior muscle, and then runs posterior to the medial malleolus into the foot, where it divides into the lateral and medial plantar arteries of the foot. The **plantar arch** is formed by the dorsalis pedis and lateral and medial plantar arteries to give off digital branches to the toes. The **fibular (peroneal) artery** descends obliquely from its origin toward the fibula, coursing along the posterior lateral aspect of the leg, supplying the popliteus muscle and muscles of the posterior and lateral compartments of the lower leg. It then passes to the anterior surface of the foot where it joins the arcuate artery.

EXAMINATION OF CARDIOVASCULAR AND RESPIRATORY STATUS

The examination of cardiovascular and respiratory status includes checking vital signs (systemic circulation) and peripheral circulation to quickly identify blood and O_2 perfusion throughout the body or body segment. Check vital signs to determine that the heart and lungs are functioning properly. Check peripheral circulation whenever you suspect an injury has compromised that circulation within an extremity. These examinations are of the utmost importance, as abnormal findings can threaten life and limb if not identified quickly and attended to.

Systemic Perfusion (Vital Signs)

Examine vital signs to quickly determine the athlete's overall condition. When a problem impairs vital organ or system function, respiration, heart rate, and blood pressure change accordingly. Any athlete whose injury or illness results in serious breathing or circulatory problems should be treated as a medical emergency.

Respirations

As previously mentioned, the brain strictly regulates respiratory function and automatically increases or decreases respiration to maintain an appropriate balance of O_2, CO_2, and H^+ in the blood. Under normal conditions, respirations typically occur without conscious thought, effort, sound, or pain. Visual, auditory, and palpation methods are used to determine respiration rate, quality, rhythm, and depth.

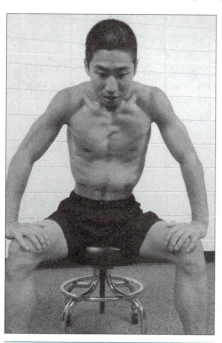

Figure 9.6 Tripod position.

A stridor is a high-pitched crowing that indicates an airway obstruction.

- **Rate.** Record the rate of respiration in breaths per minute by counting the number of breaths in a 30-second time period and multiplying by 2. Count breaths by watching the chest or abdomen rise and fall, placing a hand on the patient's back to feel the rise and fall, or listening to the breaths if they are clearly audible. You may count respirations over a longer (60-second) window, but counting less than 30 seconds reduces the accuracy of your measurement. This is particularly important with conditions that suppress the breathing rate (e.g., hypothermia), as counting over a shorter time period might lead you to believe patients are not breathing when in fact they are simply breathing at a very slow rate. Normal respiration rates under resting conditions are 12 to 20 breaths per minute for adults and 20 to 30 breaths per minute for children.

- **Quality.** Respiration quality is a subjective examination that identifies abnormal breathing. Determine breath quality by watching and listening as the patient breathes. The athlete exhibits **labored breathing** when he has difficulty speaking or exerts unusual effort to inhale. Leaning forward with the hands on the knees (tripod position) and using the accessory muscles of the neck and upper chest indicate increased effort to draw more air into the lungs (figure 9.6). Unusually noisy breathing may indicate partial airway obstruction (audible wheezing or stridors) or fluid in the lungs (gurgling or bubbling).

- **Rhythm and depth.** To examine the rhythm and depth of respirations, watch the patient's chest or listen to their breaths. Determine if respirations are steady or if they speed up and slow down without reason, and if they are shallow, suggesting minimal oxygen delivery, or deeper, suggesting oxygen deprivation. Abnormal findings may indicate head injury, respiratory distress, or compromise. **Cheyne-Stokes respirations**, characterized by a rhythmic fluctuation between rapid, deep breathing (hypernea) and slow or absent breathing (apnea), is an abnormal rhythm and depth sometimes found with head injury.

Pulse

The **pulse** indicates the rate and strength of the heartbeat, or more specifically, the surge of blood circulating through the vessels with each beat of the heart. To examine an athlete's pulse rate, gently place the flat portions of the pads of your index and third fingers over one of the patient's superficial arteries (usually the carotid, brachial, or radial artery) to palpate and count the number of beats per minute (bpm) (figure 9.7). Do not use your thumb to palpate, as it also has a fairly strong pulse that may confound your examination. Count the number of beats over 10 or 15 seconds and multiplied by 6 or 4, respectively. For greater accuracy when the pulse rate is unusually slow, count over a longer period.

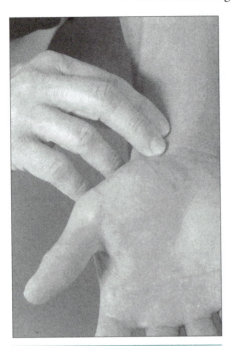

Figure 9.7 Proper technique for palpating pulse.

During your palpation, note the pulse strength and regularity. Changes in pulse strength suggest a change in pumping quality or demands on the heart. A bounding pulse is stronger than normal and a weak or thready pulse is weaker and more difficult to feel.

The rhythm of the pulse should be regular. A **dysrhythmia** is a disturbance in the normal rhythm, such as a premature or late beat. While some patients may have a chronically benign dysrhythmia (recurring irregular beats with no associated pathology), an irregular pulse rate in patients with signs and symptoms of cardiovascular or respiratory complications suggests an electrical disturbance in the heart. A variety of factors can cause electrical disturbances leading to dysrhythmias, including cardiac muscle ischemia, electrolyte disturbances, hypothermia, drugs, direct trauma to the chest, and electrical shock (Taylor, Key, and Trach 1998). **Sinus dysrhythmia**, however, is a common occurrence in which pulse rate varies with the respiratory cycle, naturally slowing with expiration and increasing with inspiration.

A heart rate under normal, resting conditions is strong and regular, typically beating 60 to 80 bpm in an adult and 80 to 100 bpm in a child. However, heart rates may be higher in untrained, sedentary athletes (80 to 100 bpm) and lower in trained athletes (40 to 60 bpm). Due to greater cardiovascular efficiency, highly trained endurance athletes often have heart rates in the low 40s and sometimes even in the 30s (Wilmore and Costill 2004). **Bradycardia** describes a heart rate that falls below the normal range and **tachycardia** describes a very rapid heart rate.

Blood Pressure

Adequate blood pressure is essential for circulating blood throughout the body. **Diastolic pressure** measures the pressure exerted against the artery walls when the heart rests (i.e., left ventricle relaxed), and **systolic pressure** measures the pressure against the artery walls when the heart pumps (i.e., left ventricle contracting). Blood pressure is measured with a stethoscope and sphygmomanometer (figure 9.8) and is recorded in millimeters of mercury (mmHg). It is reported as a fraction, with the systolic written over the diastolic (e.g., 120/80 mmHg). To accurately record blood pressure, you should use a quality stethoscope and blood pressure cuff in the correct size. A normal cuff fits the arms of most adults, while a large cuff fits athletes with well-developed arm musculature. You may also use a large cuff in the rare event it is necessary to measure blood pressure over the thigh (e.g., pressure over the arms is contraindicated). A pediatric cuff is intended for younger patients but may also be appropriate for exceptionally small adults.

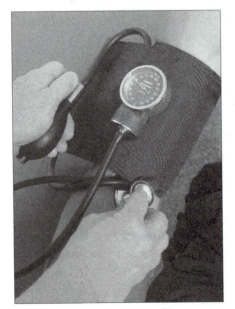

Figure 9.8 Taking blood pressure with a sphygmomanometer and stethoscope.

To take blood pressure, position the cuff just above the patient's elbow, aligning the arrow (center of the bladder) with the brachial artery (see figure 9.8). The cuff should be snug but not tight. The arm should be relaxed, with the elbow and forearm level with the heart. Place the stethoscope over the brachial artery in the antecubital fossa. Palpate the brachial artery just medial to the biceps tendon, then place the bell of the stethoscope directly over the artery, holding it firmly with the fingers of your nondominant hand. Making sure the valve to the bladder is closed, with your other hand pump up the bladder of the cuff until the pressure gauge reads approximately 200 mmHg. Listen for the pulse and increase pressure until the pulse sounds are absent. Then, gradually open the bladder valve to *slowly* release the air from the cuff and gradually drop the pressure (at a rate of 3-5 mmHg/second) so you can accurately determine the pressure at which you hear the first strong "thump." The value at which this first sound occurs indicates the systolic pressure. Memorize this value and continue to listen as the pressure falls until you can no longer hear the pulse. The diastolic pressure is the value at which you heard the last audible pulse. As soon as you have obtained the diastolic value, open the valve completely to release the pressure. If you are unsure of your recordings and need to take the blood pressure again, allow the cuff to fully deflate and the patient a moment to rest before reinflating the cuff.

In some noisy athletic environments, it may be difficult to hear the pulse through the stethoscope (auscultation method). If it is not possible to move the athlete to a quieter area, you may need to record blood pressure via palpation. To do so, palpate the radial pulse on the same arm as the cuff. Keeping your fingers in a fixed position putting fixed pressure on the radial artery, inflate the cuff above 200 mmHg. Then, as the valve is released and pressure gradually drops, record the gauge pressure when you first feel the radial pulse return (systolic). You will not be able to obtain the diastolic value using this method, so you will report only the systolic, as "BP is ___ by palpation," with the underlined space replaced by the systolic value obtained.

Normal blood pressure in adults ranges between 90/60 mmHg and 130/85 mmHg. Pressures up to 140/90 are considered high-normal or borderline hypertension, while exceeding values indicate hypertension. Hypotension (low blood pressure) is indicated by a value below the normal ranges. While it is not uncommon for trained athletes to have pressures near or below the normal limit, systolic pressures below 80 to 90 mmHg for adults and 70 mmHg for children are critically low. Critically low systolic pressure accompanied by injury or illness suggests that the body is not sufficiently compensating for changes in the circulatory system and is unable to maintain adequate perfusion (AAOS 1999).

Skin

Examining the skin provides valuable information on O_2 perfusion throughout the system, the status of peripheral circulation, and body temperature. Always examine the skin for color, temperature, and moisture, as signs and symptoms of various conditions affect these characteristics in a combination of ways (see table 9.1).

Pink skin is normal, while pale, ashen, or grayish skin indicates poor perfusion and conditions such as heat exhaustion, hypothermia, or shock. Red skin may be found in athletes who are exercising or suffering hypertension, heat stroke, or CO_2 poisoning. Skin that is blue or

Table 9.1

Interpretation of Skin Color for Circulatory Status

Color	Indication	Likely conditions
Pink	Good perfusion	Normal
Pale, ashen	Poor perfusion	Heat exhaustion, hypothermia, shock
Red	Increased perfusion	Exercise, hypertension, heat stroke, CO_2 poisoning
Blue	Cyanotic (lack of O_2)	Tissue hypoxia

cyanotic suggests hypoxia, or lack of tissue oxygenation. Skin that has a yellowish tint is a sign of liver disease or dysfunction. In patients with darker skin, color changes may be difficult to determine, in which case you will need to check the color of the skin in the nail bed, the mucosa of the mouth, around the lips, in the palms, and under the arms.

Examine temperature and moisture with the back of your hand. Normally, skin is warm and dry to the touch. You will note very cold skin with hypothermia, while wet, pale, and cold skin is associated with shock. Cool and clammy skin is found with heat exhaustion. Skin will feel hot with conditions such as fever, burns, and heat stroke. With moderate to intense exercise, skin will be hot and wet.

Examination Considerations for the Exercising Athlete

When providing medical coverage during athletic practices and events, you will frequently need to examine vital signs of an injured athlete who was exercising at the time of injury. In these cases, remember that heart rate, blood pressure, and respirations are naturally elevated due to the greater oxygen demands of exercise. Heart rate during exercise can increase to as much as 180 to 200 bpm. Systolic blood pressure can increase to 150 to 250 mmHg, but diastolic pressure should remain relatively unchanged (Brooks, Fahey, and White 1996). However, given the strength of the pulse, you may be able to hear the diastolic longer than normal during auscultation. After moderate to intense exercise, labored breathing may also be present. The skin will also have a reddish appearance and will be warm and moist due to increased circulation and sweating.

You must be able to distinguish between abnormal findings that are the result of exercise versus the injury you are examining. This also highlights the importance of monitoring vital signs over time. If you are unsure whether abnormal findings are a result of exercise versus injury or illness, repeat your tests 3 to 5 minutes later. If the abnormal findings are due to exercise, you should see a return to near-normal levels within this time. If abnormal findings remain or worsen, you should suspect underlying pathology.

Expected Findings for the Exercising Athlete

Heart Rate: 150 to 200 bpm (depending on intensity)
Blood Pressure: Increase in systolic to 150 to 250 mmHg
Respirations: Increased (>30) breaths per minute
Skin: Red, hot, moist

Peripheral Circulation

When a patient injures an extremity (limb), examine it for changes in circulation and perfusion. You should examine peripheral circulation in both injured and uninjured limbs so you can compare them. Always examine peripheral circulation distal to the suspected injury. Factors that characterize peripheral circulation are skin color and temperature, distal pulse, and capillary refill.

- **Skin color and temperature.** In light-skinned athletes, skin that feels cool and appears whitish suggests reduced perfusion, while cold, bluish, or mottled skin indicates a lack of O_2 in the tissues. In dark-skinned athletes, check for skin coloration changes in the fingernail beds, in the mucosa of the mouth, around the lips, and in the palms of the hands.

- **Distal pulse.** Several pulse points for the upper and lower extremities represent a major artery that can be superficially palpated for pulse presence, strength, and rate. Figure 9.9 shows the primary pulse points. While you can palpate pulses over any superficial arterial structure, these locations are the most common. First, palpate for pulse. If you are unable to

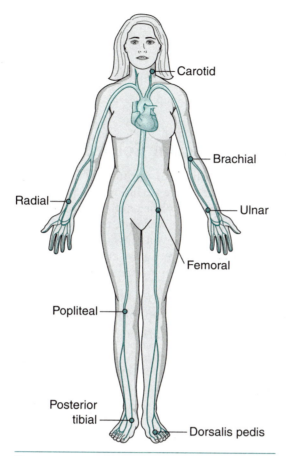

Figure 9.9   Peripheral pulse points.

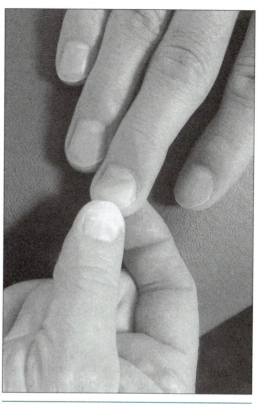

Figure 9.10   Capillary refill test.

feel the pulse, suspect a complete occlusion of the artery and that no blood or O_2 is reaching the distal tissues. If the pulse is present but weaker than in the opposite extremity, suspect a partial occlusion due to pressure from a displaced joint or bone or due to excessive swelling.

• **Capillary refill.** To test capillary refill, depress the tip of the athlete's fingernail or toenail bed firmly enough to blanch it (figure 9.10). Once you release the pressure, watch for the blood to return. If the tissue is receiving enough blood and O_2, the skin should quickly turn from white back to pink. If the color return is slow or absent, the cause is likely poor circulation and oxygen perfusion. Check capillary refill whenever you suspect fractures and dislocations.

Chapter 21 covers a variety of medical conditions that can result in cardiovascular compromise.

CARDIOVASCULAR COMPROMISE

The body is highly sensitive to alterations in oxygen levels and blood pressure. When it senses a lack of O_2, it immediately prioritizes O_2 demands to the heart, brain, lungs, and then kidneys to sustain life.

In the event of bleeding or reduced O_2 flow to vital organs and tissues, the body compensates for the lost volume by

- manufacturing additional red blood cells;
- absorbing excess fluid from interstitial tissue into the blood stream;
- forming clots by accumulating platelets;
- proliferating white blood cells to collect and control infection; and
- adjusting pulse rate, respirations, and blood pressure to maintain perfusion and O_2 delivery.

Causes and Types of Cardiovascular Collapse (Shock)

Shock is a state of circulatory collapse in which the cardiovascular system does not circulate enough blood to the body. To maintain adequate perfusion, the heart must properly pump blood into the periphery, blood volume must be sufficient to maintain pressure in the vessels, and the vessels must be intact and regulate their wall tone to respond to changes in volume and output. Shock can occur with any injury, so you must understand the mechanisms that produce shock. You should be able to quickly recognize the signs and symptoms of shock so you can efficiently and effectively treat it when it occurs. Shock may occur for any of the following reasons:

1. The heart is damaged and ineffectively pumps blood (cardiogenic shock).
2. Blood volume is lost so that there is an insufficient quantity to flow through the system (hypovolemic, metabolic shock).
3. The blood vessels dilate so that there is ineffective perfusion of fluid through the system (neurogenic, psychogenic, anaphylactic, septic shock).
4. The O_2 supply is inadequate.

Suspect serious bleeding and possible shock whenever you observe any of the following:

- Significant injury
- Deep, penetrating injury, even with limited external bleeding
- Displaced fracture or dislocation
- Poor general appearance
- Signs and symptoms of shock
- Uncontrollable external bleeding
- Significant blood loss
- Suspected internal injury or blunt trauma

There are seven types of shock:

1. Cardiogenic shock occurs when the heart fails or works very ineffectively. Any condition that interferes with the heart's ability to pump can lead to cardiogenic shock; common causes include myocardial infarction (heart attack), viral myocarditis (inflammation of the myocardium due to a viral infection), dysrhythmia (disturbed heart rhythm), pulmonary embolism (blood clot obstructing the pulmonary artery), valvular heart disease (disease affecting function of the heart valves), and other myocardial inflammatory diseases. These conditions prevent the heart from contracting strongly enough to generate enough pressure to circulate blood to all the organs.

Myocardial refers to the muscle of the heart.

2. Hypovolemic shock, also known as hemorrhagic shock, results when significantly decreased blood volume lowers blood pressure. Decreased volume signals the sympathetic nervous system to maintain blood pressure by making the following adjustments:

- Increasing vessel tone to constrict the vessel walls, decrease their diameter, and increase blood volume in the system

- Shunting blood away from nonvital areas to maintain perfusion to vital organs
- Increasing heart rate

If these changes compensate for the reduced volume, the body has sufficiently adjusted to the reduced blood volume. However, if volume continues to drop, the peripheral vessels constrict even more and begin to deprive nonessential tissues of O_2. This deprivation can result in **metabolic acidosis** in the tissues due to anaerobic by-product buildup and increased permeability of the capillary walls. Metabolic acidosis exacerbates the condition, as more fluid leaks out of the vessels, reducing volume even further. When volume decreases to the point that the cardiovascular system cannot maintain sufficient pressure through compensatory mechanisms, blood pressure falls, and cardiovascular collapse (shock) occurs, and ultimately death ensues. Hypovolemic shock occurs secondary to blood loss due to bleeding, injury to internal organs, or a severe, large fracture such as a femoral or pelvic fracture. Hypovolemic shock can also result from plasma loss sufficient to reduce blood volume (e.g., burns that cause plasma loss).

Table 9.2 lists the stages of hemorrhage (blood loss) and the signs and symptoms associated with each stage. Moderate shock occurs with 15% to 20% loss of blood volume, and life-threatening shock occurs with a loss of 30% or more. Note that blood pressure does not fall until the very late stages of shock. A more sensitive indication of shock is mental status, which indicates blood perfusion through the brain. Confusion, anxiety, and disorientation indicate inadequate brain perfusion.

Table 9.2
Stages of Hemorrhage

Stage	Vascular response	Signs and symptoms
Stage 1 (≤15% blood loss; equivalent to donating a pint of blood)	• Vasoconstriction to maintain blood pressure	• Normal blood pressure • Normal or slightly elevated pulse • Normal respirations • Normal skin color and temperature
Stage 2 (15% to <30% blood loss; equivalent to 1-2 pints)	• Vasoconstriction • Shunting of blood to vital organs (brain, heart, lungs) and away from extremities, skin, and intestines	• Confusion, anxiety, or restlessness • Pale, cool, dry skin • Narrow pulse pressure (systolic pressure unchanged, diastolic pressure ↑) • Weak and rapid pulse (>100 bpm) • Increased respirations • Delayed capillary refill • Reduced urine output
Stage 3 (30-35% blood loss)	• Loss of vasoconstriction • Decreased cardiac output • Decreased tissue perfusion	• Increased confusion, restlessness, and anxiety • Rapid pulse (>120 bpm) and respirations (>30/minute) • Decreased systolic pressure • Cool, clammy, and pale skin
Stage 4 (>35% to 40% blood loss)	• Vascular collapse • Lack of adequate blood flow to brain and other vital organs	• Pulse and respirations remain elevated • Pulse pressure narrows further • Lethargy, drowsiness, stupor • Increasingly abnormal vital signs • Organ failure • Death

From B.Q. Hafen, K.J. Karren, and K.J. Frandsen, 1999, *First aid for colleges and universities,* 7th ed. (Boston: Allyn and Bacon), 95; and N.L. Caroline, 1995, *Emergency care in the streets,* 5th ed. (Boston: Little, Brown), 194.

3. Metabolic shock is a form of hypovolemic shock that occurs when the blood volume drops secondary to loss of body fluid due to a chemical imbalance. Body fluid can be lost when illness causes diarrhea, excessive urination, or vomiting. Insulin shock and diabetic coma also fall under this category. Like hypovolemic shock, cardiovascular collapse is due to content failure, or lack of blood. There is simply not enough volume in the system to maintain adequate blood pressure and circulation.

4. Neurogenic shock becomes a danger when blood vessels lose their tone and ability to constrict. Vessel tone is essential for maintaining consistent blood pressure and perfusion. Blood vessels are constantly changing in response to signals from the sympathetic nervous system. For example, to prevent you from fainting when you move from lying down to standing up, the vessels in the legs constrict to divert more blood to the head and vital organs. Damage to the spinal cord and nerves innervating the smooth muscle lining the blood vessels may cause neurogenic shock from excessive dilation of those vessels and the consequent severe drop in blood pressure. Although there is no fluid loss, the blood vessel, or the container holding the blood, expands dramatically, increasing so greatly that the volume of fluid is no longer sufficient to maintain blood pressure and adequate circulation.

5. Psychogenic shock is a transient condition that occurs when a person faints. A sudden, involuntary nervous system reaction causes temporary, generalized vasodilatation and blood pooling in the peripheral vessels, reducing blood flow to the brain and causing the person to faint. Since the condition is transient, circulation soon returns to normal. Causes of psychogenic shock include fear, severe mental anguish, and unpleasant sights (e.g., blood or gross deformity).

6. Anaphylactic shock occurs when the body violently reacts to an allergen. Common causes are injection, ingestion, and inhalation of an allergen. Anaphylactic shock occurs rapidly and affects multiple systems. The initial signs are often allergic, including flush skin, itching, sneezing, and watery eyes. These signs may be accompanied by skin rash and swelling of the airways. Victims may also complain of gastrointestinal upset. These allergic symptoms quickly progress to signs and symptoms of cardiovascular and respiratory compromise. As part of the allergic reaction, the blood vessels dilate rapidly, severely decreasing the volume of circulating blood. Fluid may also leak out of vessel walls due to increased permeability, further reducing blood volume and decreasing blood pressure. Acute respiratory obstruction from swelling of the airways is also common, and without prompt medical care will result in anxiety, cyanosis, wheezing, altered consciousness, cardiac irregularity, and death.

7. Septic shock results when a bacterial infection causes severe dilation of the blood vessels and reduced circulating blood volume. The bacterial infection also damages blood vessels, causing loss of blood volume through vessel walls.

Recognition of Shock

Signs and symptoms of shock progress and can eventually lead to loss of consciousness and even death if left untreated (see table 9.2). Early signs include cold, wet skin; profuse sweating; paleness that may change to cyanosis in later stages; shallow, rapid, labored, or irregular breathing; a weak, rapid pulse; nausea or vomiting; anxiety or restlessness; dull, lusterless eyes; dilated pupils; and gradually falling blood pressure. Once blood pressure drops, the patient is well into the later stages of shock. Shock is usually irreversible once blood is shunted away from the liver and kidneys in an effort to maintain perfusion to the heart and brain. At this stage, organ systems begin to fail and death is imminent.

Immediately transport the shock victim to an emergency care facility. Prior to and during transport, maintain an adequate airway and control bleeding with compression and elevation. Also, splint fractures to minimize bleeding, maintain the patient's body temperature, keep the patient comfortable, don't allow her to eat or drink, and continually monitor her vital signs. Shock is an emergency situation that you must attend to with efficiency, calm, and appropriate care.

Signs and Symptoms Associated With Shock

1. Restlessness
2. Anxiety
3. Thirst
4. Nausea and vomiting
5. Cold, clammy, and pale skin (wet, white)
6. Weak, rapid pulse
7. Shallow, rapid respirations
8. Decreased level of consciousness (anxiety, restlessness, confusion, dizziness)
9. Decreased blood pressure (late stages only)
10. Dilated pupils

For additional information on shock care and treatment, refer to *Introduction to Athletic Training, Second Edition,* (Hillman 2005).

External Bleeding

The source and severity of external bleeding should be quickly determined, as bleeding can lead to inadequate perfusion and shock if not quickly controlled. Sources of severe bleeding include arteries, veins, and capillaries. Arterial blood is bright red, since it is highly oxygenated, and it is easy to distinguish from other vessel bleeds because it spurts with each heartbeat due to the artery's high pressure. An arterial bleed can quickly reduce blood volume. Conversely, venous blood is dark red (low oxygenation) and flows steadily (low vessel pressure). Capillary blood is red and flows with a small, steady drop. Capillary and venous bleeding usually result in little blood loss because they can quickly form a clot to stop the bleeding. Arterial bleeding, on the other hand, does not spontaneously clot (because of the high vessel pressure) and requires emergency care to control bleeding.

For more information on the control of external bleeding, refer to *Introduction to Athletic Training, Second Edition,* (Hillman 2005).

Hemophilia is a genetic condition in which the blood does not clot. Known hemophiliacs are rarely involved in sport activity because of the risk of injury and internal bleeding, but if you work in a clinic or industrial setting you may encounter an athlete with this condition. Hemophilia is characterized by a platelet deficiency, where one or more hormones (prothrombin, thrombin, fibrinogen, fibrin) in the clotting cascade are missing. This condition is very serious, as a person with hemophilia can bleed to death with even minor trauma. Whenever an injured athlete presents with this condition, you should summon EMS as soon as possible and provide supportive care.

SUMMARY

1. Identify the functional components of the cardiorespiratory system necessary for adequate blood perfusion.

The cardiorespiratory system contains the heart, lungs, arteries, veins, and capillaries, which sustain life by delivering blood to the tissues to meet the cells' needs for O_2, nutrients, and waste removal.

2. Identify the components and functional importance of the peripheral vascular system.

The peripheral circulatory system includes a series of arteries, arterioles, capillaries, venules, and veins that communicate with the tissues of the body. Peripheral circulation begins at the aorta, the sole vessel that arises from the heart's left ventricle to supply blood to the primary arteries. The arterial branches serve as the primary blood conduits, giving rise to smaller branches (arterioles), which ultimately terminate in a network of capillaries (capillary bed) where nutrient exchange with the surrounding tissues occurs. Following nutrient exchange, the blood returns to the heart through a reverse series of venules and veins. The venous system begins at the capillary beds as venules that converge to form larger and larger veins leading back to the heart. Blood enters the heart through the superior and inferior vena cava. The deep veins typically have the same name as their accompanying artery. The venous system plays a critical role in cardiovascular function, controlling approximately 80% of the blood volume and acting as a blood reservoir.

3. Identify the primary vessels and pulse points of the upper and lower limbs.

The primary vessels of the upper extremity include the axillary artery, which supplies the shoulder and axilla; the brachial artery, a continuation of the axillary that courses down the medial upper arm into the cubital fossa; the radial and ulnar arteries, branches of the brachial artery that supply the structures of the forearm; and the deep and superficial palmar arches and digital arteries formed by the radial and ulnar arteries to supply the hand and fingers. Pulse is readily palpable over the brachial artery at the cubital fossa and the radial and ulnar arteries on the ventral surface of the wrist.

Blood supply enters either lower limb from the femoral artery, which courses along the anterior medial aspect of the thigh and branches to supply the thigh. The femoral artery becomes the popliteal artery at the posterior knee, where it branches to supply the knee joint. The popliteal artery then divides into the anterior and posterior tibial arteries. The anterior tibial artery courses through the anterior compartment of the lower leg, supplying the compartment and contributing branches to the knee and ankle joints. It gives rise to the dorsalis pedis artery at the anterior ankle, supplying the foot. The posterior tibial artery passes deep in the posterior compartment of the lower leg and runs along the posterior medial surface of the tibia and into the foot, where it divides into the lateral and medial plantar arteries of the foot. In the foot, the dorsalis pedis and lateral and medial plantar arteries form the plantar arch that branches to the toes. A branch off the posterior tibial nerve called the fibular (peroneal) artery courses along the posterior lateral aspect of the leg, supplying the popliteus muscle and posterior and lateral compartments of the lower leg. Pulse is readily palpable over the femoral artery in the anterior medial groin, popliteal artery in the posterior knee, posterior tibial artery behind the medial malleolus, and dorsalis pedis on the top of the foot.

4. Examine systemic cardiovascular and respiratory status by recording vital signs.

Examine vital signs to quickly determine the athlete's overall condition. Changes in respiration, heart rate, blood pressure, and skin color, temperature, and moisture reflect impaired vital organs or systems. Treat any athlete who sustains an injury or illness that results in serious breathing or circulatory problems as a medical emergency. Examine and record vital signs as a baseline, then reexamine every 5 to 15 minutes to monitor the athlete's general condition. Remember that exercise naturally elevates heart rate, blood pressure, and respirations due to its greater O_2

demands. If you are unsure whether abnormal findings are the result of exercise or injury or illness, repeat your tests 3 to 5 minutes later. If abnormal findings are due to exercise, you should see a return to near-normal levels within this time. If abnormal findings remain or worsen, you should suspect underlying pathology.

5. Examine peripheral circulation and vascular status.

If extremities are injured, examine for changes in circulation and O_2 perfusion. Examine peripheral circulation in both injured and uninjured limbs and compare your observations. Always examine peripheral circulation at a location distal to the suspected injury. The primary tests to determine peripheral vascular status are the presence and strength of distal pulses, capillary refill, and skin color and temperature.

6. Identify the etiology, stages, and signs and symptoms of shock.

Shock is a state of circulatory collapse in which the cardiovascular system does not circulate enough blood to the body. Shock occurs when the heart is damaged and ineffectively pumps blood (cardiogenic shock), blood volume is lost so that there is an insufficient quantity to flow through the system (hypovolemic and metabolic shock), or when blood vessels dilate or increase in permeability, causing volume and blood pressure to drop to the point that perfusion is inadequate (neurogenic, psychogenic, anaphylactic, and septic shock). Signs and symptoms of shock are progressive and can lead to loss of consciousness and even death if left untreated. Early signs include cold, wet skin; profuse sweating; paleness that can change to cyanosis in later stages; shallow, rapid, labored, or irregular breathing; a weak, rapid pulse; nausea or vomiting; anxiety or restlessness; dull, lusterless eyes; dilated pupils; and gradually falling blood pressure. Once signs of decreased blood pressure are evident, the athlete is well into the later stages of shock.

REVIEW QUESTIONS

1. How is cardiorespiratory function controlled? Are changes in respirations, heart rate, and blood pressure conscious or unconscious?

2. What qualities of respirations should you examine and what are their normal parameters?

3. Why should you not measure an athlete's pulse with your thumb?

4. How would you examine the blood pressure of an injured basketball player during a game in a noisy gym?

5. What are normal ranges for pulse, respirations, and blood pressure in a 10-year-old athlete? A 70-year-old athlete?

6. What does cyanotic skin suggest?

7. When the body senses a lack of O_2, it shunts blood away from _____ to shift more blood and O_2 to _____, _____, _____, and _____.

8. When examining blood pressure, how do you determine systolic and diastolic pressure?

9. What vital signs might you expect in a football player who has just come off the field after an offensive effort that went 90 yards in 15 plays.

10. At what stage of shock is each of the following signs or symptoms evident?
    - Weak, rapid pulse
    - Cool, clammy, pale skin
    - Decrease in blood pressure
    - Confusion

CRITICAL THINKING QUESTIONS

1. How does the venous system "blood reservoir" help compensate for hypovolemic conditions?

2. You see an athlete who appears to have a dislocated elbow. What would you examine to assess potential vascular compromise? If you were concerned that this athlete was going into shock, what vital signs would you monitor and what initial signs would you look for?

3. A highly trained endurance runner walks into the athletic training room complaining of feeling faint. She reports a history of recent flu symptoms including vomiting and diarrhea. You record her vital signs, and her pulse is 37 bpm and blood pressure is 90/50 mmHg. Would you consider these values normal or abnormal for this athlete? If you are unsure, how would you determine that the values are normal or abnormal?

4. Consider the opening scenario. Frank did not understand the purpose behind taking the athlete's vital signs. What do you think caused the athletic trainer to monitor the athlete's vital signs? Which potential conditions that characterize severe bleeding and potential shock do you believe caused the athlete's condition?

CITED REFERENCES

American Academy of Orthopaedic Surgeons (AAOS). 1999. *Emergency care and transportation of the sick and injured.* 7th ed. Eds. B.D. Browner, L.M. Jacobs, and A.N. Pollak. Boston: Jones and Bartlett.

Brooks, G.A., T.D. Fahey, and T.P. White. 1996. *Exercise physiology: Human bioenergetics and its applications.* 2nd ed. Mountain View, CA: Mayfield Publishing.

Caroline, N.L. 1995. *Emergency care in the streets.* 5th ed. Boston: Little, Brown.

Hafen, B.Q., K.J. Karren, and K.J. Frandsen. 1999. *First aid for colleges and universities.* 7th ed. Boston: Allyn and Bacon.

Wilmore, J.H., and D.L. Costill. 2004. *Physiology of sport and exercise.* 3rd ed. Champaign, IL: Human Kinetics.

Taylor, R.V., C.B. Key, and M. Trach. 1998. *Advanced cardiac care in the streets.* Philadelphia: Lippincott-Raven.

ADDITIONAL RESOURCES

Hillman, S. 2005. *Introduction to athletic training.* 2nd ed. Champaign, IL: Human Kinetics.

Moore, K.L. 1992. *Clinically oriented anatomy.* 3rd ed. Baltimore: Williams & Wilkins.

Putting It All Together: General Examination Strategies

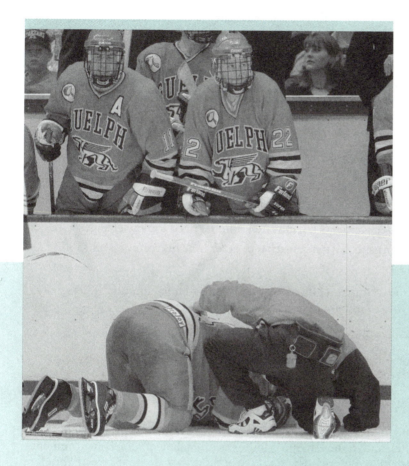

Objectives

After completing this chapter, the reader will be able to do the following:

1. Describe when to perform an on-site examination

2. Identify the goals and purpose of an on-site examination

3. Explain the factors involved in a primary survey of an unconscious athlete

4. Discuss the situations that indicate immediate medical referral

5. Describe the goals of an on-site examination once the primary survey has been performed

6. Explain the purpose of an acute (sideline) examination

7. Identify how a clinical examination differs from an acute examination

It was the final 3 minutes of the conference football championships. The score was tied and Paula's team was within scoring position. Paula was just finishing taping the ankle of a defensive lineman when one of the players on the sideline ran up to her and exclaimed, "Keith just got plowed by one of their halfbacks, and now he's not moving or getting up!" As Paula ran on to the field to tend to the injured tight end, several thoughts ran through her mind. During her entire approach, she did not see any movement from Keith, so Paula had to make some quick decisions.

You have now learned all the elements of an injury examination: the subjective portion that includes the history, and the objective portion that includes observation, palpation, special tests and testing for range of motion, strength, neurological status, circulatory status, and functional capacity. How you will use the various elements of an examination depends on the patient's situation and the severity of the injury. Occasionally, you will not complete an entire examination because the patient's injury is so serious that completion is unnecessary, counterproductive, or impossible.

Now that you understand the nature and importance of each element of the examination, this chapter puts the elements together to demonstrate how each contributes to the final goal: diagnosis and direction for treatment or referral.

You will examine patients at various times following an injury and for various purposes:

- At the time of injury to determine first aid, emergency care, disposition (i.e., return to play, removal from play, medical referral, emergency medical services [EMS] referral), and transportation needs
- Before initial treatment to determine general and specific treatment
- During treatment to determine its effectiveness and the need for any changes
- Before the patient returns to full participation to determine his readiness and ability to return

Other texts cover specific techniques for patient treatment and rehabilitation. This section deals with the different types of initial injury examination.

To learn the examination techniques for treating and rehabilitating a patient, refer to *Therapeutic Exercise for Musculoskeletal Injuries, Second Edition,* (Houglum 2005), chapter 4.

An initial injury examination occurs in three different environments: on the field (onsite), on the sideline (acute), and in the athletic training facility (clinical). Each environment demands a different examination. Before looking at each of these environments, we will briefly consider the documentation you must perform for all examinations. As mentioned in chapter 2, documentation must be accurate and concise. Each examination record is an official legal document and should be treated as such. Two common errors clinicians make are being too verbose and using incorrect abbreviations. Notes need not be written in complete sentences but should be very specific. Many facilities provide their own forms that make taking notes simple and efficient.

Standard abbreviations are those accepted by the medical community. Do not use locally accepted or individually designed abbreviations. Table 10.1 lists acceptable abbreviations and symbols.

Table 10.1
Accepted Abbreviations and Symbols

A	Anterior	BM	Black male
A:	Assessment	BOS	Base of support
Ⓐ	Assistance	BP	Blood pressure
ā	Before	bpm	Beats per minute
AAROM	Active assistive range of motion	BS	Blood sugar; breath sounds; bowel sounds
a.c.	Before meals	BUN	Blood urea nitrogen
abd	Abduction	Bx	Biopsy
ABG	Arterial blood gases	c̄	With
AC joint	Acromioclavicular joint	C	Celsius; centigrade
ACL	Anterior cruciate ligament	CA	Carcinoma; cancer
add	Adduction	C&S	Culture and sensitivity
ADL	Activities of daily living	CABG	Coronary artery bypass graft
ad lib.	As desired; at discretion	CAD	Coronary artery disease
adm	Admitted; admission	cal	Calories
AFO	Ankle foot orthosis	cap	Capsule
AIDS	Acquired immunodeficiency syndrome	CAT	Computerized axial tomography
AE	Above elbow	CBC	Complete blood count
AK	Above knee	cc	Cubic centimeter
A-line	Arterial line	CC, C/C	Chief complaint
ALS	Amyotrophic lateral sclerosis	CGA	Contact guard assist
AMA	Against medical advice	CHF	Congestive heart failure
AMB	Ambulation; ambulates; ambulating	CHI	Closed head injury
amt	Amount	cm	Centimeter
ANS	Autonomic nervous system	CNS	Central nervous system
ant	Anterior	CO_2	Carbon dioxide
AP	Anterior-posterior	c/o	Complains of
ARF	Acute renal failure	cont.	Continue
AROM	Active range of motion	CMC	Carpometacarpal
ASA	Aspirin	COPD	Chronic obstructive pulmonary disease
ASAP	As soon as possible	CPAP	Continuous positive airway pressure
ASHD	Arteriosclerotic heart disease	CPR	Cardiopulmonary resuscitation
ASIS	Anterior superior iliac spine	CSF	Cerebrospinal fluid
AT	Athletic trainer	CT	Computed tomography
ATC	Certified athletic trainer	CTR	Carpal tunnel release
Ⓑ	Bilateral	cu mm	Cubic millimeter
BE	Below elbow	CV	Cardiovascular
b.i.d.	Twice a day	CVA	Cerebrovascular accident
BK	Below knee	CXR	Chest X ray

(continued)

Table 10.1

(continued)

d	Day	FROM	Functional range of motion
Ⓓ	Dependent	ft	Foot; feet
DC, D/C	Discharge	FUO	Fever of unknown origin
DC	Doctor of chiropractic medicine	FWB	Full weight bearing
DDS	Doctor of dental surgery	Fx	Fracture
DIP	Distal interphalangeal (joint)	G	Good muscle strength (grade 4)
DJD	Degenerative joint disease	GB	Gall bladder
DO	Doctor of osteopathic medicine	GH joint	Glenohumeral joint
DOB	Date of birth	GI	Gastrointestinal
DOE	Dyspnea on exertion	gm	Gram
DM	Diabetes mellitus	g, gr	Grain
dr	Dram	GTT	Glucose tolerance test
Dr.	Doctor	h	Hour
DTR	Deep tendon reflexes	HA, H/A	Headache
DVT	Deep vein thrombosis	H&P	History and physical
Dx	Diagnosis	HBV	Hepatitis B virus
ECG	Electrocardiogram	HCT, Hct	Hematocrit
ECHO	Echocardiogram	HEENT	Head, eyes, ears, nose, throat
ED	Emergency department	HEP	Home exercise program
EEG	Electroencephalogram	HGB, Hgb	Hemoglobin
EKG	Electrocardiogram	HIPS	History, inspection, palpation, special tests
EMG	Electromyogram	HIV	Human immunodeficiency virus
ENT	Ear, nose, throat	HOPS	History, observation, palpation, special tests
ER	Emergency room	HR	Heart rate
ETOH	Ethyl alcohol	hr.	Hour
eval.	Evaluation	hs	At bedtime
ext	Extension	Ht	Height
F	Fahrenheit; fair muscle strength (grade 3)	HTN	Hypertension
f	Female	Hx	History
FACP	Fellow of the American College of Physicians	I&O	Intake and output
FACS	Fellow of the American College of Surgeons	Ⓘ	Independent
FBS	Fasting blood sugar	ICU	Intensive care unit
FH	Family history	IDDM	Insulin-dependent diabetes mellitus
flex.	Flexion	IM	Intramuscular
fl oz	Fluid ounce	IMP	Impression

in.	Inches	MVA	Motor vehicle accident
IP	Inpatient	MVP	Mitral valve prolapse
IV	Intravenous	N	Normal muscle strength (grade 5)
kg.	Kilogram	neg	Negative
KUB	Kidney, ureter, bladder	NG	Nasogastric
L	Left; liter	NIDDM	Non-insulin dependent diabetes mellitus
Ⓛ	Left	NKA	No known allergy
lat	Lateral	NKDA	No known drug allergy
lb	Pound	nn	Nerve
LBP	Low back pain	noc	Night
LCL	Lateral collateral ligament	NPO	Nothing by mouth
LE	Lower extremity	NSR	Normal sinus rhythm
LLQ	Left lower quadrant	NWB	Non-weight bearing
LOC	Loss of consciousness	O	Objective; oriented
LP	Lumbar puncture	O_2	Oxygen
LTG	Long-term goal	OA	Osteoarthritis
LUQ	Left upper quadrant	OX4	Oriented to time, place, person, situation
m	Murmur; meter; male	OBS	Organic brain syndrome
max	Maximum	OH	Occupational history
MCL	Medial collateral ligament	OP	Outpatient
med	Medial	OR	Operating room
meds	Medications	ORIF	Open reduction, internal fixation
MFT	Muscle function test	OT	Occupational therapy; occupational therapist
MD	Muscular dystrophy; medical doctor	oz	Ounce
mg	Milligram	$\bar{p}$	After
MI	Myocardial infarction	P	Plan; posterior; pulse; poor muscle strength (grade 2)
ml	Milliliter	PA	Posterior anterior; physician assistant
min	Minutes; minimum	pc	After meals
mm	Millimeter	PCL	Posterior cruciate ligament
MMT	Manual muscle test	PE	Physical examination
mo	Month	per	By
mod	Moderate	PET	Positron emission tomography
MP, MCP	Metacarpophalangeal	PFT	Pulmonary function test
MRI	Magnetic resonance imaging	PID	Pelvic inflammatory disease
MS	Musculoskeletal; multiple sclerosis	PIP	Proximal interphalangeal

(continued)

Table 10.1

(continued)

PM, p.m.	Afternoon	resp	Respiratory; respiration
PMH	Past medical history	RLQ	Right lower quadrant
PNF	Proprioceptive neuromuscular facilitation	RN	Registered nurse
PNI	Peripheral nerve injury	R/O	Rule out
PNS	Peripheral nervous system	ROM	Range of motion
p.o.	By mouth	ROS	Review of symptoms
pos	Positive	RROM	Resistive range of motion
poss	Possible	RT	Respiratory therapy; respiratory therapist
postop	Postoperation	RTC	Return to clinic
PRE	Progressive resistive exercise	RTO	Return to office
preop	Preoperation	RUQ	Right upper quadrant
prn	As needed	RSD	Reflex sympathetic dystrophy
pro	Pronation	Rx	Recipe; prescription; therapy; intervention plan
PROM	Passive range of motion	$\bar{s}$	Without
PSIS	Posterior superior iliac spine	S	Subjective
pt	Patient	SAQ	Short arc quad
PT	Physical therapy; physical therapist	SBA	Standby assistance
PT/PTT	Prothrombin time; partial thromboplastin time	SCI	Spinal cord injury
PVD	Peripheral vascular disease	SC joint	Sternoclavicular joint
PWB	Partial weight bearing	SH	Social history
Px	Physical examination	SI(J)	Sacroiliac (joint)
q	Every	Sig	Instruction to patient; directions for use; give as follows
qd	Every day	SLE	Systemic lupus erythematosus
qh	Every hour	SLR	Straight leg raise
q2h	Every 2 hours	SOAP	Subjective, Objective, Assessment, Plan
q.i.d.	Every other day	SOB	Shortness of breath
qt	Quart	SOC	Start of care
R	Right; respiration	SpGr	Specific gravity
Ⓡ	Right	S/P	Status post
RA	Rheumatoid arthritis	sq	Subcutaneous
RBC	Red blood cell count	SR	Systems review
RD	Registered dietician	S/S	Signs and symptoms
re:	Regarding	STAT	Immediately
rehab	Rehabilitation	STD	Sexually transmitted disease
reps	Repetitions	STG	Short-term goal

sup	Supination; superior	wt	Weight
Sx	Symptoms	x	Number of times performed (x2 = twice; x3 = three times)
T	Temperature; trace muscle strength (grade 1)	+1 (+2)	Assistance of 1 person (2 persons) required
T&A	Tonsillectomy and adenoidectomy	y.o.	Year old
tab	Tablet	yd	Yard
TB	Tuberculosis	yr	Year
TBI	Traumatic brain injury	♂	Male
tbsp	Tablespoon	♀	Female
TEDS	Thromboembolic disease stockings	↓	Down; downward; decrease
TENS, TNS	Transcutaneous electrical nerve stimulator	↑	Up; upward, increase
THR	Total hip replacement	Δ	Change
TIA	Transient ischemic attack	⊥	Perpendicular to
t.i.d.	Three times a day	↔	To and from
TKR	Total knee replacement	←	From; regressing backward
TM(J)	Tempromandibular (joint)	→	To; progressing forward, approaching
Tx	Treatment; traction	1°	Primary
UA	Urinalysis	2°	Secondary
UMN	Upper motor neuron	~	Approximately; about
URI	Upper respiratory infection	@	At
US	Ultrasound	>	Greater than
UTI	Urinary tract infection	<	Less than
UV	Ultraviolet	=	Equals
VC	Vital capacity	+, (+)	Plus; positive
VD	Venereal disease	-, (-)	Minus; negative
v.o.	Verbal orders	#	Number (when placed before the number: #1); pound (when placed after the number: 1#)
vol	Volume	/	Per
VS	Vital signs	%	Percent
WBC	White blood cell count; white blood count	+, &, et.	And
w/c	Wheelchair	°	Degree
W/cm^2	Watts per square centimeter	√	Flexion
WDWN	Well developed, well nourished	/	Extension
wk	Week	±, +/-	Plus or minus
WFL	Within functional limits	//	Parallel to
WNL	Within normal limits	// bars	Parallel bars

ON-SITE EXAMINATION

Perform an on-site examination when the patient goes down during athletic practice or competition or while performing his job. You may examine the patient on an outdoor field, cross-country course, indoor floor, or warehouse, construction site, or any other work location. Before performing an on-site examination, put in place an emergency plan for managing and transporting the patient. Such plans are beyond the scope of this book, but whatever the emergency care plan, instruct all athletes and coaching staff or coworkers not to move the patient before you have attended to him. Instruct anyone who suffers a significant injury to remain down and still until adequately examined.

> For details of emergency plans and procedures, refer to *Introduction to Athletic Training, Second Edition,* (Hillman 2005) and *Management Strategies in Athletic Training, Third Edition,* (Ray 2005).

When caring for athletes in game situations, you should know the rules regarding on-site examination for each sport for which health care coverage is provided. Many sports have specific rules for injuries. Some sports won't allow you onto the field or court until the official has beckoned you, and other sports have very specific time frames within which a decision for care must be made before the team or athlete is penalized (charged with a time-out, removed from play, or disqualified). While such rules should never compromise your care of and attention to the athlete, knowing them will help you avoid unnecessary conflicts.

Goals and Purposes

Use on-site examinations to rule out life-threatening and serious injuries, determine the severity of the injury, and ascertain the most appropriate method of transporting the athlete or worker from the scene. Your goals are to make a quick, accurate examination and to treat the injury in order to minimize its effects. These initial decisions are among the most critical you must make, since an incorrect decision can have dire, even deadly, consequences. For example, allowing a patient with a spinal cord injury to move may cause permanent paralysis, and ignoring the signs of shock can result in death.

Even though an on-site examination often demands rapid decision making, you must stay calm, take your time, and yet be focused and efficient. Good examination skills and judgment along with knowledge and experience are essential, and you must make all decisions with the athlete's safety in mind. If you are ever unsure of the severity or nature of the athlete's condition, it is better to err on the side of caution and refer the athlete rather than assume referral is unnecessary. Always remember to stay within the scope of your practice and training. Hippocrates said that those in medicine should do no harm. Adhere to that advice and never hesitate to call for assistance if the best course of action is unclear or the demands of the situation exceed your training or knowledge.

You will see two types of athletes in an on-site examination: conscious and unconscious. On-site examination of an unconscious athlete is one of the most serious situations in which you may find yourself. Unconsciousness is an emergency situation that requires specific steps to assure an optimal outcome.

On-Site Examination of the Unconscious Athlete

During your career, you will likely encounter an unconscious athlete and not know the etiology of her condition. Although unconsciousness may result from traumatic injury, it may also result from a variety of general medical conditions or drug interactions (see chapters 21-23).

Systematically examine patients who are unconscious for no known reason, proceeding from searching for life-threatening conditions to identifying potential signs and symptoms that may reveal the cause for unconsciousness. Most of the examination techniques you will use in general examination of the unconscious patient are described in other chapters.

Therefore, in this section you will read about the general framework of the examination and be referred to the appropriate chapters for details.

Primary Survey

Your first goal is to look for unconsciousness and life-threatening conditions by examining vital signs and checking for severe bleeding. Attempt to arouse the patient by calling her name. Check airway, breathing, and circulation for respirations and pulse. Because you do not know the cause for unconsciousness, you must use spinal precautions until you have ruled out cervical spine injury (chapter 11). If pulse or breathing is absent, call EMS and begin cardiopulmonary resuscitation. There is no need to continue the examination. If respirations and pulse are present, check for signs of severe bleeding and if these are present, control the bleeding before proceeding.

Secondary Survey

In your secondary survey, continue to look for life-threatening conditions and signs of the cause of unconsciousness. However, considering the number of conditions that may cause abnormal findings, your primary goal is not so much to determine the nature of the injury or illness as to identify positive signs that will help you make decisions about referral and emergency care or first aid. Your main examination tools include history taken from bystanders, observation, and palpation.

History

Obviously, an unconscious patient will not be able to give you any information. However, you may gain valuable information from the environment, bystanders, or both. As you look at the surroundings, check for evidence that indicates a traumatic event. Ask bystanders if they have any idea what caused the unconsciousness. Did they witness an accident or event, or was there no apparent trauma or injury mechanism? Did they note whether the loss of consciousness was gradual or rapid? Sudden onset is common with such conditions as syncopal episodes, concussion, and epilepsy, whereas gradual onset is common with increasing intracranial hemorrhage, shock, heat illness, and diabetic coma. Ask how long the athlete has been unconscious. If bystanders observed her losing consciousness, try to determine her level of consciousness or behavior before losing consciousness and the activity in which she was engaged. Was she confused or disoriented, or did she seem fine just before losing consciousness? Did she complain of any pain, illness, or other symptoms? Abdominal pain may be a clue to internal hemorrhage, and chest pain may indicate cardiorespiratory pathology.

Finally, ask bystanders if they know of any aspects of the patient's medical history that may have contributed to her unconsciousness. For instance, does she have diabetes or epilepsy? Has she lost consciousness before, and if so, what was the cause of the previous episode? Friends may also know whether she is taking medications or abusing drugs or alcohol. The more information you can obtain from bystanders, the more precisely you can define the patient's condition and the more information you will be able to provide to emergency medical personnel when they arrive.

Observation and Inspection

Inspect the patient for any signs indicating a life-threatening condition as well as clues to the type of trauma or illness. As you approach the unconscious athlete, for example, observe the head, neck, and extremities for deformities or unusual positioning. Note any unusual body posturing (decorticate or decerebrate rigidity; see chapter 19) that indicates head trauma or brain injury. An athlete who appears relaxed and is positioned normally usually has a less serious condition. Note any evidence of seizure activity and take the appropriate actions to protect the patient from further injury.

Although you have already checked for breathing, recheck respirations for presence, rate, depth, and rhythm (chapter 9). Aside from the fact that he may have been performing physical activity before the injury, observe if his respirations are rapid and shallow (shock, syncope) or slow, shallow, or irregular (head injury). Normal respiration immediately following activity may be rapid, but the breaths will be deep, not shallow. Note any signs of respiratory distress such as wheezing or difficulty exchanging air. Chapters 19 through 21 cover conditions that could alter respiration.

Inspect the skin for temperature, coloration, and moisture. Is the skin hot and dry, indicating a heat-related illness? Or is it cool, pale, and clammy, which might indicate shock and internal hemorrhage? Is the athlete cyanotic around the lips and face? This could indicate inadequate oxygenation.

Next, check pupils for size, equality, and reaction to light (chapter 19). Someone who has simply fainted will have equal and reactive pupils. Pupils that are equal and dilated may indicate a grand mal seizure or shock. Pinpoint pupils indicate drug overdose. Dilation, inequality, or lack of reactivity in one pupil indicates a space-occupying brain lesion.

Inspect the mouth for bleeding and evidence of an unusual odor. The hyperglycemic patient has a sweet, fruity breath odor (see the discussion of diabetes in chapter 22). A patient who has suffered a seizure may have bitten the tongue, and bleeding may be observable.

Inspect the patient head to toe for evidence of trauma. First inspect around the head, scalp, and neck for any swelling, deformity, or discoloration that would indicate a skull fracture or head injury. Check the nose for **rhinorrhea**, or fluid coming from the nose, and check the ears for **otorrhea**, or fluid coming from the ear (chapter 19). Inspect for swelling, deformity, or discoloration of the chest wall, trunk, and abdomen that may indicate a rib fracture or underlying internal pathology (chapter 20).

Finally, inspect the extremities for swelling, deformity, or discoloration. Although injuries to the extremities usually do not cause loss of consciousness, these signs may indicate the severity of trauma and other conditions (i.e., shock and internal injuries). If this inspection reveals any positive signs, call EMS at once.

Palpation

Use palpation to confirm the presence and strength of vital signs and to screen the patient head to toe for evidence of trauma. First palpate the pulse for presence, rate, and strength (chapter 9). Take and record blood pressure. Hypertension and bradycardia may indicate intracranial hemorrhage (chapter 19), whereas a rapid, weak pulse and low blood pressure indicate shock and internal hemorrhage (chapters 9 and 20). The pulse is also fast and weak secondary to a variety of medical conditions (chapters 21-23).

After examining vital signs, palpate the body head-to-toe. Palpate the head, neck, and scalp for deformity, crepitus, depressions, or swelling for possible bleeding, fracture, or dislocation. Palpate the chest, trunk, and extremities for deformity (fracture and dislocation), crepitus (fracture), unusual contours, and swelling that would indicate trauma. Palpate the abdomen for distension and rigidity to discern internal injury.

Level of Consciousness

Finally, examine the level of consciousness if you have not already done so. You should also constantly reexamine vital signs throughout the examination to monitor for worsening or improving conditions. Use the Glasgow Coma Scale described in chapter 19 to determine whether the athlete is drowsy, stuporous, or comatose. An athlete is drowsy if she can be aroused with verbal stimuli and stuporous if she can be aroused with painful stimuli such as a pinch to the trapezius or the inner arm or thigh. If there is no response to either stimulus, she is comatose.

Use the Examination of an Unconscious Athlete checklist to guide your examination. You may use this checklist to help you develop your own routine.

When to Refer

Do not use any special or functional tests to examine an unconscious athlete unless she regains consciousness and you get a better sense of the cause. The history, observation, and palpation should give you sufficient information for determining the need to summon EMS and provide emergency first aid. In almost all cases of unconsciousness the patient should be referred to a physician for medical examination and diagnosis. Immediate emergency referral is warranted in any of the following situations:

- The athlete fails to regain consciousness within a few minutes.
- You cannot determine the cause of unconsciousness, even if consciousness is regained.
- You observe any abnormal vital signs.
- You note any signs of serious or limb-threatening or life-threatening injury or illness.

Checklist for the Examination of an Unconscious Athlete

▷ Primary Survey

As with any emergency situation, you should begin your examination with a *primary survey:*
- ☐ Attempt to arouse athlete; call name
- ☐ Check airway (cervical spine precautions)
- ☐ Check breathing (look, listen, feel)
- ☐ Check circulation

▷ Secondary Survey

If you rule out the need to call EMS, you may proceed to your *secondary survey:*

▷ History

Try to obtain from bystanders or the surroundings as much information as possible about the following:
- ☐ The cause (trauma or no apparent trauma)
- ☐ Whether loss of consciousness was gradual or rapid in onset
- ☐ Duration of unconsciousness
- ☐ Level of consciousness or behavior prior to loss of consciousness
- ☐ Any complaints made by the athlete prior to losing consciousness
- ☐ Any medical history that might have contributed to the loss of consciousness

▷ Observation and Inspection

- ☐ Note position of head, neck, and extremities for deformities
- ☐ Note any unusual body posturing (decerebrate or decorticate rigidity)
- ☐ Note presence of seizure and take appropriate action to protect the athlete
- ☐ Determine presence of and note any irregularities in rate, depth, and rhythm of respirations
- ☐ Inspect skin for temperature, color, and moisture
- ☐ Check pupils for size, equality, and reaction to light
- ☐ Check mouth for bleeding (seizures) or unusual odors (diabetes)
- ☐ Inspect for swelling, deformity, or discoloration around the head, neck, or scalp
- ☐ Inspect for otorrhea and rhinorrhea
- ☐ Inspect for swelling, deformity, or discoloration of the chest wall, trunk, and abdomen
- ☐ Inspect for swelling, deformity, or discoloration of the extremities

▷ Palpation

- ☐ Determine presence, rate, and strength of pulse
- ☐ Record blood pressure
- ☐ Palpate head, neck, and scalp for deformity, crepitus, and swelling
- ☐ Palpate chest, trunk, and extremities for deformity, crepitus, and swelling.
- ☐ Palpate abdomen for distension and muscle rigidity

▷ Determine Level of Unconsciousness (Glasgow Coma Scale)

Does the athlete exhibit any of the following:
- ☐ Drowsiness (athlete is aroused by verbal stimuli)

(continued)

(continued)

☐ Stupor (athlete is aroused by painful stimuli such as a pinch to the trapezius or inner arm or thigh)

☐ Coma (no response to any stimulus, verbal or painful)

▷ *Functional Tests*

☐ None

▷ *Referral*

Refer the athlete when any of the following occurs:

☐ Athlete does not regain consciousness

☐ Cause for unconsciousness cannot be determined even if consciousness is regained

☐ Any abnormal vital signs are present

☐ Any positive signs are noted on exam

On-Site Examination of the Conscious Athlete

If your primary survey finds the patient breathing, conscious, and coherent without severe bleeding, use the secondary examination to determine injury severity and the most appropriate method for removing the patient from the area of play or work (see the On-Site Examination checklist).

History

When taking an on-site history, quickly determine the mechanism, location, and severity of the injury. In some cases questioning the athlete may be a challenge, but it may also calm him and shift his focus off the pain or fear, allowing you to proceed more easily with your examination. To establish the mechanism, ask how the injury occurred and what happened. If you were an eyewitness to the injury, you may have discerned vital information regarding the injury mechanism and forces. Seeing the patient's initial response to the trauma firsthand can provide valuable information as well. You may find that the athlete has a different perspective from your own or from that of other bystanders. For example, although observers on the sideline may not have heard a sound, he may have experienced a pop or snap. Torque or rotational forces may also be experienced without being readily observed.

Questions regarding the location and intensity of symptoms help you determine injury severity and decide on the method of transport off the field. Does the athlete experience pain? Does she complain of neck or back pain so that you suspect a spinal injury? If so, ask if there is any numbness or tingling. If these symptoms are present, your examination should proceed accordingly (see chapters 8, 11, and 15). Is there any complaint of being dizzy, lightheaded, or nauseated? This type of questioning helps you quickly focus on the area of injury and make appropriate decisions about the direction of your examination.

Completing the history on-site is unnecessary. Gather the information you need to determine the general nature and extent of the injury and the best course of immediate action, and defer the rest of the history to the acute examination.

Observation

As you approach the patient on the ground, check to see if he is moving. Check for abnormal positioning of the head, neck, or extremities. How is he reacting to the injury? Is he able to move the injured part, is he protecting it, or is he not moving it at all? Do his facial expressions show pain, fear, or panic? Does he show no expression? Is his skin pale, flushed, or normal? Is he bleeding from the head or showing other signs of head trauma? (See chapter 19 for more on head trauma.) If he suffered a severe blow to the trunk, especially the abdomen and chest, immediately suspect internal injuries and evaluate the athlete as outlined in chapter 20. Check the extremities for obvious deformity indicating fracture or dislocation. Also examine the athlete for signs of shock.

Monitor for Shock

Patients with severe injuries, severe pain, first-time injuries of any severity, or poor tolerance for injury are most susceptible to shock. You must understand the signs and symptoms of shock, monitor them throughout the exam, and be prepared to take immediate action if necessary. Look for pale, cool, clammy skin; rapid, shallow breathing; and a weak, rapid pulse (think of "**W**et, **W**hite, and **W**eak" to help you remember these signs). Also look for nausea and falling blood pressure. Treat patients exhibiting any of these signs immediately and transport them to an emergency medical facility. For a complete discussion of shock, see chapter 9.

Screening

Before moving the patient, you must initially examine the severity of the injury in order to select the appropriate transportation. If you suspect a spinal injury, stabilize the patient's head while bilaterally examining peripheral nerves for sensory and motor innervations. Chapters 8, 11, and 15 of this book and other texts in this series (Hillman 2005) cover these specific screening techniques in more detail.

If you suspect a peripheral nerve injury, perform sensory and motor testing for the specific nerve involved. For a suspected head injury, proceed with a head injury examination and ask the patient to ascertain his orientation to time, place, and person, which helps you determine the seriousness of the condition (see chapter 19).

If the injury involves a bony region, palpate for possible fractures or dislocation. With confirmation of either, proceed with proper immobilization and splinting. If the limb exhibits deformity, test for neurovascular compromise. Muscle injuries require a quick palpation for muscular defects and a gross examination of range of motion (ROM) and strength. For suspected ligament injury, perform immediate stress tests before transporting the athlete, as muscle spasm quickly sets in and precludes accurate stress tests, especially once you move the athlete and pain increases. You may use other special tests to determine the athlete's disposition or whether it is safe to move him off the field. These tests depend on the body region and are discussed in part II.

Immediate Action Plan

If the previous steps reveal any serious or life-threatening signs or symptoms, refer the patient for further examination and treatment as needed. If you find that her injury does not require immediate medical care, appropriately transport her off the field or out of the work environment and proceed with a more detailed examination in a quieter environment such as the sideline or treatment facility.

Select the method of transporting the patient on the basis of the injury, its severity, and the patient's response. Choose the method that aggravates the injury the least and optimizes the outcome with efficient and safe removal of the athlete from the field. The staff responsible for transport must be well-rehearsed in the various methods so that transportation proceeds efficiently and effectively. Procedures for immediate treatment to minimize and control the injury, procedures for immediate medical referral when indicated, and appropriate communication systems must be in place in advance so that the patient's care is optimal, efficient, appropriate, and correct. All facilities should have an Emergency Operating Plan (EOP) to assure clear role delineations and smooth execution when speed is essential.

For more information on emergency operating plans, refer to *Management Strategies in Athletic Training, Third Edition,* (Ray 2005).

General Checklist for On-Site Examination

▷ Goals

- Rule out emergency conditions
- Assess severity of injury
- Determine transport method

▷ Primary Survey

Begin every on-site examination with a primary survey. Sometimes it will be immediately obvious that there is or is not a problem in one or all of these areas, but whether examination simply involves moving through a checklist in your head or involves a more thorough process, never shortchange assessing

1. consciousness,
2. ABCs (airway, breathing, circulation), and
3. bleeding severity.

▷ Secondary Survey

Once you have examined and cared for any immediate life-threatening problems, you may proceed with a secondary survey.

▷ Essential History

- ☐ From athlete, if conscious
- ☐ From bystanders, if athlete is unconscious

▷ Observation

- ☐ Position or posturing
- ☐ Respirations (rate, depth, rhythm)
- ☐ Trauma
  - ☐ Observable signs of head injury
  - ☐ Gross deformity, swelling, or discoloration of the extremities
  - ☐ Signs of shock (wet, white, weak)
- ☐ Athlete's response to injury

▷ General Screening

- ☐ Sensory and motor testing for suspected spinal or nerve injury
- ☐ Neurovascular tests for suspected fracture or dislocation
- ☐ Assessment for head injury if suspected
- ☐ Orthopedic assessment
  - ☐ Palpation
  - ☐ ROM
  - ☐ Strength examination
  - ☐ Special tests
- ☐ Continued monitoring for shock

Communicating On-Site Examination Results

If you suspect that an injured athlete requires stretcher transport off the field, it may take several minutes to prepare the equipment and personnel for transport. Although most officials understand this fact, occasionally an official may pressure you to move more quickly. You should either address the official or ask someone involved in the examination but not in the transportation to explain to him the importance of careful preparation and transport. The value of ensuring safety before resuming work or athletic play is often readily apparent when calmly explained.

If the patient does not require emergency transport to a medical facility but is brought to the sideline or another location out of the way, complete a more thorough examination. Once you determine the extent of the injury, inform the patient of her status, the plans for her care and treatment, and whether or not she will be able to return to participation that day.

In athletic situations, both players and parents may want to forego the treatment and resume play, especially when the game is important for the team or the athlete. It is imperative that you convey the consequences of such a choice and document the discussion. If the team physician is present, you should also inform her of your findings, impressions, and plans for treatment and disposition. When referring the athlete to a medical facility or specialist for care, you should communicate, either in writing or verbally, the findings of the initial examination and subsequent treatments provided.

Even when a coach is so involved in ongoing game play that he appears uninterested in an injured athlete, you should inform him of the player's status once you complete the examination. He will want to know whether the athlete is able to resume participation. If the situation is a close or important competition, the coach may express a desire for the injured athlete to return to play. This can be stressful for you, but your first responsibility lies with the athlete's health, not with the results of the competition. Allow an athlete to return to participation only if your professional judgment deems it safe. If there is a risk of further injury or later development of health complications, you are obligated to restrict the athlete from returning to competition until it is safe to do so.

ACUTE EXAMINATION

The acute examination either follows the on-site examination or is the initial examination of an injured patient who has walked off the field or from the workplace on his own. The purpose of the acute examination is to determine more precisely the nature and severity of the injury so that you can administer appropriate treatment or return the patient to full function. As with an on-site examination, you may have seen the injury occur and already know what segment was injured and if the symptoms are referred from the injury site or are localized. For this reason, you usually perform palpation early in the acute examination. Because you already have a good idea of the segment injured, you also use special tests early in the examination to confirm or disconfirm your suspicions and to determine injury severity (see the Acute Examination checklist). Depending on injury severity, special tests can be used before or after ROM tests.

Perform an acute examination in the following order:

1. History
2. Observation
3. Palpation
4. Special tests
5. ROM tests
6. Strength tests
7. Neurological and circulatory tests (if necessary)
8. Functional tests (if necessary)

Subjective Segment

During the subjective segment of the acute examination, you should gather more information from the patient and other observers than you first obtained during the on-site examination. By the time the patient seeks care, she is often less agitated and is able to recall information that she could not remember while on the field. Also obtain relevant medical information and previous injury history at this time. Details of taking a history are provided in chapter 3.

The purpose of the history is to provide you with information about the severity and possible nature of the injury as well as the patient's reaction to it. The history will help you focus on specific segments and determine how much vigor you should use when performing tests.

Objective Segment

While the patient is reporting his history, use your observation skills to notice how he moves and holds the injured part and to check for any evidence of swelling, deformity, and abnormal skin coloration. Chapter 4 discusses the observation in greater detail. Once you have completed the history and observed the injury, palpate the area (chapter 5) and then perform the necessary tests to confirm or refute suspicions you formed while taking the history. Such tests include special tests (see general principles of stress tests in chapter 6 and region-specific chapters in part II), active and passive ROM tests (chapter 6), strength tests (chapter 7), neurological tests (chapter 8), vascular tests (chapter 9), and functional tests (chapter 2 and part II).

If the objective tests do not confirm the hypotheses you formed during the subjective segment, reexamine and retest for other possible injuries or refer the patient to another medical professional for further examination and diagnosis. Use common sense when deciding how aggressively you will perform the objective examination. If the patient is in severe pain, perform only one or two tests to establish the most appropriate immediate treatment or referral and defer further examination until the pain lessens. Tests that need to be performed as soon as possible, however, are those that pain or swelling will later obscure, such as ligament, capsule, and muscle strain tests. If the patient is able to tolerate a more extensive examination, proceed, but only as necessity and pain level dictate. Otherwise you will aggravate the injury and lose the patient's confidence in your ability.

Special tests by themselves do not completely profile the injury. During the examination, every question, observation, and test progressively focuses the picture and narrows the injury possibilities. Be careful not to make unfounded assumptions or rush the investigation by prematurely focusing on one or two special tests. Since special tests are numerous and unique to each body segment, they are discussed in part II in the chapters that deal with the various body segments.

Deciding on the degree of stress or which special test to use requires good judgment. It is sometimes neither necessary nor appropriate to use a special test to stress an injury. This is true, for example, in the case of a patellar dislocation. The patient may feel too much pain to undergo a stress test, in which case it is better to defer the special test than to further aggravate the injury. If, on the other hand, the athlete experiences moderate pain with palpation over the lateral ligament structures of the elbow, you should use ligament stress tests to determine if the injury involves the collateral ligaments of the elbow and to examine the degree of injury. Likewise, when examining a patient who has moderate shoulder pain and weakness on active and resistive motion, special tests will help you ascertain whether the injury involves the rotator cuff, biceps, or other muscular support around the shoulder joint.

The special tests presented throughout this text are those clinicians most commonly use because of their accuracy and demonstrated reliability. Sometimes there is more than one test that can be used for a specific injury. For example, the Lachman test and anterior drawer test can both be used to stress the ACL. There may be times when you may use both tests and other times when you may use only one. The specific situation, athlete, and injury are some of the factors that will guide you in deciding the best test or tests to use.

Always remember that negative or positive results of a single special test do not necessarily confirm or rule out a specific injury. A test may falsely yield a positive result and you may need other tests for confirmation. Therefore, your conclusions are based on the total injury profile you have created from all the subjective and objective information; this total image provides your diagnosis. Your skills and ability to perform the tests reliably can influence test results; thus your experience plays an important role in the accuracy of special tests. A special test should reproduce the athlete's symptoms, so unless you require further confirmation, a test or two per structure is usually adequate and better tolerated by the patient.

Perform functional tests during acute examination only if there is a possibility that the patient may return to full function. These tests, which include agility and skill activities that test the injury, are discussed in chapter 2 and individual chapters in part II. Return the athlete to participation only if he successfully completes these tests.

General Checklist for Acute Examination

▷ *Goals*
- Determine nature of injury
- Determine severity of injury

▷ *Subjective Segment*
- ☐ History
    - ☐ Current
    - ☐ Past

▷ *Objective Segment*
- ☐ Observation
    - ☐ Skin coloration
    - ☐ Swelling, deformity, ecchymosis
- ☐ Palpation
- ☐ Special tests
- ☐ ROM
    - ☐ Active
    - ☐ Passive
- ☐ Strength tests
    - ☐ General isometric manual muscle tests
    - ☐ Specific manual muscle tests
- ☐ Neurological tests (as appropriate)
    - ☐ Sensory
    - ☐ Motor
    - ☐ Reflex
- ☐ Circulatory tests
    - ☐ Pallor
    - ☐ Distal pulse
    - ☐ Capillary refill
- ☐ Functional tests (as appropriate)

CLINICAL EXAMINATION

Often, you will not evaluate an injury immediately after it happens. Commonly, a patient reports to the treatment facility complaining of an injury that occurred within the past few hours or days, or an injury that had no acute onset but has progressively worsened over time. Without witnessing an injury, your detective work must be broader and more detailed, as the injury's severity, irritability, nature, and stage can be much more complicated. An injury's profile changes over time, so findings at the onset may change upon reexamination, making accurate examination more difficult.

General Principles of the Clinical Examination

Although the procedures for a clinical examination follow a specific routine and include many of the same components as the acute examination, some components are slightly altered and others are added. In both examinations you should look for a comparable sign. Both the acute and clinical examinations include subjective and objective segments. The following discussion covers only those components that differ from the acute examination. Keep in mind that the clinical examination does include all the components of the subjective and objective segments. Refer to the previous chapters for a complete discussion of these components. Note that the sequence of the clinical examination differs from that of the acute examination, mainly in that you palpate much later in the clinical examination than in the on-site or acute examination (see General Checklist for Clinical Examination).

The clinical examination proceeds in the following order:

1. Subjective segment (history)
2. Observation
3. Differential diagnosis
4. ROM tests
5. Strength tests
6. Neural tests
7. Vascular tests
8. Special tests
9. Joint mobility tests
10. Palpation
11. Functional tests

Subjective Segment

You will ask many of the same questions during the clinical examination that you ask at the sideline regarding the mechanism of the injury and any history of prior injury and treatment. You must first decide whether the injury is acute or chronic, so ask questions about its onset. For chronic injuries, inquire about onset, symptoms, pain profile, and treatments in addition to the usual history questions (see chapter 3 for more details). Use medical questions to rule out general medical problems and internal injuries, some of which could be serious and refer pain to the extremities. Chapters 21, 22, and 23 describe the signs and symptoms of common general medical conditions with which you should be familiar.

Objective Segment

Before conducting the objective examination on a post-acute or chronic injury, caution the patient that the examination may aggravate the symptoms. It is not unusual for a patient's symptoms to increase following the examination; assure the patient that these effects should quickly subside. Instruct the patient to inform you at the next visit whether or not symptoms increased.

Differential Diagnosis

When you do not witness an injury you may find it difficult to pinpoint its mechanism and nature, even after learning the patient's history. For example, if a weekend warrior comes to you complaining of shoulder pain since colliding with another athlete at her last soccer game, you need to eliminate the neck as the injury site before you can identify the shoulder as the problem area. It could be that during the collision she suffered a cervical nerve injury and her only subsequent symptom is pain in the lateral shoulder. If you are examining an older athlete, you should also consider the cardiac system as a source of shoulder pain, especially if the athlete's history indicates the possibility. The source of symptoms can sometimes be difficult to discern, since more than one injury can cause the same profile. You must be able to delineate the possible causes and eliminate as many factors as possible. This process is called a **differential diagnosis**.

Differential diagnosis should be part of any clinical examination in which the injury is not obvious. You should eliminate possible involvement of adjacent joints early in the examination before focusing on the area of complaint. For example, the cervical region can refer symptoms to the shoulder, elbow, and wrist; the lumbar region can refer to the hip, knee, and ankle; any upper-extremity joint can refer to another upper-extremity joint; and any lower-extremity joint can refer to another lower-extremity joint. Therefore it is necessary to eliminate referrals as the source of the complaint.

Quick tests can often eliminate possible sources of symptoms. For example, if a patient has hip and back pain, have him perform a squat. If he reports no difficulty and performs the move smoothly through a full ROM, the problem may be related to the lumbar spine and not the hip. If the patient reports anterior thigh pain but is unable to recall a specific quadriceps injury, have him perform lumbar flexion, extension, side-bending, and rotation movements while standing. If he reports pain during any of these movements, investigate the lumbar spine to eliminate the possibility of a lumbar injury with nerve root dysfunction. If he reports symptoms in the shoulder but you are unsure whether they relate to a shoulder or cervical problem, quickly screen cervical passive and active ROM before focusing on the shoulder. If the symptoms are related to the cervical region, they may be reproduced by these tests.

Range of Motion

Examine active and passive ROM in the clinic using a goniometer to accurately measure physiological motions. Refer to chapter 6 for details of ROM examination. During the clinical examination capsular tightness may cause ROM deficits, so also examine accessory motions at this time. On-site and acute examinations do not include passive motion tests for joint accessory motion since capsular patterns do not occur immediately.

As mentioned in chapter 6, prolonged immobilization or inflammation can result in loss of normal capsular mobility. A capsular pattern occurs when the joint's capsule becomes adherent. If a capsular pattern was noted during active motion, passive joint accessory motion can identify where the restrictions exist in the capsule. Capsular restriction is progressive. The more restricted the joint, the less motion available. Although early capsular restriction may exhibit only slight loss of motion in one or two directions, more progressive restriction includes greater loss of motion in all directions. For example, in early capsular restriction of the shoulder, only lateral rotation may be limited, but in later stages, lateral rotation, abduction, and flexion will all be limited, with lateral rotation having the greatest limitation and flexion the least.

Joint mobilization tests are the ROM tests used to identify or rule out possible capsular restriction. These are discussed in chapter 6 and presented in detail in the region-specific chapters in part II.

Strength

As in acute examinations, strength tests in the clinic begin with isometric screening for gross discrepancies and proceed to specific muscles or muscle groups exhibiting bilateral differences. As with the acute examination, manual muscle tests are the most convenient method of examining strength. However, clinical examination may also incorporate instrumented equipment to provide more objective outcomes. Equipment selection depends upon availability, your preference, the muscle or muscle group being tested, and the patient's condition. Equipment can range from isometric tensiometers to free and machine weights to isokinetic equipment, all of which are presented in chapter 7. While manual muscle tests are the most efficient and readily available means of examining muscle strength, instrumented strength testing provides a more objective and reproducible measure.

Neural Tests

Although clinical neural tests are the same as those used during the acute examination, they serve a dual purpose in the clinical examination. Since you did not witness the injury, it may be difficult to determine if the injury is segmental or neural. As a rule of thumb, if an athlete presents in the facility with complaints below the acromion in the upper extremity or below the gluteal fold in the lower extremity, perform a neural examination to rule out neural causes.

General Checklist for Clinical Examination

▷ *Goals*

- Determine severity of injury
- Determine irritability of injury
- Determine nature of injury
- Determine stage of injury

▷ *Subjective Segment*

- ☐ History
    - ☐ Current: Acute
    - ☐ Current: Chronic
    - ☐ Past

▷ *Objective Segment*

- ☐ Observation
    - ☐ Skin color
    - ☐ Swelling, deformity, ecchymosis
    - ☐ Posture and gait
- ☐ Differential diagnosis tests
- ☐ ROM
    - ☐ Active
    - ☐ Passive
- ☐ Strength tests
    - ☐ General isometric manual muscle tests
    - ☐ Specific manual muscle tests
    - ☐ Instrumented assessment
- ☐ Neurological tests (as appropriate)
    - ☐ Sensory
    - ☐ Motor
    - ☐ Reflex
- ☐ Circulatory tests (as appropriate)
    - ☐ Pallor
    - ☐ Distal pulse
- ☐ Special tests
- ☐ Joint mobility tests
- ☐ Palpation
- ☐ Functional tests

Special Tests

Many of the special tests used during the acute examination are also used in the clinic. Other tests may also be appropriate, depending on the patient's history and your preliminary findings from other objective tests. Because clinical examination is more likely to reveal chronic injuries, additional tests may be necessary to confirm your preliminary impression of the chronic nature of the injury. These joint-specific special tests are discussed in relation to the clinical examination in the chapters on the various body segments.

Palpation

You will palpate later in the clinical examination than in the acute examination, after you have already identified the source of the patient's pain. Waiting to palpate until completing the motion and special tests narrows the possible nature of the injury and allows you to concentrate on a specific area. If you perform palpation early in the clinical examination, you may palpate uninvolved tissue because the pain may actually be referred from another source, something you will not know until you have performed other portions of the examination.

As with the acute examination, palpation in the clinic proceeds systematically, moving from superficial to deep structures and traversing the body segment in a specific routine such as from anterior to posterior or superior to inferior. Likewise, palpation of the structures is the same in both the acute and clinical examinations. Carefully note differences between the involved and uninvolved sides in soft tissue tension, spasm, restriction, temperature, moisture, swelling, thickness, texture, bony and soft tissue contours, and tenderness. Palpation is covered in detail in chapter 5.

Functional Tests

As with the acute examination, clinical functional tests identify the patient's readiness to return to participation. If previous segments of the examination have determined that the patient will not be able to participate in her sport, defer functional tests until after the patient has been treated for the injury.

SUMMARY

1. Describe when to perform an on-site examination.

   Perform an on-site examination when the patient goes down during practice or competition or while working on the job.

2. Identify the goals and purpose of an on-site examination.

   The on-site examination rules out life-threatening and serious injuries, determines the injury's severity, and ascertains the most appropriate method of transporting the patient off the field or out of the work area. The goals are to examine the patient quickly and accurately and to initially treat the injury in order to minimize its effect.

3. Explain the factors involved in a primary survey of an unconscious athlete.

   Check airway, breathing, and circulation. Because you do not know the cause of unconsciousness, you must use spinal precautions until you have ruled out cervical spine injury. If pulse or breathing is absent, stop the examination, call EMS, and begin cardiopulmonary resuscitation. If respirations and pulse are present, check immediately for severe bleeding, and if present, control the bleeding before proceeding.

4. Discuss the situations that indicate immediate medical referral.

   Immediate emergency referral is warranted in any of the following situations: (1) the patient fails to regain consciousness within a few minutes, (2) you cannot determine the cause for the unconsciousness, even if consciousness is regained, (3) you observe any abnormal vital signs, or (4) you note any serious or life-threatening injury or illness.

5. Describe the goals of an on-site examination once the primary survey has been performed.

   If the primary survey finds the patient breathing and conscious without severe bleeding, use the secondary examination to determine the injury's severity and the most appropriate method of removing the patient from the field of play or work environment.

6. Explain the purpose of an acute (sideline) examination.

The acute examination follows the on-site examination or serves as the initial examination of an injured athlete who has walked off the field on his own. It allows you to precisely determine the injury's nature and severity so that you can administer appropriate initial treatment or allow the patient to return to participation.

7. Identify how a clinical examination differs from an acute examination.

Although clinical examination follows a specific routine and includes many of the same components as the acute examination, it also alters some of those components and adds others. Since you did not witness the injury, you may find it difficult to pinpoint the mechanism and nature of the injury. In such cases you must make a differential diagnosis, investigating adjacent or related areas in a clinical examination. Capsular restriction of motion may be present in more chronic injuries, so any joint that exhibits a capsular pattern during ROM testing should be examined with joint mobilization techniques to identify areas of capsular tightness. Strength examination in a clinical examination can be more objective when specialized equipment is used rather than manual muscle tests. If a patient presents in the treatment facility with complaints below the acromion in the upper extremity or below the gluteal fold in the lower extremity, perform a neural examination to rule out neural causes. Because the clinical examination is more likely to reveal chronic injuries, additional special tests may be necessary to confirm the preliminary impression of a chronic injury. You will palpate later in the clinical examination than in the acute examination, after other portions of the examination have identified the source of pain. Waiting to perform palpation until after completing the motion and special tests helps determine the nature of the injury so you can concentrate on a specific area.

REVIEW QUESTIONS

1. Describe the steps of an on-site examination. At which points do you decide to refer or transport the patient from the area?

2. What is involved in a secondary examination of an unconscious athlete on the field or in the workplace?

3. During an acute examination, what tests would you perform on a conscious patient that you did not perform on-site?

4. If a basketball player collides with another player and suffers what you suspect is a midhumeral fracture, what will you say to the player, coach, and team physician?

5. A grocery employee suffers a knee sprain while loading heavy flats and is brought to you for an examination. What tests would you perform that you would not have performed if you had seen the injury occur?

CRITICAL THINKING QUESTIONS

1. A 400m-hurdler reports to the athletic training facility stating that at yesterday's meet he stumbled over one of the hurdles and feels like he sprained his ankle. He stated that this morning the ankle was a lot more swollen and sore, and he is concerned about being ready for the next meet. What history, observation, palpation, and tests will you perform to examine his injury?

2. A lacrosse player suddenly collapses on the field. As you move toward her you see that she is moving on the ground, holding her right knee with both hands. She is not hysterical but is in obvious pain. What should you do once you reach her side? If you determine that she has injured her anterior cruciate ligament, how will you transport her off the field? What factors are you basing your decision on?

3. Looking back at the scenario at the beginning of the chapter, what do you think is running through Paula's mind as she goes to Keith on the field? Once Paula is at Keith's side and sees that he is still not moving, what should Paula include in her immediate examination?

4. You are on the sideline with a softball shortstop who reports that during the last play she lunged for a line drive and rolled over on her ankle. She has injured the ankle before but not in the past year. She is sure it is the same injury as before and wants to get the ankle taped to go back on the field when the team's turn at bat is over. What questions will you ask to form a better picture of the injury? Identify what you will look for during your observation. What areas will you palpate? What ranges of motion will you test? If you find minor results indicating a mild lateral ankle sprain, will you allow her to return to the game? What functional tests will you perform to assist your decision?

5. A gymnast enters your treatment facility and reports that for the past month she has had pain in her Achilles tendon whenever she practices the floor exercise or vault. What would you observe in your clinical examination to help you identify the problem?

ADDITIONAL RESOURCES

Hillman, S.K. 2005. *Introduction to athletic training.* 2nd ed. Champaign, IL: Human Kinetics.

Houglum, P.A. 2005. *Therapeutic exercise for musculoskeletal injuries.* 2nd ed. Champaign, IL: Human Kinetics.

Ray, R. 2005. *Management strategies in athletic training.* 3rd ed. Champaign, IL: Human Kinetics.

II

Region-Specific Examination Strategies

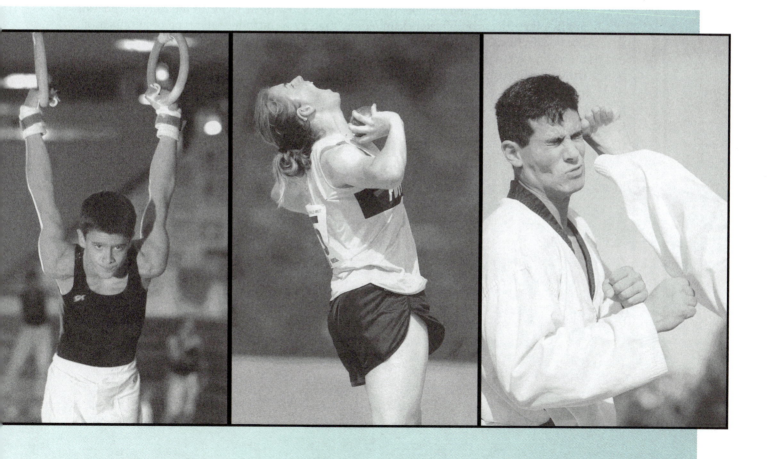

Part I of this text presented the foundational principles and individual components of the orthopedic examination process. Part II of this text applies these general principles to the recognition and examination of injuries and conditions specific to each body region. Body regions are as follows:

- Cervical and upper thoracic spine
- Shoulder and arm
- Elbow and forearm
- Wrist and hand
- Lower thoracic and lumbar spine
- Leg, ankle, and foot
- Knee and thigh
- Hip, pelvis, and groin
- Head and face
- Thorax and abdomen

Chapters addressing each body region consist of four primary sections. Each chapter opens with a section on functional anatomy, reviewing the anatomical characteristics of the region to be examined. Recognition of injuries specific to the region are presented next, focusing on the definition, etiology, and signs and symptoms of acute and chronic injuries commonly incurred by the physically active. Specific objective tests for the region follow, including those for palpation, range of motion, strength, neurovascular, special tests, and joint mobility examinations. Each chapter concludes by incorporating these tests into specific injury examination strategies for injuries examined immediately at the site of injury, shortly following the injury, and at some time later in the treatment facility. One to two scenarios precede the discussion of each examination strategy to introduce the type of examination. Because the history and observation portions will vary considerably based on injury acuity and the environment in which the examination is performed, these components will be discussed with injury examination strategies.

Cervical and Upper Thoracic Spine

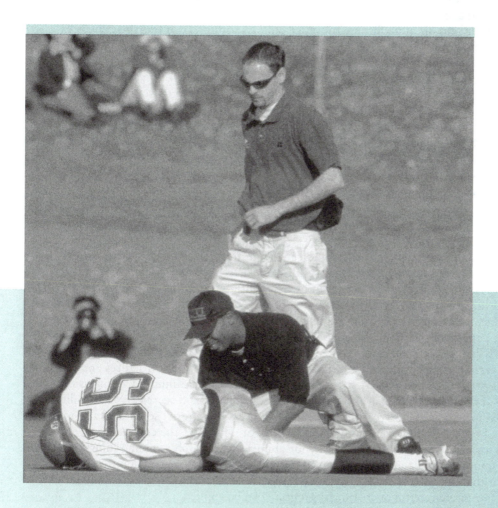

Objectives

After completing this chapter, the reader will be able to do the following:

1. Identify the causes of cervical strain
2. Identify the types of fractures in the cervical spine and the potential for spinal cord injury associated with each
3. Discuss the causes of neuropathy in the upper extremity relative to cervical spine pathology
4. Conduct a neurological exam for the upper extremity, including sensory, motor, and reflex testing

5. Perform an on-site examination for a suspected spinal cord injury and determine when the injury is serious
6. Perform an acute examination for the cervical spine region
7. Perform a clinical examination for the cervical spine region

oug was the starting linebacker for his high school football team. He never missed a game and the team relied heavily on his talent. During a game one evening, he went to make a tackle, using the top of his shoulder to make contact. Upon contact, he felt a shooting pain down his arm. He was able to get up and walk off the field under his own power but immediately sought out Jeff, the certified athletic trainer who was covering the game.

"Jeff, I need your help, man," Doug said, holding his arm.

Jeff was already on his way toward Doug—he had seen the tackle. He had also observed that Doug was a little slow to get up and that as he walked off the field he was leaning to the right with his arm hanging, appearing to be in pain. "What happened?" Jeff asked, already having a good idea from what he had seen.

"I went to make this tackle and hit him with my shoulder. All of a sudden I got this shooting and burning pain going down my arm. It's kinda hard to lift my arm," Doug said.

"Do you have pain in your neck?" Jeff asked.

"No, just my arm—but you know what, the pain is letting up now. . . . Yeah, I think I'm all right. I'm ready to go back in," Doug said, as he had stopped feeling concerned and was anxious to get back in the game. As he spoke, he started to head for the coach to say he was good to go.

"Hold up a minute," Jeff said. "We need to take a look first and make sure you have your full strength back. You can wait a couple more plays." Doug was impatient, but cooperative.

Upon completing his full examination, Jeff found that Doug's pain had not resolved. He also noted some sensory changes in Doug's lateral arm and weakness with shoulder abduction and biceps strength. Until these signs and symptoms subsided, Doug would remain a spectator.

Injuries to the cervical and thoracic spine can range from relatively minor to severe and life threatening. Traumatic injuries that result from severe whiplash, hyperflexion, or axial loading forces through the head can result in spinal instability and injury to the spinal cord. Faulty posture and work or study mechanics, poor sleeping positions, degenerative changes in the spine, athletics-related trauma, and even auto accidents frequently cause a variety of soft tissue pathologies in the physically active. Chronic conditions involving the neck can be particularly troublesome, becoming more severe over time. Prolonged stress and repetitive force (as seen in contact sports) can eventually affect joint and bony structures and weaken soft tissue structures, making an area more susceptible to acute injury. Compression and irritation of the nerve roots may also result from both chronic and acute cervical conditions, causing symptoms in the extremities such as radiating pain, altered sensation, and muscle weakness. Because of the varied nature and severity of injuries to the cervical spine and the potential for catastrophic consequences, your ability to accurately examine injuries in this area is paramount. Your examination must correctly decipher causes, identify preexisting conditions that may set the athlete up for an injury, and discern tissue structures involved so that an appropriate referral or treatment program can be applied.

FUNCTIONAL ANATOMY

The vertebral column includes 33 vertebrae: 7 cervical, 12 thoracic, 5 lumbar, 5 fused sacral, and 4 coccyx. The typical vertebra has a body, a vertebral arch consisting of two pedicles and two laminae, a spinous process, superior and inferior articular processes, and transverse processes (figure 11.1a-b). Note that the first (**atlas**) and second (**axis**) cervical vertebrae are specialized for head movement. The arch and body surround the vertebral foramen, creating a space along the entire vertebral column known as the **vertebral canal**. The canal houses and protects the delicate spinal cord. Vertebra fracture or dislocation can traumatize the spinal cord and partially or completely paralyze the structures innervated below the injury site. Each two adjacent vertebrae create an opening known as the intervertebral foramen. It is through these openings that the paired spinal nerves leave the vertebral column to innervate the trunk and extremities (figure 11.2). Between the bodies of each two adjacent vertebrae lies

Nucleus pulposus is the soft, inner substance of the intervertebral disc.

the intervertebral disc, which consists of outer fibrous rings known as the annulus fibrosus and a soft inner mucoid material known as the nucleus pulposus (figure 11.3). A bulging or herniation of the nucleus pulposus against or through the annulus fibrosus can apply pressure to a spinal nerve where it exits the vertebral column through the intervertebral foramen. This pressure causes the burning, numbness, and muscular weakness and atrophy commonly associated with a ruptured disk. Such injuries are most commonly seen in the cervical and lumbar regions, resulting in symptoms in the upper and lower extremities, respectively.

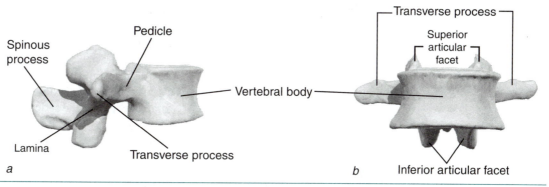

Figure 11.1 Anatomical landmarks of the typical vertebra in *(a)* lateral and *(b)* anterior views.

Images courtesy of Primal Pictures, Ltd.

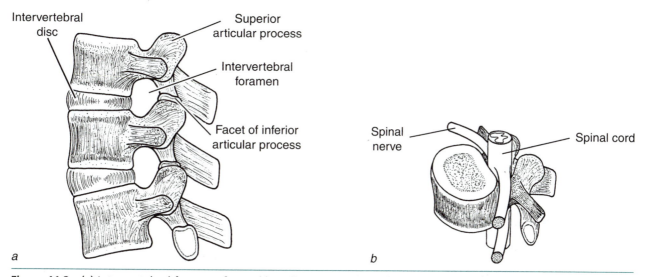

Figure 11.2 (a) Intervertebral foramen formed by adjacent vertebrae; (b) spinal cord enclosed in the vertebral canal and spinal nerve exiting through intervertebral foramen.

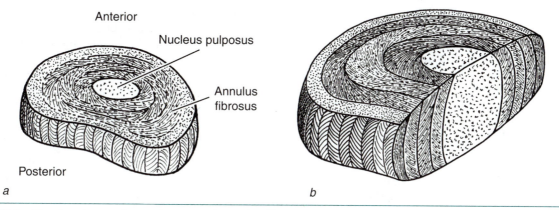

Figure 11.3 Disc showing nucleus pulposus and annulus fibrosus.

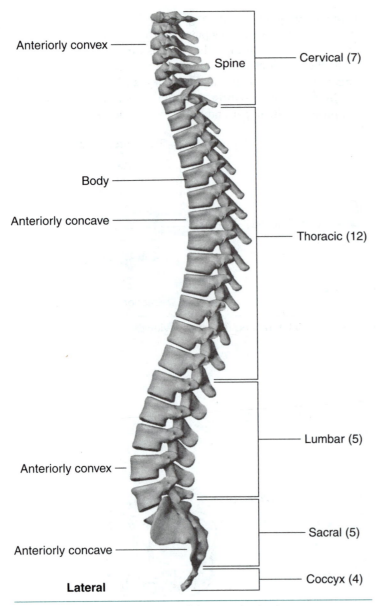

Anteriorly convex

Spine

Cervical (7)

Body

Anteriorly concave

Thoracic (12)

Lumbar (5)

Anteriorly convex

Sacral (5)

Anteriorly concave

Coccyx (4)

Lateral

Figure 11.4   Normal curvature of the vertebral column.

The vertebral column bends in four normal curves: the cervical, thoracic, lumbar, and sacral (figure 11.4). These curves enhance the vertebral column's ability to bear weight. Flexion of the head and neck as in diving and illegal spear tackling in football straightens the cervical curve and increases the axial loading forces that result from contact with the top of the head. This is one reason spear tackling and diving in shallow water carry the potential for catastrophic injuries (fractures and dislocations) to the cervical spine.

Cervical spine movements include flexion, extension, lateral flexion and extension, and rotation. Specialized articulations between the skull and atlas (**atlantooccipital joint**) and the atlas and axis (**atlantoaxial joint**) permit remarkable head mobility. The atlantooccipital joint permits flexion and extension, and the atlantoaxial joint permits rotation. The least amount of movement of the spine occurs in the thoracic region, largely because that is where the ribs attach to the vertebral column. The muscles that move the cervical spine are numerous and complex. In general, the posterior muscles (rectus and obliquus capitis, longissimus, splenius, semispinalis, iliocostalis, spinalis, multifidi, and rotator muscles) contribute to extension, rotation, and lateral flexion of the cervical spine and skull. The trapezius muscle assists with extension and rotation of the skull. The sternocleidomastoid muscle produces flexion, lateral flexion, and rotation of the skull to the side opposite the acting muscle.

The nerve roots of the brachial plexus originate from the fifth cervical to first thoracic vertebrae (see figure 8.6, page 128). The C5 and C6 roots converge to form the upper trunk, C7 becomes the middle trunk, and the C8 and T1 roots become the lower trunk. (Note that the C5 root exits the column above C5 and the C8 nerve root exits below C7). The trunks give rise to anterior and posterior divisions. The anterior divisions of the upper and middle trunks become the lateral cord, the anterior division of the lower trunk becomes the medial cord, and the posterior divisions of all three trunks become the posterior cord. From the cords continue the terminal nerves that innervate the muscles and skin of the upper extremity. You must have a thorough understanding of the brachial plexus to examine injuries of the cervical spine and upper extremity (see chapter 8, pages 127-131 for more information on the structure, function, and innervations of the brachial plexus).

CERVICAL AND UPPER THORACIC SPINE INJURIES

Cervical and upper thoracic spine injuries can range from minor to catastrophic. Because the cervical spine sacrifices stability for greater mobility, it is more prone to injury than the relatively stable thoracic spine. This section focuses on the etiology and signs and symptoms of common traumatic injuries and chronic dysfunctions of the cervical and upper thoracic spine. Catastrophic cervical injuries are discussed later in this chapter.

Acute Soft Tissue Injuries

Acute soft tissue injuries can result from direct contact, acute overstretch, or mechanical overload mechanisms. Sprains and strains make up the majority of injuries seen in the cervical and thoracic spine. Because the injury mechanisms and resulting symptoms are often similar, you may find it difficult to differentiate a sprain from a strain. Both commonly occur with traumatic injury.

Contusions

Contusions can result from a direct blow to either the soft tissue or the bony prominences of the neck. Although cervical contusions are uncommon, they can cause considerable pain and other symptoms. Signs and symptoms include pain, muscle spasm and decreased range of motion (ROM). A blow to the base of the neck can also traumatize the brachial plexus, resulting in numbness and weakness in the upper extremity.

Sprains

Cervical and upper thoracic sprains involve the ligamentous and capsular structures that stabilize and connect the vertebrae and their facet joints. Sprains to the cervical and upper thoracic region most often result from compression, or jamming, of the spine into extension. However, cervical sprains may also occur during forceful hyperflexion, hyperextension, or rotational movements. Sudden, forced extension followed by sudden, forced flexion is referred to as **cervical whiplash**. This mechanism can occur in sports and motor vehicle accidents and can result in a combined sprain–strain injury. Typical signs and symptoms include neck or interscapular pain, or both, depending on the location of injury. Particularly during muscle activity, pain may also be noted in the muscles attaching near the injured joint. ROM will be restricted and painful in the direction that stresses either the injured muscle or ligament. Neurological symptoms are rarely associated with acute cervical sprains. Any muscular weakness is usually secondary to an unwillingness to fully exert the neck musculature because of pain.

Strains

Acute strains of the cervical and upper thoracic musculature are common. Frequently involved muscles include the levator scapula, trapezius, rhomboid, sternocleidomastoid, scalene, and the extensor muscle group. Isolated muscular strains often result from a single episode of mechanical overload or from violent stretching into flexion, extension, or rotation, as in a whiplash injury. Chronic overuse or poor posture can precipitate what appear to be acute strains, as chronic stress can fatigue postural muscles, making them more susceptible to mechanical overload.

Signs and symptoms of cervical and thoracic strain include muscular pain, point tenderness, spasm, and decreased ROM. These symptoms are commonly delayed or gradually worsen up to 24 hours following injury as soft tissue swelling and muscle spasm increase. Pain is reproduced with either stretching or contraction of the involved musculature. Depending on the severity of the symptoms, the patient is often seen splinting, or stiffening the neck, rotating or flexing at the trunk rather than the neck to avoid painful cervical motion. Although cervical and thoracic strains are usually not serious, when poorly managed or left untreated they can lead to muscular weakness or dysfunction and make the muscle more susceptible to recurrent injury.

Chronic or Overuse Soft Tissue Injuries

Many chronic or overuse soft tissue injuries in the cervical and thoracic spine are caused by joint and muscular dysfunction resulting from poor posture and recurrent sprains or strains. The mobile cervical region is particularly susceptible to chronic soft tissue injuries. These injuries can lead to permanent **degenerative** changes if left untreated, so refer any patient complaining of chronic neck pain, decreased ROM, or any hint of neurological symptoms for a thorough cervical spine examination.

Degenerative Disc Disease

Annulus fibrosis *is the outer fibrous covering of the intervertebral disc that withstands tension and prevents distortion of disc material.*

Degenerative disc changes can occur with recurrent sprains and chronic joint dysfunction. The annulus fibrosis can be weakened or damaged with repetitive injury or stress, reducing disc height and shock-absorbing capability. While the degenerative disc may be asymptomatic and unrecognized for some time, secondary problems resulting from the diminished disc space include impingement of the facet joints, degenerative changes of the bony surfaces, and increased susceptibility to nerve impingement within the intervertebral foramen (Wroble and Albright 1986).

Facet Syndrome

Chronic inflammatory and degenerative changes can affect the facet joints. Chronic inflammation, scarring, and fibrosis of the capsule can result from extension overload, repetitive sprains, and impingement secondary to disc degeneration. Signs and symptoms include pain and decreased motion at the facet joints. Pain is usually exacerbated with extension and rotation to the involved side. Chronic inflammation of the facet joint can also cause irritation of the nearby nerve root.

Chronic Cervical Joint Instabilities

As with any joint, a potential complication of cervical sprains is chronic joint instability. Instability of the cervical spine has serious implications in that hypermobility can increase the neurological structures' risk for injury. Instabilities are not easily identifiable during injury examination and typically require radiographic examination in flexion and extension views, so always refer patients who sustain a cervical sprain to a physician in order to rule out resulting instabilities.

Bone and Joint Pathologies

Bone and joint pathologies are among the most potentially serious and life-threatening injuries of the cervical spine. These structures are intimately associated with and serve to protect the spinal cord and nerve roots. When forces exerted on the cervical spine are sufficient to displace bone and joint structures, catastrophic injury may result.

Cervical Spine Fractures, Dislocations, and Subluxations

The primary cause of cervical fractures, dislocations, and subluxations is headfirst contact, which compresses and buckles the cervical spine as it is forced to decelerate the still-moving torso (figure 11.5). The mechanisms that contribute to various cervical spine pathologies are not necessarily based on head movement, but rather on the direction of the impact and resulting buckling or bending forces acting on the spinal segments (Winkelstein and Myers 1997).

Regardless of mechanism, immediate recognition of the signs and symptoms associated with cervical fracture or dislocation is paramount to avoiding further injury. Signs and symptoms may include central spine pain, tenderness with palpation of the involved spinous processes, muscle spasm, position deformity, and an unwillingness to move the neck. Neurologic symptoms of associated cord injury include bilateral sensory deficits (burning hands, paresthesia, numbness, or loss of sensation), motor weakness, and paralysis in the upper and lower extremities. The level of spinal injury may be determined by examining the patterns

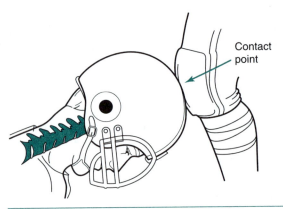
Contact point

Figure 11.5 Spearing with the head may buckle the cervical spine.

of sensory and motor weakness. Respiratory difficulty may be noted with fractures involving C3 or C4.

Compression Mechanisms

Impact to the top of the head poses the greatest risk for catastrophic spine injury. These injuries are seen most often in motor vehicle accidents and football but can also occur in any activity or sport that involves head contact, such as ice hockey, wrestling, rugby, and gymnastics. Diving into shallow water and striking the head during recreational water activities is a frequent cause of activity-related injury. The cervical spine in its normal posture has a lordotic curve that increases its capacity to absorb energy. However, when the cervical spine is flexed to about 30°, it becomes a straight, segmented column. When an athlete makes contact with an opponent or immovable object with the top of the head and the spine in this flexed position (e.g., axial compression or "spearing"), stress is absorbed primarily by the vertebral bodies rather than by the neck musculature. Because the compressive force acts perpendicular to the cervical spine, the head is unable to move to one side or the other and escape the compressive force (Winkelstein and Myers 1997). Once the spinal column reaches its maximum energy-absorbing capacity, it will fail and fracture or buckle.

Depending on the resulting bending or rotational forces acting on the spinal segment, a variety of fractures or dislocations may occur. Figure 11.6 provides a graphic example of the relationship between resulting forces and type of cervical spine injury typically produced. Burst, wedge, and compression fractures of the vertebral bodies may occur at any level in the cervical spine.

Burst Fracture

A **burst fracture** at C1, also known as a **Jefferson fracture**, rarely results in spinal cord damage, unless displacement is severe, because the spinal canal is rather large at this level.

Hangman's Fracture

Similarly, a fracture of the pedicle or pars of C2 (**hangman's fracture**) can also occur without spinal cord injury. Signs and symptoms associated with C1 and C2 fractures without neurologic involvement include cervical pain and limited ROM. Because the spinal canal narrows as it descends, burst fractures of vertebral bodies C3 and below commonly involve some level of cord pathology, resulting in quadriplegia. When spinal cord injury does occur above C3, the injury is fatal, since innervation for respiratory muscle function is lost.

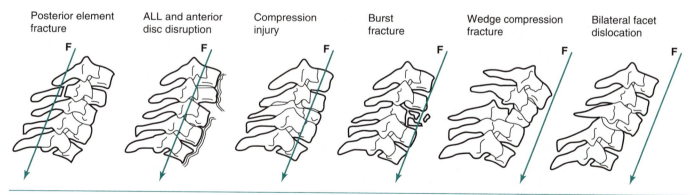

Posterior element fracture | ALL and anterior disc disruption | Compression injury | Burst fracture | Wedge compression fracture | Bilateral facet dislocation

Figure 11.6   Cervical spine injuries resulting from various forces.

Reprinted, by permission, from B.A. Winkelstein and B.S. Myers, 1997, "The biomechanics of cervical spine injury and implications for injury prevention," *Medicine and Science in Sports and Exercise* 29(7 Suppl): S246-255.

Cervical Vertebral Dislocation

Dislocation of the cervical vertebrae can occur with or without fracture because of the **transverse** orientation of the facet joints (figure 11.7). Typically, the superior vertebra translates anteriorly, causing the superior facets to ride forward and lock anterior to the inferior facets. Isolated unilateral facet dislocations occur most often when axial loading is combined with rotational and forward flexion moments. Neurological involvement is likely and may involve both the nerve root and spinal cord. Bilateral facet dislocation typically results from flexion buckling of the spine with axial loading and almost certainly causes some level of spinal cord injury, particularly in the absence of an associated fracture.

Hyperflexion and Hyperextension Mechanisms

Although impact to the face or the posterior head poses a substantially lower risk to the cervical spine than impact to the top of the head, it can nevertheless cause significant injury. Pure hyperflexion injuries can compress the anterior body and tear the posterior ligaments. Since contact of the chin with the chest limits flexion, dislocation and neurological involvement are less common with pure flexion mechanisms (Marks, Bell, and Boumphrey 1990). With hyperextension mechanism, resulting from face first contact, patients who have normal cervical spines are at a low risk for fractures or neurologic injury. However, patients with spinal stenosis or osteophytes may have an increased risk for neurologic compression with pure extension mechanisms.

Spinous Process Fractures

Although uncommon, spinous process fractures of the cervical and thoracic spine can result from either hyperflexion or extension mechanisms. Contact or impingement of adjacent spinous processes can cause a push-off fracture with hyperextension mechanisms. Avulsion fractures secondary to traction of attaching ligaments may occur with hyperflexion injuries (figure 11.8). Signs and symptoms associated with spinous process fractures include localized pain, tenderness to palpation, and pain with extreme flexion and extension movements. Neurological injury is not typically associated with these fractures.

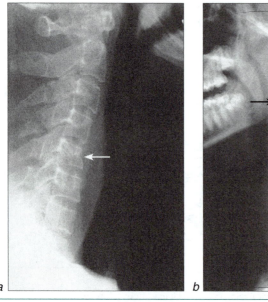
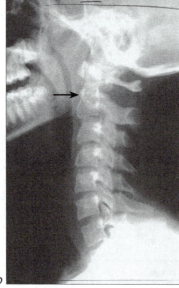

Figure 11.7 *(a)* Compression fracture of C5 and dislocation of C3 and C4, and *(b)* subluxation of C2 on C3.

Courtesy of Theodore E. Keats.

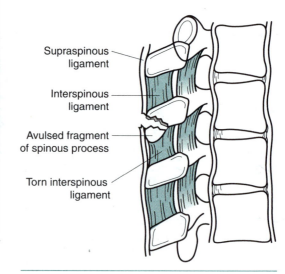

Supraspinous ligament

Interspinous ligament

Avulsed fragment of spinous process

Torn interspinous ligament

Figure 11.8 Spinous process avulsion fracture.

Defects and Abnormalities Secondary to Trauma or Repetitive Stress

Although degenerative joint conditions are more commonly seen in older adults, younger people can also exhibit degenerative bony changes due to traumatic injury or repetitive insult. These changes are most commonly seen in athletes involved in contact and collision sports such as football and rugby. Complications associated with the degenerative bony changes include structural malalignment, narrowing of the spinal canal or intervertebral foramen resulting in nerve compression, and increased risk of nerve injury.

Osteophytes

Osteophytes, or **bone spurs,** can arise from the **uncinate processes** of the vertebral bodies secondary to degenerative disc changes that increase wear and compression of the joint surfaces. Osteophytes are most commonly found posterolaterally but can also be found anteriorly. Posterolateral osteophytes can narrow the intervertebral foramen, resulting in nerve root compression and increased susceptibility to brachial plexus neuropraxia (figure 11.9). Osteophytes can also straighten the spinal column, reducing its capacity for axial loading. Signs and symptoms associated with osteophytic changes include decreased ROM, postural changes, neck discomfort that increases with lateral rotation and extension, and neurological symptoms that increase as intervertebral narrowing progresses.

Spinal Stenosis

Spinal stenosis is more often found in older adults and is characterized by a developmental or congenital narrowing of the cervical spinal canal. Spinal stenosis can be disabling for anyone, but it is of particular concern in contact sports and may disqualify an athlete from participation because of the greater risk of spinal cord injury. The narrowed spinal canal increases the risk for cord compression and injuries resulting from hyperextension or hyperflexion mechanisms. When these factors are coupled with secondary complications such as cervical spine instability or disc herniation, the risk for spinal cord injury is further increased.

Nerve and Vascular Injuries

Nerve and vascular injuries associated with the cervical spine are typically caused by bone or soft tissue encroaching into the spinal canal or intervertebral foramen spaces, causing compression of the neurovascular structures that run through that space (figure 11.10).

Spinal Cord Injury and Transient Neuropraxia

Although the spinal cord is well protected within the spinal column, neurological complications can result from either acute trauma or chronic degenerative changes.

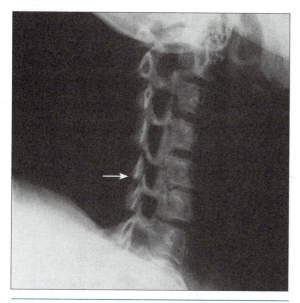

Figure 11.9   Posterolateral osteophytes and narrowing of the intervertebral foramen.

Courtesy of Theodore E. Keats.

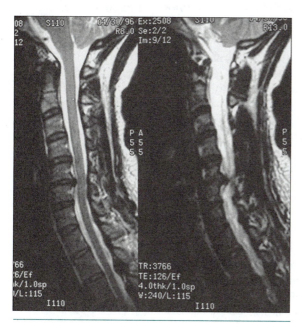

Figure 11.10   Encroachment and compression of the spinal cord and nerve root by a herniated disc.

Transient Neuropraxia

As previously discussed, spinal cord injury can be a consequence of acute fractures and dislocation of the cervical and upper thoracic spine and range from contusions to complete severance of the cord. Central cord compression and **transient neuropraxia** can also result secondary to posterior disc herniation, spinal stenosis, congenital fusion, or instability in the cervical spine. Signs and symptoms of transient neuropraxia include sensory changes, such as burning, tingling, or numbness, and motor changes ranging from weakness to temporary paralysis in both the upper and lower extremities (Torg et al. 1996). These symptoms usually subside within a few minutes but may persist for 1 to 2 days. Regardless of the cause, bilateral neurological symptoms in either the upper or lower extremities and bowel or bladder dysfunctions indicate central cord involvement, and you should refer anyone presenting with any of these symptoms for further examination.

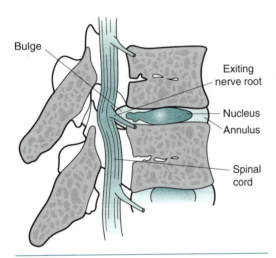

Figure 11.11 Posterolateral disc herniation compressing the exiting nerve root.

Labels: Bulge; Exiting nerve root; Nucleus; Annulus; Spinal cord

Nerve Root Injury and Compression Syndromes

Nerve root injury can be caused by either stretch or compressive mechanisms resulting from acute trauma or chronic mechanical stress. Injury may involve a single nerve root due to encroachment of a herniated disc or osteophyte formation, or may involve multiple nerve roots with brachial plexus traction injuries.

Intervertebral Disc Herniation

Cervical disc **herniation** can result from acute trauma causing compression, flexion, or extension of the cervical spine. More often, it is caused by a gradual weakening or failure of the annulus fibrosis secondary to chronic or repetitive mechanical stress. Examples of mechanical stress conditions include poor posture, poor body mechanics, and excessive or limited segmental mobility. The cervical levels most often affected are C4-C5 and C5-C6 (involving the C5 and C6 nerve roots, respectively) because of their exceptional mobility and susceptibility to everyday stress. Because the disc is stronger anteriorly and the posterior longitudinal ligament is firmly attached to the central-posterior body of the vertebrae and disc, most herniations occur posterolaterally (figure 11.11). As a result, the herniated disc material typically protrudes into the intervertebral foramen, compressing and irritating the exiting nerve root. Occasionally, if the posterior longitudinal ligament is disrupted, the disc material may protrude centrally into the spinal canal, causing cord compression.

Symptoms associated with neurological compression typically cause the patient to seek medical care. Signs and symptoms of cervical disc herniation and associated nerve compression include pain and discomfort that improves with cervical distraction and worsens with extension and rotation to the side. Rotational pain may be ipsilateral or contralateral, depending on the location of the herniation relative to the nerve root. The patient exhibits decreased ROM and muscular splinting, tilting the head away from or toward the involved side to avoid compressive and painful positions.

Nerve root compression refers pain along the distribution of the involved nerve. Neurological deficits such as sensory deficits, motor weakness, or diminished reflex may also be present. Muscle atrophy may be observed in chronic cases. The disc protrusion may also cause additional signs and symptoms associated with spinal cord compression, including bowel and bladder dysfunction, sensory or motor changes in the lower limbs, and episodes of decreased coordination or tripping with no apparent cause. Disc herniation and neurological encroachment are typically confirmed with radiographic examination such as computed tomography, magnetic resonance imaging, or myelogram studies.

Brachial Plexus Injury

Brachial plexus injury involves mechanical deformation of the C5 through T1 nerve roots as they exit the cervical spine (see figures 8.6 and 12.4). Injury to the brachial plexus occurs most frequently in sports such as football and less often in wrestling, rugby, and water skiing. Brachial plexus injury can result from either traction or compression mechanisms. A pinch type of injury occurs when the neck is rotated, laterally flexed, and compressed or extended to the same side, closing down the intervertebral foramen and impinging the nerve roots. Compression injuries can also occur secondary to a direct blow to the base of the neck, particularly when the neck is flexed away from the involved side and the brachial plexus is stretched. Conversely, a stretch injury occurs when the head is forced laterally away from the shoulder while at the same time the shoulder is forced downward. Although these forces can be sufficient to seriously disrupt the integrity of the nerve **(neurotmesis),** typically the injury transiently blocks nerve function (due to mechanical deformation) but causes little or no structural disruption (neuropraxia).

Brachial plexus injuries are often termed **stingers** or **burners** because of the classical symptom of immediate sharp, burning pain radiating into the arm at the time of injury. The patient will also complain of temporary weakness or inability to move the arm. Symptoms may be reproduced with lateral flexion away from the stabilized shoulder, or with flexion and extension toward the involved side. Symptoms associated with brachial plexus injury are usually short-lived and the extremity typically regains full function within minutes. However, neurological symptoms may persist for a few days or even months, depending on the severity of nerve disruption. In rare cases involving sufficient trauma to cause a neurotmesis, permanent neurological deficits and muscle wasting result.

The distribution of motor and sensory weakness localizes the level of the nerve root lesion. Since injury most often involves the upper trunk, or nerve roots C5 and C6, residual numbness and motor weakness will most often be noted in the deltoid, biceps, and medial and lateral shoulder rotators. Wrist and thumb extensor weakness is also common. Note an important distinction between brachial plexus injury and cervical spine injury: Brachial plexus injuries typically do not result in central cervical spine pain or loss of cervical motion. Therefore, when you find these symptoms associated with a suspected brachial plexus injury, further examine for possible cervical spine involvement before allowing the athlete to return to activity. In a patient who experiences repeated or recurrent brachial plexus injuries, carefully evaluate the cervical spine for spinal stenosis or other degenerative conditions that may increase the potential for nerve traction or impingement.

> ⚠ Carefully evaluate the cervical spine in patients who suffer repeated or recurrent brachial plexus injuries to rule out spinal stenosis or other degenerative conditions that may increase the potential for nerve tension or impingement.

Vascular Compression

Thoracic outlet syndrome (TOS) describes compression of the neurovascular structures as they exit through the thoracic outlet.

Thoracic Outlet Syndrome

The thoracic outlet is marked by the anterior scalene muscle anteriorly, the middle scalene posteriorly, and the first rib inferiorly. Structures that exit through the thoracic outlet into the upper extremity include the brachial plexus and the subclavian artery (figure 11.12). As these neurovascular structures proceed into the axillary region, there are three primary locations where compression may occur due to encroachment of either bony or soft tissue structures. The most proximal and common site of compression is the interscalene triangle, where compression can be caused by hypertrophy, tightness, or fibrotic bands within the anterior or middle scalene muscles or, in rare cases, by the presence of a cervical rib. Moving further distally, compression may occur within the costoclavicular space between the first rib and the posterior clavicle. Narrowing within this space can result from hypertrophy of the subclavian muscle or from an encroaching posterior angulation or callous formation following a clavicular fracture. The third common location of compression is the insertion of the pectoralis minor at the coracoid process. As the neurovascular structures pass under the tendon, compression can occur between the tendon and the coracoid process, particularly when the arm is abducted.

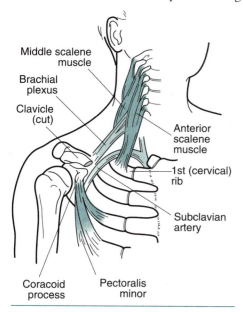

Middle scalene muscle
Brachial plexus
Clavicle (cut)
Anterior scalene muscle
1st (cervical) rib
Subclavian artery
Coracoid process
Pectoralis minor

Figure 11.12 Location and structures involved in TOS.

Incidence of TOS is more common in women than in men. TOS also prevails in patients with postural imbalances, such as rounded or depressed (drooping) shoulders, which can strain the scapular stabilizing muscles and further traction the neurovascular bundle. In many cases, TOS occurs secondary to a previous trauma or injury that results in residual swelling, muscular imbalance, or altered shoulder or scapular mechanics.

TOS involves neurological structures more often than vascular structures, with compression of the lower trunk of the brachial plexus being the most common pathology. Because of the multiple anatomical sites where compression can occur and the neurovascular structures that can be involved, symptoms can vary considerably. Therefore, signs and symptoms may include pain anywhere between the neck, face, and occipital region or into the chest, shoulder, and upper extremity. The patient may also complain of altered or absent sensation, weakness, fatigue, or a feeling of heaviness in the arm and hand. There may be swelling and discoloration. Signs and symptoms are typically worse when the arm is abducted overhead and externally rotated with the head rotated to the same or the opposite side. As a result, activities such as overhead throwing, serving a tennis ball, or painting a ceiling may exacerbate symptoms. Because of the complexity of symptoms and their similarity to other cervical conditions, you may find it difficult to determine TOS.

Structural and Functional Abnormalities

Postural deviations are commonly seen in the cervical and thoracic spines. Postural deviations may be functional, resulting from pain, muscular imbalance, or poor posture, or they may involve permanent structural changes that can be debilitating and disfiguring.

Forward Head Posture

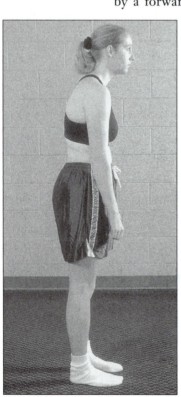

The most common acquired postural deviation is a forward head posture, characterized by a forward alignment of the head relative to the shoulders, rounded shoulders, and increased extension of the lower cervical spine in order to maintain an upright head position (figure 11.13). This posture can be caused by pain avoidance secondary to cervical injury but more commonly results from muscle imbalances developed over time or from poor postural mechanics. Muscle imbalances can occur when a patient strengthens the anterior pectoral muscles and ignores the upper back muscles. This results in tight pectoral muscles and lengthened and weakened rhomboid and trapezius muscles. Other contributing factors include poor sitting posture (slouching) and study habits.

Regardless of the contributing factor, the posterior postural muscles have to work much harder against gravity in order to keep the head upright as compared to the situation with a neutral posture. Therefore it is common for affected patients to report muscular discomfort secondary to chronic overuse and muscular fatigue. If the underlying postural mechanics and muscular imbalances are not recognized and corrected, degenerative disc and joint changes can result from increased mechanical stress over time.

Torticollis

Torticollis is a soft tissue condition in the neck that draws the head to one side and usually rotates it to the opposite side. It is also referred to as **wryneck** or **stiff neck.** This condition affects the sternocleidomastoid muscle and can be either congenital or acquired. Congenital torticollis is due to a fibrous tumor in one of the sternocleidomastoid muscles that may either subside as the infant ages or shorten the muscle. More commonly, the condition is caused by spasm of the sternocleidomastoid muscle. The patient presents with a stiff neck and pain with attempts to align the head to the midline.

Figure 11.13   Forward head posture.

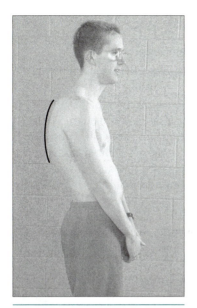

Figure 11.14   Kyphosis.

Kyphosis and Scheuermann's Disease

Kyphosis is an excessive posterior curvature of the thoracic spine (figure 11.14). The upper thoracic spine normally has a rounded contour, but this curve can be accentuated secondarily to congenital factors, compensatory changes, muscular imbalance, joint disease, compression fractures, osteoporosis in older adults, and Scheuermann's disease in youth. **Scheuermann's disease** is a growth disorder characterized by inflammation and osteochondritis of the thoracic vertebrae. This degenerative condition wedges or narrows the anterior vertebral body at three or more levels secondary to axial and flexion overload. An active condition may contraindicate sport participation and often increases pain with activity and forward flexion movements. Patients with a history of Scheuermann's disease may complain of occasional pain, muscular fatigue, and spasm associated with the increased kyphosis.

OBJECTIVE TESTS

Objective tests for the cervical and upper thoracic spine include observation, palpation, ROM, strength, neurological, and special tests that examine nerve compression, brachial plexus neuropathy, and cervical disc and neurovascular dysfunction. Pertinent tests and strategies for history and observation are discussed specific to on-site, acute, and clinical examinations later in this chapter.

Palpation

Begin to palpate superficially and proceed from the superficial muscles to deep muscles, noting any restricted skin or fascia movement. Use a systematic approach to avoid accidentally omitting any muscle. You can begin palpation in the superior posterior neck at the occiput and move distally to the upper thoracic region. Systematically examine the lateral neck and then the anterior neck from a superior to an inferior approach.

- **Posterior structures.** The spinous processes can be palpated posteriorly. C2, C6, C7, and the upper thoracic spinous process are usually easily palpated, but C3, C4, and C5 usually lie more anterior and can be difficult to differentiate. Palpate the spinous processes for point tenderness and palpate the base of the occiput and ligamentum nuchae for tenderness and restriction. Palpate the upper trapezius, levator scapulae, spleni group, and paraspinal muscles for soft tissue restriction, trigger points, muscle spasm, and areas of tenderness.

- **Lateral structures.** Palpation of lateral structures includes lateral fibers of the upper trapezius and sternocleidomastoid muscles. The C1 transverse processes can be palpated slightly inferiorly and laterally from the mastoid process behind the ear. These slight nubs are commonly tender, but the right and left transverse processes should feel balanced, with the same degree of protrusion and tenderness on each side.

- **Anterior structures.** The main anterior bony structures to palpate are the hyoid bone, thyroid cartilage, and first cricoid ring. These structures are most prominent when the patient is supine and the anterior muscles are relaxed. The hyoid bone is superior to the thyroid cartilage, at the level of C3 vertebral body. Move inferiorly until you feel the Adam's apple, which is the superior portion of the thyroid cartilage at the level of C4. Next is the first cricoid ring, located at the base of the lower edge of the thyroid cartilage at the level of C6. The first cricoid ring is just superior to the site for performing an emergency tracheostomy. Other structures to be palpated include the distal insertion of the sternocleidomastoid, the scalenes, the first rib, the anterior lymph nodes, and the carotid arteries. The scalenes, which lie lateral to the sternocleidomastoid and superior to the clavicle, are often tender to palpation in persons with a forward head posture. The lymph nodes will only be palpable if they are enlarged.

Range of Motion

ROM testing includes active, passive, and goniometric examinations.

Active ROM

Full active motion should be available in all cervical motions. As the patient performs the motions, there should be no hesitation of movement. Watch for changes in the patient's facial expressions for indications of pain or difficulty with the motion. Full cervical flexion allows the chin to touch the chest (figure 11.15a); full extension lets the eyes point straight to the ceiling and produces a straight vertical line from the chin down the throat (figure 11.15b); lateral flexion creates a 45° angle between a vertical line and a line through the nose and chin in both left and right end motions (figure 11.15c); and rotation places the chin almost in line with the tip of the shoulder (figure 11.15d). Watch forward and lateral flexion from the posterior view to observe spinal motion during these movements. These motions should create a uniform roundness of the cervical spine. If the cervical spine appears flat in any portion, there may be facet blockage or muscle spasm restrictions.

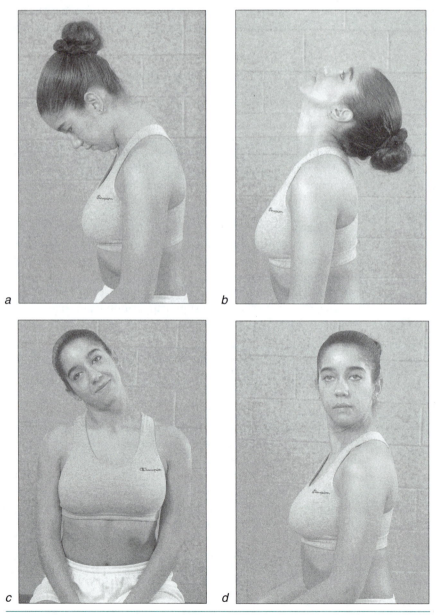

a   b   c   d

Figure 11.15   Cervical ROM: *(a)* flexion, *(b)* extension, *(c)* lateral flexion, and *(d)* rotation.

Passive ROM

Perform passive motion tests either after the patient completes all active motions or after each active motion test. If the patient experiences no pain with the active movement, follow each active motion with a gentle but full-motion passive movement. For example, after the patient fully flexes the neck, ask whether the motion causes pain. If the answer is no, apply force to the top of the head to further flex the neck. Ask whether pain occurs with this movement while you examine the motion's end feel. Before applying passive motion, observe whether a bulge occurs in the upper posterior spine during cervical flexion. If it does, you should not apply passive overpressure, since this bulge signals a possible atlas subluxation (figure 11.16). In this case you should end the examination and refer the patient to the physician.

Passive overpressure motion tests attempt to reproduce the patient's pain. Passive **overpressure** motion is applied gently on the head to move the neck in the desired direction. The motion is not quick or severe but is controlled, slow, and gentle, continuing until an endpoint is felt. However, if the patient complains of pain in the neck or of pain or sensation changes in the extremities with active motion, do not perform passive overpressure motions. Likewise, if you suspect that the cervical spine itself may have an injury such as a fracture or subluxation or may be unstable, do not perform passive overpressure motion tests.

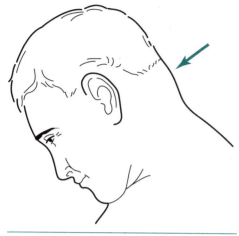

Figure 11.16   Atlas subluxation.

Goniometric Examination of ROM

Objectively measuring the active motions is easiest with a tape measure. The process is described in table 11.1 and demonstrated in figures 11.17, a through d. However, you can

Table 11.1
Tape Measure Examination of Cervical ROM

Motion	Location of tape measure	Movement	Measurement	Normal range
Forward flexion	Tip of chin to tip of sternal notch	Neck flexion (moving chin toward chest); instruct athlete to slightly tuck the chin before initiating the movement (watch for anterior jutting of the jaw)	Distance (mm) between chin and sternal notch at end range	Chin touching chest (watch for mouth opening to help chin reach chest)
Extension	Same as forward flexion	Extension of neck (looking toward the ceiling)	Same as forward flexion	Eyes pointing straight to the ceiling
Lateral flexion	Mastoid process to tip of the acromion process	Direct movement of ear toward shoulder; watch for cervical rotation and the shoulder rising to achieve motion	Distance (mm) between mastoid and acromion at end range	Head tilts bilaterally at approximately 45°
Lateral rotation	Tip of chin to tip of acromion process	Head rotation to left and right as far as possible, without contributing motions into extension, flexion, or lateral flexion	Distance (mm) between chin and acromion at end range	Approximately 90° of rotation bilaterally; chin nearly in line with acromion

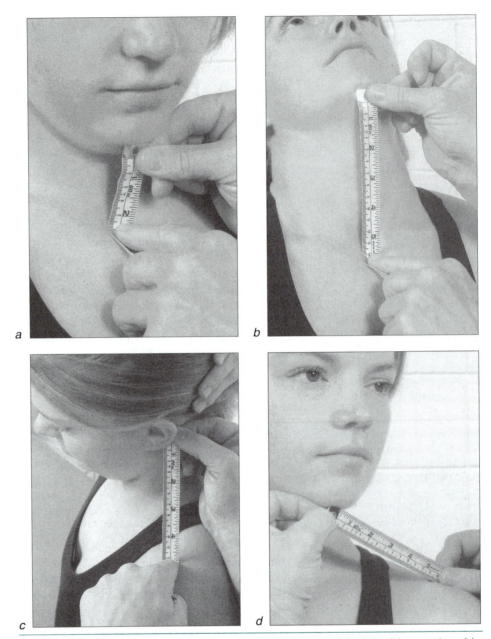

Figure 11.17   Tape measurement examination of *(a)* forward flexion, *(b)* extension, *(c)* lateral flexion, and *(d)* lateral rotation.

measure cervical ROM equally well using a goniometer, tape measure, or inclinometer. You should develop your examination skills using a single measurement method. When performing these measurements, seat the patient with the back supported. Watch for compensatory movements such as jutting the jaw (forward flexion), raising the shoulder to the ear (lateral flexion), and back extension (extension).

Strength

Isometric strength tests are performed against cervical flexion, extension, lateral flexion, and rotation with resistance provided at the head (table 11.2).

To test flexion, place the resistive hand on the forehead (figure 11.18a). To test extension, place the resistive hand on the posterior head (figure 11.18b). For lateral flexion place the resistive hand on the side of the head and the stabilizing hand on the opposite shoulder (seated)

Table 11.2
Manual Strength Tests for Cervical Motions

Motion	Athlete position	Stabilizing hand placement	Resistance hand placement	Instruction to athlete	Primary muscles tested
Cervical flexion	Supine	Thorax	Forehead	From neutral position, tuck the chin and flex the head and neck toward the chest	Sternocleidomastoid, anterior scalenes, rectus capitus anterior, longus capitus, longus colli bilaterally
Cervical extension	Prone, arms at sides, head off table	Thorax to discourage trunk extension	Posterior aspect of head	From neutral position, lift and extend head against resistance	Paravertebral extensor muscle groups (spenius, semispinalis, capitis), upper trapezius bilaterally
Lateral flexion	Seated or sidelying	Ipsilateral shoulder (sidelying) Contralateral shoulder (seated)	Lateral aspect of head	From neutral position, attempt to move ear toward shoulder	Sternocleidomastoid, scalenes, upper trapezius, and small intrinsic muscles unilaterally
Lateral rotation	Seated	Contralateral shoulder	Open palm along the lateral forehead and cheek	From neutral position, rotate the head against applied resistance	Sternocleidomastoid unilaterally

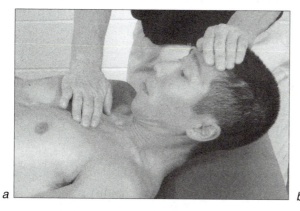
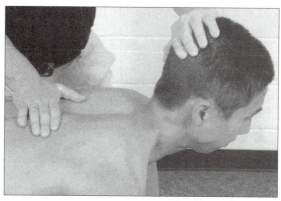
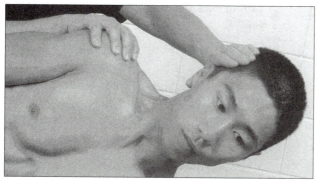
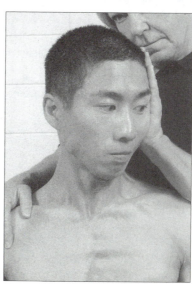

Figure 11.18 Manual strength tests for the cervical spine: *(a)* flexion, *(b)* extension, *(c)* lateral flexion, and *(d)* lateral rotation.

or same shoulder (sidelying) (figure 11.18c). Place your hands on the sides of the forehead or lateral cheek, not the jaw, since resistance at the jaw can aggravate any temporomandibular joint dysfunction the athlete may have. To test rotation strength, provide resistance with one hand and stabilize the opposite shoulder with the other hand (figure 11.18d). With each test, stabilize the athlete's upper trunk by placing a hand on the shoulder, chest, or back. You can perform these motions in a midrange position. Slowly build force until you create a maximum resistance; also be sure to release the force slowly. Be sure to tell the patient what to expect before executing each movement.

Neurological Examination

Once you have examined ROM and strength, perform neurological tests.

Neurological Tests for the Cervical Spine

The dermatome, myotome, and reflex parameters of the cervical and brachial plexus that you test depends on the level of suspected injury and whether the patient reports any sensory disturbances or weakness distal to the acromion. Examinations for the upper cervical region (C1-C4) are detailed in chapter 8 (see table 8.3 and figures 8.3-8.5). Examinations for the lower cervical region (C5-C8) are described in table 8.4 and figures 8.7, 8.9, and 8.11. These tests are summarized in table 11.3. If the patient reports no numbness, tingling, burning, or weakness distal to the acromion, a neurological examination is not necessary.

Special Tests

As previously mentioned, special tests for the cervical spine and upper thoracic region are designed to reveal neurovascular compromise secondary to nerve compression, brachial plexus pathology, disc pathology, and TOS.

Table 11.3

Dermatome, Myotome, and Reflex Testing for the Upper and Lower Cervical Spine

Nerve root	Dermatome	Myotome	Reflex
C1	Top of head	(Contributes to cervical flexion)	None
C2	Temporal, occipital regions of the head	Cervical flexion (longus colli, sternocleidomastoid, rectus capitus)	None
C3	Posterior cheek, neck	Lateral neck flexion (trapezius, splenus capitis)	None
C4	Superior shoulder, clavicle area	Shoulder shrug (trapezius, levator scapulae)	None
C5	Deltoid patch, lateral upper arm	Shoulder abduction (deltoid), elbow flexion (biceps)	Biceps (brachioradialis)
C6	Lateral forearm, radial side of hand, thumb and index finger	Elbow flexion (biceps, supinator), wrist extension	Brachioradialis (biceps)
C7	Posterior lateral arm and forearm, middle finger	Elbow extension (triceps), wrist flexion	Triceps
C8	Medial forearm, ulnar border of hand, ring and little finger	Ulnar deviation, thumb extension, finger flexion and abduction	None

Nerve Compression Tests

Compression Test

A compression test is performed in various positions. First, seat the patient and apply a downward compressive force to the top of the head with the neck in a neutral position. If this test is negative, have the patient bend the neck to the side. Apply a downward compressive force, not a lateral force, as in the first test (figure 11.19). If this test is negative, have the patient position the neck in extension and rotation to the side of complaint. Apply a direct downward compressive force as in the other tests. This last test position is also known as **Spurling's test**. With any of these positions, symptoms down the arm on the side of the cervical concavity indicate nerve root compression. In the neck, pain referred down the arm from nerve root compression is known as **cervical radiculitis**. If the patient reports pain or sensory changes on the convex side, the problem is probably muscle or soft tissue related. If the patient reports pain in the neck without radiation, the injury is probably related to soft tissue in the neck and so it is a negative test result.

Nerve Root Compression Relief Test (Shoulder Abduction Test)

If you suspect a nerve root compression or disc injury, use a relief test. Once the patient is seated, she places the hand that is on the side of the symptoms on top of her head (figure 11.20). This position decreases the nerve root pressure by reducing the traction caused by the weight of the hanging limb. A reduction in the patient's symptoms is a positive sign for nerve root compression or disc injury. If the symptoms increase, they may be secondary to TOS. This test is also known as the shoulder abduction test.

Cervical Distraction Relief Test

If the patient complains of burning, tingling, numbness, or weakness into the upper extremity, a cervical distraction relief test will confirm a nerve root compression injury. Seat the patient and place one hand at the base of the skull and the other under the chin. Gradually apply an upward distractive force to the neck by slowly lifting the head (figure 11.21). A positive sign occurs if the symptoms subside. Nerve root pressure can be further reduced and symptoms decreased if you have the patient abduct the shoulder during the test.

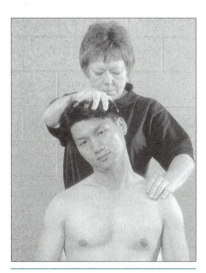

Figure 11.19 Compression test with downward compressive force to the side of the head.

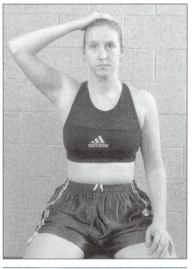

Figure 11.20 Nerve root compression relief test.

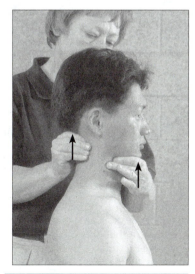

Figure 11.21 Cervical distraction relief test.

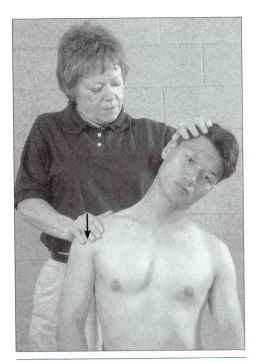

Figure 11.22   Shoulder depression test.

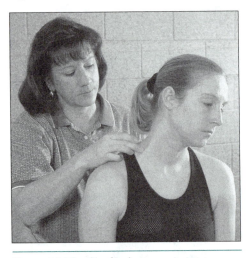

Figure 11.23   Tinel's sign.

Remember, the objective of the special tests is to reproduce the patient's symptoms during the examination. Tests that reproduce the patient's symptoms are positive. Positive tests help determine type of injury, tissue involved, and whether referral to a physician is necessary.

Brachial Plexus Neuropathy Tests

If the patient reports nerve pain, brachial plexus neuropathy tests are indicated. Nerve pain is any pain likely to be caused by nerve irritation and presents as complaints of numbness, tingling, burning, or shooting. Nerve pain is usually constant or persistent, with few episodes of relief. Results of a nerve tension test are positive when the right and the left differ in symptoms and the test reproduces or changes the symptoms. Since other soft tissue structures are stretched along with the nerve, it is common for the patient to complain of a stretch sensation or ache in the anterior shoulder, cubital fossa, wrist, or forearm during the test. Since the nerve is stretched, a normal response may be a tingling sensation in the fingers, but this sensation is different from the symptomatic results of a positive test and is usually noted bilaterally.

Shoulder Depression Test

If you suspect a brachial plexus stretch, have the patient sit down. Ask the patient to laterally flex the neck to the shoulder opposite the side with symptoms. Apply a downward pressure to the involved shoulder while applying a lateral pressure to the head (figure 11.22). A positive sign (comparable sign) confirms a brachial plexus injury.

Tinel's Sign

Pain or radiation of symptoms reproduced with nerve percussion (**Tinel's sign**) indicates pathology in the brachial plexus. To perform the test, have the patient sit with the neck slightly flexed. Then use a finger to tap each nerve root at the transverse processes (figure 11.23).

Passive Upper-Limb Tension Tests

Neuropathy tests also include upper-limb tension tests. Various limb positions are used to stetch each nerve of the brachial plexus. Although the position also stretches other soft tissue, symptoms elicited indicate the tissue affected. If the patient reports an increase in symptoms since their onset or if the injury is very acute, do not use these tests because they can aggravate the condition. The patient is supine for these tests, with the shoulder at the edge of the examination table. Passively depress the patient's shoulder girdle for each test by placing your hand on the top of the shoulder and pulling caudally. Test the median, ulnar, and radial nerves by passively placing the elbow, wrist, and hand in different positions to place the nerve on its bias, or stretch:

- To place the median nerve on bias, place the shoulder in slight abduction, lateral rotation, and full extension; the elbow in full extension; the wrist in extension; and the fingers in extension (figure 11.24a).
- To place the radial nerve on bias, place the shoulder in slight abduction, medial rotation, and extension; the elbow in full extension; the wrist in flexion and ulnar deviation; and the fingers in flexion (figure 11.24b).
- To place the ulnar nerve on bias, place the shoulder in abduction and lateral rotation; the elbow in flexion; the wrist in extension and radial deviation; and the fingers in extension (figure 11.24c).

Once you have completed each nerve bias test and the patient reports minimal or no symptoms, ask the patient to laterally flex the neck to the opposite side. Apply each joint position one at a time for each nerve bias, each time asking the patient if any symptoms are reproduced. There is no need to continue the nerve bias test if positive results occur at any time during the test.

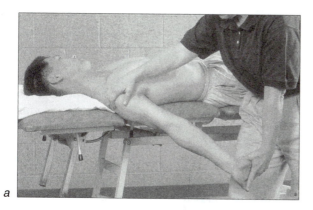

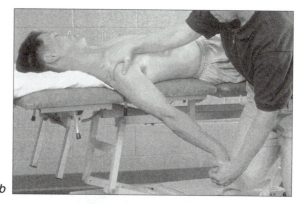

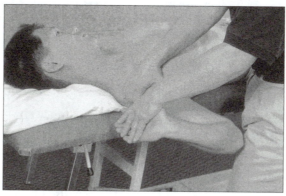

Figure 11.24   Nerve bias tests of the (a) median nerve, (b) radial nerve, and (c) ulnar nerve.

Active Upper-Limb Tension Tests

These nerve tension tests can also be performed actively as a quick examination prior to the passive bias tension tests:

- For the ulnar nerve, seat the patient and have him abduct the shoulder and place the hand of the involved side behind his head with the shoulder in full lateral rotation. The elbow is kept behind the body's mid line (figure 11.25a).

  - For the median nerve, have the patient place his arm in 90° abduction with his elbow in full extension. Then, fully laterally rotate the shoulder and move it posteriorly into horizontal extension (figure 11.25b).

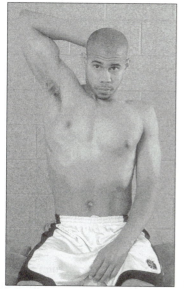

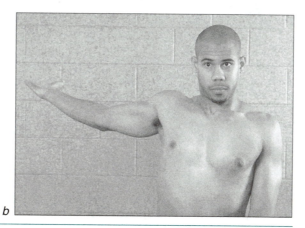

Figure 11.25   Correct position for the (a) active ulnar nerve tension test and the (b) active median nerve tension test.

Intrathecal pressure is pressure within the spinal canal.

Cervical Disc Pathology Test

If the physician has seen the patient and diagnosed a cervical disc pathology, you may perform these tests before beginning treatment so you will have a baseline by which to assess your treatment results. If the patient has not yet seen a physician and any of these tests produce positive results, refer the patient to a physician for medical tests before performing further tests or treatment.

Valsalva Maneuver

In a **Valsalva maneuver,** the patient takes a deep breath, holds it, and then bears down or blows into a closed fist (figure 11.26). These activities increase intrathecal pressure, so if swelling or a disc bulge has reduced the intervertebral space, the increase in pressure will cause a radiation of symptoms down the distribution of the compromised nerve root.

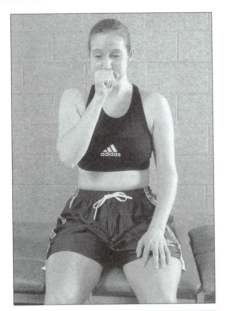

Figure 11.26 Valsalva maneuver.

Vascular Dysfunction Test

The vertebral artery test evaluates compression of the vertebral artery.

Vertebral Artery Test

Perform this test with the patient sitting or supine. Passively move the patient's neck into extension and lateral flexion, and then rotate it to the same side (figure 11.27). Hold this position for 30 seconds. The test is positive if the patient reports dizziness or if nystagmus occurs. **Nystagmus** is an involuntary lateral oscillatory movement of the eyes.

Thoracic Outlet Syndrome Tests

As has been mentioned, TOS can result from brachial plexus or subclavian artery compression from a number of primary causes. In examining TOS you should attempt to either reproduce the patient's symptoms (comparable sign) or reduce circulation, so you must observe for the presence of either of these signs. Since there are several causes of TOS, there are also several tests for identifying it. Some of the more common tests are presented here.

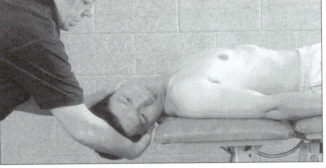

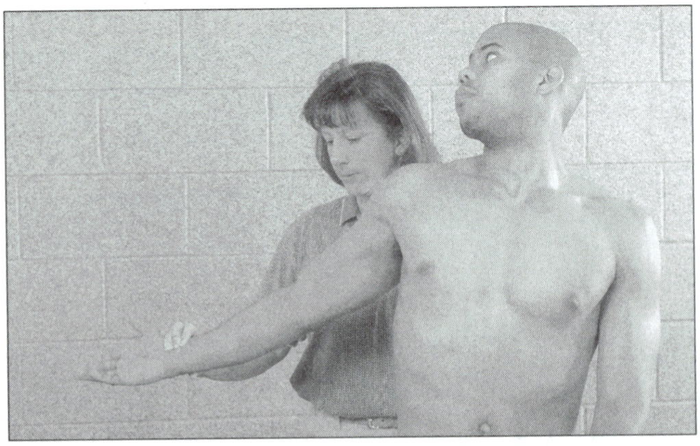

Figure 11.27 Vertebral artery test.

Adson's Test

Palpate the radial pulse of the involved side and instruct the patient to rotate the head to the same side. As he extends his neck, extend and externally rotate his shoulder (figure 11.28). In this position, have the patient take a deep breath and hold it while you palpate for a pulse. If the pulse is diminished or gone, the test is positive.

Allen Test

Locate the patient's radial pulse and then position the upper extremity with the elbow at 90° flexion and the shoulder in lateral rotation and horizontal abduction. Have the patient rotate the head away from the tested arm (figure 11.29). The test is positive if the pulse is diminished or absent.

Figure 11.28 Adson's test.

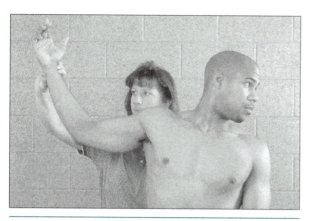

Figure 11.29   Allen test.

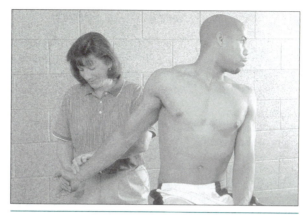

Figure 11.30   Military brace position.

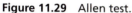

Military Brace Position

The military brace position test is also called the **costoclavicular syndrome test.** Palpate the patient's radial pulse with the elbow and shoulder in full extension. Position the shoulder into hyperextension and lateral rotation and have the patient rotate the head away from the side being tested (figure 11.30). A positive test occurs if the pulse is diminished or absent.

INJURY EXAMINATION STRATEGIES

As with any injury, your choice of tests and the comprehensiveness of your examination are dictated by the severity of the injury and the environment in which it occurred. As an allied health care professional, sometime in your career you will likely perform an on-site examination of a serious neck injury. Although these injuries don't occur often, your ability to accurately and efficiently determine the nature and extent of the injury could mean the difference between life and death or full recovery and permanent paralysis. Therefore, you should periodically practice your on-site examination skills to keep sharp and ready for when the time comes.

Most of the time, however, you will evaluate a postacute or chronic cervical injury. Examination of these injuries is sometimes difficult, as they may result from chronic postural or repetitive stresses that are unrelated to physical activity. In all cases, knowledge of which symptoms and findings dictate immediate medical referral versus conservative care is essential for the on-site, acute, and clinical examination procedures.

On-Site Examination

Consider a football player who lowers his head and makes contact with a player's chest using the top of his head, then falls to the ground, face down. He does not appear to be moving.

It is important to observe the downed athlete as you approach. Noting the position of the head and neck and observing whether the athlete is moving or lying motionless are among the most important things you do before reaching the athlete.

Primary Survey

Upon arriving at the athlete's side, do a **primary survey** to check for consciousness as well as airway, breathing, and circulation. If the athlete is facing down and not breathing, you will need to carefully logroll the athlete to a supine position, while supporting and protecting the cervical spine, in order to initiate cardiopulmonary resuscitation. If the athlete is unconscious, assume that he has a spinal cord injury.

Secondary Survey

If the primary survey is cleared and the athlete conscious, place a reassuring hand on a shoulder to keep the athlete calm, quiet, and still and to help him focus on your immediate questions. When you suspect a cervical injury, examine the athlete in the position found. An assistant should immediately stabilize the head while you examine the athlete. Until you have made your examination and proven otherwise, you must assume that the athlete has suffered a spinal cord injury.

Before moving the athlete, it is crucial to know whether there is any neck pain or any numbness, burning, or tingling in any extremity. Is the athlete having any difficulty moving the extremities? Is there any difficulty breathing or swallowing? A quick sensory test for light touch over the hands and lower legs, with comparisons of right and left sides, can confirm any suspicions. Areas to test on the hand are over the lateral thumb for C6, over the middle finger for C7, and over the little finger for C8. In the lower extremity, a light touch test can be performed over the distal anterior thigh for L3, over the anteromedial lower leg for L4, over the lateral lower leg for L5, and over the posterolateral lower leg for S1. See chapter 8 for details on these tests. If any of these signs are positive, you must assume a serious neck injury.

If all tests to this point are negative and the athlete has only neck pain, check for tenderness and deformity in the cervical region and perform a quick muscle test for strength and function. Ask the athlete to squeeze your hands, and look for good and equal strength left to right. Can the athlete dorsiflex the ankle against manual resistance equally left to right? If these motor tests are positive for weakness, assume the neck injury is serious.

If all findings so far are negative, have the athlete demonstrate slow, active cervical ROM. It sometimes happens that the athlete has no pain as long as he lies quietly but once he moves, pain appears. If the athlete is unwilling to move, if neck pain is increased, or if there are sensory changes, cease your examination and assume serious neck injury.

If at any time in your examination a serious neck injury is assumed, no further examination is necessary; emergency medical services (EMS) should be notified and the athlete should be properly stabilized and secured to a spine board for transportation. Even if the symptoms appear minor (i.e., the athlete has only minimal sensation or strength deficits), you must follow procedures for a serious spine injury. In other words, any positive test should be regarded as indicative of a possible spinal cord injury, and the athlete should be transported accordingly. Before EMS arrives, monitor vital signs and use a reassuring voice to help keep the athlete calm during the waiting period and during transport.

> ⚠ If at any time in your examination you suspect a serious neck injury, do not proceed with the examination; notify EMS at once, and see that the patient is properly stabilized and secured to a spine board for transportation.

For further discussion of transportation procedures for a serious spine injury, refer to *Introduction to Athletic Training, Second Edition,* (Hillman 2005), chapter 8.

Only if the on-site examination (i.e., sensory, motor, palpation, cervical motion, strength) is negative can the athlete leave the field without assistance for further examination on the sideline.

Acute Examination

Here's a look at the components of cervical and upper thoracic spine examination as you would apply them in an acute examination.

Consider the opening scenario where Doug, the starting linebacker for his high school football team, made a tackle using the top of his shoulder to make contact. Upon contact, he felt a shooting pain going down his arm. He was able to get up and walk off the field under his own power but as he did so, the athletic trainer noted he was leaning to his right side with his arm hanging, appearing to be in some pain.

Consider how your examination would proceed from the on-site examination, once you determined it safe for Doug to leave the field under his own power.

Checklist for On-Site Examination of Cervical and Upper Thoracic Spine

▷ Primary Survey

As you approach:

- ☐ check surroundings and environment
- ☐ gain history of event from bystanders if you did not witness
- ☐ note position of head and neck

Necessary checks:

- ☐ Consciousness
- ☐ Airway, breathing, and circulation
- ☐ Severe bleeding

▷ Secondary Survey (Evaluate Athlete in the Position Found)

If athlete is unconscious, assume a serious spinal injury. If conscious, examine the following:

- ☐ Presence of neck pain
- ☐ Sensations of numbness, tingling, or burning
- ☐ Difficulty with breathing
- ☐ Difficulty in moving extremities

If any of the above are positive, assume serious spine injury. If neck pain only:

- ☐ Palpate for tenderness and deformity
- ☐ Check for grip and dorsiflexion strength

If signs are positive, assume serious neck injury. If signs are negative:

- ☐ Examine slow active ROM of cervical spine
- ☐ Examine for sensory changes with motion

If positive, assume serious neck injury. If negative, move off-site for further examination.

Throughout primary and secondary surveys:

- ☐ Continue to monitor vitals and check sensory and motor function in extremities

History

Once the patient comes off the field, obtain a thorough history. Appropriate questions can determine the mechanism, symptoms, location of the involved tissue, and severity of the injury. You can even sometimes judge from the history alone whether or not referral to a physician is necessary. Can the person describe the mechanism of injury? Were any noises heard at the time of injury? Where was the pain at the time of injury, and has it changed? Have the person describe the pain in terms of type and intensity using the 10-point scale. Does the patient have any unusual sensations now? Has there been any prior injury to the area? Is there any dizziness, light-headedness, or headache?

Headaches can originate from the cervical spine or may result from an associated head injury if the mechanism involved contact with the head. You should suspect a neck-related headache if the pain is in the suboccipital region at the base of the neck, if neck motion changes the headache pain, or if the patient reports sensory changes in the suboccipital area. Cervical muscle-related headaches can also create symptoms in the occipital, temporal, and frontal areas of the head. Occasionally eye, ear, or jaw pain is related to cervical muscle dysfunction. It is important to differentiate these symptoms from those caused by a head injury (see chapter 19).

Observation

In your observation, note how the patient holds her head and arm and the patient's posture and general body alignment (see chapter 4 for details on postural examination). Is there a normal concave curve of the cervical spine, or is the spine flattened from muscle spasm? Note how the patient moves the head. Are movements slow or guarded, or are they normal and without hesitation? Does the head move freely, or does the patient look side to side by turning the trunk rather than the head (an indication of pain and muscle guarding)? Does upper- and lower-extremity movement occur normally, or is any guarding or weakness noticeable? Is the gait normal? Is she able to sit, stand, and move normally?

Palpation

Acute palpation is a cursory palpation to determine the presence and intensity of muscle spasm. Pain referred to the head, base of the skull, and posterior scapular areas can be secondary to muscle spasm. Muscle spasm is palpated as a rigidity of the muscle, and the muscle in spasm exhibits tenderness to pressure. Muscle spasm can also be confirmed with a reduced active cervical ROM. Palpated muscle spasm should receive immediate treatment of ice and rest with the patient lying supine. An in-depth palpation sequence for both soft tissue and bony structures are described earlier in this chapter (see page 199).

Objective Tests

A positive result for any of these tests indicates referral to a physician. If any test produces a positive sign, there is no need to continue testing:

- Compression test (figure 11.19)
- Nerve root compression relief (shoulder abduction) test (figure 11.20)
- Cervical distraction relief test (figure 11.21)
- Shoulder depression test (figure 11.22)
- Valsalva maneuver (figure 11.26)

Perform ROM, strength, and neurological tests in the order described earlier in this chapter. When testing ROM, if the patient complains of pain or sensation changes in the neck or extremities with active motion, do not perform passive overpressure motions. Perform strength examinations bilaterally to ensure equal strength and function. Conduct sensory, motor, and reflex tests for suspected neurological compression or distraction injuries.

Functional Tests

Only if all previous tests are negative should the patient undergo functional tests to determine physical and psychological readiness to return to participation. These functional tests should include some basic test and some activity-specific tests. Basic tests might include a functional sensory examination such as having the patient tie shoes with the eyes closed. This requires adequate sensory feedback from the fingers and tests balance when the person is in a standing position with the foot up on a bench or chair.

Activity-specific functional activities are skill-execution drills that mimic the patient's sport or activity. A drill may involve agility, coordination, power, and flexibility from the extremity (upper, lower, or both), depending on the athlete's sport and position within the sport. Observe for flow of movement without hesitation, coordination and agility during the execution, and demonstration of adequate flexibility, movement, and strength throughout the drill. It is important in functional examination of cervical injuries to observe carefully whether the athlete moves the head easily and naturally in all directions without guarding.

Checklist for Acute Examination
of Cervical and Upper Thoracic Spine

▷ *History*

☐ Mechanism of injury
☐ Unusual sensations experienced at time of injury and currently
☐ Symptoms of headache, dizziness, or lightheadedness
☐ Previous injury

▷ *Observation*

☐ Presence of cervical lordosis
☐ Spasm, swelling, discoloration
☐ Bilateral asymmetry
☐ Evidence of pain or restricted movement
☐ Position of head

▷ *Palpation*

☐ Evidence of bony tenderness
☐ Evidence of muscle tenderness, spasm, trigger point
☐ Bilateral comparison

▷ *Special Tests*

☐ Valsalva test
☐ Compression test
☐ Shoulder depression test
☐ Nerve root compression relief test
☐ Cervical distraction test

▷ *Range of Motion*

☐ Active ROM: cervical flexion, extension, lateral flexion, and rotation
☐ Passive ROM: end-range cervical flexion, extension, lateral flexion, and rotation

▷ *Strength Tests*

☐ Manual resistance to cervical flexion, extension, rotation, and lateral flexion

▷ *Neurological Tests*

☐ Dermatome (C1-C4; C5-T1)
☐ Myotome (C5-T1)
☐ Reflex (biceps, brachioradialis, triceps)

▷ *Functional Tests*

☐ Basic skills (e.g., tie shoes with eyes closed)
☐ Activity or sport-specific tasks
☐ Upper extremity movements
☐ Note ease of cervical movement with trunk and upper extremity movement

Clinical Examination

It is common for a patient to have a cervical injury but no complaints at the time it occurs, especially if the injury involves cervical muscles or ligaments. In these cases, however, muscle spasm and other symptoms will often surface later. In a typical example, a football receiver is tackled from the side as he makes a sudden cut into the unseen opponent. As he falls to the ground the opponent's impact forces him in one direction but his momentum continues to move his neck in the opposite direction, causing a cervical whiplash. The athlete feels a brief pain in his posterolateral neck, but not enough pain to interrupt his participation. His neck may feel slightly stiff after the game, but he thinks little of it and continues in his normal activities. The next morning, his neck is stiff, painful, and difficult to move because muscle spasm has become predominant.

Consider a 35-year-old computer analyst who comes into your facility complaining of an increasing amount of pain and discomfort in her neck and an ache in her left arm. She does not remember any specific injury but states that over the past 6 months she has often awakened in the morning with a stiff neck and experiences an increasing amount of discomfort at work when sitting at the computer for long periods. She also is an avid swimmer and weightlifter who spends 5 hours a week in the gym.

The clinical examination is more complex than the acute examination for several reasons. There are more potential conditions to consider, there are complications that occur with untreated symptoms, and masking of original symptoms and overriding of new symptoms occur after the initial injury incident. The patient may present with a post-acute injury (first scenario) or an injury caused from repetitive stress (second scenario). Causes and effective treatment of repetitive stress injuries can be difficult to identify and frustrating to resolve. Acute injuries that are not immediately treated usually develop additional symptoms, and the severity of the symptoms increases. This can change the injury's profile and can complicate the examination. As an allied health care provider you must be aware of additional possible injuries and changes in the symptoms of acute injuries, and you must make an accurate and total examination so you do not overlook these potential problems. To ensure adequate treatment, you must take a careful history and attempt to reproduce the patient's symptoms using objective tests to clearly identify the injury's SINS (Severity, Irritability, Nature, and Stage).

History

Any patient entering your treatment facility warrants a complete history. The patient may be able to recall the injury incident but may or may not be able to identify factors since its occurrence that may have contributed to the condition. In other cases, a specific onset of symptoms is unclear. There also may be preexisting factors adding to the problem (e.g., previous unresolved injury) or additional problems that have developed secondary to the injury and subsequent lack of treatment.

If the patient is able to recall the injury specifically, ask for the details related to the occurrence. The mechanism of injury, sensations experienced in the neck and surrounding area at the time of injury, postinjury activity, and previous injuries are all important factors to glean from the athlete. The history should identify the location of the patient's pain and symptoms. Is there any radiation of the pain, or is it localized? What kind of sensation is it? A sensation of burning, stinging, tingling, or heaviness may indicate a nerve-related problem. An ache or sharp pain may indicate a muscle, joint, or ligament injury. Does the pain increase with coughing, laughing, or sneezing? These activities increase intrathecal pressure and can signal disc dysfunctions. Does the pain change with activity or time of day? What activities aggravate

Tinnitus is a sensation of ringing or a similar noise in the ear.

the symptoms, and what activities ease them? Does the patient have headaches, tinnitus, or blurry vision? These signs can indicate either a cranial nerve injury that affects the sympathetic system or myofascial referred pain. Does the pain awaken the patient, and is there difficulty returning to sleep? Sleep disturbances with difficulty returning to sleep indicate an irritable injury. What position does the patient sleep in? Prone sleeping is very stressful on the neck, especially an injured neck. How many pillows does the patient use? More than one pillow under the head can increase cervical curvature and maintain a poor cervical alignment to add to the cervical stress. As with other injuries, the patient's pain profile will provide insight into the intensity, irritability, and possible tissue involved. If the patient is unable to identify when, how, or why the symptoms started, a good history can also point to the stage of the injury: Is it acute, subacute, or chronic?

If the patient complains of pain or sensory changes distal to the acromion process, perform a neurological examination, since the changes may result from nerve root compression or injury. If the pain is severe, ranked 7 or higher on a 10-point scale, the injury may be easily irritated, which may warrant an abbreviated examination. If the patient indicates the pain is less than a 7, you may use a more aggressive examination. If you detect neurological changes (sensory, motor, or reflex), you should refer the patient to a physician.

Observation

Throughout the history taking process, note the patient's movements and watch for hesitation in cervical or extremity movement, incomplete motions, restricted motions in one or more directions, and grimacing or facial expression changes with movements; also note whether or not the patient changes positions frequently and seems unable to find a comfortable position. Watching the patient remove a sweatshirt or shirt will also indicate how guarded and painful movement is.

Lordosis is a curvature of the spine characterized by an anterior convexity.

Observe the patient's posture (chapter 4). Some cervical lordosis is normal, but excessive lordosis or a flat cervical spine can indicate either poor cervical posture or muscle spasm. In normal cervical posture, the earlobe aligns with the acromion process from a lateral view, and the nose lines up with the manubrium and xiphoid process of the sternum from a frontal view. A forward head position with the earlobe anterior to the acromion process is frequently combined with rounded shoulders and can indicate poor posture, muscle spasm, or pain that restricts the athlete's normal posture. Head tilt to one side can indicate pain or spasm. Reduced mobility or guarded movements are also possible signs of muscle spasm, pain-restricting movement, or both. If the patient supports an upper extremity, there may be a nerve root irritation that is aggravated if the arm is allowed to hang at the side normally.

Differential Diagnosis

There are many common referral patterns that both emanate from and centralize into the cervical area. Whenever a patient presents in the treatment facility with cervical complaints, you must eliminate other possible sources of pain. This is especially true if the patient reports symptoms distal to the acromion process. Other causes that you must eliminate include nerve root lesions, disc injuries, brachial plexus lesions, peripheral nerve injuries, upper-extremity joint or muscle injuries, and myofascial irritations. Special tests for these injuries are discussed in the special test and palpation subsections of this chapter.

Range of Motion

Test range of motion of the cervical spine in all planes with the patient sitting. Examine the quantity and quality of cervical movement as well as the presence or absence of a capsular pattern or movement. The capsular pattern for the cervical spine is equal limitation of lateral flexion and rotation, with less restriction into extension. The patient should perform active motion slowly and smoothly through a full ROM; note changes in the patient's facial expressions that indicate pain or difficulty with the cervical movement.

After each pain-free active cervical motion, apply a passive overpressure and ask whether the motion reproduces the patient's pain. If all positions with overpressure are negative,

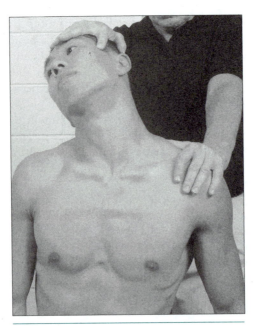

Figure 11.31   The quadrant position.

then place the head into a **quadrant position** with the neck in end-range extension and rotation, side-bending to the same side as the symptoms. Then apply an overpressure force to the head in this position (figure 11.31). If the patient reports pain in the neck or into the upper extremity, these are positive signs and an indication of a facet syndrome or a nerve root pathology.

Strength

Test cervical muscle strength with the patient positioned so that the muscle is working against gravity for each cervical movement (table 11.2 and figure 11.18a-d). Stabilize the trunk with the patient lying on the examination table. With the patient supine, resist neck flexion. Lateral flexion is typically performed with the patient seated but can also be performed with the patient lying on the side for maximal resistance against gravity. Cervical extension is tested with the patient prone and the head over the end of the table. It is important that the neck begin in good alignment. For example, to test cervical extension, the patient first places the head in proper posture alignment (i.e., without a forward head or excessive lordosis) and then moves the neck into extension against manual resistance. The resistance is gradually built up to a maximum with the neck in proper alignment and in a midrange position for each motion tested.

Manual resistance to scapular elevation and retraction movements may also be indicated to examine the upper and middle trapezius muscles (see chapter 12). Because of the possibility of injury with machine resistance, isokinetic and other instrumented strength examinations are not usually used for cervical strength testing, and manual muscle tests are the examination of choice.

Neurological Tests

If the patient reports symptoms distal to the acromion, perform neurological tests. These symptoms may range from a subtle dull muscle ache to sharp, radiating pain down the extremity. Perform sensory, motor, and reflex tests (chapter 8) to eliminate neural injury as the cause of peripheral symptoms. If the tests are negative, the tissue involved is probably not neural, but if any of the tests are positive, neural structures are probably involved. Remember, not all neurological tests need to be positive to indicate pathology. Except in severe or prolonged cases, it is not usual for all three types of neurological tests to be positive at the same time, and sensory deficits are often noted before motor deficits.

Sensory tests can be for temperature, deep pressure, and pain, but most often light touch or pinprick is used. Compare sensation responses between the left and right extremities. If the patient reports a difference between the two sides, refer her to a physician for a more detailed neurological investigation. Myotome tests can be quickly and efficiently performed with the athlete sitting. When testing, move from proximal to distal innervation.

Special Tests

Since an injury examined in the treatment facility may have originated from additional factors other than the acute injury mechanism, special tests besides those used in the acute examination will be necessary for differential diagnosis to rule out other types of injuries (see also chapter 12 for tests to rule out upper extremity injury). You will have narrowed the possibilities through the history and objective examination, so not all tests will be necessary. Tests performed during the acute examination may also be indicated in the clinical examination (refer to the special test section of the acute examination). These tests include the Valsalva maneuver, compression tests, shoulder depression test, nerve root compression relief test, and cervical distraction relief test. In addition to these tests, you should include tests for neuropathy (Tinel's sign, passive and active limb tension tests) and vascular compromise in the clinical examination, as indicated.

Palpation

Palpation is best performed with the patient supine for enhanced relaxation of supporting muscles. If the patient is uncomfortable in this position, you can perform palpation with the patient prone on a table that has a face hole or with the patient sitting and leaning forward with the head and arms supported on a structure of appropriate height. Cervical muscles in spasm or with active trigger points can refer pain into other areas such as the head, base of the skull, and posterior scapular areas, thus mimicking nerve pain. Figure 11.32 illustrates some of the more common referral patterns of cervical muscles. In the presence of referred pain symptoms, you must investigate whether the pain is secondary to neural or muscular dysfunctions. A precise examination can help determine the injury source. If palpation of muscle structures produces a comparable sign, it is likely that the pain is soft tissue related. If, however, the pain is reproduced by some of the special tests discussed previously, the pain is likely neurological in origin.

Functional Tests

Functional tests were discussed in connection with the acute examination. If the patient complains that any daily work or sport-related activities are difficult because of the injury, examine the patient's performance. If previous examination tests were positive, defer functional tests. Functional tests should be part of the final examination before the patient is allowed to resume full participation.

Specific functional tests depend upon the athlete's specific sport and position within the sport or upon the nonathlete's specific activities or work responsibilities. Since the cervical and upper thoracic spine can affect upper and lower extremities as well as the trunk, the patient should perform functional tests for both extremities and for those movements that require stabilization of the upper trunk. Also include activities that require full ROM of the cervical spine.

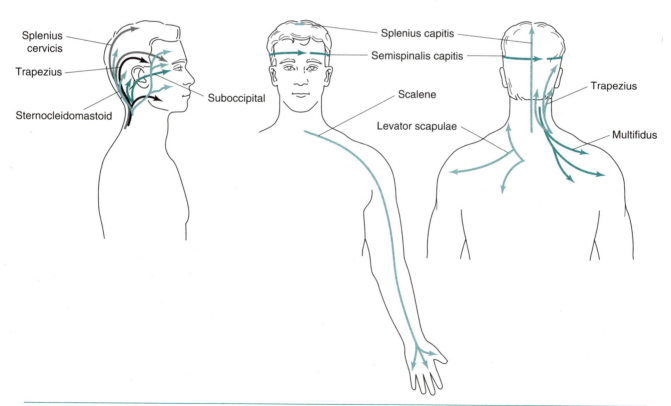

Figure 11.32 Common referral patterns of cervical muscles.

Checklist for Clinical Examination of Cervical and Upper Thoracic Spine

▷ *History*

- ☐ Mechanism of injury
- ☐ Unusual sensations at time of injury
- ☐ Previous injury
- ☐ Type and location of pain
- ☐ Numbness and tingling
- ☐ Chief complaint

If chronic, ascertain:

- ☐ Aggravating and easing factors
- ☐ Onset and duration of symptoms
- ☐ Effects of time of day or activity on symptoms
- ☐ Night pain
- ☐ Sleeping position

▷ *Observation*

- ☐ Posture (head and upper body)
- ☐ Restriction, guarding, or hesitation in movement
- ☐ Facial expressions
- ☐ Visible swelling, discoloration, spasm, asymmetry

▷ *Differential Diagnosis*

Refer to palpation procedures and special tests listed below to rule out:

- ☐ Nerve root lesions
- ☐ Disc injury
- ☐ Brachial plexus lesions
- ☐ Peripheral nerve injury
- ☐ Upper extremity joint or muscle injury
- ☐ Myofascial irritations

▷ *Range of Motion*

- ☐ Active ROM: cervical flexion, extension, lateral flexion, and rotation
- ☐ Passive ROM: end-range cervical flexion, extension, lateral flexion, and rotation
- ☐ Shoulder motion as appropriate

▷ *Strength*

- ☐ Manual resistance to cervical flexion (supine), extension (prone), lateral flexion (seated or sidelying), and rotation (seated)

▷ *Neurological Tests*

- ☐ Dermatome (C5-T1)
- ☐ Myotome (C5-T1)
- ☐ Reflex (biceps, brachioradialis, triceps)

▷ Special Tests

- ☐ Valsalva test
- ☐ Compression test
- ☐ Shoulder depression test
- ☐ Nerve root compression relief test
- ☐ Cervical distraction relief test
- ☐ Tinel's sign
- ☐ Upper limb tension tests
- ☐ Vertebral artery test
- ☐ TOS tests (Adson's, Allen, Military Brace)

▷ Palpation

- ☐ Soft tissue mobility
- ☐ Cervical and upper thoracic spinous processes
- ☐ Transverse processes
- ☐ Posterior, lateral, and anterior cervical and upper back muscles

▷ Functional Tests

Check for normal unrestricted movement with:

- ☐ Sport-specific or work-specific activity
- ☐ Overhead and upper-extremity movements
- ☐ Trunk movements
- ☐ Tasks that require full ROM or cervical spine

SUMMARY

1. Identify the causes of cervical strain.

   Cervical strains, common in physically active persons, can result from both acute trauma and chronic stresses. Acute causes are sudden mechanical overload or violent overstretching into rotation, flexion, or extension (i.e., whiplash). Chronic overuse, postural faults, and poor mechanics can make the cervical spine susceptible to acute strains. Signs and symptoms include muscular pain and spasm, tenderness, and decreased ROM.

2. Identify the types of fractures in the cervical spine and the potential for spinal cord injury associated with each.

   Fractures in the cervical spine can result from hyperflexion, hyperextension, and axial loading mechanisms. The primary cause of cervical fractures resulting in catastrophic spinal cord trauma is headfirst contact with or without the spine flexed, resulting in axial loading and buckling of the cervical spine. Compression fractures, burst fractures, fracture dislocations, and facet dislocations are the most serious spinal fractures and have a high probability for spinal cord involvement. Contact to the back of the head and face can also result in avulsion fractures of the spinous processes, but these rarely have associated neurological pathology.

3. Discuss the causes of neuropathy in the upper extremity relative to cervical spine pathology.

   Neurological symptoms into the upper extremity can result from a variety of mechanisms that either tense or compress the spinal cord and nerve roots. Spinal cord compression, caused by acute fractures and dislocations as well as severe degenerative conditions (stenosis), can result in bilateral neurological symptoms. Nerve root compression, which causes radiating symptoms, sensory impairment, and motor weakness in one extremity, can result from brachial plexus stretch and compression mechanisms, thoracic outlet syndromes, degenerative disc disease, acute disc herniations, and osteophytes, that lead to stenosis in the intervertebral foramen. These conditions can be differentiated by special tests that examine sensory, motor, and reflex responses, as well as tests for various compression syndromes.

4. Conduct a neurological exam for the upper extremity, including sensory, motor, and reflex testing.

A neurological exam consists of sensory, motor, and reflex testing. Each nerve root exiting the cervical spine has a specific sensory, motor, and reflex distribution (table 11.3). Sensory testing typically examines sensory acuity using a light touch applied over the dermatome for each nerve root. Motor tests are performed with manual muscle testing of specific muscles that have a single nerve root as their primary innervation. Reflex testing of the biceps, brachioradialis, and triceps muscle also provides information on the type and location of nerve pathology. Depending on the nerve pathology, one or all of these tests may be positive. Refer an athlete with any positive neurological sign to a physician for further examination.

5. Perform an on-site examination for a suspected spinal cord injury and determine when the injury is serious.

Acute cervical injuries can be life threatening or can cause paralysis. Immediate on-site examination must establish the severity of the injury, including whether or not possible spinal cord injury exists. Begin with a primary survey for level of consciousness, ABC (**A**irway, **B**reathing, **C**irculation) examination, and body position and follow with tests for cervical spine pain, sensation impairment, motor weakness, and palpable defects to determine the nature of the injury and to ascertain whether you should suspect a serious spine injury. If these tests reveal any positive signs, call EMS and transport the athlete off the field with a spine board. See page 215 for an examination checklist.

6. Perform an acute examination for the cervical spine region.

If emergency transportation is not warranted, conduct a more complete examination on the sideline or in the treatment facility. This examination includes continued observation of the patient's movements; a more detailed history of the injury; testing of ROM, strength, and neurological parameters; and special tests. These special tests include the Valsalva maneuver and compression test for disc or nerve root injury, shoulder depression test for brachial plexus stretch, and nerve root compression test and relief tests for nerve root injuries. Palpate the cervical and upper thoracic areas to determine specific areas of tenderness, muscle spasm, active trigger points, and soft tissue restriction. If there are no positive results on any of these tests, perform a functional examination to determine the patient's ability to return to full activities. See page 217 for an examination checklist.

7. Perform a clinical examination for the cervical spine region.

When the patient enters the injury treatment facility complaining of a neck injury or neck pain, examination must be more thorough since there are additional possible causes and injury types. There can also be other injuries that you must eliminate through differential diagnosis. Additional objective examination tools include examination of active and passive ROM, strength, and neurological parameters if symptoms are present distal to the acromion process, as well as special tests that include those performed in the acute examination. Additional special tests are those for cervical neuropathy (Tinel's sign, upper-limb tension tests), the vertebral artery test, and tests for TOS. Palpation then determines the precise location of pain and examines bony and soft tissue structures. Functional tests are not commonly performed when the patient is initially examined, but they are necessary before the patient's return to full participation. See page 222 for an examination checklist.

REVIEW QUESTIONS

1. What are the dangers associated with spearing in football?

2. Describe some of the degenerative changes that can occur in the cervical spine and the symptoms and potential complications such changes may cause over time.

3. What is TOS? Describe the etiology and signs and symptoms associated with this injury. What other cervical spine conditions may result in similar symptoms?

4. During an on-site examination of a cervical spine injury, when can you determine that it is safe for the athlete to move and leave the field under her own power?

5. What is considered the normal posture and active ROM of the cervical spine?

6. What contraindicates performing passive overpressures for cervical spine motions?

7. Describe the special tests used in the clinical examination to evaluate for nerve root compression.

8. Describe the special tests used in determining brachial plexus injury. What would a positive result for each of these tests indicate?

CRITICAL THINKING QUESTIONS

1. Think back to the scenario at the beginning of the chapter. What injury did Doug likely have? Based on the location of his symptoms, what specific structures were likely involved? Finding that Doug was not being completely honest in reporting his pain, what specific tests did Jeff use to determine that Doug had weakness and sensory changes? If you were Jeff, how would you have gone about your examination, and what other tests would you have performed to rule out related conditions?

2. Assume that Doug's symptoms subsided within a few minutes and Jeff's examination revealed that Doug had regained full ROM and strength with no evidence of neurological deficits. What functional tests would you have Doug perform to ensure he is ready to return to action?

3. Revisit the scenario of the 35-year-old computer analyst who comes into the clinic complaining of an increasing amount of pain and discomfort in her neck and some achiness in her left arm. She does not remember any specific injury but states that over the past 6 months she has often awakened in the morning with a stiff neck and experiences an increasing amount of discomfort at work when sitting at the computer for long periods. She also is an avid swimmer and weightlifter who spends 5 hours a week at the gym. Given her chief complaint, how would you go about taking a history of this physically active patient? Given the type of work and training that she does, what are some questions you could ask and observations you could make to obtain some clues to possible overload stresses that may be causing her pain?

4. How might you differentiate between referred pain into the arm caused by a chronic muscle condition and a nerve compression syndrome? Discuss some of the special tests you would use to make this determination.

CITED REFERENCES

Marks, M.R., G.R Bell, and F.R. Boumphrey. 1990. Cervical spine injuries and their neurologic implications. *Clin Sports Med* 9: 263-278.

Torg, J.S., R.J. Naranja, H. Palov, B.J. Galinat, R. Warren, and R.A. Stine. 1996. The relationship of developmental narrowing of the cervical spinal canal to reversible and irreversible injury of the cervical spinal cord in football players. *J Bone Joint Surg* 78A: 1308-1314.

Winkelstein, B.A., and B.S. Myers. 1997. The biomechanics of cervical spine injury and implications for injury prevention. *Med Sci Sports Exerc* 29: S246-255.

Wroble, R.R., and J.P. Albright. 1986. Neck and low back injuries in wrestling. *Clin Sports Med* 5: 295-325.

ADDITIONAL RESOURCES

Cantu, R.C. 1998. Neurologic athletic head and neck injuries. *Clin Sports Med* 17: 1-210.

Durham, J.R., J.S. Yao, W.H. Pearce, G.M. Nuber, and W.J. McCarthy. 1995. Arterial injuries in the thoracic outlet syndrome. *J Vasc Surg* 21: 57-69.

Hershman, E.B. 1990. Brachial plexus injuries. *Clin Sports Med* 9: 311-329.

Hillman, S.K. 2005. *Introduction to athletic training*. Champaign, IL: Human Kinetics.

Houglum, P.A. 2005. *Therapeutic exercise for athletic injuries*. Champaign, IL: Human Kinetics.

Nichols, A.W. 1996. The thoracic outlet syndrome in athletes. *J Am Board Fam Prac* 9: 246-55.

Spencer, C.W. 1986. Injuries to the spine. *Clin Sports Med* 5: 213-410.

Torg, J.S. 1987. Cervical spinal stenosis with cord neuropraxia and transient quadriplegia. *Clin Sports Med* 6: 115-133.

Shoulder and Arm

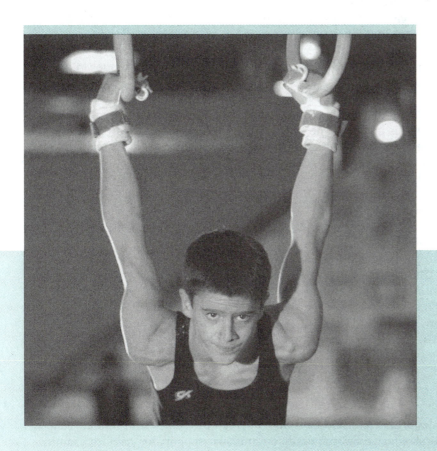

Objectives

After completing this chapter, the reader will be able to do the following:

1. Discuss the types of overuse injuries that commonly result from repetitive overhead throwing activities

2. Identify the signs and symptoms associated with various stages of rotator cuff impingement

3. Explain the purpose of and demonstrate the appropriate use of objective tests for the shoulder and arm

4. Describe and perform the special tests for examining joint instabilities

5. Describe and perform the special tests for examining muscle and tendon pathologies

6. Perform an on-site examination of the shoulder and upper arm, and discuss criteria for immediate referral and mode of transportation from the field

7. Perform an acute examination of the shoulder and upper arm, and discuss criteria for determining return to activity

8. Perform a clinical examination of the shoulder and upper arm, including differential diagnosis from cervical pathologies

Janet was a senior athletic training student who was looking forward to taking her certification exam in six months and getting her first job. One day, Darin, her clinical supervisor, asked her to perform a shoulder examination on Kevin, one of the swimmers. After Janet finished the examination, she and Darin sat down to discuss her impressions of the injury.

"Well, Janet, what did you think?" Darin asked.

"It seems pretty clear to me that Kevin is having some shoulder impingement. All the impingement tests I performed reproduced his pain." Janet felt pretty confident in her examination.

"What do you think is causing it?" Darin asked.

"Causing it? Well, uh . . . I guess his swimming? But he didn't report any unusual changes in his swim workouts." Janet was not so confident now.

"Did you notice his posture?"

"Uh, no, not really—what would that have to do with it?"

"Well," Darin explained, "I noticed his posture is not the greatest. His head is forward and his shoulders are rounded; a posture like this can be a result of muscle imbalance and can also contribute to impingement. How about his weight training? Any problems there?"

"His weight training? I didn't really ask him about that, but I see him in the weight room all the time. Oh, he did say it hurts a bit on bench press, but I don't think strength is an issue."

Now Janet wasn't sure what Darin was looking for.

"It may not be a strength issue as much as a muscular balance issue. It is not unusual for athletes to work hard on bench press and other chest exercises but not be so faithful when it comes to exercises for the back. I saw his weight program last week. He has about one back and posterior shoulder exercise for every three chest and anterior shoulder exercises. Between that and being a breaststroker, I would bet he is pretty tight anteriorly and weak posteriorly, and that's probably contributing to his problem," Darin suggested.

"Okay, I see what you mean now," Janet said thoughtfully. "I guess I got so focused on his pain and symptoms, I really didn't look at the big picture to see what might be causing it. I'll keep that in mind next time. Thanks for the pointers!"

The shoulder complex is characterized by a high degree of mobility with limited skeletal stability. Because the shoulder relies so heavily on muscular support for stability, examination of muscle weakness, dysfunction, and imbalance is key to the examination of shoulder dysfunction and injury. Because the soft tissues of the shoulder complex are chronically exposed to repetitive high velocity and eccentric forces over a large range of motion, the joint is particularly susceptible to chronic instability and repetitive stress injuries.

FUNCTIONAL ANATOMY

The shoulder is a highly mobile joint that allows a large range of motion in all planes to perform a variety of overhead activities. Statically, the glenohumeral joint is supported by the capsule, capsular ligaments, and glenoid labrum. However, to allow freedom of movement, these ligaments have to be relatively lax. As a result, the glenohumeral joint relies on the deltoid and rotator cuff muscles for dynamic stabilization. The cost of the shoulder joint's mobility is that it is relatively unstable and dislocations of the joint are relatively common.

The shoulder complex as a whole is unique in that it relies very little on bony and ligament structures for stability, with the majority of support coming from the 18 muscles acting on the shoulder complex. The only direct attachment of the upper extremity to the axial skeleton is through the sternoclavicular (SC) joint. The scapula, completely suspended by muscles, serves as a mobile yet stabilizing platform to facilitate glenohumeral motion. When scapular muscles are weak or atrophied, normal scapular motion is affected, which can have a significant effect on shoulder mechanics and function. This dysfunction, combined with the stress placed on the shoulder's static and dynamic stabilizing structures by repetitive overhead throwing activities, is a common cause of soft tissue injuries and instability in the shoulder region. Therefore, it is important to consider the shoulder complex as a whole when performing a shoulder examination.

The shoulder complex includes both the shoulder (glenohumeral) joint and girdle (scapula) (figure 12.1). The movements of the glenohumeral joint include flexion and extension, abduction and adduction, inward (medial) and outward (lateral) rotation, horizontal extension (abduction) and flexion (adduction), and circumduction. The movements of the scapula include abduction and adduction, elevation and depression, upward (outward) and downward

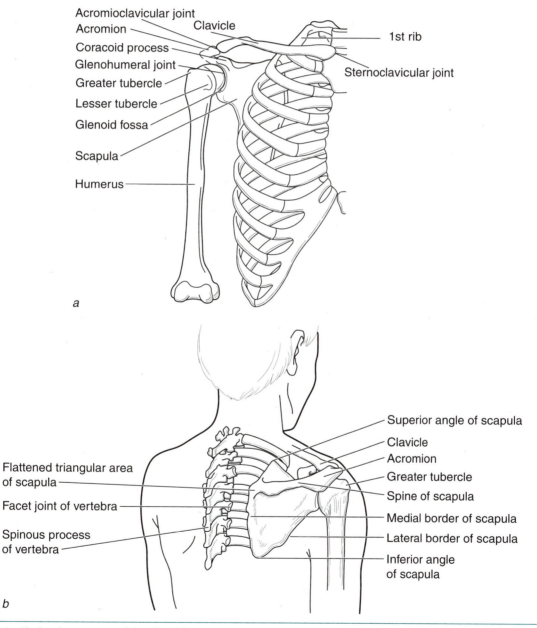

Figure 12.1   Skeletal anatomy of the shoulder complex: *(a)* anterior and *(b)* posterior views.

(inward) rotation, and forward (protraction) and backward (retraction) tilt. For full mobility of the upper extremity, the motions of the shoulder joint and scapula must be unrestricted and occur in a coordinated fashion. For example, abduction of the shoulder joint is accompanied by upward rotation of the scapula in a 2:1 relationship after the first 30° of shoulder abduction. Likewise, flexion of the shoulder is accompanied by upward rotation of the scapula in a 2:1 ratio after the first 60° of shoulder flexion. If the scapula is unable to move freely through its full range of motion, motion of the shoulder joint is restricted. This is why it is necessary to examine the entire shoulder complex as part of your upper-extremity examination.

A force couple is equal and opposite forces created by two muscles to create torque at the joint.

Eleven muscles act on the shoulder joint, including the deltoid, supraspinatus, infraspinatus, teres minor, subscapularis, pectoralis major, latissimus dorsi, teres major, coracobrachialis, and the biarticulate muscles (biceps brachii and triceps brachii) (figure 12.2). The

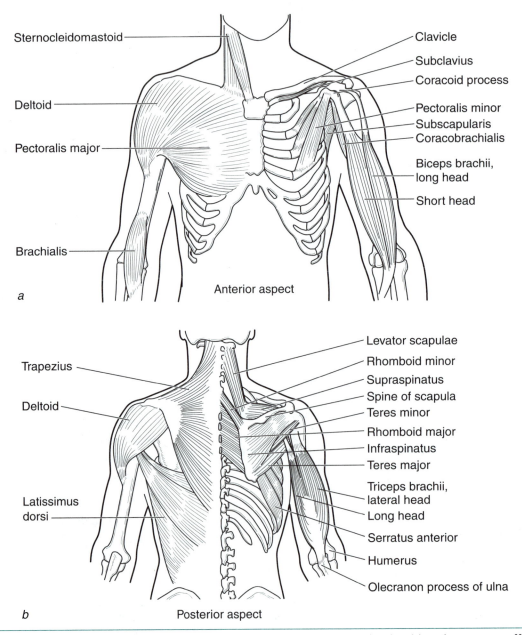

Figure 12.2 *(a)* Anterior and *(b)* posterior aspects of the muscles that act on the shoulder. The rotator cuff includes the subscapularis (anterior aspect), teres major, teres minor, and infraspinatus (posterior aspect) muscles.

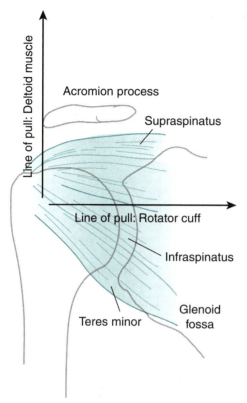

supraspinatus, infraspinatus, teres minor, and subscapularis make up the rotator cuff muscles. While the rotator cuff muscles internally and externally rotate the shoulder, an equally important function is to depress the head of the humerus into the glenoid fossa so the deltoid muscle has the mechanical ability to abduct the shoulder joint (**force couple**) (figure 12.3). Six muscles act on the scapula, including the subclavius, pectoralis minor, serratus anterior, levator scapulae, trapezius, and rhomboids.

The brachial plexus innervates all muscles of the upper limbs except the trapezius and levator scapulae. A thorough understanding of the motor and sensory innervations of the brachial plexus is necessary to comprehensively examine the upper extremity. The superficial nature of the peripheral nerves emanating from the brachial plexus render them susceptible to injury through compression or contusion, and the plexus can be compressed or stretched anywhere along its roots, trunks, divisions, or cords. The signs and symptoms of these injuries include numbness and muscle weakness and atrophy, with the magnitude of involvement depending on the level of injury within the brachial plexus. Figure 12.4 depicts the common points of injury to the brachial plexus and the corresponding muscle involvement.

Figure 12.3 Force couple of the rotator cuff and deltoid in shoulder abduction.

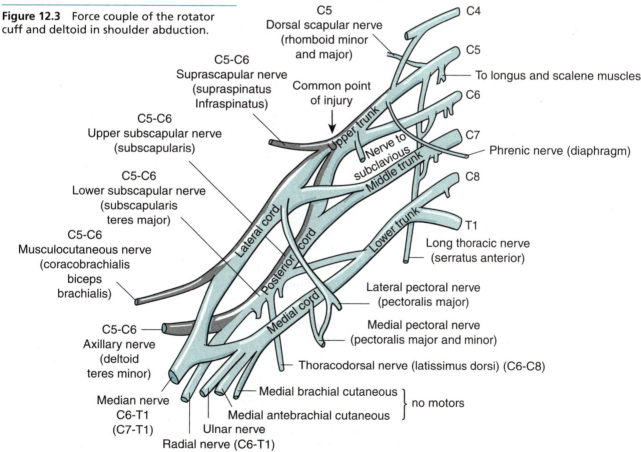

Figure 12.4 Peripheral nerve consequences of injury to the brachial plexus.

Reprinted, by permission, from C.D. Schneck, 1983, Neck injuries. In *Athletic injuries to the head, neck, and face*, edited by J.S. Torg (Philadelphia: Lippincott, Williams & Wilkins), 212.

INJURIES OF THE SHOULDER COMPLEX AND UPPER ARM

The shoulder joint is particularly susceptible to injuries because of its great mobility and inherent instability. The heavy reliance on soft tissue structures and balanced muscular control for stabilization through a large ROM places considerable demands on these structures, resulting in both acute and chronic injuries. Injury recognition is sometimes difficult because of the interplay of the muscles acting on the shoulder during functional activity.

Acute Soft Tissue Injuries

Acute soft tissue injuries can result from direct trauma, movements forcing the joint beyond its normal range, and forceful muscle contraction during activity.

Contusions

During sports such as football, wrestling, and soccer, direct contact with other players and the ground can result in contusions to superficial bony anatomy and the surrounding musculature. The clavicle, acromion, and lateral arm are bony structures with little soft tissue protection.

Bone Contusions

Contusion of the acromion is often referred to as a "shoulder pointer." **Blocker's exostosis** (also known as **tackler's exostosis** or **blocker's spur**), on the other hand, results from repetitive insult and irritation of the bone, causing excessive bone formation and at times a palpable spur on the anteriolateral surface of the humerus. Contusions to these isolated bony structures are rarely disabling, with signs and symptoms typically limited to localized swelling, pain, and point tenderness.

Muscle Contusions

Contusions to the musculature can be more disabling, since hematoma formation and pain can severely limit muscular function. A complication of biceps muscle contusion is **myositis ossificans**, or calcification within and around the biceps. Myositis ossificans can result from an unresolved hematoma in cases with large hematoma formation, repetitive insult, or continued use following the initial contusion. In most cases, this can be prevented with proper rest and treatment.

Sprains and Dislocation

Sprains involving the ligaments and capsule of the shoulder complex vary in frequency and severity, depending on the structure involved. Ligamentous and capsular disruption can result from both compressive and tractional forces that force the joint beyond its normal range of motion. Sprains of the glenohumeral and acromioclavicular (AC) joint occur more frequently than sternoclavicular (SC) joint sprains.

Glenohumeral Joint Sprains

In order to provide the mobility inherent in the glenohumeral joint, the joint's capsule and ligaments are comparatively lax throughout most of glenohumeral motion. This means the capsule and ligaments are minimally involved in maintaining joint stability throughout most of the range, with tensioning and potential injury to these structures occurring at the extreme ranges of motion. As a result, mild to moderate (first- and second-degree) glenohumeral sprains are fairly uncommon. However, forces exerted at the end ranges of motion that are sufficient to tear the glenohumeral ligaments can cause subluxation or dislocation of the humeral head because of its shallow articulation with the glenoid.

Acromioclavicular Joint Sprains

Within the shoulder complex, the acromioclavicular (AC) joint is the most commonly sprained or "separated" joint. Ligament injuries to this joint typically result from a fall or from direct contact to the point of the shoulder, driving the acromion caudally into the clavicle. Forces transmitted through the arm with a fall on an outstretched hand may also produce an AC sprain. **First-degree** sprains are characterized by localized pain, point tenderness, and swelling over the joint. The patient may complain of mild to moderate pain during shoulder motion, particularly with abduction above 120° and horizontal adduction. **Second-degree** injuries involve partial tearing of one or both of the AC and coracoclavicular ligaments. The patient will have increased complaints of pain, swelling, and disability with arm motion above horizontal. The distal end of the clavicle may or may not be elevated, depending on the extent of disruption of one or both of the associated ligaments (AC and coracoclavicular). **Third-degree** injuries are characterized by complete disruption of the AC and coracoclavicular ligaments. The patient will complain of severe pain at the time of injury and demonstrate an unwillingness to raise the arm, typically protecting it at his side. You will also note obvious swelling and elevation of the distal clavicle relative to the acromion (figure 12.5).

Sternoclavicular Joint Sprains

The SC joint is quite stable, and sprains are infrequent. SC joint injury involves disruption of both the SC and costoclavicular ligaments. Injury can result from an anteriorly directed force, or direct blow, but more commonly results from forces transmitted along the long axis of the clavicle. Signs and symptoms of SC sprains include localized pain, swelling, and point tenderness directly over the joint. Pain increases with forward rotation of the shoulders and horizontal adduction, which act to compress the joint. With a first-degree sprain there is minimal ligament tearing, with no laxity or joint displacement. Second-degree sprains involve partial tearing of both the SC and costoclavicular ligaments, resulting in some displacement of the proximal clavicle from the sternum.

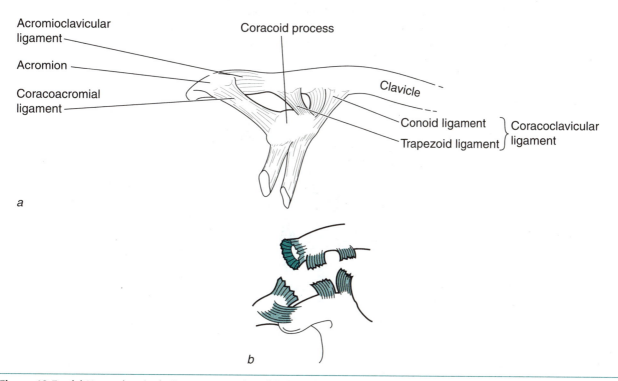

Figure 12.5 *(a)* Normal articulation compared to *(b)* third-degree AC separation.

> **!** When posterior dislocations of the clavicle on the sternum with a third-degree SC separation are accompanied by difficulty breathing or signs of vascular collapse (i.e., shock, decreased or absent radial pulse), you should suspect injury to the underlying neurovascular structures and immediately refer the patient to emergency medical care.

Third-degree sprains are readily observed and are characterized by complete separation of the SC joint with complete rupture of both ligaments. In most cases, the proximal clavicle is displaced anteriorly and superiorly in relation to the sternum secondary to its bony joint contour at the articular surface. However, on occasion, an anteriorly directed force displaces the clavicle posteriorly. With posterior displacement, secondary injury to the trachea, esophagus, and vascular structures (subclavian artery and brachiocephalic vein) underlying the proximal end of the clavicle may occur, causing potentially life-threatening breathing and vascular complications (figure 12.6). Specific signs and symptoms to watch for include difficulty breathing, vocal changes, difficulty swallowing, signs of vascular compromise in the upper extremity on the affected side (i.e., white or mottled skin coloration, reduced or absent distal pulses), and shock.

Strains

The muscles of the shoulder complex provide much of the stability for the shoulder through most of its normal ROM. Consequently, acute muscle and tendon strains frequently occur with overstretch during ballistic arm activities, forceful concentric contractions during limb acceleration, and excessive eccentric loading during limb deceleration. Improper warm-up, poor conditioning, and muscular fatigue can also make the muscles more susceptible to acute strain. Any of the 18 muscles acting within the shoulder complex may be injured. Signs and symptoms are typical of any first-, second-, or third-degree muscle injury, and you should identify the specific muscle involved through isolated manual muscle testing.

Rotator Cuff

The rotator cuff muscles are among the most commonly injured. A rotator cuff injury can significantly disable an athlete. In addition to the mechanisms previously mentioned, acute rotator cuff injuries can result from a fall on the shoulder or an outstretched hand that forces the humeral head into the acromion. These compressive injuries result in contusion and inflammation of the underlying surface of the rotator cuff tendons. Conversely, falling on the top of the shoulder and driving the humeral head downward can traction and tear the supraspinatus near the myotendon junction. Signs and symptoms of acute rotator cuff injury resulting from these mechanisms include anterolateral shoulder pain, point tenderness, decreased ROM, and loss of strength consistent with the severity of injury. Pain may radiate

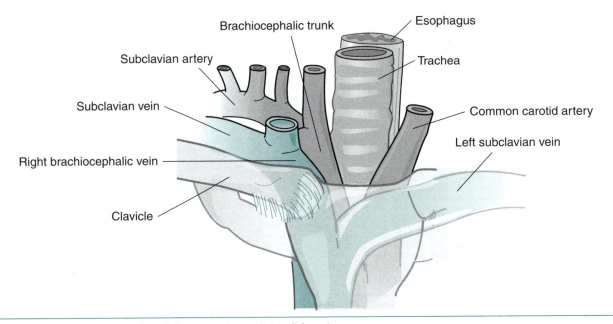

Figure 12.6   Structures at risk with a posterior SC joint dislocation.

down the lateral arm but usually stops at midhumerus. Pain is often increased at night while the patient is lying on the affected side.

Only rarely does acute trauma fully tear the rotator cuff. More often, complete tears are secondary to an underlying cumulative microtrauma. In young athletes, complete tears rarely occur without bony avulsion, since the myotendinous structures are often stronger than the bone.

Biceps Tendon Injuries

Acute rupture may be caused by a single traumatic event, such as rapid, forceful elbow flexion against heavy resistance, or by repetitive microtrauma over time. Proximal tendon ruptures typically involve the **long head of the biceps** and result from repetitive microtrauma and degeneration (e.g., repetitive overhead throwing motion) that weakens the biceps' tensile strength over time. Consequently, you will see this injury more commonly in older athletes. Rupture of the proximal biceps tendon is easily observed as a bulging of the muscle in the anterior arm, particularly when contracted. When the proximal biceps tendon is ruptured, the athlete complains of experiencing a sudden sharp pain in the anterior shoulder and may experience a "pop" or snapping sensation. You will note palpable tenderness in the anterior shoulder, along with muscular weakness and eventual swelling and discoloration.

Subluxation or dislocation of the biceps tendon (long head) can occur within the bicipital groove if there is tearing of the transverse humeral ligament or the portion of the subscapularis tendon that stabilizes the tendon within the groove. The mechanism most often associated with dislocation of the biceps tendon is a rapid and abrupt lateral rotation of the humerus while the biceps is under tension. The patient complains of anterior shoulder pain located over the tendon in the bicipital groove and a painful popping or snapping sensation as the tendon slips in and out of the groove during medial and lateral rotation. Tenderness is present directly over the biceps tendon.

Chronic or Overuse Soft Tissue Injuries

Given the repetitive nature of overhead motions that physically active athletes typically perform, the rotator cuff, biceps tendon, and associated bursa are particularly susceptible to chronic inflammatory and degenerative conditions.

Biceps Tendinitis

The long head of the biceps can be involved in a number of pathologies. Tendinitis can result from repetitive overloading and friction as the long head of the biceps passes through the bicipital groove and under the transverse humeral ligament on its way to its proximal attachment on the superior glenoid labrum (figure 12.7). Traction of the tendon's attachment on the glenoid labrum can also occur with forceful contraction during deceleration phases of throwing. In cases of glenohumeral instability, the biceps and the subscapularis may be overloaded as they are called on to provide more of the anterior restraint to glenohumeral motion. This can cause inflammation and pain within the substance of the tendon and at its attachment to the superior glenoid labrum. Biceps tendinitis occurs infrequently as an isolated injury and is typically associated with a shoulder impingement syndrome. Signs and symptoms may include diffuse anterior shoulder pain with point tenderness specifically over the bicipital groove and proximal tendon. Pain can

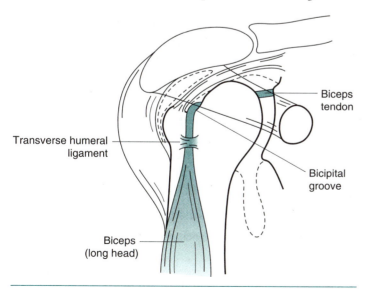

Biceps tendon

Transverse humeral ligament

Bicipital groove

Biceps (long head)

Figure 12.7 The biceps tendon passing through the bicipital groove to its attachment on the glenoid rim.

be elicited with passive stretching of the biceps tendon and with contraction of the biceps while resisting supination. The throwing motion may also be painful, particularly during late cocking and acceleration phases.

Rotator Cuff

As previously mentioned, the rotator cuff acts both as a prime mover for shoulder rotation and as a primary stabilizer for normal glenohumeral function, so it is prone to overuse. In cases of glenohumeral instability, the increased demands on the rotator cuff as a glenohumeral stabilizer make it susceptible to chronic strains and inflammatory conditions. With overhead throwing activities, repetitive forceful muscle contraction during deceleration phases of throwing can eccentrically injure the midsubstance and undersurface of the supraspinatus and infraspinatus portions of the cuff (Meister and Andrews 1993). Signs and symptoms include pain during throwing, tenderness over the supraspinatus or infraspinatus, and mild weakness of the lateral rotators. You may also note infraspinatus atrophy in long-standing chronic cases. Other chronic rotator cuff tendon pathologies and strains typically result secondary to an impingement syndrome.

Impingement Syndrome

Impingement syndrome is caused by encroachment in the subacromial space that decreases the area through which the supraspinatus and subacromial bursa pass underneath the subacromial arch (figure 12.8). Impingement is most commonly seen in occupations and sporting activities involving repetitive overhead shoulder motions. The rotator cuff in older adults is also more prone to injury as it becomes less vascular with age. Impingement, which has been categorized as either primary or secondary, can result from a variety of mechanisms including acute injury, glenohumeral instability, muscle weakness, inflammation secondary to chronic overuse, and bony abnormalities. Primary impingement is caused by direct encroachment within the subacromial space and is most often seen in adults. Anatomical or bony encroachment can occur with variations in the contour of the acromion. A more curved or hooked acromion is often found in association with rotator cuff pathologies. Weakness in the rotator cuff, particularly the infraspinatus and subscapularis, can disrupt the deltoid and rotator cuff force couple, causing the head of the humerus to ride too far superiorly and compress the supraspinatus tendon against the coracoacromial arch. Weakness of the supraspinatus lessens its ability to hug and depress the humeral head against the glenoid fossa, which also may cause the humeral head to ride too far superiorly. In older adults, the more likely cause of primary impingement is degenerative changes to the bony surface and soft tissue structures caused by chronic inflammation that decrease the subacromial space. These degenerative changes include scarring and weakness in the avascular zone of the supraspinatus tendon, spur formation on the undersurface of the acromion, and thickening of the subacromial bursa. Acute injuries with unresolved inflammation and resultant scarring and weakness can also cause muscular dysfunction and decrease the subacromial space.

Secondary impingement results from encroachment due to other shoulder pathologies such as glenohumeral instability. It is the most frequent mechanism associated with impingement in the young athlete. Jobe and Pink (1993) describe an instability continuum in which anterior instability leads to subluxation, which in turn leads to impingement and eventual rotator cuff tears. Many times the instability is not noted until symptoms of impingement and rotator cuff pathology occur. Glenohumeral instability increases the demands on the rotator cuff,

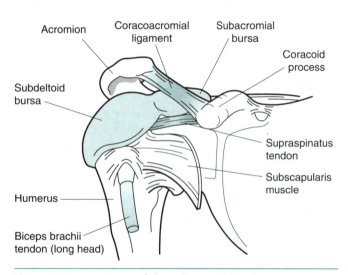

Figure 12.8   Anatomy of the subacromial arch.

increasing its role in shoulder stabilization. This can lead to overuse, fatigue, and repetitive microtrauma, which may inflame the rotator cuff and disrupt its normal functioning. With anterior glenohumeral instability, ROM is often lost with medial rotation secondary to posterior capsule tightness.

In 1973, Neer described three stages of impingement:

- **Stage I** is found most often in younger athletes and is characterized by edema and hemorrhage within the rotator cuff. Symptoms include pain only with activity and little or no weakness; ROM is unrestricted. If impingement is recognized and treated during this early stage, permanent tissue injury can be avoided.
- **Stage II** is characterized by thickening and fibrosis of the subacromial bursa and supraspinatus tendon. There will be pain both during and after activity, including activities of daily living, and perhaps also at night. Because degenerative changes have occurred, stage II impingement is not thought to be reversible with conservative treatment.
- **Stage III** degeneration has progressed to partial- or full-thickness tears of the rotator cuff tendons; there are also bony changes to the surface of the humerus and anterior acromion located within the subacromial space. The patient complains of continuous pain and restricted ROM.

Biceps tendinitis often occurs secondary to impingement because of the close proximity of the proximal biceps tendon to the joint capsule and rotator cuff insertion. The subacromial bursa, which separates the coracoacromial arch from the underlying rotator cuff, also becomes inflamed (subacromial bursitis) and further diminishes the subacromial space. As impingement progresses, the bursa will thicken and become fibrotic. Pain and weakness associated with impingement is most pronounced midrange, from 60° to 120° of abduction and flexion. The patient typically complains of a dull or deep pain underneath or near the acromion. Point tenderness may be noted just anterolateral to the acromion and at the insertion of the supraspinatus tendon. The patient may also complain of pain radiating down the anterior (biceps) and lateral (supraspinatus) aspects of the upper arm.

Traumatic Fractures

Fractures within the shoulder and upper arm are usually caused by traumatic forces; stress fractures are rare. Traumatic fractures can result from both direct contact and indirect forces. Because of the relatively weak ligamentous and capsular support of the glenohumeral joint, dislocation typically occurs before fracture. However, in the young athlete, fractures are more of a concern because of the weakness and immaturity of the growth plate.

Clavicle

Within the shoulder complex, the clavicle is the most commonly fractured bone. The clavicle can fracture as a result of a direct anterior blow—or more often as a result of a force transmitted through the shoulder. Forces transmitted through the shoulder include those resulting from a fall on an outstretched hand or from landing on the shoulder with the arm adducted. The fracture usually occurs at the distal one-third where the contour of the bone changes. Signs and symptoms include pain, localized swelling, and point tenderness. The bone may or may not be displaced. However, since the clavicle is so superficial, any deformity is easily noted. Suspect a fracture any time force is transmitted through the shoulder and there is localized point tenderness over the clavicle.

> ⚠ Because of the close proximity of the neurovascular structures to the shoulder joint and humerus, always check neurovascular status in the upper extremity with any suspected fracture.

Humerus

Fractures of the proximal humerus and humeral shaft are usually caused by a direct blow but may also result from a fall on an outstretched hand. Fractures caused by this type of fall are more commonly seen in older adults. In young adults, the ligament and capsular structures usually fail first, resulting in dislocation rather than fracture. In some cases, both glenohumeral dislocation and anatomical neck fracture may result. Signs and symptoms include severe pain, swelling, and disability. There may also be deformity and crepitus near the fracture site. In cases of anatomical neck fracture, the deformity may resemble a glenohumeral dislocation.

Epiphyseal fractures of the proximal humeral growth plate, or **Little Leaguer's shoulder**, are usually associated with skeletally immature throwing athletes. These injuries occur most often during the deceleration phase of throwing. The primary sign of impending epiphyseal injury is severe shoulder pain during hard throwing. Spiral fractures of the humeral shaft can result from torsional forces associated with the throwing mechanism, particularly during the acceleration phase (Ogawa and Yoshida 1998). Throwing fractures are most prevalent in young adult pitchers. At the time of injury, the fracture is often audible enough to be heard by others. Pain may be experienced anywhere in the midshaft and may extend to the elbow or shoulder. Deformity may be noted if displacement occurs.

A potential complication of humeral shaft fractures is injury to the radial nerve, or **radial nerve palsy** (figure 12.9). Anatomically, the radial nerve exits the axilla and passes posteriorly from medial to lateral along the radial groove of the humeral shaft. If the fracture is displaced, the radial nerve can be contused or injured. In cases of radial nerve involvement, there will be numbness or tingling down the distribution of the nerve into the dorsal forearm and hand. Weakness or paralysis may be noted in the wrist and thumb extensors.

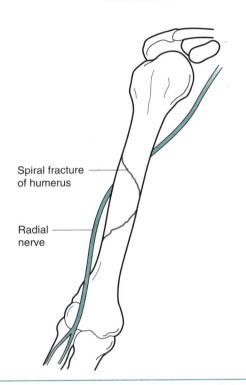

Spiral fracture of humerus

Radial nerve

Figure 12.9 Spiral fracture with potential radial nerve compression.

Scapula

The scapula is one of the least commonly fractured bones of the upper extremity, primarily because of the numerous muscles protecting the bony surfaces, as well as the scapula's mobility on the posterior chest wall. Because the scapula is so protected, fracture usually does not occur unless there is a significant and direct trauma, so scapular fractures are often associated with other, more serious injuries to thoracic structures. On very rare occasions, less traumatic mechanisms such as intensive and prolonged muscular action can result in stress fractures (Deltoff and Bressler 1989). Initial signs and symptoms include diffuse aching over the posterior shoulder region and musculature and an unwillingness to move the arm. The pain may become more localized, with tenderness and swelling over the scapula. Patients with this injury typically hold their arm to the side and demonstrate significant weakness when attempting abduction. Because of the overlying musculature, stress-related scapular fractures may mimic signs and symptoms of rotator cuff and other muscular injuries, depending on the location of the fracture.

Bony or Cartilaginous Lesions Secondary to Repetitive Stress

Athletes complaining of pain and a sensation of clicking or catching with overhead throwing motions may have sustained an injury to the glenoid labrum.

Glenoid Labrum Tear

The glenoid labrum deepens the glenoid fossa to increase glenohumeral stability (figure 12.10). Glenoid labral tears are usually associated with glenohumeral instability and

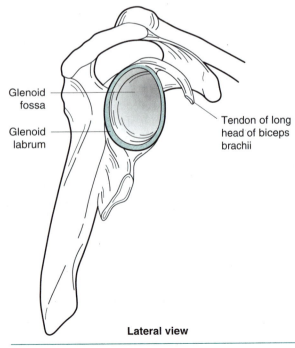

Glenoid fossa

Glenoid labrum

Tendon of long head of biceps brachii

Lateral view

Figure 12.10 Glenoid labrum.

can result from either acute trauma or dislocation or chronic instability. Stresses related to throwing can also disrupt the labrum, particularly near the attachment of the biceps tendon. Swimmers, softball and baseball players, javelin throwers, and volleyball players are all susceptible to labral tears.

Dislocation and Subluxation

Glenohumeral dislocations are named according to the direction in which the humeral head is displaced in relation to the glenoid (figure 12.11a-c). Dislocations and subluxations can result from both acute traumatic events and chronic shoulder instability.

Anterior Dislocation

Anterior glenohumeral dislocations represent the large majority of all glenohumeral dislocations. Anterior subluxations and dislocations typically occur with the arm in an abducted and laterally rotated position. Hyperextension of the joint in this position, or a force applied to the posterior or lateral aspect of the humerus, can stress the anterior and inferior glenohumeral ligaments and capsule and cause them to fail. At lower applied forces the capsular ligaments may be partially stretched, and the athlete feels a slipping or giving sensation that indicates a subluxation or spontaneous relocation. As these static restraints are further stretched and torn, the humeral head is displaced anteriorly and usually lodges between the anterior inferior glenoid rim and the coracoid process (see figure 12.11b). A patient with an anterior dislocation typically presents with the arm slightly abducted and supporting the injured extremity. The acromion is prominent, and the deltoid appears flattened. The humeral head appears as a prominence in the anterior-inferior aspect of the shoulder or may be palpable in the axilla. The patient complains of pain and is unwilling to move the extremity. In cases of subluxation or spontaneous reduction, the patient will be apprehensive and complain of pain when the arm is abducted and laterally rotated. Because of its close proximity to the humeral head in the axilla, the axillary nerve may also be injured. In this case, there is impaired sensation and motor function in the deltoid.

Posterior Dislocation

Posterior dislocations are less frequent but can occur if a posteriorly directed force is applied along the length of the humerus while the arm is flexed forward. Straight-arm blocking and falling on the elbow with the shoulder in a forward and flexed position are examples of this type of mechanism. This mechanism drives the humeral head through the posterior capsule, allowing it to dislodge between the posterior glenoid and the posterior cuff muscles (see figure 12.11c). Posterior dislocations are not as obvious as anterior dislocations, as they often spontaneously reduce so the deformity associated with humeral head displacement is not as

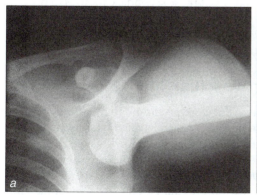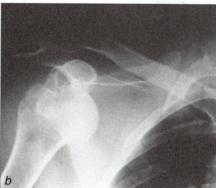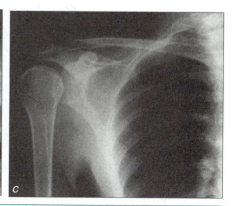

Figure 12.11 Three directions of glenohumeral dislocations: *(a)* anterior-inferior, *(b)* anterior, and *(c)* posterior.
Courtesy of Theodore E. Keats

pronounced. Patients with a posterior dislocation typically present with the arm adducted and medially rotated. The anterior-lateral portion of the deltoid may or may not appear flattened, and the coracoid process may be prominent. The humeral head may be palpable posteriorly. There will also be signs and symptoms of pain and swelling and an unwillingness to move the extremity.

Inferior Dislocation

Displacement of the humeral head directly inferior to the glenoid is fairly uncommon. More often, the displacement is anterior-inferior (see figure 12.11a). Mechanisms associated with inferior dislocation include forced abduction with stress applied to the inferior joint capsule.

Chronic Instability

Chronic glenohumeral instability is commonly seen in physically active persons because of the inherent mobility and weak static stabilizing structures of the shoulder. **Chronic instability** is also classified by the direction of excessive humeral head translation (anterior, inferior, posterior, and multidirectional). Chronic instability can result from an initial traumatic event but also may be unrelated to any previous trauma or dislocation. Repetitive overload caused by overhead activities can also stress and slacken the anterior and inferior ligaments and capsule.

Young athletes involved in overhead activities such as baseball, swimming, javelin, tennis, volleyball, and even golf can place tremendous stress on the anterior structures of the glenohumeral joint. If the musculature (pectoralis major, subscapularis, latissimus dorsi, and teres major) that supports the anterior capsule becomes fatigued, weakened, or injured, the anterior capsule can become stretched and lax, allowing the humeral head to translate anteriorly. Over time, this anterior laxity can result in tightening or shortening of the posterior capsule and subsequent impingement syndrome (Jobe and Pink 1993). This posterior tightening further encourages anterior translation.

Athletes with chronic instability are most susceptible to episodes of subluxation or dislocation when the arm is abducted and laterally rotated. Signs and symptoms include pain and a sensation of joint slippage while the glenohumeral joint subluxes during overhead activity. The athlete may also complain of weakness, numbness, and tingling following the subluxating event. Resultant from the glenohumeral instability, secondary injuries involving degeneration of the glenoid labrum, overuse syndromes of the dynamic stabilizers (rotator cuff muscles and biceps tendon), and shoulder impingement syndromes are common. Signs and symptoms of these secondary injuries may be more pronounced than those associated with the instability and may represent the first indication of a possible instability.

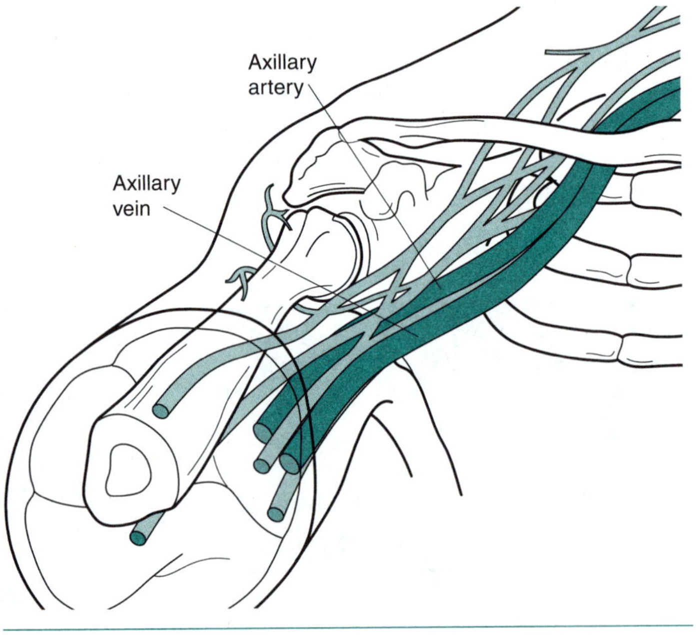

Neurovascular Injuries

Because of the close proximity to the shoulder of the brachial plexus and axillary vessels, neurovascular injury is a concern with significant shoulder trauma (figure 12.12). Associated nerve injuries are more common than vascular injuries at the shoulder. However, any time

Axillary artery

Axillary vein

Figure 12.12 Note the close proximity of the brachial plexus (light green) and axillary vessels (dark green) to the shoulder joint.

there are changes in skin coloration, diminished distal pulses, numbness, tingling, weakness, and loss of motor function, you should suspect neurovascular trauma or compression. Axillary and radial nerve palsy associated with fractures and dislocations of the humerus have been previously discussed (pages 237-238). Brachial plexus injuries and thoracic outlet syndrome were discussed in chapter 11 (pages 200-202) but are equally pertinent in the examination of shoulder injuries. Other peripheral nerves that may be involved in trauma at the shoulder include the suprascapular, long thoracic, and spinal accessory nerves.

Suprascapular Nerve Injury

The suprascapular nerve is vulnerable to injury through both direct blow and traction mechanisms. Signs and symptoms include diffuse posterior shoulder pain and weakness of the supraspinatus and lateral rotators. Pain and a burning sensation may also be produced with horizontal arm adduction across the front of the body (Silliman and Dean 1993). For these reasons, the signs and symptoms of suprascapular nerve injuries may be confused with those of rotator cuff injuries. Entrapment of the suprascapular nerve occurs most often as it passes through the suprascapular notch. Direct pressure or percussion over the notch often elicits suprascapular nerve pain and symptoms. You may note atrophy of the supraspinatus or infraspinatus, depending on the duration of symptoms and the location of nerve compression or injury.

Long Thoracic Nerve Injury

The long thoracic nerve is also prone to both traction and compression injuries. It is particularly vulnerable to direct blows as it runs superficially along the lateral chest wall to innervate the serratus anterior muscle. Long thoracic nerve injury may or may not be associated with pain in the posterior shoulder and scapular regions. Injury may remain unrecognized until serratus anterior weakness and subsequent winging of the scapula are noted. (See the section on scapular winging on page 242.)

Spinal Accessory Nerve Injury

The spinal accessory nerve innervates the trapezius muscle and runs near the posterior triangle of the neck. Injury to this nerve can result from a direct blow to the base of the lateral neck or with shoulder traction and depression. Signs and symptoms include pain, weakness with shoulder elevation, and rotatory winging of the superior angle of the scapula (Silliman and Dean 1993). The trapezius muscle may also show atrophy with time.

Structural and Functional Abnormalities

Structural deformities are usually congenital, whereas functional deformities result from prior injury or musculoskeletal dysfunction. Although these conditions are rarely seen in people who are physically active, it is important to be able to recognize them, as they can significantly affect the normal mechanics of the shoulder.

Adhesive Capsulitis

A concern with immobility following any shoulder injury is **adhesive capsulitis**, or frozen shoulder syndrome. If the arm is volitionally held or purposely immobilized for an extended period of time, the inflamed shoulder capsule may develop adhesions and subsequent contractures, severely limiting ROM. Adhesive capsulitis can usually be avoided through proper treatment and rehabilitation following shoulder injury.

For more information on adhesive capsulitis, refer to *Therapeutic Exercise for Musculoskeletal Injuries, Second Edition,* (Houglum 2005), chapter 17.

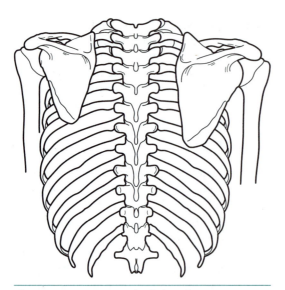

Figure 12.13 Sprengel's deformity.

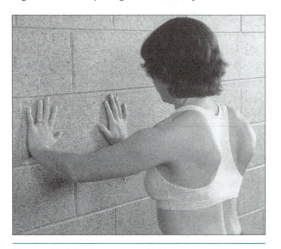

Figure 12.14 Scapular winging.

Sprengel's Deformity

Sprengel's deformity is the most common congenital deformity of the shoulder. It is characterized by an underdeveloped scapula that sits high on the posterior chest wall (figure 12.13). Often the scapula will be medially rotated and the scapular muscles poorly developed. This deformity is caused by a failure of the scapula to descend properly and may be associated with other congenital abnormalities. Sprengel's deformity may be found both unilaterally and bilaterally. Depending on severity, it may affect shoulder abduction ROM. Muscle imbalance or dysfunction created by underdevelopment of the scapular muscles may precipitate other shoulder joint pathologies.

Scapular Winging

Scapular winging is characterized by a protrusion of the vertebral border away from the posterior chest wall (figure 12.14). The scapula is stabilized against the posterior chest wall primarily by the combined function of the serratus anterior and trapezius muscles. If the serratus anterior or trapezius muscles are weak because of deconditioning or muscle imbalance, slight to moderate scapular winging may be present. Severe winging can occur with injury to the spinal accessory (trapezius) or long thoracic (serratus anterior) nerve. Given that scapular stabilization is imperative for proper glenohumeral function, scapular winging may be an important finding in the examination of glenohumeral joint pathology.

OBJECTIVE TESTS

Objective tests for the shoulder are numerous and include observation and palpation of the bony and soft tissue structures of the shoulder, scapular, and distal neck regions; ROM and strength examinations for the muscles that control glenohumeral and scapular motions; tests for neurovascular status; and special tests for examining joint instability (glenohumeral, AC, and SC) and muscle and tendon (rotator cuff and biceps brachii) pathologies. Of course, you will always precede these tests with a history, which guides your choice of objective tests in a given situation. The objective examination begins with observation of not only the injured site but also posture and movement, which further guides your selection of the other objective elements of your examination. Because of this, observation will be discussed later under Injury Examination Strategies (p. 260).

Palpation

Palpation is best performed with the patient sitting. This allows you to move from the anterior to the lateral to the posterior aspect of the shoulder without requiring the patient to change positions. If she has a difficult time relaxing during palpation, it may be advantageous for her to recline and move from supine to prone as you palpate.

- **Anterior structures.** Anterior shoulder palpation begins at the SC joint and moves laterally along the clavicle to the AC joint. The coracoid process is located about 1 in. (2.5 cm) inferior to the junction of the lateral one-third and medial two-thirds of the clavicle where it is most concave. Palpate the sternum, costocartilage, and ribs if the patient complains of anterior chest tenderness or symptoms or has received an anterior impact injury. Palpate the pectoralis major on the anterior chest wall and the biceps and biceps tendons on the anterior arm.

- **Lateral structures.** Palpate the lateral shoulder beginning with the acromion process. Directly inferior to the acromion process is the greater tubercle, and immediately medial to the

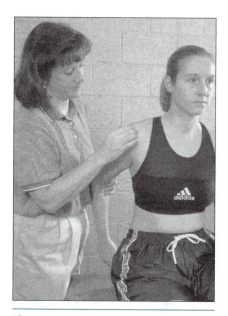

Figure 12.15 Palpation of the sub-acromial bursa.

greater tubercle is the bicipital groove. The lesser tubercle is immediately medial to the bicipital groove. The bicipital groove and lesser tubercle are sometimes easier to palpate if the arm is laterally rotated. In full lateral rotation, the bicipital groove lies directly under the acromion. The rim of the lesser tubercle is the attachment site of the subscapularis tendon. If the patient places a hand at the small of the back, you can palpate the supraspinatus tendon about 0.8 in. (2 cm) inferior to the anterior acromion. If you position the shoulder passively in end hyperextension, you can palpate the subacromial bursa immediately anterior to the anterior acromion (figure 12.15). Palpate the deltoid muscle (anterior, mid, and posterior fibers).

- **Posterior structures.** Palpation of the posterior shoulder begins with bony structures: the spine of the scapula, the lower cervical and upper and middle thoracic spinous processes, and the inferior and superior angles of the scapula. Muscles to palpate include levator scapula, trapezius, rhomboids, teres major, and latissimus dorsi. The triceps tendon can also be palpated. If the patient lies prone with the elbows slightly medial to the shoulder and medially rotated, you can palpate the infraspinatus tendon immediately inferior to the most lateral aspect of the scapula.

- **Axillary structures.** When you passively abduct the patient's shoulder 30° to 40°, you can palpate the axillary structures. The muscles must remain relaxed for this palpation. The anterior wall is formed by the pectoralis major; the posterior wall is the latissimus dorsi; and the medial wall consists of the ribs and anterior serratus. Palpate each of these structures for tenderness and abnormalities. You can also palpate the brachial artery in the axilla.

Range of Motion

Peform shoulder ROM first actively and then passively. Observe for full motion that is controlled, painless, and smooth.

Active ROM

Active ROM consists of both glenohumeral and scapular motions. In addition, functional motion tests allow you to quickly examine motion in more than one plane.

- **Glenohumeral motion.** Test active motion in all planes: flexion and extension (figure 12.16a-b), abduction and adduction (figure 12.16c-d), horizontal adduction and abduction (figure 12.16e-f), and medial and lateral rotation (figure 12.16g-h). These motions can be performed with the patient sitting unless the patient displays less than grade 3 (against gravity) strength.

- **Scapular motion.** Scapular motions to assess during active ROM testing of the shoulder include elevation and depression (figure 12.17a-b), protraction and retraction (figure 12.17c-d), and upward and downward rotation (figure 12.17d-f). See Muscles Involved in Scapular Movement and figure 12.2, a and b, on page 230 for the muscles involved in these scapular movements.

- **Combined movements.** You can use Apley's scratch test to examine a combination of movements. For example, placing the hand behind the back and up on the spine requires shoulder extension, adduction, and medial rotation (figure 12.18a), while placing the hand behind the head involves shoulder flexion, abduction, and lateral rotation (figure 12.18b).

Passive ROM

Perform passive movements when the active motion is less than normal in order to assess full ROM and end feel. Normal end feel for shoulder motions is most often a sensation of a soft tissue stretch. However, it is not abnormal to feel a bony restriction at the end of shoulder abduction. Note any abnormal restriction either in end feel or motion. Passive motions for the shoulder are best performed with the patient supine while passive motions of the scapula are performed with the patient lying on their side.

End feel can identify abnormal tissue restriction that may be limiting ROM. At the end of each active motion, move the patient's arm into the end degrees of the motion. This is usually a few more degrees than the patient is able to move actively (see chapter 6, Types of End Feel Encountered With Passive Overpressure).

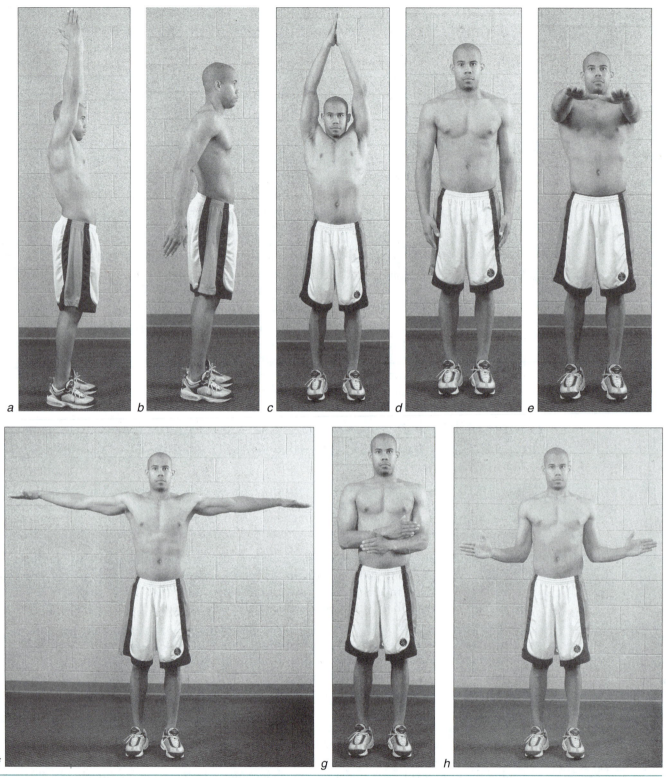

Figure 12.16   Active ROM for *(a)* flexion, *(b)* extension, *(c)* abduction, *(d)* adduction, *(e)* horizontal adduction, *(f)* horizontal abduction, *(g)* medial rotation, and *(h)* lateral rotation.

Goniometric Examination of ROM

The goniometric techniques for measuring the shoulder with and without scapular motion are listed in table 12.1 and demonstrated in figure 12.19.

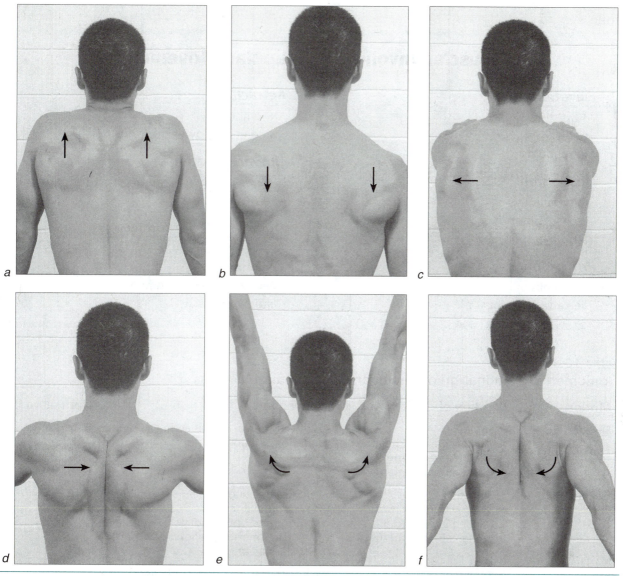

Figure 12.17 Active scapular motions include *(a)* elevation, *(b)* depression, *(c)* protraction, *(d)* retraction, *(e)* upward rotation, and *(f)* downward rotation.

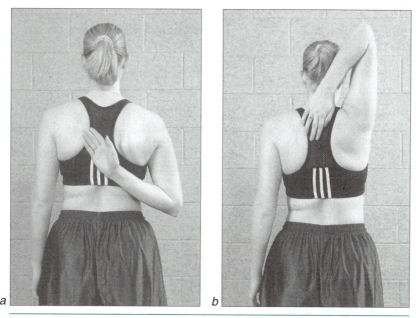

Figure 12.18 Apley's scratch test for *(a)* shoulder extension, adduction, and medial rotation, and *(b)* shoulder flexion, abduction, and lateral rotation.

Muscles Involved in Scapular Movement

Elevation
Trapezius
Levator scapula
Rhomboids

Depression
Pectoralis minor
Lower trapezius
Subclavius

Protraction
Pectoralis minor
Serratus anterior

Retraction
Rhomboids
Medial and lower trapezius

Upward rotation
Upper and lower trapezius
Serratus anterior

Downward rotation
Levator scapula
Rhomboids
Pectoralis major and minor
Latissimus dorsi

Table 12.1

Goniometric Examination of Shoulder and Scapular Motions

Motion	Location of goniometer	Movement	Normal range
Flexion	P: Supine A: Central humeral head S: Midline lateral trunk M: Long axis of humerus	Humerus moves overhead in an anterior and upward direction	0° to 180°
Flexion with scapula fixed	P: Seated A: Central humeral head S: Midline lateral trunk M: Long axis of humerus	While stabilizing the scapula and clavicle, move the humerus in an anterior and upward direction until no further motion is allowed without scapular elevation	0° to 120°
Extension	P: Supine or seated A: Central humeral head S: Midline lateral trunk M: Long axis of humerus	While stabilizing the scapula and trunk, move the humerus posteriorly	0° to 45-60°
Abduction	P: Supine or seated A: Midposterior (seated) or anterior (supine) GH joint S: Parallel to sternum M: Long axis of humerus	Humerus moves in a lateral and an upward direction	0° to 150-180°
Abduction with scapula fixed	P: Supine or seated A: Midposterior (seated) or anterior (supine) GH joint S: Parallel to sternum M: Long axis of humerus	While stabilizing the scapula and clavicle, move the humerus in a lateral and an upward direction until no further motion is allowed without scapular elevation	0° to 90-120°
Horizontal abduction	P: Seated A: Superior acromion process S: Perpendicular to trunk M: Long axis of humerus	With arm abducted to 90°, move the arm in a posterior direction	0° to 30-45°
Horizontal adduction	P: Seated A: Superior acromion process S: Perpendicular to trunk M: Long axis of humerus	With arm abducted to 90°, move the arm in an anterior direction across the chest	0° to 135°

Motion	Location of goniometer	Movement	Normal range
Medial rotation	P: Supine A: Olecranon process S: Perpendicular to table/floor M: Long axis of ulna	With arm abducted to 90°, move the palm of the hand inferiorly toward the table	0° to 70-90°
Lateral rotation	P: Supine A: Olecranon process S: Perpendicular to table/floor M: Long axis of ulna	With arm abducted to 90°, move the back of the hand in a superior direction toward the head of the table	0° to 80-90°

P = athlete position; A = goniometer axis; S = stationary arm; M = movable arm; GH = glenohumeral joint.

Figure 12.19 Goniometric examination of shoulder for *(a)* flexion with and *(b)* without scapular motion; *(c)* extension and abduction *(d)* with and *(e)* without scapular motion; *(f)* horizontal abduction; *(g)* horizontal adduction; *(h)* medial rotation; and *(i)* lateral rotation.

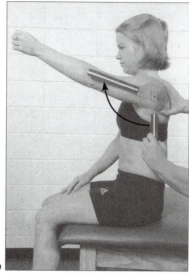
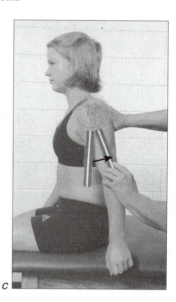
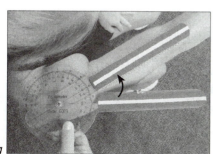

a

b

c

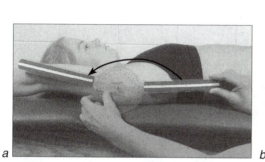
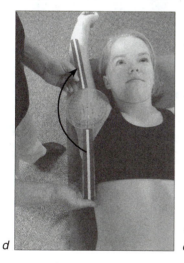
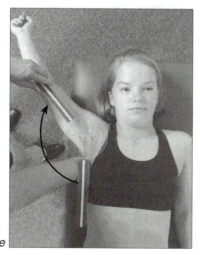
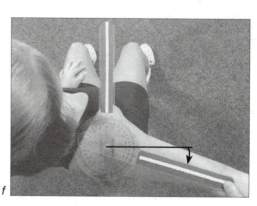

d

e

f

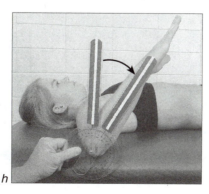
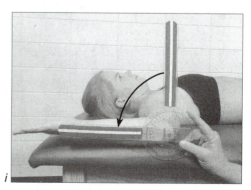

g

h

i

Strength

Both manual and instrumented tests should be used to test strength in the shoulder.

Manual Muscle Tests for Glenohumeral Motion

Glenohumeral motions of flexion and extension (figure 12.20a-b), abduction and adduction (figure 12.20c-d), medial and lateral rotation (figure 12.20e-f), and horizontal adduction and abduction (figure 12.20g-h) are ideally tested against gravity (table 12.2). Since the biceps and triceps also influence the shoulder and can be involved in shoulder injuries, they should also be tested for strength deficiencies (see figures 13.26a-b in chapter 13).

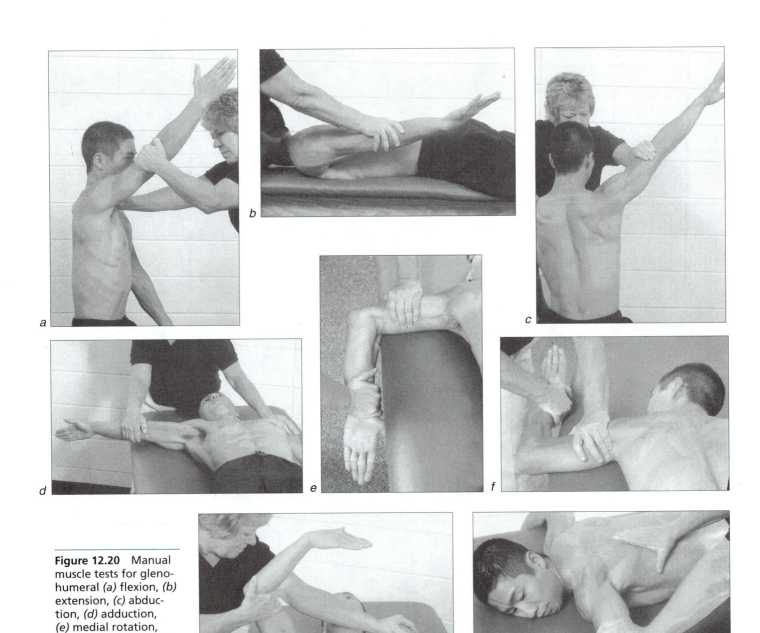

Figure 12.20 Manual muscle tests for glenohumeral *(a)* flexion, *(b)* extension, *(c)* abduction, *(d)* adduction, *(e)* medial rotation, *(f)* lateral rotation, *(g)* horizontal adduction, and *(h)* horizontal abduction.

Table 12.2
Manual Muscle Tests for Glenohumeral Motion

Motion	Athlete position	Stabilizing hand placement	Resistance hand placement	Instruction to athlete	Primary muscles tested
Flexion	Seated	Scapula and clavicle	Distal humerus	Leading with the thumb, raise arm forwardly (anteriorly)	Anterior deltoid
Extension	Prone	Trunk	Distal posterior–medial aspect of humerus	Raise palm toward the ceiling	Latissimus dorsi and teres major
Abduction	Seated	Superior scapula	Distal lateral aspect of humerus	Palm down, raise arm out to the side (laterally)	Middle deltoid and supraspinatus
Adduction	Supine	Scapula	Distal aspect of humerus	Palm down, move arm toward side (medially)	Pectoralis major, latissimus dorsi, teres major
Medial rotation	Prone	Humerus	Ventral aspect of distal forearm	Move palm toward the ceiling	Subscapularis
Lateral rotation	Prone	Humerus	Dorsal aspect of distal forearm	Move back of hand toward ceiling	Infraspinatus, teres minor
Horizontal adduction	Supine, shoulder abducted and elbow flexed to 90°	Opposite shoulder	Distal anterior aspect of humerus	Pull arm across the body toward opposite shoulder	Pectoralis major
Horizontal abduction	Prone, shoulder abducted and elbow flexed to 90°	Scapula	Distal posterior aspect of humerus	Raise elbow toward the ceiling	Posterior deltoid
Elbow flexion	Seated	Distal humerus	Ventral surface of distal forearm	Move palm toward shoulder	Biceps brachii
Elbow extension	Prone	Shoulder	Dorsal surface of distal forearm	Straighten elbow, move back of hand toward ceiling	Triceps brachii

Although isometric tests can be performed with the muscle in any position, they are usually performed with the muscles at midlength. If you find a deficiency, you can test the muscle at other joint angles or against resistance through its full ROM.

Manual Muscle Tests for Scapular Motion

You should also test scapular motions (table 12.3). These motions are elevation (figure 12.21a), depression and upward rotation (figure 12.21b), retraction (figure 12.21c), protraction (figure 12.21d), and downward rotation (figure 12.21e).

Instrumented Strength Examination

In cases where machine strength examination is appropriate, isokinetic testing is frequently used to obtain objective results. Isokinetic machines can quantify muscle function (concentric and eccentric) in a variety of motions and joint positions at different speeds (figure 12.22). You can obtain other objective strength measures with 1RM examination using dumbbells or weight machines. If you use these, you should indicate on the examination form the position in which you tested the patient, since different positions may produce different results. For example, when the patient performs shoulder flexion with a dumbbell while standing, maximum resistance will occur at 90° flexion, whereas in the supine position maximum resistance occurs at the start of the motion, leading to different results with the same weight lifted.

Table 12.3
Manual Muscle Tests for Scapular Motion

Motion	Athlete position	Stabilizing hand placement	Resistance hand placement	Instructions to athlete	Primary muscles tested
Scapular elevation	Seated, arm in neutral	Posterior thorax	Superior border of scapula	Shrug the shoulder	Trapezius, levator scapula
Scapular depression and upward rotation	Prone, arm overhead	Posterior thorax	Scapula	Elevate the shoulder	Pectoralis minor, lower trapezius, subclavius, levator scapula, rhomboids
Scapular retraction	Prone, shoulder abducted and laterally rotated	Posterior thorax	Medial border of scapula	Squeeze shoulder blade (adduct scapula) toward midline	Rhomboids, medial and lower trapezius
Scapular protraction	Seated, shoulder flexed to 90-120°	Posterior thorax	Elbow	Push arm forward and upward	Pectoralis minor, serratus anterior, rhomboids
Scapular downward rotation	Prone, hand behind back	Posterior thorax	Medial inferior border of scapula	Elevate hand toward the ceiling	Upper and lower trapezius, serratus anterior, pectoralis major and minor

Figure 12.21 Scapular motion strength tests for *(a)* elevation, *(b)* depression and upward rotation, *(c)* retraction, *(d)* protraction, and *(e)* downward rotation.

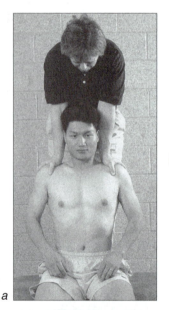

a

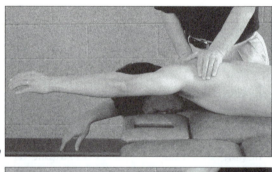

b

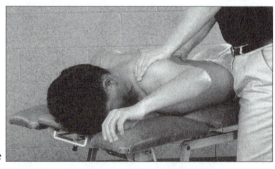

c

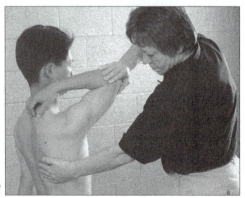

d

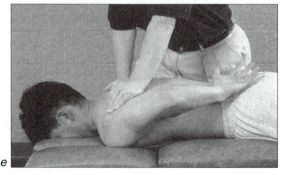

e

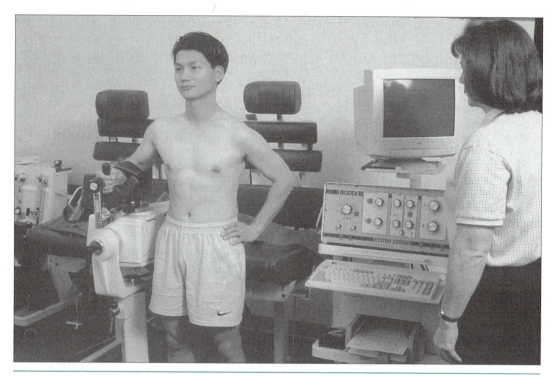

Figure 12.22 Isokinetic machines effectively test shoulder muscle strength. If the injury is very irritable or severe enough to prevent an accurate test, it may be prudent to defer the strength tests until the injury has improved sufficiently to produce accurate results.

Neurovascular Examination

Examine for neurovascular compromise with any fracture or dislocation and whenever a patient reports numbness, tingling, burning, or referred pain. Neurological examination for the shoulder includes sensory, motor, and reflex testing for the brachial plexus. These tests are covered in detail in chapter 8 (see table 8.6 and figures 8.7-8.11). Use distal pulses (brachial and radial) and capillary refill tests to assess vascular compromise (see chapter 9).

Special Tests

Special tests for the shoulder joint complex are organized in this section by joint instability tests (glenohumeral, AC, SC) and muscle and tendon pathology tests (rotator cuff, biceps, other).

Glenohumeral Instability Tests

The glenohumeral joint can be unstable anteriorly, posteriorly, inferiorly, and in multiplanar directions. There are different tests for each of these instabilities; the more commonly used tests are presented here.

Load and Shift Test

Anterior shoulder pain indicates you should use the load and shift test to assess anterior and posterior instability. Unless you are an experienced examiner, perform each test separately to get a clear result—that is, separate the anterior and posterior movements rather than gliding from one to the other. Although anterior instability is a common problem among throwing athletes, it can also occur in other patients. You can perform the load and shift test with the patient sitting or supine. In sitting, the patient's arm rests on the thigh while you stand at his side and slightly behind him. To perform the test, use one hand to stabilize his scapula and clavicle and use the other as your test hand. Place your test hand on the shoulder with your thumb over the posterior humeral head and your fingers over the anterior humeral head. Load the humerus by pushing the humeral head into the glenoid fossa to seat it in its proper neutral position. While maintaining the humeral head in a seated position, shift the humerus forward by applying an anterior force to assess anterior instability. Apply a posterior force to assess posterior instability (figure 12.23). Some movement in each direction is normal, but it should not be more than 25% of the humeral head size. Grade I instability is present if the humeral head moves 25% to 50% in either direction; grade II is present with more than 50% movement with spontaneous reduction when the force is stopped; and grade III is present when the humeral head shows more than 50% movement without spontaneous reduction and remains dislocated (Hawkins and Mohtadi 1991). A combination of laxity and reproduction of the symptoms determines whether or not the test is positive.

Relocation Test and Apprehension Test

The relocation test is also known as the **Fowler test** or the **Jobe relocation test**. It also examines anterior instability. The apprehension test, also called the **crank test**, assesses anterior shoulder dislocation (figure 12.24a). With the patient supine, position the shoulder in 90° abduction and maximum lateral rotation. It is when the patient is in this position that the test is referred to as the crank test, or apprehension test. A positive apprehension test occurs if the patient either looks apprehensive or resists further movement. To continue with the relocation test, create the position slowly to minimize the patient's apprehension and the risk of dislocation (figure 12.24b). If the position is painful, apply an anterior–posterior force to the shoulder to relocate the humerus in the glenoid; the pain will diminish if the test is positive.

Anterior Drawer Test

There are many variations of the anterior drawer test. The primary feature is the application of a posterior-anterior (PA) **glide force** to the shoulder to stress the joint's anterior structures. With the patient supine and the involved shoulder over the edge of the table, place the patient's hand between your upper arm and your side to support the arm. The patient's arm should be relaxed. Position it in midrange abduction with some forward flexion and lateral rotation, about 20° to 30° each. Place your stabilizing hand on the scapula so that your fingers and thumb secure the scapula at the spine of the scapula and the coracoid process.

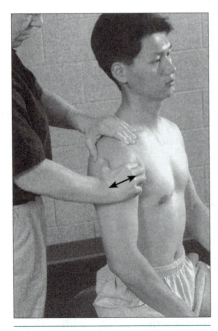

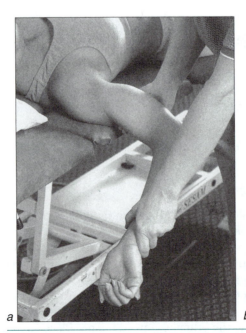

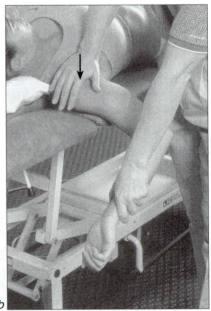

a

b

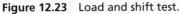

Figure 12.23   Load and shift test.

Figure 12.24   *(a)* Crank, or apprehension, test and *(b)* relocation test.

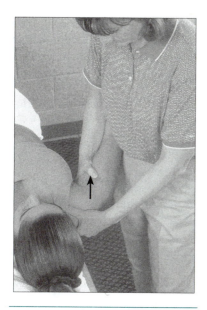

Figure 12.25   Anterior drawer test.

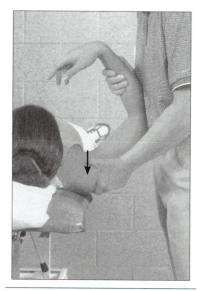

Figure 12.26   Posterior drawer test.

With the test hand supporting the posterior upper arm, pull the patient's arm anteriorly to apply a PA glide force to the glenohumeral joint (figure 12.25). If you hear a click during the maneuver, the glenoid labrum may be torn, or the joint may be sufficiently lax to allow the humeral head to glide over the glenoid labrum rim.

Posterior Drawer Test

The posterior drawer test assesses posterior glenohumeral laxity. As with the anterior drawer test, there are several variations. The intent with each is to apply a force sufficient to stress the soft tissue structures that stabilize the posterior joint, enabling you to determine the presence and degree of laxity. The patient lies supine with the arm relaxed. Use one hand to support the arm and position the shoulder in midrange abduction and about 30° flexion. Place your other hand on the humerus, just off the acromion. As you move the patient's shoulder into greater flexion, apply an anterior-to-posterior force to the humeral head (figure 12.26). A positive test may not produce pain but demonstrates obvious laxity. The patient may show signs of apprehension.

Inferior Drawer Test (Feagin Test)

The inferior drawer (Feagin) test assesses inferior subluxation or glenohumeral joint instability. Have the patient sit on the table with the shoulder abducted 90°, elbow in full extension, and arm resting on your shoulder. Place your clasped hands over the proximal one-third of the humerus. Apply an inferiorly and slightly anteriorly directed force to the humerus and palpate for inferior movement (figure 12.27). Excessive joint play and apprehension indicate glenohumeral joint inferior instability.

Sulcus Sign

The **sulcus sign** assesses inferior instability. The patient sits or stands with the arm hanging relaxed at the side. Palpate the shoulder by placing your thumb and fingers on the anterior and posterior aspects of the humeral head. Your testing hand grasps the elbow and applies a distal distraction force (figure 12.28). As you apply the force, observe the skin over the surface inferior to the acromion. If the sulcus sign is positive, dimpling may occur between the acromion and humeral head as the humeral head moves inferiorly with distraction force. The distance between the humeral head

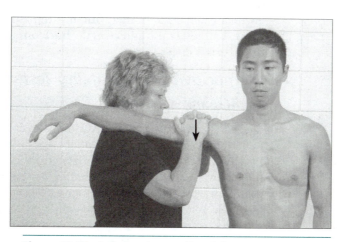

Figure 12.27   Inferior drawer (Feagin) test.

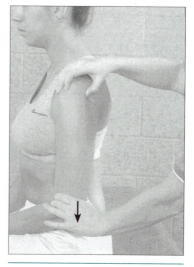

Figure 12.28   Sulcus sign test.

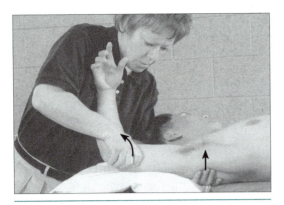

Figure 12.29   Clunk test.

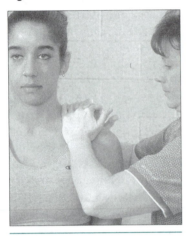

Figure 12.30   Shear test.

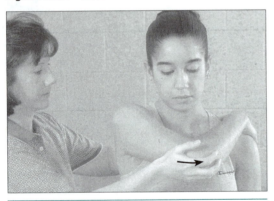

Figure 12.31   AC compression test.

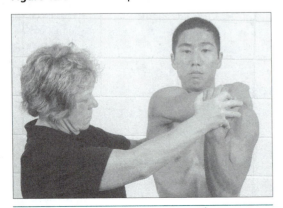

Figure 12.32   SC compression test.

and acromion—and thus the amount of dimpling—depends on the degree of laxity. Movement of the humeral head less than 1 cm distally is a grade +1 sulcus sign; movement of about 1 cm is grade +2; and movement of 1.5 cm or more is grade +3. If the shoulder demonstrates laxity inferiorly, it may also be multidirectionally unstable, so you should also perform anterior and posterior stability tests.

Clunk Test

The clunk test assesses glenoid labrum integrity. With the patient supine, position the involved shoulder in full flexion overhead. Place one of your hands under the shoulder and your other hand on the distal upper arm. As you apply an anterior force with your hand under the patient's humeral head, use your distal hand (hand on the upper arm) to move the shoulder into lateral rotation (figure 12.29). A positive test produces a grinding or clunk in the shoulder.

Acromioclavicular Instability Tests

There are two tests to assess stability of the AC joint: the shear test and the compression test. Use these tests when you suspect an AC joint injury that is not severe enough to disrupt or displace the joint such that abnormal joint position is readily apparent.

Shear Test

Perform the shear test with the patient sitting and the shoulder relaxed with the forearm supported in her lap. Stand at her side and place your hands over the top of the involved shoulder. The heel of one of your hands is on the distal clavicle, and the heel of the other hand is on the lateral scapular spine. Squeeze the bases of your hands together to move the distal clavicle and spine of the scapula toward each other (figure 12.30). A positive test produces pain or laxity in comparison to the other side.

Compression Test

The patient should be sitting for the AC compression test. She places the hand from the involved side on the opposite shoulder, with the elbow positioned at shoulder level (figure 12.31). To perform the test, horizontally adduct the shoulder by passively moving the elevated elbow toward the opposite shoulder to further compress the AC joint. A positive sign is elicited if pain occurs either with or without the passive movement. This test is also known as the **horizontal adduction test** or the **cross chest test**.

Sternoclavicular Instability Tests

Compression Test

The compression test for the AC joint also compresses the SC joint. It is performed with the patient seated. The patient pulls the elbow of the involved side horizontally across the body, with the elbow positioned at shoulder level (figure 12.32). Apply passive overpressure into horizontal adduction of the shoulder by passively moving the elevated elbow toward the opposite shoulder to compress the SC joint. A positive sign is elicited if pain occurs either with or without the passive movement.

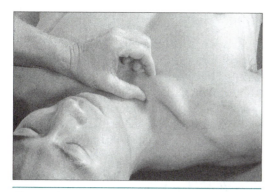

Figure 12.33 SC joint integrity test.

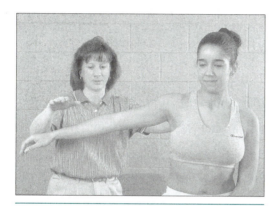

Figure 12.34 Drop arm test.

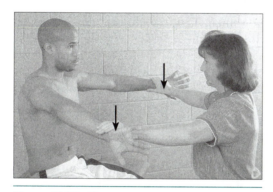

Figure 12.35 The empty can test.

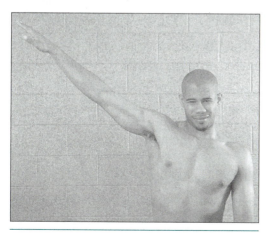

Figure 12.36 Active impingement test.

Sternoclavicular Joint Integrity Test

Test the integrity of the SC and costoclavicular ligaments with the patient supine. Grasping the proximal head of the clavicle, attempt to move it superiorly and inferiorly, then anteriorly and posteriorly, being very careful not to apply too much pressure posteriorly (figure 12.33). Excessive joint play or laxity with associated pain as compared to the uninvolved side indicates SC joint instability.

Rotator Cuff Pathology Tests

Rotator cuff injuries can result from inflammation, instability, and acute stress. The drop arm test examines for an acute rotator cuff injury and is commonly used in the acute examination. Problems due to inflammation or instability are more commonly seen in nontraumatic situations in which the athlete reports to the athletic injury treatment facility because of repeated or prolonged pain, discomfort, or performance interference.

Drop Arm Test (Supraspinatus Test)

The **drop arm test** assesses the integrity of the rotator cuff. A positive sign indicates a rotator cuff tear. Place the athlete's arm passively in 90° of abduction. Then instruct the athlete to slowly lower the arm to the side (figure 12.34). Normal movement is precise and controlled. A rotator cuff tear will produce pain during movement, or the athlete will be unable to control movement throughout a slow motion. Acute tears of the rotator cuff are unusual in young athletes; they are more common in older athletes. A young throwing athlete may experience a rotator cuff tear, but it is usually secondary to instability and impingement.

Empty Can Test

This test, also called the **supraspinatus strength test**, assesses the integrity of the supraspinatus. A positive result indicates a possible muscle tear or, more likely, tendon or suprascapular nerve pathology. Perform the test with the athlete sitting. Place the shoulder in a position of **scaption** (abduction to 90° in a scapular plane, about 30° anterior to the frontal plane). Apply a downward force against the athlete's arm, who attempts to prevent shoulder motion (figure 12.35). A positive result occurs when the athlete is unable to resist the force.

Impingement Tests

The tests described here are for suspected inflammation-based injuries. Since inflammatory conditions (tendinitis and bursitis) can be secondary to impingement of the rotator cuff, impingement tests are discussed here.

Active Impingement Test

This test identifies impingement of the active structures in the shoulder with the presence of a painful arc of motion. The athlete stands and actively abducts or flexes the shoulder through a full ROM (figure 12.36). A positive test occurs when the athlete reports pain in the middle of the motion's arc.

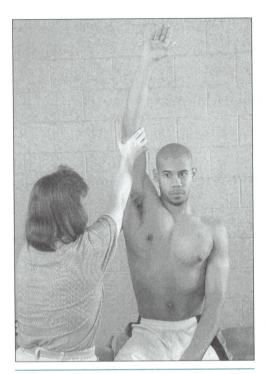

Figure 12.37　Neer impingement test.

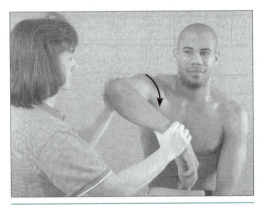

Figure 12.38　Hawkins-Kennedy Test.

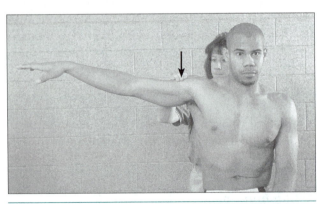

Figure 12.39　Impingement relief test with inferior glide for shoulder abduction.

Neer Impingement Test

The Neer impingement test is named after the orthopedic surgeon who first described it. It compresses the supraspinatus and biceps tendons and the subacromial bursa between the anterior acromion and greater tubercle. The athlete flexes the shoulder as far as possible, and then you passively flex the shoulder to its end motion (figure 12.37). A positive sign occurs if the athlete experiences pain with the test, indicating impingement of either the biceps or supraspinatus tendon.

Hawkins-Kennedy Test

This impingement test is also referred to as the **Hawkins test**. It compresses the supraspinatus tendon against the coracoacromial ligament. With the athlete's arm flexed to 90°, forcefully move the shoulder into medial rotation (figure 12.38). A positive sign occurs when the athlete reports pain with the test, which indicates impingement of the supraspinatus tendon.

Impingement Relief Test

If other active and passive impingement tests are positive, the impingement relief test (Corso 1995) can help you identify the involved structures. The athlete repeats the active impingement test 3 to 5 times and reports where the painful arc of motion begins with each movement, as well as how much pain is present on a 0- to 10-point scale. The active impingement test is then repeated: Immediately at the onset of the painful arc, apply an inferior glide for an abduction movement (figure 12.39) or a posteroinferior glide for a flexion movement. If the glide completely resolves the painful arc, the source of the injury is deficiency within the contractile tissues. The muscles that depress the humerus in the glenohumeral joint or the scapulothoracic muscles that rotate the scapula or create scapulohumeral rhythm are weak, imbalanced, or uncoordinated in their firing patterns. If the athlete experiences some but not complete relief of the painful arc, both contractile tissue and inert tissue may be involved. In addition to the deficiencies already listed, you should suspect inert tissue tightness, especially in the inferior or posteroinferior capsule. If the test does not relieve pain, you should suspect inert tissues as the source of the athlete's painful arc of motion. Tightness of the capsule and glenohumeral ligaments may be the primary source of restriction.

Biceps Tendon and Pectoralis Major Muscle Pathology Tests

Other myotendinous tests are those for the biceps tendon and pectoralis major muscle. Tests to examine integrity of the biceps tendon include those for acute tear, chronic tendinitis, or both. The pectoralis major is examined for tightness that may contribute to chronic shoulder impingement.

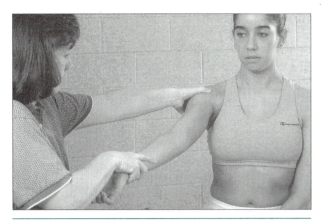

Figure 12.40   Speed's test.

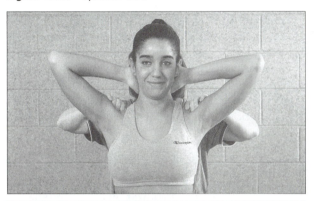

Figure 12.41   Ludington's test.

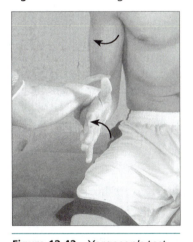

Figure 12.42   Yergason's test.

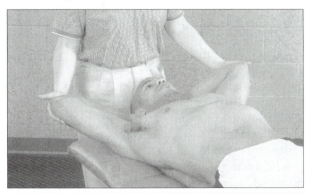

Figure 12.43   Pectoralis major contracture test.

Speed's Test

Speed's test (biceps test or straight arm test) examines the integrity of the biceps tendon. Since the biceps is an integral part of the shoulder joint, it can often be the site of injury in the athletic shoulder. A positive result can indicate either tendinitis or rupture of the biceps tendon, depending on the severity of the response. If the test reveals significant weakness, the tendon may be ruptured. If the primary test result is pain, the injury is probably bicipital tendinitis. Have the athlete sit with the elbow in full extension and palpate the bicipital groove; use your other hand to resist the athlete's attempt to forward flex the shoulder (figure 12.40). Perform the test with the forearm in supination and repeat with the forearm in pronation.

Ludington's Test

A positive result from Ludington's test indicates a tear of the tendon of the long head of the biceps. With the athlete sitting, instruct her to place both hands behind the head and to relax the arms by letting the interlocked hands support both arms in this position. Stand behind the athlete and palpate the bicipital groove (figure 12.41). Then instruct the athlete to alternately contract the right and left biceps as you palpate the tendons. In a positive test, the uninjured tendon can be palpated, but the involved one cannot. If you do not readily observe a biceps tear, Ludington's test is the preferred test to assess for one.

Yergason's Test

Yergason's test assesses bicipital tendinitis and subluxation. It is not as effective as Speed's test for tendinitis, since the tendon does not move within the bicipital groove as much during this test. Position the elbow in 90° flexion, with the forearm pronated. Resist the athlete's attempt to supinate the forearm and laterally rotate the shoulder (figure 12.42). A positive test produces bicipital pain during the resistive movement. If the transverse humeral ligament is torn, an audible or palpable pop may occur as the biceps tendon subluxes over the lesser tuberosity.

Pectoralis Major Contracture Test

This test identifies tightness of the pectoralis major. Tightness in this muscle can affect shoulder impingement, so you should examine chronic shoulder injuries for pectoralis major tightness. The athlete lies supine with both hands behind the head. With your assistance, the athlete then attempts to lower both elbows to the table (figure 12.43). A positive test occurs if the elbows do not reach the table.

Thoracic Outlet Syndrome Tests

TOS was covered in chapter 11 but also applies to the shoulder, as brachial plexus or subclavian artery compression can result from a number of causes in the shoulder region. Because of this, multiple tests are used to isolate the source of impingement. In examining for TOS you should attempt to either reproduce the athlete's symptoms or reduce circulation, so you must observe for the presence of either of these signs. Refer to chapter 11 for the descriptions and illustrations of the following tests:

- Adson's Test (figure 11.28)
- Allen Test (figure 11.29)
- Military Brace Position (figure 11.30)

Joint Mobility Examination

As noted in chapter 6, joint mobility is divided into two types: physiological and accessory (see pages 81-83). Whereas physiological movements are examined earlier, during ROM testing, accessory movements are examined by using joint mobilization techniques after completing the special tests if a capsular pattern of motion was observed during examination of physiological motions. The shoulder's capsular pattern of motion is more limitation of motion in lateral rotation (LR) than in abduction (Abd), more limitation of abduction than flexion (flex), and more limitation of flexion than medial rotation (MR) (LR>Abd>flex>MR).

Examine accessory joint mobility of the glenohumeral, scapulothoracic, and clavicular joints with the athlete reclined in a comfortable position. Most of the techniques are performed with the patient supine, but in a few the patient is side-lying or prone. Supine positioning is preferred for most glenohumeral motions because it permits stabilization of the scapula and relaxation of the surrounding muscles, increasing the chances of an accurate examination. Examine joint play in various directions by comparing the involved side to the uninvolved side for each of the joints. A positive result occurs if the injured shoulder has different joint play than the uninvolved side or if movement reproduces the athlete's symptoms. These tests determine joint capsule mobility in the various planes. Joint capsular restriction will limit shoulder ROM. For example, if the inferior posterior capsule is limited, the athlete will have limited shoulder flexion and medial rotation. On the other hand, if the anterior capsule has excessive mobility, the joint will have anterior instability that can affect shoulder stability during follow-through in throwing. If the anterior capsule is lax, it is also likely that the athlete's symptoms may include shoulder impingement.

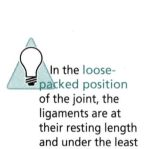

In the loose-packed position of the joint, the ligaments are at their resting length and under the least amount of tension.

Glenohumeral Joint Mobility

The resting position of the glenohumeral joint is 55° flexion and 20° to 30° horizontal abduction, so many of the joint examination techniques are initially performed in this position. This position allows the greatest passive movement possible and provides a reference point for comparison with the uninvolved shoulder and with future examinations.

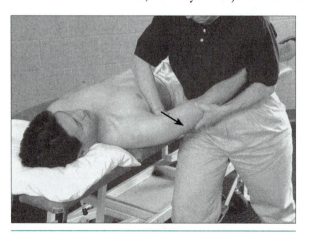

Figure 12.44   Glenohumeral distraction test.

Distraction

Distraction is typically used to provide an overall impression of mobility, or tightness or looseness in the joint. With the athlete supine, stand between his side and arm. Support the arm with one hand while placing your mobilizing hand high in the axilla with your fingers on the posterior arm and your thumb on the anterior arm just distal to the shoulder joint (figure 12.44). Apply a distraction force perpendicular to the joint's surface to move the humerus away from the glenoid fossa, and compare the quality and quantity of mobility to that of the opposite shoulder.

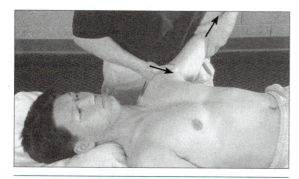

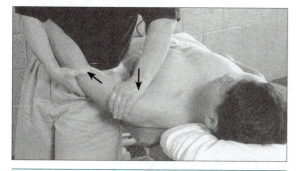

Figure 12.45 Glenohumeral caudal (inferior) glide.

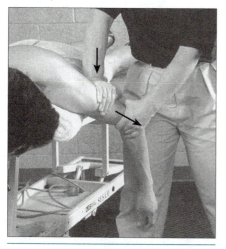

Figure 12.46 Posterior glide test.

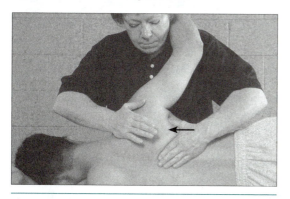

Figure 12.47 Anterior glide test.

Figure 12.48 Scapulothoracic joint mobility test.

Caudal (Inferior) Glide

This maneuver, also called an inferior glide, examines inferior capsule mobility. Limited abduction, caused by a restricted capsule, will display tightness in this test. A glenohumeral joint with a history of inferior dislocations may have an abnormally loose glide. With the athlete lying supine, stand at his side lateral to the arm. Passively place the arm in the shoulder's resting position. Place your mobilizing hand on top of the athlete's shoulder immediately lateral to the acromion. Your stabilizing hand applies a slight distraction of the glenohumeral joint, and your mobilizing hand applies a caudally directed force (figure 12.45).

Posterior Glide

The posterior glide examines posterior capsule mobility. If the athlete's posterior capsule is restricted, physiological motions of horizontal abduction, medial rotation, and flexion will be limited. The athlete lies supine with the involved shoulder over the edge of the table. Standing between the athlete's side and arm, support the shoulder in a resting position with the athlete's arm secured between your side and your stabilizing arm (figure 12.46). Place your mobilizing hand over the anterior shoulder just distal to the acromion. As you apply some joint distraction with your stabilizing hand, apply a downward force with your mobilizing hand to assess posterior capsule movement.

Anterior Glide

This maneuver assesses anterior capsule mobility. An athlete with a restricted anterior capsule will present limited shoulder extension, horizontal abduction, and lateral rotation. A lax anterior capsule indicates a profile of impingement, anterior instability, or glenoid labrum tear. The athlete lies prone with the involved shoulder over the edge of the table. Stand alongside the athlete, facing toward the top of the table; with your supporting hand, position the arm in a resting position. Place your mobilizing hand on the posterior shoulder just distal to the posterior acromion. As your stabilizing hand applies a slight distraction force, your mobilizing hand applies a posterior-anterior force to the glenohumeral joint (figure 12.47).

Scapulothoracic Joint

The scapula rests against the rib cage, separated from the ribs by muscles. It is not a true joint in the sense of two bones supported by ligaments, but restricted glenohumeral movement can limit normal scapular motion on the thorax. If the athlete demonstrates reduced glenohumeral physiological motion, examine the mobility of the scapula on the ribs. The scapula moves on the thorax in several planes. It glides superiorly and inferiorly, glides laterally and medially, and rotates. To assess these motions, have the athlete lie on her side with the shoulder that will be examined on top. Support the arm by the scapula at its superior aspect and inferior angle. Alternate your hands in applying the mobilizing force and examining the scapular movement. For example, when examining scapular inferior mobility, your mobilizing hand is the superior hand. It pushes the scapula inferiorly as the hand at the inferior angle palpates for degree and quality of movement. To assess superior mobility, the inferior hand applies the force while the superior hand assesses the lateral-medial and rotational scapular movements (figure 12.48).

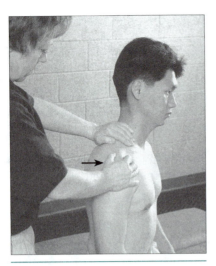

Figure 12.49 AC joint mobility test.

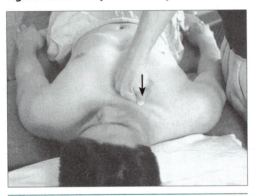

Figure 12.50 SC joint mobility test.

Clavicular Joints

Examine joint mobility of both the AC and SC joints if glenohumeral physiological motions display a capsular pattern. These joints should also be examined if you suspect an injury to either one.

Acromioclavicular Joint

Stand behind the athlete, who should be seated, and place a stabilizing hand over the glenohumeral joint. Place the thumb of your mobilizing thumb on the posterior aspect of the lateral clavicle (figure 12.49). Apply an anteriorly directed force to the posterior clavicle just medial to the AC joint.

Sternoclavicular Joint

To examine the SC joint, have the athlete lie supine and stand either at the head or side of the table facing the athlete. Although the joint can be examined in various maneuvers, a commonly used technique is the posterior glide. To perform this glide, place the pads of one or both of your thumbs directly over the anterior surface of the clavicle, just lateral to the sternum (figure 12.50), and apply an anterior-to-posterior force.

INJURY EXAMINATION STRATEGIES

By now you should have an appreciation for the acute and chronic conditions commonly seen in people who are physically active. This knowledge, along with a strong background in anatomy, will help you interpret the findings of your examination.

On-Site Examination

You are covering the senior women's tennis tournament when you observe one of the athletes lunge for a ball, trip, and attempt to break her fall by putting her arm out in front of her. She is now clearly in agony and holding her arm.

You see a receiver who is tackled and lands on his right shoulder. As you run onto the field, you notice that he has rolled onto his back and is grasping the top of the shoulder with his left hand.

On-site examination can be the most efficient when you have observed the injury occur. You can glean much from seeing the mechanism of injury, including an immediate impression of the severity and the athlete's immediate physical and emotional response. As you approach the athlete, observe the surroundings as well as the position and response of the athlete. Is she moving, holding her arm to protect the shoulder, or keeping her arm in the position of injury? Is the shoulder in abduction or held close to the side? Does it appear deformed? Is she in excessive pain or able to control her response?

Once you are at the athlete's side, check the ABCs and look for obvious signs of deformity or severe bleeding. Touching the athlete with a reassuring hand will calm her while taking a history regarding the location and severity of the pain. Routinely palpate for a distal pulse

Remember, the patient does not have to experience a severe injury to suffer shock. You should always be aware of his reaction to the injury and observe for signs of shock. If he appears to be going into shock, stabilize the injury and arrange for immediate emergency care.

and sensory and motor perception (C5-T1 nerve roots) with more severe injuries, particularly with suspected fractures or dislocations that may compromise the neurovascular structures. If signs of neurovascular compromise are present, activate emergency medical services (EMS) and immediately refer the athlete for emergency care. If not, continue the examination. Palpate the shoulder's bony and soft tissue structures, comparing them to the structures on the uninvolved side to reveal any gross deformities and areas of tenderness around the shoulder (see the following section on acute examination for the complete palpation sequence). Check for any flattening of the deltoid that would indicate a dislocation or subluxation. If there is no deformity, ask the athlete to slowly move the arm. You can place a hand on the shoulder during active motion to palpate for any crepitus or abnormal movement.

If the athlete is able to move the arm, shows no sign of serious injury, and is not in extreme pain, assist him to a seated position and then to a standing position, being careful not to pull on the injured arm. Be sure to support the arm or have the athlete support it with the uninvolved hand before standing and ambulating off the field. The athlete then moves to the sideline for a more detailed examination.

For most upper-extremity injuries, athletes will be able to move to the sidelines under their own power, without the need for passive transport. However, passive transport may be necessary in the case of fracture or dislocation or if the athlete is in severe pain, light-headed, or nauseous. If you suspect a fracture or dislocation, immobilize the arm before moving the athlete. The athlete's safety is always the primary concern when deciding the mode of transportation from the field. Although efficiency is also a concern, it should never compromise the athlete's health and welfare.

Checklist for On-Site Examination of the Shoulder and Arm

▷ *Primary Survey*

- ☐ Consciousness
- ☐ Airway, breathing, and circulation
- ☐ Severe bleeding

▷ *Secondary Survey*

  ▷ *History*

- ☐ Mechanism, location, and severity of pain
- ☐ Information from bystanders

  ▷ *Observation*

- ☐ Deformity, swelling, discoloration
- ☐ Athlete's response to injury
- ☐ Unusual limb positioning

  ▷ *Palpation*

- ☐ Deltoid contour
- ☐ Bony tenderness
- ☐ Bone and joint deformity or crepitus

  ▷ *Neurovascular examination*

- ☐ Sensory (C5-T1)
- ☐ Motor (C5-T1)
- ☐ Distal pulse (radial)

  ▷ *Active ROM*

Determine mode of transportation from site

Acute Examination

The star quarterback is injured while attempting to throw a forward pass as an oncoming linebacker makes contact with his arm and chest. As you approach, the quarterback is now standing, holding his arm at his side, and in obvious pain. On the field, you palpate under his shoulder pads and note that the contour of the shoulder joint seems equal bilaterally. He states his pain is located more in the anterior upper chest and increases when he tries to move his arm. Your neurovascular examination revealed no signs of compromise. From your cursory field examination, you determine it is safe to remove him from the field for further examination.

A female basketball player with a history of shoulder subluxations reports to you at halftime that she experienced another subluxation when she was blocked on a lay-up right before the end of the half. This time, however, she feels like it is still out of joint, and she can't get it back in place like she usually does.

Once the athlete is off the field and you have determined that the injury is not severe enough to warrant emergency transport from the field, an acute examination enables you to determine the severity of the injury, the specific tissue or structure involved, and the ability of the athlete to return to participation.

History

Remember to ask open-ended, non-leading questions when taking a history from an injured athlete.

Ask the athlete to provide a more detailed history of the injury even if you saw the injury happen. Many times he can provide information about the direction of forces applied that people on the sideline cannot observe. The athlete also has information about the sounds and sensations heard or felt at the time of injury and immediate sensations after the injury. Specific questions may include the following: How did you land? Did you hear or feel anything (i.e., a snap or pop) at the time of the injury? Was there immediate pain? Has the pain changed? Ask him to describe the location, quality, and intensity of the pain. Do the symptoms radiate (e.g., up to the neck or down the arm)? If so, what sensations is he feeling? This is also the time to ask about any previous injuries to the shoulder. If he was previously injured, what was the nature of the injury and what treatment, if any, did he receive? Were there any problems with the shoulder before that, and have there been any since? Also inquire about prior injuries to the uninjured shoulder to help you interpret your bilateral comparisons.

Observation

Throughout the history portion of the examination, observe the athlete's actions and response to the injury. Observe for signs of swelling, discoloration, deformity or abnormal contours, pain, and guarding. Does he gesture freely with the arm or hold and support it? Does he remove his shirt without difficulty, or does he require assistance or is he hesitant to move the arm overhead?

If you suspect a severe injury, cut his clothing and equipment away rather than move the shoulder into positions that might cause further injury or pain. Once the shirt is removed, observe the shoulder for contour and balance in comparison to the uninvolved side. Check for any flattening of the deltoid that may indicate a subluxation or dislocation, and check for deformity and swelling over the clavicle that may indicate a clavicular fracture or SC separation. Also assess the posture of the shoulder, neck, and upper back, since poor posture can either aggravate or be caused by an injury. The head should be in the midline position in an anterior and posterior view. The acromions, SC joints, inferior border of the scapulae, and scapular spines should be level bilaterally. However, it is common for the dominant shoulder to be slightly lower than the nondominant, so this difference, if it is not exaggerated, is not considered abnormal. The shoulders should be rounded and have equal contour left to right. In normal shoulder alignment, the inferior tip of the scapula is in line with T7, and the superior medial ridge is in line with T2. The medial border of the scapula is 2 to 3 in. (5.1 to 7.6 cm) from the thoracic spinous processes. Since it is usually difficult to hide pain through facial expressions, observe the patient's facial expressions throughout the examination to help determine his level of discomfort.

Palpation

Look for areas of tenderness or differences between the right and left sides in bony and soft tissue contour, muscle tone, and soft tissue mobility. Palpate along the clavicle from the SC joint to the AC joint for signs of swelling, crepitus, and tenderness. Superficial muscles to palpate are the pectoralis major anteriorly; the trapezius and supraspinatus superiorly; the trapezius, rhomboids, levator scapula, teres major, latissimus dorsi, and posterior cuff muscles posteriorly; and the deltoid laterally. Palpate the muscles for tenderness, spasm, and defect.

Special Tests

Since several joints and soft tissue structures constitute the shoulder complex, you must examine many elements in order to examine the shoulder thoroughly. The special tests you select will be based on the cumulative results of your examination thus far. It may be useful to briefly pause in the examination to consider your impressions before proceeding. For example, if you have eliminated the possibility of AC injury, then there is no need to perform the special tests for it. Special tests that you will typically perform in the acute examination are for joint instability and musculotendinous strains and ruptures.

Range of Motion

Perform shoulder ROM testing actively and then passively. Glitches in the movement because of pain or difficulty with the motion are abnormal and call for further examination. Incomplete motion or substituted motions are also abnormal and require further investigation.

It is often best if the athlete performs the motions simultaneously with right and left arms. This will allow you to more easily compare flow of movement and ranges of motion. Substitutions are more obvious, too. Observe motions from anterior, lateral, and posterior views for complete comparisons. From the posterior view, you should also observe scapular motion during these movements. Although the scapula does not act alone, you should observe scapular movement bilaterally during the shoulder motions just described, checking for smooth and equal movement. Asymmetrical movement may indicate muscle substitution (compensatory movement) or may even be secondary to chronic dysfunction.

You may note that the dominant arm has slightly less motion than the nondominant arm. This is normal. Some athletes may also exhibit excessive motion in specific planes (**hypermobility**), which may also be considered normal. For example, pitchers will have more than the "normal" 90° of lateral rotation—less than 90° would be considered abnormal for them. Pain through the arc of motion into shoulder flexion is pathological. There is pathology in the subacromial soft tissue structures (biceps tendon, bursa, or rotator cuff) if the pain occurs during the midarc of the motion, and there is AC pathology if the pain occurs at the end of the motion. If pain occurs with horizontal adduction, the AC joint is likely involved.

Strength

The athlete can perform the strength tests outlined in table 12.2 in sitting unless there is less than grade 3 strength. Apply resistance with the scapula stabilized. The resistance should gradually build to a maximum and then gradually decrease; it should not be suddenly released. Resistance to medial and lateral rotation on the sideline is more commonly performed sitting (rather than prone) with the athlete's elbow stabilized at his side.

Neurovascular Tests

Distal pulse should be periodically checked with all dislocations and fractures. If the athlete reports numbness, tingling, burning, or shooting pain distal to the acromion, perform a neurological examination. The neurological tests include examination of sensory, motor,

Checklist for Acute Examination of the Shoulder and Arm

▷ *History*

Ask questions pertaining to the following:

- ☐ Chief complaint
- ☐ Mechanism of injury
- ☐ Unusual sounds or sensations
- ☐ Type and location of pain or symptoms
- ☐ Previous injury
- ☐ Previous injury to opposite extremity for bilateral comparison

▷ *Observation*

- ☐ Visible facial expressions of pain
- ☐ Swelling, deformity, abnormal contours, or discoloration
- ☐ Does athlete let arm hang and swing, or does athlete hold or splint the arm?
- ☐ Overall position, posture, and alignment (anterior, lateral, and posterior)
- ☐ Muscle development—are there areas of muscular atrophy?
- ☐ Bilateral comparison of acromions, SC joints, inferior border of scapula, and scapular spine
- ☐ Is the inferior tip of scapula level with T7 and the superior medial ridge level with T2?

▷ *Palpation*

Bilaterally palpate for pain, tenderness, and deformity over the following:

- ☐ SC joint, clavicle, AC joint, acromion, coracoid process, subacromial bursa, greater tuberosity, lesser tuberosity, bicipital groove
- ☐ Spine, superior and inferior angles of scapula, lower cervical and upper thoracic spinous processes
- ☐ Rotator cuff insertion
- ☐ Sternocleidomastoid, pectoralis
- ☐ Biceps tendon and muscle
- ☐ Trapezius, rhomboid, latissimus dorsi, serratus anterior
- ☐ Axillary structures

▷ *Special Tests*

- ☐ Glenohumeral stability tests
- ☐ AC and SC stability tests
- ☐ Rotator cuff pathology tests
- ☐ Biceps tests

▷ *Range of Motion*

- ☐ Active ROM for shoulder flexion and extension, abduction and adduction, horizontal adduction and abduction, and medial and lateral rotation
- ☐ Observe scapular elevation and depression, retraction and protraction, upward and downward rotation with active motions listed above
- ☐ Passive ROM for shoulder motions listed
- ☐ Passive ROM for scapular motions listed
- ☐ Bilateral comparison

▷ *Strength Tests*

- ☐ Perform manual resistance against same motions as performed in active ROM
- ☐ Check bilaterally and note any pain or weakness

▷ *Neurovascular Tests*

- ☐ Sensory (C5-T1)
- ☐ Motor (C5-T1)
- ☐ Distal pulse (radial)

▷ *Functional Tests*

and reflex components of the brachial plexus. These tests were discussed in chapter 8 and described in table 8.6 and figures 8.7 through 8.11.

Functional Tests

If the athlete's symptoms subside during the course of the examination and you determine that the injury was minor, you should perform functional tests before allowing him back into the game or practice. Functional tests for the injured shoulder, as for other injured body segments, should accurately demonstrate readiness to return to activity. These tests, then, should include activities particular to the athlete's sport. For example, in this section's opening scenario, you would have the athlete hold the football and mimic the throwing motion and then have him throw the ball with increasing velocity and accuracy. If the athlete is a wrestler, functional tests can include handstands, resisted push-ups, and full-motion activities against resistance. If the athlete is a volleyball player, then overhead hitting, quick lateral overhead movements, and blocking shots will be part of the functional tests.

Clinical Examination

Consider the swimmer with anterior shoulder pain that was discussed in the opening scenario. The swimmer comes to you complaining of increasing pain in the anterior shoulder that is exacerbated by the butterfly stroke as well as the bench and military press. You observe a forward head and rounded shoulder posture.

A 42-year-old female factory worker comes in complaining of shoulder and right arm pain that is waking her up at night. The pain worsens when sitting and working at her computer terminal for extended periods of time.

Often an athlete with shoulder pain will not seek treatment or examination immediately following injury. Soreness may not set in until hours later or even the next day. Signs and symptoms related to repetitive stress also appear gradually over time. Therefore it is likely that the majority of shoulder examinations will be for postacute and chronic injuries.

History

Gaining a thorough history from the patient is essential in the clinical shoulder examination, particularly when the patient presents with chronic conditions. In addition to the typical questions about the mechanism, nature, and severity of the injury, you will cover activity history, especially if there was no specific injury and the pain has progressed over time. Does the patient recall when and under what circumstances the pain was first noticed? If it occurred during activity, did the pain last through the entire activity or part of the activity? When does the pain occur now? Does it last all the way through the activity, persist after the activity, or interfere with other areas of daily life? Have there been any abrupt changes in training or weightlifting practices? Do other activities aggravate or ease the symptoms? If there is a previous history of injury, when was the first and last occurrence, how often does the injury recur, what treatment was provided, and what was the outcome of treatment? Even if previous injuries were different from the current complaint, they can provide insight into potential causes of this new injury. For example, if the patient's only prior injury was a clavicular fracture and the present injury seems to be related to the rotator cuff, perhaps the shoulder was never strengthened after a period of immobilization following the clavicular injury, resulting in weakness in cuff muscles that makes them more susceptible to injury. Also inquire about previous injuries to the uninjured side. These and other questions for postacute, chronic, or overuse injuries can help you identify the stage of the injury, its severity, and its irritability.

By the time you have finished taking the athlete's history, you should have a good idea of how severe the injury is (**s**everity), how irritable the injury is (**i**rritability), what structure is probably involved (**n**ature), and whether the injury is acute, subacute, or chronic (**s**tage). Once you have determined these SINS, you will have a better sense of the special tests that you should perform and how aggressive you can be.

Observation

Observe how the patient moves her shoulder, holds her arm, and removes her jacket or shirt; also note her general posture (chapter 4). As discussed previously, a forward head posture with rounded shoulders can contribute to shoulder impingement and thoracic outlet syndromes. Observe her facial expressions both during relaxed sitting and during active movement. The best observations of the injured shoulder are made with both shoulders exposed. Compare shoulder symmetry from anterior and posterior views. Clavicle, scapular levels, and the balance, contour, and position of other structures as discussed for the acute examination are also observed in the clinical examination. Muscle atrophy indicates a more chronic problem, whereas discoloration indicates acute injuries. Atrophy can indicate either muscle disuse or neural damage resulting in weakness.

Differential Diagnosis

The shoulder and cervical regions are closely related, and it is sometimes difficult to identify whether the source of the injury is in the shoulder or the cervical area. The brachial plexus can also be a site of shoulder-related symptoms, since the complex runs through the axilla and can be damaged during a shoulder injury (fracture or dislocation) or secondary to cervical trauma. You should eliminate these sources of shoulder symptoms any time the patient's pain is distal to the acromion and you did not witness the injury.

Quick tests can eliminate the cervical and brachial plexus as sources of shoulder symptoms. These tests include cervical ROM with overpressure at each end range (see chapter 11). If the symptoms are not reproduced with overpressure of these motions, you can perform an additional quick test in the cervical quadrant position (figure 11.31). Place the patient's head in lateral flexion, rotation, and extension to the side of symptoms and apply overpressure in the end position. She may experience some discomfort in the neck, but a positive sign occurs only if any of the symptoms are reproduced.

Thoracic outlet syndrome (TOS) is another condition that you should eliminate if signs and symptoms lead you to suspect this injury. Specific tests for TOS were discussed in chapter 11.

Range of Motion

In the athletic treatment facility, use the same ROM tests used for the acute examination, checking for both quality and quantity of movement. Follow these tests with passive ROM and goniometric examination as indicated. Note whether the limitation is due to stiffness or pain. Note any capsular patterns of movement if the athlete's motion is incomplete. As previously mentioned, the shoulder's capsular pattern includes more limitation in lateral rotation than in abduction, more limitation in abduction than in flexion, and more limitation in flexion than in medial rotation. If the patient's reduced ROM follows a capsular pattern, you must perform a joint mobility examination (see page 258) to establish locations and quantity of capsular restriction. If, for example, the patient has no restriction of lateral rotation motion but is limited in abduction and flexion, a capsular pattern is not present, and reduced ROM is caused by another factor.

Strength

While manual muscle break tests with the athlete in a seated position are quicker and more conducive to the acute examination, you should use full manual muscle tests against gravity in the clinical examination (table 12.2). In addition, instrumented tests can more objectively define strength deficiencies. Use of instrumented strength tests depends on the injury's severity and irritability, as maximal strength tests can aggravate an easily irritated injury.

Neurovascular Tests

The aim of neurological tests is to establish any differential diagnosis or evidence of neurological compromise. These tests include examination of sensory, motor, and reflex components. As mentioned for the acute examination, these tests should be performed on any patient who reports symptoms of nerve pain including pain radiating down the arm, burning, tingling, sharp or dull pain, or numbness. The specific tests are described in chapter 8. Neurovascular tests associated with thoracic outlet syndrome should also be performed (see chapter 11).

Special Tests

By the time you reach this point in the examination, you should have an idea which special tests are necessary to confirm or disprove your preliminary impressions. The special tests used in the acute examination are also performed in the clinical examination. In addition, you may include other special tests to examine chronic inflammatory and overuse conditions of the muscle and surrounding soft tissues:

- Rotator cuff and impingement tests
- Active impingement test
- Neer impingement test
- Hawkins-Kennedy test
- Empty can test
- Impingement relief test
- Yergason's test
- Pectoralis major contracture test
- Other muscle and tendon pathology tests
- Joint mobility tests

Palpation

Perform palpation as outlined in the section on objective tests (p. 242). Compare right and left structures for symmetry, atrophy, nodules, and areas of tenderness or crepitus. Even though the patient's injury may not be recent, spasm may still be present. You may also find active trigger points with palpation. Follow a systematic routine to palpate all aspects of the shoulder region and its related structures. As with the acute examination, a logical progression would be to start at the anterior shoulder, progress laterally, and finish palpation in the posterior aspect. If the area of pain is the anterior shoulder, however, it may be better to begin at the posterior shoulder and progress to the anterior shoulder to complete the palpation in the region of primary complaint.

Functional Tests

Functional tests are critical for the shoulder region. Because of the high velocity and strong eccentric actions inherent in overhead throwing motions, pain and symptoms may occur during these dynamic activities that were not present, or were relatively mild, during your examination. For this same reason, functional tests for the overhead athlete should be conducted in a gradual progression of skill complexity and velocity. For example, you may ask the gymnast to perform a regular push-up. If this activity does not reproduce any symptoms, an inverted push-up may be the next test. If the gymnast performs these exercises without symptoms, instruct the athlete to perform an activity such as a front walkover or a more aggressive activity such as a running tumbling pass with multiple handsprings or other maneuvers.

Remember to tailor your functional tests to the specific demands of the patient's sport or work. Consider the different forces and stresses that the sport places on the shoulder (i.e., breaststroke versus butterfly specialist), as well as between sports (i.e., gymnast versus thrower versus tennis player versus lineman). Understanding the physical demands of work (e.g., office or computer work versus factory work versus firefighting) will guide you in tailoring functional tests to assist you in determining the patient's readiness to return.

For guidelines and examples of functional tests to use before the return of an athlete to full participation, refer to *Therapeutic Exercise for Athletic Injuries, Second Edition*, (Houglum 2005), chapter 1.

Checklist for Clinical Examination of the Shoulder and Arm

▷ *History*

Ask questions pertaining to the following:

☐ Chief complaint

☐ Mechanism of injury

☐ Unusual sounds or sensations

☐ Type and location of pain or symptoms

☐ Previous injury

☐ Previous injury to opposite extremity for bilateral comparison

If chronic, ascertain:

☐ Duration of onset

☐ Aggravating and easing activities

☐ Training history

▷ *Observation*

☐ Visible facial expressions of pain

☐ Swelling, deformity, abnormal contours, or discoloration

☐ Does athlete let arm hang and swing, or does athlete hold or splint the arm?

☐ Overall position, posture, and alignment (anterior, lateral, and posterior)

☐ Muscle development bilaterally—are there areas of muscular atrophy?

☐ Bilateral comparison of acromions, SC joints, inferior border of scapula and scapular spine

☐ Scapular position (inferior tip of scapula is level with T7, superior medial ridge is at T2)

▷ *Differential Diagnosis*

☐ Clear cervical region with overpressure tests—quadrant position

☐ Eliminate thoracic outlet and brachial plexus pathologies

▷ *Range of Motion*

☐ Active ROM for shoulder flexion and extension, abduction and adduction, horizontal adduction and abduction, and medial and lateral rotation

☐ Observe scapular elevation and depression, retraction and protraction, upward and downward rotation with active motions listed above

☐ Passive ROM for shoulder motions listed

☐ Passive ROM for scapular motions listed

☐ Bilateral comparison

▷ *Strength Tests*

☐ Perform manual resistance against same motions as in active ROM

☐ Check bilaterally and note any pain or weaknesses

▷ *Neurovascular Tests*

☐ Sensory

☐ Motor

☐ Reflex

☐ Distal pulse

☐ Thoracic outlet tests for neurovascular compromise

▷ Special Tests

- ☐ Glenohumeral stability tests
- ☐ AC stability tests
- ☐ Rotator cuff pathology and impingement tests
- ☐ Biceps tests (Speed's and Yergason's)
- ☐ Pectoralis major contraction test
- ☐ SC stability tests

▷ Joint Mobility (as appropriate)

Note capsular restriction and end feel:

- ☐ Glenohumeral joint
- ☐ Scapulothoracic joint
- ☐ Clavicular joint

▷ Palpation

Bilaterally palpate for pain, tenderness, and deformity over the following:

- ☐ SC joint, clavicle, AC joint, acromion, coracoid process, subacromial bursa, greater tuberosity, lesser tuberosity, bicipital groove
- ☐ Scapular spine
- ☐ Rotator cuff
- ☐ Sternocleidomastoid, pectoralis
- ☐ Biceps tendon and muscle
- ☐ Trapezius, rhomboid, latissimus dorsi, serratus anterior
- ☐ Axillary structures

▷ Functional Tests

SUMMARY

1. Discuss the types of overuse injuries that commonly result from repetitive overhead throwing activities.

   The considerable velocity and eccentric forces that occur repetitively over a large range of motion during overhead throwing activities are a common cause of chronic shoulder conditions. Strains in the rotator cuff and biceps tendon that decelerate the arm during throwing are common. Traction forces of the biceps tendon attachment to the glenoid labrum during deceleration can cause bicipital tendinitis and tear the glenoid labrum. Glenoid labral tears can also result from chronic instability. In addition, throwing athletes often experience chronic instability and shoulder impingement.

2. Identify the signs and symptoms associated with various stages of rotator cuff impingement.

   Rotator cuff impingement is caused by encroachment in the subacromial space that has decreased the area through which the supraspinatus and subacromial bursa pass underneath the subacromial arch. Impingement is most commonly seen in occupations and sporting activities involving repetitive overhead motions. Signs and symptoms for impingement range from mild pain with activity and no loss of strength or ROM (stage I) to degenerative changes and full thickness tears of the rotator cuff that cause considerable pain and disability (stage III).

3. Explain the purpose of and demonstrate the appropriate use of objective tests for the shoulder and arm.

Objective tests for the shoulder include observation and palpation of the bony and soft tissue structures of the shoulder, scapular, and distal neck regions; ROM and strength examinations of the muscles that control glenohumeral and scapular motions; tests for neurovascular status; and special tests for joint instability (glenohumeral, AC, and SC) and muscle and tendon (rotator cuff and biceps brachii) pathologies. Equally important to mastering special tests is knowing which tests to include in your examination. You will always precede these tests with a thorough history, which will guide the objective tests you use.

4. Describe and perform the special tests for examining joint instabilities.

Several tests are used to determine glenohumeral joint instability, which can occur in anterior, inferior, posterior, or multiplanar directions. The more frequently used tests include the load and shift test, relocation and apprehension test, anterior drawer test, posterior drawer test, sulcus sign, and clunk test. Tests for AC and SC instability include compression and shear tests.

5. Describe and perform the special tests for examining muscle and tendon pathologies.

Special tests for rotator cuff and biceps tendon pathology include those for acute strains and those for chronic impingement and overuse syndromes. For acute injuries, the drop arm test examines tears in the rotator cuff, and the Speed's, Ludington's, and distal biceps tendon rupture tests indicate biceps tendon tears and ruptures. Shoulder impingement tests include the active impingement, Neer impingement, Hawkins-Kennedy, empty can, and impingement relief tests. The Yergason's test examines bicipital tendinitis and subluxation.

6. Perform an on-site examination of the shoulder and upper arm, and discuss criteria for immediate referral and mode of transportation from the field.

As with other injuries, on-site examination of a shoulder injury requires that you be observant in approaching the athlete. Following a primary survey, palpate the injured part to determine obvious signs of fracture or dislocation. You must determine the injury's severity, examine the level of pain, examine for shock, and establish neurovascular integrity of the limb before deciding how to transport the athlete off the site.

7. Perform an acute examination of the shoulder and upper arm, and discuss criteria for determining return to activity.

In the acute examination, you can perform a more specific and detailed examination of the severity of the injury in order to determine the athlete's ability to return to sport participation. The acute examination includes a thorough palpation, an investigation of the shoulder's active and passive ROM, strength testing, neurovascular status testing, and examination of specific structures. Palpation determines the presence of spasm, deformity, and tissue restriction. Special tests of these structures address tissue integrity, joint stability, and pathology that would warrant excluding the athlete from immediate return to participation. Only if findings are negative or the injury is deemed minor are functional tests performed.

8. Perform a clinical examination of the shoulder and upper arm, including differential diagnosis from cervical pathologies.

Athletes will commonly report to you with an injury that occurred at some delay following acute trauma or with a gradual onset over a period of time. In either case, you must thoroughly examine the athlete's shoulder to define the SINS of the injury. These results will determine the treatment program. Obtain a complete history from the athlete, including information on training and activities of daily living. Closely observe the athlete throughout the process to note any abnormal posture or any restricted use of the shoulder or arm. Differential diagnoses to eliminate other sources of the symptoms that may emanate from the cervical region should be part of the clinical examination. Tests in addition to those used in the acute examination, as well as joint accessory examination, are incorporated to investigate chronic overuse and inflammatory conditions.

REVIEW QUESTIONS

1. What is the difference between primary and secondary impingement? Which is more commonly seen in the young athlete?

2. Why would glenohumeral instability contribute to an impingement syndrome?

3. What is the role of the scapula in glenohumeral motion, and what affect could scapular dysfunction have on shoulder injuries?

4. Name three peripheral nerve injuries that may occur with trauma to the shoulder. What are the signs and symptoms associated with each? How would you test for them?

5. What are the primary conditions that you would want to check in an on-site shoulder examination before moving the athlete from the field?

6. What tests determine glenohumeral joint mobility? How do you determine whether instability or restriction exists?

7. What potential complications might result from a posterior SC dislocation and what special tests would you use to examine these complications?

CRITICAL THINKING QUESTIONS

1. In a clinical examination, how would you differentiate between a primary and secondary impingement? Discuss what special tests you would use to distinguish between these conditions and what findings you would expect for each.

2. Consider a scenario similar to the one where the quarterback had his arm cocked back to throw when he was hit. You palpate underneath his shoulder pads and in this case, you feel a flattening of the deltoid muscle. What injury might you suspect, and how would you proceed with your examination?

3. A 15-year-old pitcher comes to you complaining of pain in his shoulder, particularly with hard throwing. He states that sometimes when he throws a fastball he gets a "twang" in the shoulder, followed by a tingling sensation down his arm. What shoulder conditions might you suspect in this young athlete? What types of questions would you ask, and how would you proceed with your examination?

4. An 18-year-old soccer player comes into the athletic training room holding his arm at his side. He states he was goofing around on the field and fell on his shoulder. He points to pain at the tip of his shoulder and is unable to raise his arm because of pain. You have already noted some swelling over his acromion. What type or types of injuries might you suspect given this history? What tests might you perform, and how would you determine the severity of the injury?

5. Consider the factory worker with shoulder pain that radiates into the arm. What types of questions would you ask this patient to get a better sense of her symptoms? How would you examine her posture, and what specific postural deviations would you observe for?

CITED REFERENCES

Corso, G. 1995. Impingement relief test: An adjunctive procedure to traditional examination of shoulder impingement syndrome. *J Orthop Sports Phys Ther* 22(5): 183-192.

Deltoff, M.N., and H.B. Bressler. 1989. Atypical scapular fracture. *Am J Sports Med* 17(2): 292-295.

Hawkins, R.J., and N. Mohtadi. 1991. Clinical evaluation of shoulder instabilities. *Clin J Sports Med* 1: 59-66.

Jobe, F.W., and M. Pink. 1993. Classification and treatment of shoulder dysfunction in the overhand athlete. *J Ortho Sports Phys Ther* 18(2): 427-432.

Meister, K., and J.R. Andrews. 1993. Classification and treatment of rotator cuff injuries in the overhand athlete. *J Ortho Sports Phys Ther* 18(2): 413-421.

Neer, C. 1973. Impingement lesions. *Clin Orthop* 173: 70-77.

Ogawa, K., and A. Yoshida. 1998. Throwing fracture of the humeral shaft. *Am J Sports Med* 26(2): 242-246.

Sallis, R.E., D.A. Zillmer, B.A. Russell, and S.T. Doberstein. 2001. Confirming a biceps brachii tendon rupture. *Phys Sportsmed* 29(2): 21.

Silliman, J.F., and M.T. Dean. 1993. Neurovascular injuries to the shoulder. *J Ortho Sports Phys Ther* 18(2): 442-448.

ADDITIONAL RESOURCES

Clarkson, H.M. 2000. *Musculoskeletal assessment: Joint range of motion and manual muscle strength.* 2nd ed. Philadelphia: Lippincott Williams & Wilkins.

Houglum, P.A. 2005. *Therapeutic exercise for musculoskeletal injuries.* 2nd ed. Champaign, IL: Human Kinetics.

Kendall, F.P, E.K. McCreary, and P.G. Provance. 1993. *Muscles: Testing and function.* 4th ed. Philadelphia: Lippincott Williams & Wilkins.

Jensen, K.L. 1999. The shoulder. In *The injured athlete.* 3rd ed. ed. D.H. Perrin, 241-280. Philadelphia: Lippincott-Raven.

Magee, D.J., and D.C. Reid. 1996. Shoulder injuries. In *Athletic injuries and rehabilitation.* eds. J.E. Zachazewski, D.J. Magee, and W.S. Quillen, 509-542. Philadelphia: Saunders.

Elbow and Forearm

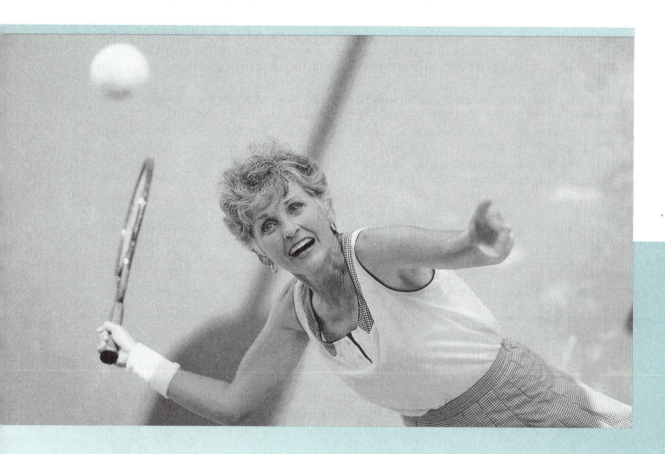

Objectives

After completing this chapter, the reader will be able to do the following:

1. Describe the etiology, signs and symptoms, and potential complications associated with acute and chronic injuries of the elbow and forearm commonly encountered in physically active people

2. Identify the common pathologies associated with repetitive valgus overload stresses in the throwing athlete

3. Identify causes of forearm compartment syndrome and the 5 Ps of neurovascular compromise

4. Identify the anatomical sites and signs and symptoms associated with nerve compression syndromes

5. Describe the normal anatomical alignment, carrying angle, and ROM of the elbow joint

6. Explain the purpose of and demonstrate the appropriate use of objective tests for the elbow and forearm

7. Perform an on-site examination of the elbow and forearm, and determine criteria for immediate medical referral and mode of transportation from the field

8. Perform an acute examination of the elbow and forearm, noting criteria for referral and return to activity

9. Perform a clinical examination of the elbow and forearm, noting considerations for differential diagnosis

Randy was a 14-year-old baseball player who lived for Saturdays, when he pitched for his Little League team. As he was warming up for a big game, he felt the same pain on the inside of his elbow that he had been noticing for months. He wasn't overly worried about it—a friend of his dad's had looked at it and said it was just some tendinitis that would eventually go away. This was someone who should know, after all, because he was an avid golfer and had once had the same symptoms.

In the second inning, Randy noticed that his arm was sorer than usual. But he was facing the toughest batter on the other team, so he decided to throw a hard, fast ball for a strikeout that would end the inning. As Randy wound up and threw the ball, he felt a snap and tremendous pain in his elbow.

The news at the emergency room wasn't good. Randy had avulsed a piece of bone off of his medial elbow and would be out of action for the rest of the season.

On Monday, he saw Jill, the athletic trainer at his high school, and told her what had happened.

"Why didn't you tell me you were having pain, Randy?" asked Jill.

"I just thought it was tendinitis. A friend of my dad's had the same thing and I figured it would just go away on its own. I didn't know something like this could happen," Randy said, dejected.

"Randy, you're young and your bones are still growing," Jill explained. "They will be weaker in certain areas than your muscles and tendons until you get a few years older. As a young athlete, you'll have different injuries than an older adult. So even though your pain may be the same, your injury probably isn't. Pain is never something you should ignore, particularly when it is near a bone. Next time something is painful, you should tell me right away—understood?"

"Yes," said Randy. "I promise to tell you right away next time—if there is a next time."

The elbow plays a critical role in positioning the hand to perform physical and daily living activities. Specifically, the elbow extends and retracts the length of the limb and rotates the forearm to effectively position the hand for particular tasks. Consider how difficult it would be to perform simple activities such as combing your hair, brushing your teeth, or opening a door without the elbow. Because of the importance of the elbow, even minor elbow injuries can be disabling.

FUNCTIONAL ANATOMY

Unlike the shoulder, the elbow is one of the more stable joints in the body. It is made up of three joints contained in a single capsule: the radioulnar, humeroulnar, and humeroradial joints. The bony configuration of the humeroulnar joint, along with the strong medial and lateral collateral ligaments, lends to its stability (figure 13.1, a-b). As a result the elbow can withstand substantial forces and usually only a significant force causes traumatic injuries such as fracture and dislocation. However, when traumatic injury does occur, neurovascular complications often arise because of the close proximity of major nerves and vessels as they pass anteriorly (brachial artery, median nerve, musculocutaneous nerve), medially (ulnar nerve), and posteriolaterally (radial nerve) to the joint on their way to the forearm.

Chronic injuries commonly occur as a result of physical activity. A variety of medial stress injuries can occur in both younger and older athletes due to valgus overload forces associated with overhead throwing activities (figure 13.2). Athletes engaging in sports such as tennis and golf also frequently experience repetitive stress injuries. As the opening scenario suggests, the young athlete presents unique pathologies that you should always consider in the evaluative process. As you read this chapter, consider the common types of repetitive stress injuries and the conditions that can be associated with each.

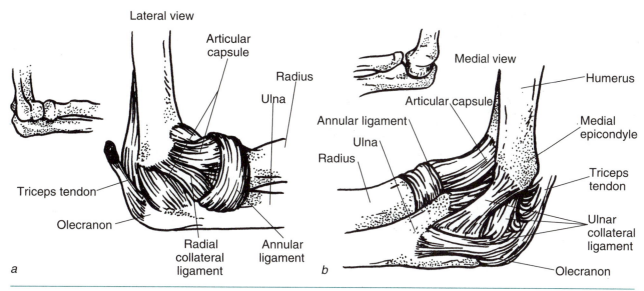

Figure 13.1 Joints and ligaments of the elbow in *(a)* lateral and *(b)* medial views.

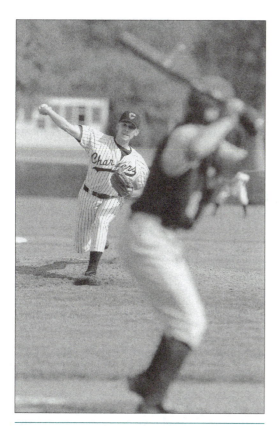

Figure 13.2 The late cocking and early acceleration phase of pitching demonstrates valgus loading of the elbow.

Flexion and extension of the elbow occur at the articulation of the trochlear notch of the ulna with the trochlea of the humerus, and the head of the radius with the capitulum of the humerus (see figure 13.1). The forearm pronates and supinates at the proximal radioulnar joint, which is the articulation of the head of the radius and the radial notch of the ulna. The elbow flexor muscles are the biceps brachii, brachioradialis, and brachialis; the triceps brachii and anconeus extend the elbow. Contraction of the pronator teres and pronator quadratus pronate the forearm, and the supinator supinates it. The biceps brachii, by virtue of its insertion into the radius, is an example of a triarticulate muscle: It assists with shoulder flexion, produces elbow flexion, and when the forearm is in the pronated position, assists with forearm supination.

As you review the muscle attachment about the elbow, note that several muscles acting on the forearm and wrist originate from either the medial epicondyle or the lateral epicondyle of the humerus. The muscles originating from the medial epicondyle are known as the flexor–pronator group because they either pronate the forearm or flex the wrist. They include the pronator teres, flexor carpi radialis, flexor carpi ulnaris, and palmaris longus muscles (figure 13.3). The muscles originating from the lateral epicondyle comprise the extensor–supinator group because they either supinate the forearm or extend the wrist. They include the supinator, extensor carpi radialis brevis, and extensor carpi ulnaris muscles (figure 13.4). Repetitive forearm pronation and wrist flexion stretch the attachment of the extensor–supinator muscles to the lateral epicondyle and can cause lateral epicondylitis. You will commonly see this condition in tennis players (tennis elbow), politicians who shake many hands, and musicians such as violinists. You will see the opposite condition, medial epicondylitis, in patients who engage in activities requiring repetitive forearm supination and wrist extension. Because one classic patient is the youth baseball player who attempts to pitch a curve ball, this condition is known as Little League elbow.

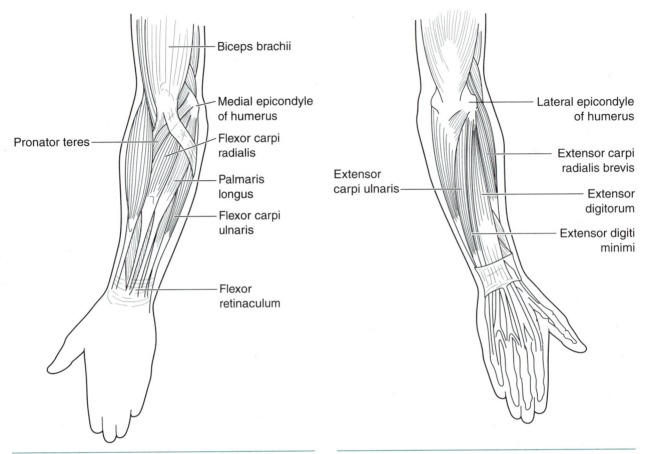

Figure 13.3 Muscles originating from the medial epicondyle of the humerus.

Figure 13.4 Muscles originating from the lateral epicondyle of the humerus.

ELBOW AND FOREARM INJURIES

The performance of the upper extremities depends on the integrity of the bones, ligaments, and muscles of the elbow and forearm that help position the hand. To allow full mobility at the elbow joint, the elbow and forearm are typically left unprotected during athletic activity and thus are exposed to a variety of contact injuries. Injuries associated with the repetitive forces inherent in overhead throwing and racket sports are also common.

Acute Soft Tissue Injuries

Acute soft tissue injuries at the elbow and forearm include contusions, ligament and capsular sprains, and muscle and tendon strains.

Contusions

During sport activity, contusions frequently occur to the muscles of the forearm and the superficial bony surfaces of the elbow as a result of direct contact with another player (blocking in football), a sport implement (lacrosse stick or pitched ball), or the ground. Signs and symptoms include point tenderness localized over the contact area and ecchymosis. Direct blows to the olecranon process of the ulna frequently cause inflammation or bleeding in the overlying olecranon bursa that results in significant bursal swelling, mild to moderate pain, and limited elbow flexion. Because of the superficial course of the ulnar nerve between the medial epicondyle of the humerus and the olecranon process of the elbow, this nerve is vulnerable to contusions. With a direct blow to the ulnar nerve, the athlete will complain of radiating pain down the medial aspect of the forearm, the hand, and into the fourth and fifth fingers. Contusions to the extensor or flexor muscle masses of the forearm may produce symptoms of decreased range of motion (ROM) and pain during muscular stretch or active motion. Although contusions to the forearm muscles are rarely serious or debilitating, severe bleeding within a muscular compartment can significantly raise intracompartmental pressure and compromise neurovascular structures. The resulting **compartment syndrome**, a serious, limb-threatening condition, is discussed later in this chapter.

Sprain

The elbow is a relatively stable joint because of its bony configuration and strong collateral ligaments. However, acute stretching or tearing of ligament and capsular structures can occur in sport due to excessive joint loading resulting from rotational, hyperextension, and varus and valgus forces imposed on the elbow. These high-level joint forces can be created internally by muscular forces and externally through contact with another player or object.

Varus is a laterally directed force or angulation of a joint.

Valgus is a medially directed force or angulation of a joint.

Ulnar (Medial) Collateral Ligament Sprains

Acute stretching or tearing of the ulnar collateral ligament (UCL) most often occurs as a result of a traumatic valgus force (figure 13.5). The anterior band of the UCL is the primary structure that limits or resists valgus forces and thus is more often injured than the posterior or transverse bands. Excessive valgus force can be created when an athlete falls on an outstretched hand; these forces also occur in sports such as wrestling or football in which the athlete bears weight on the hands when contact is made to the lateral aspect of the elbow. Acute UCL ruptures can also result from overhead throwing motions such as baseball pitching and javelin throwing. However, these ruptures typically occur secondary to an underlying chronic condition of repetitive valgus loading during the late cocking or early acceleration phases of the throwing motion. This repetitive traction force on the medial structures weakens the ligament over time until it eventually fails. In such cases, the athlete typically will have experienced medial elbow pain for months before the acute injury (Jobe, Stark, and Lombardo 1986). It is important to recognize UCL injuries, particularly in throwers, to ensure adequate healing and to avoid chronic instability problems.

Signs and symptoms of UCL sprains include sudden pain following a valgus force to the elbow. The patient may report a sensation of a "pop." There is point tenderness over the anterior band of the UCL. Depending on severity, there may be significant swelling and decreased ROM, with the athlete holding the elbow in a flexed position for comfort. Valgus stress reproduces pain and you may or may not note instability with second- and third-degree sprains. Because of the close communication of the ulnar nerve with the medial elbow, it is not uncommon to find associated symptoms of ulnar nerve irritation.

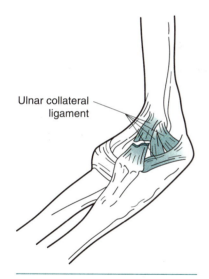

Ulnar collateral ligament

Figure 13.5 Ulnar collateral ligament (UCL) tear.

Radial (Lateral) Collateral Ligament Sprains

Lateral collateral ligament injuries occur much less frequently than medial collateral ligament injuries, since direct traction or varus forces to the lateral aspect of the elbow are rare during athletic activity. Isolated injuries to the lateral collateral ligament are thought to occur most often with the elbow hyperextended and forearm supinated (Tyrdal and Olsen 1998). This mechanism can occur with a fall on an extended elbow or when an athlete stretches out his arm to stop a ball or an opponent. Although infrequent, lateral traction forces at the elbow during the extension follow-through or deceleration phases of throwing can also injure the lateral collateral ligament (Andrews and Whiteside 1993). Signs and symptoms associated with injuries to the lateral collateral ligament include pain, point tenderness, and swelling to the lateral aspect of the elbow. Varus stress and forced hyperextension and supination of the forearm may reproduce pain. Instability is rarely noted with straight varus stress testing. If left unchecked, lateral collateral ligament tears can lead to posterolateral rotary instability of the elbow, and the athlete may complain of painful and recurrent locking or snapping with activity (Behr and Altchek 1997).

Anterior Capsular Sprains

Anterior capsular sprains can occur with forced hyperextension of the elbow (Andrews and Whiteside 1993). Typical mechanisms for forced hyperextension include using an outstretched arm to stop a ball or an opponent and falling with the arm outstretched and elbow extended. Young athletes with joint hyperlaxity and insufficient muscular strength may be more prone to hyperextension injuries than other athletes are (Andrews and Whiteside 1993). Signs and symptoms include pain and tenderness in the anterior compartment, with the athlete often apprehensive of fully extending the joint. The athlete may also complain of pain posteriorly where the olecranon process has been jammed or forced into the olecranon fossa. Severe hyperextension force mechanisms can also result in collateral ligament sprains, elbow dislocations, and fractures.

Strains

Acute muscle and tendon strains around the elbow joint can result from a one-time episode of excessive overload or stretch.

Flexor–Pronator and Extensor–Supinator Mass Strains

Strains to the wrist flexor–pronator muscle mass can occur with any activity that produces a forceful snapping of the wrist into flexion and pronation, such as a tennis serve, javelin throw, or racquetball forehand. Excessive eccentric loads that force the wrist into extension and supination during active wrist flexion and pronation movements, such as the impact of the ball against the racket, can also strain this muscle mass. Similarly, wrist extensor–supinator muscle mass strains typically result from forceful wrist extension movements and eccentric loads forcing the wrist into flexion and pronation while the wrist is concentrically extending or supinating. These extension injuries are often associated with backhand stroke mechanics in racket sports. Signs and symptoms of acute strains in the forearm muscles include acute pain and tenderness over the involved muscle mass, typically near its proximal attachment and the myotendon junction. Consequently you may find it difficult to distinguish a strain near the muscle origin from an acute tendinitis or epicondylitis (see the section on Tendinitis and Epicondylitis on page 280). The athlete will complain of pain with active and resistive motion and with passive stretch. Severity of symptoms and disability will be consistent with those of a first-, second-, or third-degree muscle strain, although third-degree strains of the wrist flexor and extensor masses are rare.

Distal Biceps Tendon

Injuries to the distal biceps tendon near or at its insertion at the radial tuberosity are rare in comparison to injuries at its proximal attachment. Distal biceps tendon strains are usually associated with a violent eccentric extension force or a ballistic flexion force against a heavy or immovable resistance. Distal biceps tendon injuries occur most often in heavy resistance training and competitive weight lifting. Injury may also occur during a football tackle or wrestling takedown when the elbow is forcibly hyperextended while the biceps is contracting. Signs and symptoms of tendon strain include immediate burning or pain in the anterior cubital area with point tenderness near the insertion on the radial tuberosity. There may be weakness and pain with active or resistive elbow flexion and supination.

A distal biceps tendon rupture (figure 13.6) may not be as obvious as proximal tendon ruptures, as other ligament or tendon attachments (e.g., brachialis and brachioradialis muscles) may limit the muscle belly from "rolling-up" and may prevent you from observing significant reductions in elbow flexion strength (Alley and Pappas 1995). Findings associated with a distal tendon rupture include palpable tenderness, swelling and a dull ache in the antecubital fossa, and weakness with forced pronation when the elbow is flexed to 90° and fully supinated. The athlete will often complain of feeling a "pop" or immediate sharp pain, or both, at the time of injury. You may observe a palpable defect and deformity anteriorly if the muscle retracts proximally into the upper arm.

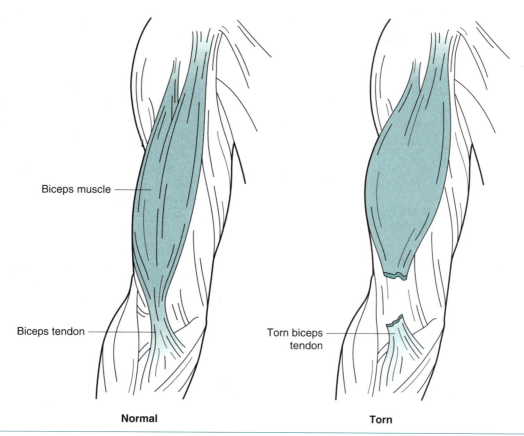

Biceps muscle

Biceps tendon

Torn biceps
tendon

Normal

Torn

Figure 13.6   Biceps tendon rupture.

Distal Triceps Tendon

Bursa is a synovial-filled membrane that lies between adjacent structures to limit friction and ease movement.

Strains and rupture of the distal triceps tendon are extremely rare but can occur with forced flexion during active extension, elbow dislocation, or a direct blow to the posterior elbow (Alley and Pappas 1995). Signs and symptoms include localized pain, swelling, and ecchymosis. The athlete will demonstrate a diminished capacity or an inability to extend the elbow against resistance. There may be a palpable defect in the distal tendon near its insertion to the olecranon.

Chronic or Overuse Soft Tissue Injuries

Chronic or overuse soft tissue injuries, the most commonly occurring elbow injuries, are typically associated with overhead throwing motions or racket sports. During these activities, the soft tissue structures of the elbow are susceptible to repetitive overuse and microtrauma that can result in chronic inflammatory conditions, fibrotic changes within the tissue, or instabilities due to stretch or weakening of the joint-stabilizing structures.

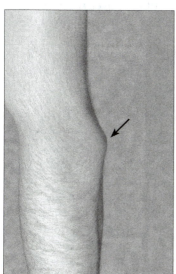

Figure 13.7   Olecranon bursitis.

Bursitis

Olecranon **bursitis** is an inflammatory condition of fluid accumulation in the subcutaneous **bursa** overlying the olecranon process (figure 13.7). Olecranon bursitis is common in sports such as football and wrestling in which the elbow is susceptible to repetitive friction and direct trauma. It is thought to occur more frequently on artificial turf than natural turf (Larson and Osternig 1974). The athlete will present with a large, localized, fluid-filled bursa; a pressure increase within the bursa during elbow flexion may limit motion. The bursa may be warm to the touch in the acute stages and is usually painless. If the athlete does not receive treatment and the condition persists, the fluid can thicken within the bursal walls and become difficult for the body to reabsorb.

Tendinitis and Epicondylitis

Tendinitis and epicondylitis are overuse injuries to the tendinous attachments of the flexor–pronator group at the medial epicondyle (figure 13.8) and to the extensor–supinator group at the lateral epicondyle. Whereas **tendinitis** is a simple inflammatory response, **epicondylitis** is a degenerative condition in which increased fibroblastic activity and granulation tissue formation occur within the tendon (Nirschl 1993). Nirschl used the term *tendinosis* to differentiate this pathological condition from simple tendinitis. Epicondylitis is often referred to as **tennis elbow** because of its high incidence in that sport. As many as 50% of tennis athletes complain of symptoms of tennis elbow at some point; the majority of cases are lateral and seen in persons over 30 years of age. However, you will also commonly see this chronic condition in golf, baseball, field throwing events, swimming, and occupational activities involving repetitive wrist motion and torque. Anyone engaged in prolonged, high-intensity, and repetitive forearm muscle use is susceptible. Contractile overloads that chronically tension or stress the tendon near its attachment on the humerus are the primary cause of epicondylitis.

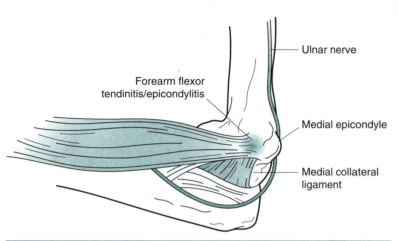

Figure 13.8 Anatomical sites of medial epicondylitis or tendinitis at the common flexor–pronator muscle origin.

- **Lateral epicondylitis (tennis elbow)**

In most cases, lateral epicondylitis involves primarily the extensor carpi radialis brevis and usually results from activities that tension and stress the wrist extensor and supinator muscles. The backhand in tennis, for example, can place tremendous stress on the wrist extensor muscle group. Factors such as faulty mechanics, inadequate muscular strength and endurance, and poor racket fit (improper string tension, grip size, or racket weight or size) may further contribute to contractile overload. Wheelchair athletes, especially marathon racers, may suffer from lateral epicondylitis due to repetitive wrist flexion and pronation as the elbow extends during the push phase. Signs and symptoms include gradual onset of pain over the anterior aspect of the lateral epicondyle with the majority of tenderness localized to the origin of the extensor carpi radialis brevis tendon. Pain can be reproduced or aggravated with gripping and wrist extensor activities, as well as passive wrist flexion with forearm pronation while the elbow is extended. Observable swelling and discoloration are rare. Pain at rest, decreased ROM, and weakened grip strength characterize severe or prolonged cases.

- **Medial epicondylitis (golfer's elbow)**

Medial epicondylitis occurs much less frequently than the lateral condition. Repetitive wrist flexor and pronator muscle activity, as in baseball pitches, golf swings, overhead tennis serve and forehand racket motions, and pull-through swimming strokes, causes medial epicondylitis (also referred to as **golfer's elbow**). Technique changes or faulty mechanics with these activities can further increase stress at the flexor–pronator origin. Signs and symptoms include pain and mild swelling over the medial epicondyle. Resisted wrist flexion and forearm pronation along with palpation just distal and lateral to the epicondyle over the flexor–pronator muscle group origin reproduce pain. Passive wrist extension and forearm supination with the elbow extended may also produce pain. Symptoms of ulnar nerve irritation are often associated with medial epicondylitis. Because of skeletal immaturity, medial epicondylitis in young athletes usually stresses or disrupts the bone rather than the tendon. Therefore, adolescents who present with symptoms of medial epicondylitis should be examined for traction avulsion apophysitis, discussed later in this chapter.

Periostitis (forearm splints)

Shin splints describes pain and inflammation of the musculotendinous unit or periosteum along the anteromedial border of the tibia.

Although **periostitis** is more commonly associated with shin splints in the lower extremity, it can also occur in the forearm. Forearm periostitis, or **forearm splints**, typically an early-season inflammatory reaction of the muscle insertion along the **periosteum**, has been seen in weight lifters, gymnasts, and pitchers prone to repetitive stress and overuse of the forearm muscles (Grossfield et al. 1998; Wadhwa et al. 1997; Weiker 1995). Signs and symptoms include diffuse aching in the forearm with pain exacerbated with activity and relieved with rest. Pain may be reproduced with repetitive or resisted action of the involved musculature, and there is tenderness with deep palpation between the ulna and radius (Grossfield et al. 1998; Weiker 1995). A bone scan can help differentiate periostitis from other forearm stress injuries by demonstrating increased uptake of a pharmaceutical agent along the bony margin, which indicates a periosteal reaction (Grossfield et al. 1998; Wadhwa et al. 1997).

Valgus Overload Instabilities

The late cocking and early acceleration phases of overhand throwing mechanics subject the medial elbow to considerable valgus forces (see figure 13.2). Repetitive and excessive valgus forces result in tractioning forces to the medial joint, causing progressive microtrauma and weakening of the UCL. Eventually, the UCL becomes stretched and valgus instability results. Chronic valgus overload, rather than acute trauma, is the major cause of medial collateral ligament ruptures in the throwing athlete. Upon examination, the athlete will complain of chronic pain with throwing that has persisted for months and of point tenderness located approximately 2 cm (0.8 in.) distal to the medial epicondyle (Caldwell and Safran 1995). There will also be pain and instability with valgus stress testing. However, undersurface tears of the UCL have been observed with little or no evidence of laxity on clinical examination (Timmerman and Andrews 1994). As a consequence of ligament instability, stress normally absorbed by the ligament is transferred to the bony articulations (compression of the humero-radial joint), injuring these structures as well (see osteochondral defects on page 283). For this reason, early recognition is essential.

Intra-articular refers to a location within the joint capsule.

Traumatic Fractures

⚠ *Because of the potential for neurovascular injury, always perform a neurovascular examination when you suspect fracture.*

Traumatic fractures at the elbow, relatively uncommon in adults, occur much more frequently in children and skeletally immature adolescents. Traumatic fractures can occur anywhere within the elbow complex from either direct or indirect forces imposed on the bony structures. Since the majority of these fractures are intra-articular, you must be concerned about their possible effects and their healing mechanisms on elbow mechanics and function. The following paragraphs deal with some of the more common or significant fractures. Signs and symptoms common to all fractures include significant pain, swelling, crepitus, and tenderness over the fracture site. You may find deformity if bony fragments are displaced. Because of the potential for neurovascular injury, always perform a neurovascular examination when you suspect a fracture.

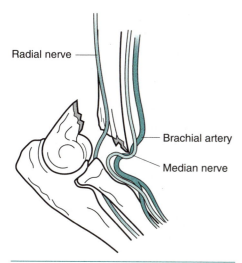

Radial nerve

Brachial artery

Median nerve

Figure 13.9 Supracondylar fracture with potential injury of neurovascular structures.

Distal Humeral Fractures

Condylar fractures can result from a direct blow, a fall on a outstretched hand, or a traumatic valgus or varus force applied to the elbow. **Supracondylar fractures** (transverse fractures just superior to the condyles), which occur more frequently in children than in others, typically result from a fall on an outstretched hand with the elbow extended. Displacement is a significant concern with these fractures. The proximal fragment of the humerus is often displaced anteriorly, greatly increasing the potential for injury to the primary neurovascular structures (brachial artery; median, ulnar, and radial nerves) (figure 13.9). Suspected injury to these structures is a medical emergency, as serious complications and permanent disability can result if the injury is not recognized and treated immediately.

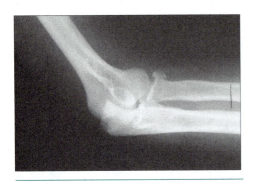

Figure 13.10   Fracture of the radial head.
Courtesy of Theodore E. Keats.

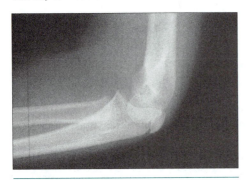

Figure 13.11   Traumatic fractures of the olecranon process.
Courtesy of Theodore E. Keats.

Radial Fractures

Radial head and neck fractures usually result from a fall on an outstretched arm with the forearm pronated, which axially compresses the radius against the capitellum (Alley and Pappas 1995; Morrey 1993). Radial head fractures may also result from traumatic elbow dislocations (figure 13.10). Signs and symptoms include swelling and pain over the lateral elbow. The athlete will complain particularly of pain with forearm pronation and supination and when you palpate the radial head.

Olecranon Fractures

A direct blow to the posterior elbow is the primary cause of traumatic olecranon fractures (figure 13.11). Fracture may also occur secondary to a violent triceps pull, although this is rare. Most fractures of the olecranon are intra-articular, and therefore joint instability may result (Cabanela and Morrey 1993). Signs and symptoms include pain, point tenderness, and swelling, as well as crepitus and deformity over the posterior elbow.

Forearm Fractures

Fractures of the forearm result from forces transmitted along or across the shaft of the radius or ulna. Axial forces, a consequence of falling on an outstretched hand, may fracture one or both bones. Transverse forces, caused by a direct blow to the forearm from an opponent or a stick, are common in contact sports such as football, hockey, and lacrosse (Griggs and Weiss 1996). In addition to the typical signs and symptoms of fracture, active wrist motion may cause pain and crepitus.

Bony Lesions Secondary to Repetitive Stress

Chronic, repetitive valgus forces at the elbow joint can result in progressive bony lesions, particularly in skeletally immature youth. As discussed previously, these forces are typically associated with throwing. Excessive valgus loading applies traction forces at the bony attachments of ligament and tendon on the medial side and compression forces on the lateral joint structures.

Traction Apophyseal and Epiphyseal Injuries (Little League Elbow)

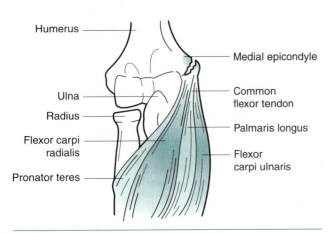

Humerus
Ulna
Radius
Flexor carpi radialis
Pronator teres
Medial epicondyle
Common flexor tendon
Palmaris longus
Flexor carpi ulnaris

Figure 13.12   Traction apophyseal fracture of the medial epicondyle.

The medial apophysis is a nonarticular growth plate in adolescent athletes that serves as the attachment site for the flexor–pronator muscle group as well as the UCL. In skeletally immature athletes, valgus traction forces applied during the late cocking or early acceleration phases of throwing stress the apophyseal plate rather than the tendon or ligament. The resulting injury, commonly known as **Little League elbow**, may start out as an inflammatory response, or **apophysitis**, and progress to an avulsion of the apophysis if the repetitive stress continues (figure 13.12). Athletes with this condition report a prolonged history of pain with throwing. Signs and symptoms include point tenderness and swelling over the medial epicondyle and pain with valgus stress localized directly over the medial apophysis (Andrews and Whiteside 1993). A flexion contracture may also be present. Other less common epiphyseal traction injuries involve the olecranon and the lateral condyle. These traction injuries can result from extension and pronation traction forces during the acceleration and follow-through phases of throwing. The athlete presents with signs and symptoms similar to those just described: prolonged pain with throwing, tenderness over the involved epiphyseal site, and decreased elbow extension (Lowery et al. 1995).

Osteochondral Defects

Osteochondritis dissecans appears to result from compressive forces that damage the vascular supply to the osteochondral surface, causing vascular insufficiency and aseptic necrosis. Osteochondritis dissecans at the elbow, most often seen in young throwing adolescents (ages

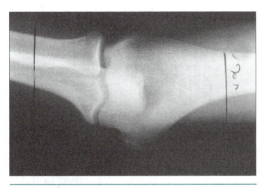

10-15), primarily affects the capitellum and radial head (figure 13.13). The main cause of this pathology is repetitive throwing that subjects the radial capitellar joint to compressive and shear forces secondary to chronic valgus overload during the late cocking and early acceleration phases. However, osteochondritis dissecans has also been observed in young gymnasts (Andrews and Whiteside 1993). Medial instability further intensifies lateral joint compression. This degenerative process is characterized by changes in the articular surface, including flattening of the subchondral bone, fragmentation of the articular cartilage, and loose body formation (see the next section). Signs and symptoms include chronic elbow pain, tenderness over the capitellum, flexion contracture, and articular changes seen on radiographic examination (Bennett 1993; Takahara et al. 1998). Intermittent locking or incomplete motion may occur if loose bodies are present (Alley and Pappas 1995). Early articular changes, thought to

Figure 13.13 Osteochondritis dissecans of the capitellum.

Courtesy of Theodore E. Keats.

precede osteochondritis dissecans of the capitellum, include impaction of the subchondral bone and alterations in ossification of the epiphysis (Takahara et al. 1998). Many regard these early changes as a distinct condition known as **osteochondrosis**.

Osteophytes and Loose Bodies

Osteophytes (bone spurs) or loose bodies (e.g., bone or cartilage fragments) may form at the posterior tip and posterior medial aspect of the olecranon as a result of medial instability and chronic valgus extension overload (figure 13.14). Valgus extension overload occurs during the late acceleration and follow-through phases of the throwing motion, causing impingement of the posterior medial aspect of the olecranon on the posterior medial surface of the olecranon fossa. This impingement and resulting bony hypertrophy of the olecranon can further result in chondromalacia of the articular surface of the olecranon fossa. The athlete's chief complaint will typically be of pain between the acceleration and follow-through phases of the pitching motion, which renders these phases ineffective (Wilson et al. 1983). Other signs and symptoms may include pain over the posterior tip or posterior–medial aspect of the olecranon process and pain with forced extension and valgus stressing. A flexion contracture may also exist.

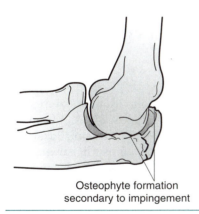

Osteophyte formation secondary to impingement

Figure 13.14 Osteophyte formation on the posterior tip and posteromedial aspects of the olecranon.

Dislocation and Subluxation

Elbow joint dislocations are among the more common dislocations seen in sport. In typical injury scenarios, a baseball player slides into base headfirst or a wrestler or gymnast stretches out his arm to break a fall. Elbow dislocations can range from simple cases involving isolated ligament disruption to more complicated cases involving associated fractures, neurovascular complications, or both. In simple cases, conservative treatment of elbow dislocations produces excellent results, and recurrent dislocation or chronic instability is rarely a concern.

Humeroulnar Joint

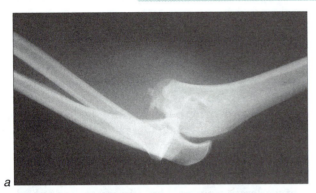

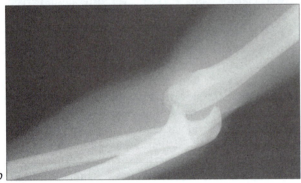

Figure 13.15 Humeroulnar dislocation (a) with a fracture and (b) without a fracture.

Courtesy of Theodore E. Keats.

In athletics, posterior dislocations of the ulna and radius on the humerus are significantly more common than anterior dislocations. The prevailing mechanism associated with a posterior dislocation of the humeroulnar joint is hyperextension during axial loading, typically resulting from a fall on an outstretched or extended elbow. This mechanism jams the olecranon process into the olecranon fossa, which acts as a fulcrum by which the trochlea is forced over the coronoid process. Because the annular ligament is usually left intact, the ulna and radius are displaced together. The displacement can be directly posterior (figure 13.15), posterolateral (most common), or posteromedial. Minimally, the medial collateral and lateral collateral ligaments are ruptured. However, if valgus and rotary forces accompany the hyperextension force, associated fractures of the radial head and neck, coronoid process, or medial epicondyle may also result (Alley and Pappas 1995). Additionally, occlusion of the brachial artery or entrapment of the median or ulnar nerves with humeroulnar dislocation (or with subsequent reduction) is a concern, indicating a medical emergency. Signs and symptoms of elbow dislocation include immediate pain, swelling, deformity, and an unwillingness to move the extremity. Signs and symptoms of associated arterial injury include excessive swelling of the forearm and hand, diminished or absent distal pulses, pale or cyanotic skin coloration, paresthesia, and pain with passive finger extension (Slowik, Fitzimmons, and Rayhack 1993). (See information on Forearm Compartment Syndrome on the next page.)

Radioulnar Joint

Isolated dislocation of the radioulnar joint is rare in adults, and subluxations are more commonly seen in children. In adults, radioulnar dislocation does not appear to result from one single mechanism, but can occur from a direct blow to the lateral elbow (Takami, Takahashi, and Ando 1997). Dislocation is typically preceded by tearing of the annular ligament, distal radioulnar joint capsule, and interosseous membrane (figure 13.16). Signs and symptoms include pain, limited ROM, elbow effusion, tenderness over the antecubital region, and inability to supinate the forearm. In young children, a traction force or longitudinal pull with accompanying pronation of the forearm can result in subluxation or dislocation of the radioulnar joint, commonly know as **nursemaid's elbow**. With this injury mechanism, the radial head is pulled down into and becomes caught in the annular ligament. Usually the annular ligament is not torn in young children, but in older children it can be. Signs and symptoms include pain, holding the forearm in a pronated position, and unwillingness to move the elbow.

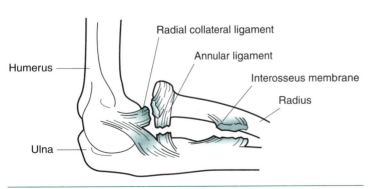

Figure 13.16 Radioulnar joint dislocation and tearing of the ligamentous structure.

Neurovascular Injuries Secondary to Trauma

As mentioned previously, a serious complication of supracondylar fractures and elbow dislocations is injury to the brachial artery and peripheral nerves, which can severely compromise blood flow and function of the forearm and hand.

General Neurovascular Injury

Always suspect and carefully examine for neurovascular injury with factures, dislocations, and other severe trauma to the elbow and forearm. Signs and symptoms of arterial injury and resulting ischemia include pain out of proportion to what is expected for the injury, diminished or absent distal pulses, poor skin coloration, and decreased skin temperature. Signs and symptoms of nerve trauma include loss of sensation and motor function over the involved nerve's distribution. There may also be additional signs and symptoms associated with ischemic complications resulting from an acute compartment syndrome.

Forearm Compartment Syndrome

Arterial injury as well as severe posttraumatic swelling can lead to a compartment syndrome in the forearm. In this condition a muscular compartment, enclosed by its relatively inelastic surrounding fascia, is subject to excessive swelling and increasing pressure (figure 13.17). As pressure exceeds that of the vessel walls within the compartment, vascular collapse occurs, compromising circulation to the muscles and nerves. Since venous pressure is lower than capillary pressure, the veins collapse first, further increasing pressure within the compartment since blood can still flow in but not out. Eventually, as pressure rises, the capillary walls collapse, causing ischemia to the surrounding muscles and nerves. If ischemia persists for more than 6 to 12 hours, tissue necrosis and permanent loss of nerve and muscular function ensue. The final complication is a **Volkmann's ischemic contracture** of the forearm that replaces the nonviable, necrotic muscle with inelastic and contracted scar tissue (figure 13.18).

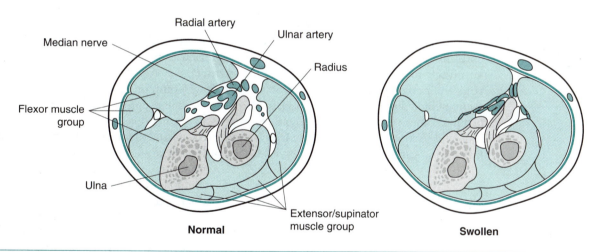

Figure 13.17 Severe forearm compartment swelling.

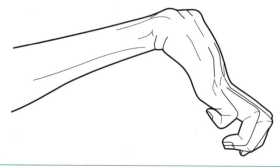

Figure 13.18 Volkmann's ischemic contracture.

Signs and symptoms of a compartment syndrome include the 5 Ps (pain, pallor, paresthesia, paralysis, and pulselessness). The earliest and most reliable symptom of a compartment syndrome is unrelenting pain, often out of proportion to the injury. Severe pain will also occur with stretching of the ischemic muscles. The compartment will be tense and tender to palpation and may take on a whitish skin color (pallor) or shiny appearance due to decreasing circulation. There will be paresthesia as the nerve becomes ischemic. As nerve ischemia progresses, the patient will experience diminished sensation (**hypoesthesia** or **hypesthesia**) and motor weakness, and eventually, numbness and complete loss of motor function (paralysis). Pulselessness may also occur if the compartment syndrome results from arterial occlusion. Otherwise, you may still observe distal pulses, since intracompartmental pressure rarely exceeds that of major arterial vessels. Any one of the foregoing signs or symptoms indicates a medical emergency. You must refer the athlete for surgical decompression and restoration of blood flow in order to avoid a Volkmann's ischemic contracture.

Nerve Compression Syndromes

Nerve compression syndromes are common around the elbow, frequently resulting from repetitive compression or traction mechanisms seen in sports such as throwing and tennis. This section deals with the more common compression syndromes of the major peripheral nerves of the forearm.

Ulnar Nerve

The elbow is the most common site for ulnar nerve compression and injury. The ulnar nerve passes the elbow superficially between the medial epicondyle and the medial border of the olecranon. Because of its superficial course and anatomical constraints as it passes the medial elbow, it is prone to contusions, subluxation, traction and frictional forces, compression syndromes, and irritation caused by surrounding chronic or degenerative conditions. Ulnar nerve contusions can result from a direct blow to the medial surface of the elbow where the nerve passes superficially, particularly when the elbow is in a flexed position. Recurrent subluxations can result when the overlying retinaculum, which holds the nerve within the epitrochlear (ulnar) groove, becomes stretched or torn. **Cubital tunnel syndrome** (ulnar neuropathy and compression) can result from a variety of conditions, such as inflammation or scarring of the nerve, muscle hypertrophy, occupying lesions, fractures, dislocations, or any pathology that narrows the nerve's passageway as it crosses the elbow. Common sites of anatomical compression include the arcade of Struthers, medial intermuscular septum, cubital tunnel, flexor carpi ulnaris aponeurosis, and the deep flexor–pronator aponeurosis (figure 13.19). Chronic traction and frictional forces resulting from valgus overload and medial instability associated with throwing can also irritate the nerves. Other inflammatory conditions such as chronic medial epicondylitis, flexor–pronator tendinitis, and UCL injuries can cause ulnar neuropathy.

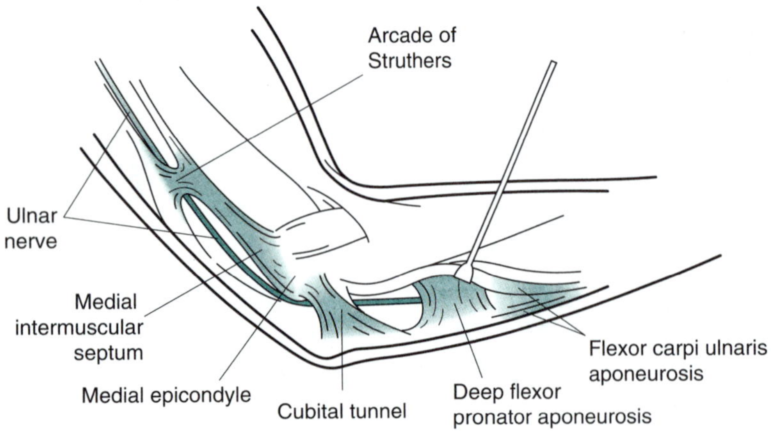

Regardless of the underlying cause, the signs and symptoms of ulnar neuropathy are similar. Symptoms may begin gradually with chronic and degenerative conditions or acutely with traumatic injury. Signs and symptoms include pain or aching originating at the medial elbow and radiating down the lateral forearm into the fifth digit and the medial surface of the fourth digit. When you palpate, the nerve may be tender just posterior to the medial epicondyle. Elbow flexion and extension can often reproduce nerve subluxation

Figure 13.19   Common anatomical sites for ulnar nerve compression syndrome.

Labels: Arcade of Struthers, Ulnar nerve, Medial intermuscular septum, Medial epicondyle, Cubital tunnel, Deep flexor pronator aponeurosis, Flexor carpi ulnaris aponeurosis

or dislocation, and the athlete may complain of "clicking" over the posteromedial aspect of the elbow. With chronic compression syndromes, the athlete presents with paresthesia over the ulnar distribution of the forearm and hand, which may advance to numbness if symptoms progress. Symptoms usually worsen when the elbow is flexed, since anatomical structures stretch over the cubital tunnel and significantly decrease the space within in this position. Radiating pain or paresthesia may be reproduced with light tapping over the inflamed nerve (**Tinel's sign**). In severe compressive or traumatic cases, the intrinsic muscles of the hand may show muscle atrophy, motor weakness, and function loss. There may also be reduction or loss of pinch or grip strength.

Median Nerve

Compression of the median nerve at the elbow, or **pronator teres syndrome**, can occur between the two heads of the pronator teres secondary to muscle hypertrophy or tight fibrous bands (figure 13.20). Pronator teres syndrome is most often seen in sports such as weight lifting, rowing, golf, tennis, and racquetball as a consequence of repetitive pronation and sustained gripping. Median nerve compression is characterized by aching and pain in the volar aspect of the forearm that flexor–pronator muscle activity exacerbates (Andrews and Whiteside 1993). Paresthesia and motor weakness over the median nerve distribution of the thumb and the second and third digits may appear in later stages. A Tinel's sign over the volar aspect of the proximal forearm may also test positive.

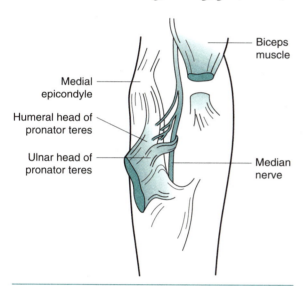

Figure 13.20   Sites for pronator teres syndrome.

Labels: Biceps muscle; Medial epicondyle; Humeral head of pronator teres; Ulnar head of pronator teres; Median nerve

Anterior Interosseous Nerve

The anterior interosseous nerve is a motor branch off the median nerve that runs along the interosseous membrane, passing between the flexor digitorum profundus and flexor pollicis longus on its way to the pronator quadratus. Occasionally this nerve is compressed by the forearm muscles or overlying fibrous bands, secondary to forceful muscle contractions. Anterior interosseous nerve compression causes pain and motor weakness in the proximal forearm. The prevailing sign is loss of pinch strength between the tips of the thumb and index finger.

Radial Nerve

The radial nerve runs from the medial to the lateral aspect of the posterior humerus and crosses the lateral epicondyle, where it passes through the radial tunnel and divides into deep and superficial branches. Radial nerve compression, or radial tunnel syndrome, can occur within the radial tunnel, which extends anteriorly from the radial head to the supinator muscle (Andrews and Whiteside 1993) (figure 13.21). Radial tunnel syndrome is typically caused by repetitive or vigorous wrist extension and forearm pronation and supination. It is often incorrectly identified as lateral epicondylitis but careful examination can differentiate the two conditions. With radial tunnel syndrome, tenderness is present several centimeters distal to the lateral epicondyle, within the supinator–extensor muscle mass of the proximal

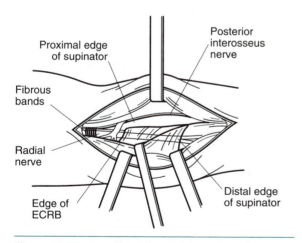

Figure 13.21   Location of radial tunnel syndrome.

Labels: Proximal edge of supinator; Posterior interosseus nerve; Fibrous bands; Radial nerve; Edge of ECRB; Distal edge of supinator

forearm (Behr and Altchek 1997). Other symptoms include pain radiating into the forearm extensors and pain reproduction with resisted supination or extension of the middle finger. You will not usually find motor weakness during clinical examination.

Posterior Interosseous Nerve

The deep branch of the radial nerve continues as the posterior interosseous motor nerve supplying the wrist and finger extensors. Just distal to the radial tunnel, the posterior interosseous nerve can be compressed under the arcade of Frohse. The **arcade of Frohse** is a fibrous band located at the proximal edge of the supinator muscle, near the edge of the extensor carpi radialis brevis and radial capitellar joint (Andrews and Whiteside 1993; Behr and Altchek 1997) (figure 13.22). Signs and symptoms include deep aching in the extensor muscle mass and proximal forearm after repetitive activities such as weight lifting, throwing, and grasping. You will note palpable tenderness approximately 2 in. (5 cm) distal from the lateral epicondyle, near the site where the nerve passes through the arcade of Frohse. What differentiates compression of the posterior interosseous nerve from radial tunnel syndrome is a primary finding of motor weakness in the wrist and finger extensors.

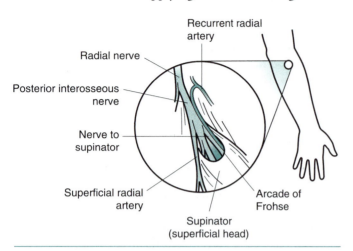

Figure 13.22   Arcade of Frohse.

Structural and Functional Abnormalities

Cubital varus and cubital valgus are two structural abnormalities of the elbow's carrying angle. The normal carrying angle of the extended elbow is slightly valgus—approximately 5° for males (figure 13.23) and 10 to15° for females.

Cubital Valgus

Cubital valgus is a carrying angle that is greater than the normal 5° or 15° valgus angulation (figure 13.24). Cubital valgus can result from an epiphyseal plate injury secondary to fracture of the lateral epicondyle. Potential complications of an increased valgus angle include decreased ROM and delayed ulnar neuropathy.

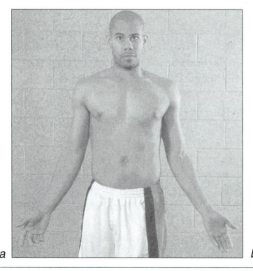
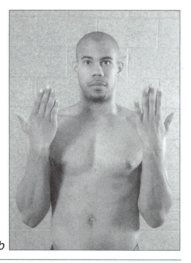
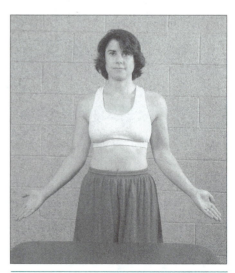

Figure 13.23   Normal carrying angle in *(a)* full elbow extension and *(b)* full elbow flexion.

Figure 13.24   Valgus carrying angle of the elbow.

Cubital Varus

Cubital varus, or **gunstock deformity**, is a carrying angle less than the normal valgus angle, with the elbow usually taking on a varus angulation (see figure 13.25). Cubital varus, which is more common than cubital valgus, is most often a result of a supracondylar fracture during childhood that either disrupts the growth plate or heals with a malalignment of the distal humerus. Little consequence or functional impairment is associated with this deformity. Note that structural abnormalities, particularly cubital valgus, are potential contributory mechanisms in chronic conditions of the elbow.

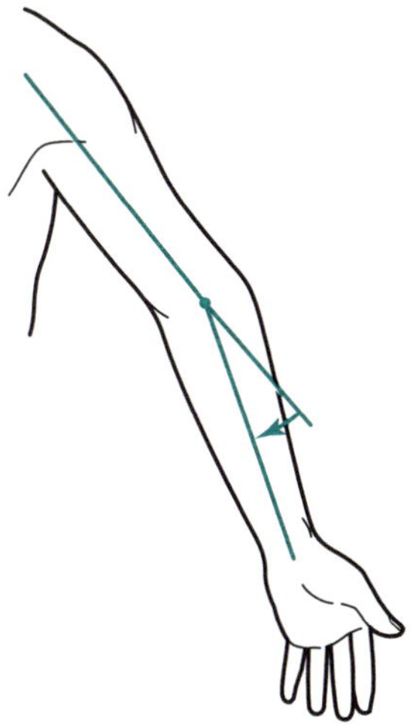

OBJECTIVE TESTS

Using your findings from the history and observation examination portions, you may perform the following objective tests depending on the environment in which you are examining the injury. Strategies for specific procedures for on-site, acute, or clinical treatment examinations will help guide your test selection.

Figure 13.25 Gunstock deformity resulting from an epiphyseal fracture.

Palpation

It is best to palpate the elbow structures with the elbow in a flexed, relaxed position. Similar to the cervical and shoulder chapters, this chapter presents elbow palpation regionally.

• **Anterior structures.** Palpate anterior structures that lie in the antecubital fossa. The antecubital fossa is bordered medially by the flexor–pronator muscle group and laterally by the brachioradialis. Proceeding from lateral to medial, you can palpate the biceps tendon, brachial artery, and median nerve within the fossa.

• **Medial structures.** Palpate for tenderness, swelling, and subtle deformities over the medial epicondyle and supracondylar ridge of the humerus. Palpate the proximal ulna just inferior to the medial epicondyle. Palpate for inflammation and tenderness of the flexor–pronator muscle mass at its origin on the medial epicondyle; the ulnar nerve within its groove; and the medial collateral ligament that fans from the medial epicondyle to the coronoid process anteriorly and the olecranon process posteriorly. Be careful as you palpate the ulnar nerve in the groove behind the medial epicondyle. Although it may not be readily palpable, it may elicit symptoms of pain or tingling if aggressively palpated.

• **Lateral structures.** To palpate the lateral structures, begin with the lateral epicondyle and supracondylar ridge. Move inferior to the epicondyle and palpate the radial head and the surrounding annular ligament that stabilizes the radial head. To facilitate palpation, move the forearm into supination and pronation so that the radial head rolls under your thumb and index fingers. In addition to the annular ligament, soft tissue structures on the lateral aspect include the extensor–supinator muscle mass and its origin on the lateral epicondyle, the brachioradialis, and the cordlike lateral collateral ligament as it runs from the lateral epicondyle to the annular ligament and proximal lateral ulna.

• **Posterior structures.** Posterior structures include the olecranon process and overlying olecranon bursa. With the elbow flexed, you can palpate the distal triceps to its insertion on the olecranon. While in a slightly flexed position, you can palpate the olecranon fossa on either side of and deep to the distal triceps tendon.

Range of Motion

As with other joints, examine elbow ROM first actively and then passively. You can quantify ROM in the athletic treatment facility using goniometric measurement techniques.

In addition to the ROM examinations presented here, you may also need to assess select motions of the shoulder (chapter 12) and wrist (chapter 14) as these motions may also affect the elbow joint.

Active ROM

Perform active ROM of the elbow for flexion and extension (figure 13.26a-b) and of the forearm for supination and pronation (figure 13.26c-d). Normal active ROM of the elbow is from 0° at full extension to 145° at flexion. Full supination should be approximately 90° and pronation slightly less, at 80° to 85°. Having the athlete grasp a pencil or pen in her hand when performing supination and pronation may help you observe the degree of motion. Observe for both quality and quantity of movement, looking for any signs of apprehension or pain with movements.

Passive ROM

Passive movement will normally be about 5° to 10° greater than active motion in elbow extension and forearm motions. It is not unusual for elbow flexion to increase as much as 15° up to a full range of 160° with passive movement. End feels vary depending on the reason for the end movement. Elbow extension should have a firm end feel as the olecranon process moves against the olecranon fossa. Elbow flexion, however, should have a soft, springy end feel as the forearm muscles contact the belly of the biceps brachii muscle.

Goniometric ROM Examination

Perform goniometric ROM examination of the elbow using the guidelines in table 13.1 and as demonstrated in figure 13.27.

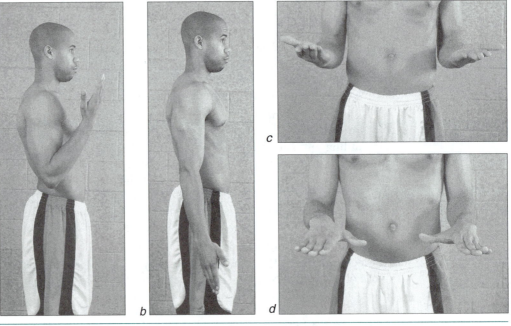

a   *b*   *c*   *d*

Figure 13.26   Active ROM of the elbow into *(a)* flexion, *(b)* extension, *(c)* supination, and *(d)* pronation.

Table 13.1
Goniometric Examination of Elbow ROM

Motion	Location of goniometer	Movement	Normal range
Flexion	P: Supine A: Lateral epicondyle S: Long axis of humerus M: Long axis of radius	Palm is moved toward shoulder	0° to 145-160° (depending on muscularity)
Extension	P: Supine, forearm off edge of table or arm placed on towel A: Lateral epicondyle S: Long axis of humerus M: Long axis of radius	Elbow is straightened as far as possible, with back of hand moving toward the table	0° (can vary from −10 to 15°)
Supination	P: Seated, arm at side and elbow flexed to 90° holding a pencil with a closed fist A: Head of 3rd metacarpal S: Perpendicular to floor M: Parallel with pencil	From neutral (pencil perpendicular to the floor), forearm is rotated externally, with palm facing the ceiling	0° to 90°
Pronation	P: Seated, arm at side and elbow flexed to 90° holding a pencil with a closed fist A: Head of 3rd metacarpal S: Perpendicular to floor M: Parallel with pencil	From neutral (pencil perpendicular to the floor), forearm is rotated internally, with palm facing downward	0° to 80-85°

P = athlete position; A = goniometer axis; S = stationary arm; M = movable arm.

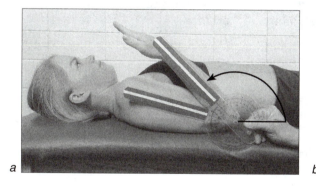
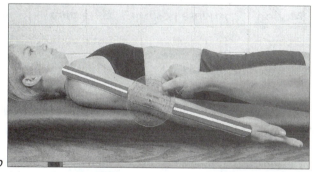
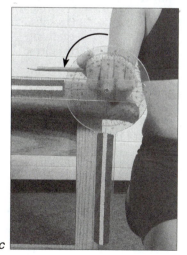
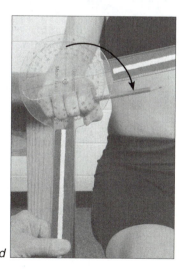

Figure 13.27 Goniometric examination of (a) elbow flexion, (b) elbow extension, (c) forearm supination, and (d) forearm pronation.

Strength

You may use manual muscle tests and instrumented strength examination to determine muscle strength.

Manual Muscle Tests

Manual muscle tests for the elbow include elbow flexion in three positions to differentially isolate the primary elbow flexors (brachioradialis, brachialis, biceps brachii), elbow extension, and forearm supination and pronation. They are described in table 13.2 and shown in figure 13.28.

Instrumented Strength Examination

Instruments for strength examination include a cable tensiometer for elbow flexion and extension and weight machines or dumbbells to determine a 1RM for strength. Dynamometers used to examine grip and pinch strength (chapter 7) can also help determine weakness emanating from an elbow injury or nerve compression, since the muscles for these activities originate at the elbow (figure 13.29). Isokinetic testing for elbow and wrist strength can further define specific strength output for elbow flexors and extensors, forearm pronators and supinators, and wrist flexors and extensors.

Table 13.2
Manual Muscle Tests for Muscles Acting on the Elbow

Motion	Athlete position	Stabilizing hand placement	Resistance hand placement	Instruction to athlete	Primary muscles tested
Elbow flexion	Seated or supine, forearm supinated	Distal posterior humerus at elbow	Ventral surface distal forearm	Move palm toward shoulder	Biceps brachii
Elbow flexion	Seated or supine, forearm pronated	Distal posterior humerus at elbow	Dorsal surface distal forearm	Move back of hand toward shoulder	Brachialis
Elbow flexion	Seated or supine, forearm neutral	Distal posterior humerus at elbow	Radial (lateral) surface distal forearm	Move thumb toward shoulder	Brachioradialis
Elbow extension	Prone with forearm off table or supine with shoulder flexed to 90° and internally rotated	Humerus	Dorsal surface of distal forearm	Straighten elbow, moving back of hand toward ceiling	Triceps brachii
Forearm supination	Seated, elbow flexed to 90°	Elbow held at athlete's side	Grasp distal forearm, resistance on dorsal aspect	From neutral position, supinate (laterally rotate) the forearm while you try to move it into pronation	Biceps brachii, supinator
Forearm pronation	Seated, elbow flexed to 90°	Elbow held at athlete's side	Grasp distal forearm, resistance on ventral aspect	From neutral position, pronate (medially rotate) the forearm while you try to move forearm into supination	Pronator teres, pronator quadratus

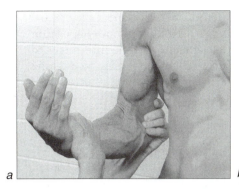
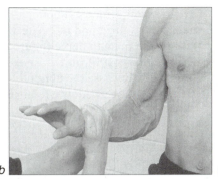
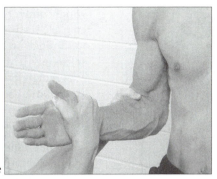

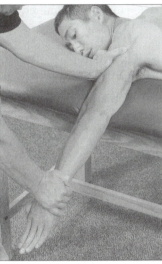
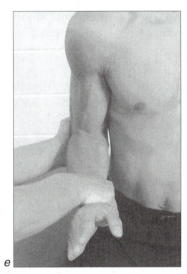
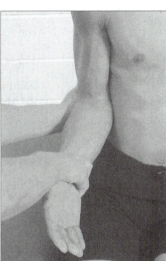

a   b   c

Figure 13.28 Manual muscle tests for elbow flexion isolating the *(a)* biceps brachii, *(b)* brachialis, and *(c)* brachioradialis; *(d)* elbow extension, *(e)* forearm supination, and *(f)* forearm pronation.

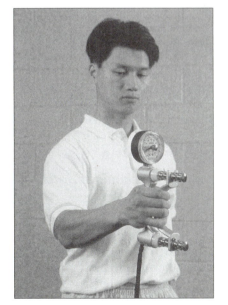

d   e   f

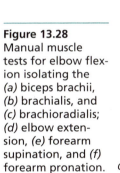

Figure 13.29 Grip strength testing in the treatment facility.

Neurovascular Examination

Because neurovascular structures lie in close proximity to the bone and joint surfaces of the distal humerus and elbow joint, you should perform neurological and vascular examinations with any significant trauma or suspected fracture or dislocation. Chronic nerve compression syndromes are common at the elbow, and certain tests help determine the extent of neuropathology. Depending on the location of injury, the neurological examination may focus on either the nerve roots or the peripheral nerve distributions of the brachial plexus.

Sensory Tests

To examine sensation around the elbow and forearm, provide light touch over sensory nerve distributions of the brachial plexus. These include the lateral aspect of the elbow (C5), lateral forearm (C6), medial forearm (C8), and medial aspect of the elbow (T1) (see chapter 8, especially table 8.6 and figure 8.3). For injuries occurring at the elbow joint or below, you should also examine sensation over the distributions of the peripheral nerves. Examine the distal lateral fifth finger (ulnar), the radial aspect of the second finger (median), the dorsal web space (radial), and the lateral forearm (musculocutaneous) (chapter 8; figures 8.7 and 8.8).

Motor Tests

Motor testing for the elbow are discussed in chapter 8 (see figures 8.9 and 8.10), including elbow flexion and wrist extension (C6), elbow extension (C7), thumb extension (C8), and finger abduction (T1). To examine motor function of the peripheral nerves, perform manual muscle testing for the median, ulnar, and radial nerves (figure 8.10). Use thumb opposition and pinch strength to test the median nerve (figure 8.10a), abduction of the fifth finger to examine the ulnar nerve (figure 8.10b), and wrist extension or thumb extension to examine the radial nerve (figure 8.10c). Because the musculocutaneous nerve does not innervate past the elbow, use elbow flexion (if injury allows) to distally examine its integrity.

Reflex Tests

Examine reflex responses over the biceps tendon (C5-C6), triceps tendon (C7-C8), and brachioradialis (C5-C6) (see chapter 8, figure 8.11). Perform these tests with the muscles relaxed and near midrange. The best way to check the biceps and brachioradialis reflexes is to place your thumb over the tendon and tap the thumbnail with a hammer. You can test the triceps reflex directly over the tendon just proximal to the olecranon process.

Vascular Tests

Examine vascular compromise using the radial distal pulse and capillary refill tests (chapter 9). Also check the skin for signs of pallor or mottled coloration and decreased temperature.

Special Tests

Special tests for the elbow include tests for joint stability, acute and chronic tendinopathies (e.g., epicondylitis), and neuropathies.

Joint Stability Tests

Joint stability tests for the elbow examine the integrity of the annular ligament and the medial and lateral collateral ligaments.

Medial and Lateral Stress Tests

Apply medial (valgus) and lateral (varus) stress tests to the collateral ligaments of the elbow joint. With the athlete's elbow in a partially flexed position (15°-20° from full extension), place your stabilizing hand on the lateral elbow and your mobilizing hand on the distal medial forearm to apply a **valgus stress** to the medial collateral ligament (figure 13.30a). Perform the lateral collateral ligament stress test similarly, but place your stabilizing hand on the medial elbow and apply a **varus stress** with the moblizing hand on the distal lateral forearm (figure 13.30b).

Radioulnar Joint Stress Test

To examine the integrity of the proximal radioulnar joint (annular ligament), apply anterior and posterior stresses to the joint. Place your stabilizing hand on the proximal aspect of the ulna, holding the athlete's forearm between your side and your arm. With your other hand, position your thumb over the anterior radial head and your

> Always test the uninvolved side first to examine quantity and quality of motion and to familiarize the athlete with the test.

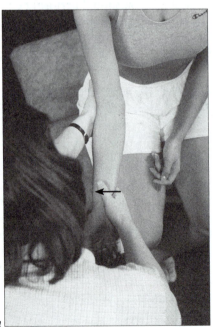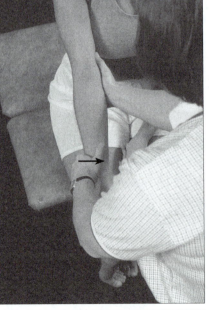

Figure 13.30 *(a)* Medial (valgus) stress test and *(b)* lateral (varus) stress test.

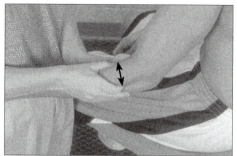

Figure 13.31   Radioulnar stress test.

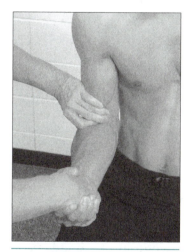

Figure 13.32   Distal biceps tendon rupture test.

index finger over the posterior aspect. Then grasp the radial head and apply stress in an anterior–posterior and posterior–anterior direction (figure 13.31).

Test for Tendon Pathologies

To assess the integrity of the tendinous attachments of the muscles acting on the elbow joint, use the following test.

Test for Distal Biceps Tendon Rupture

To examine for a distal biceps tendon rupture, you must isolate the biceps muscle and prevent substitution from the other elbow flexors. Position the athlete in 90° of elbow flexion and full supination. Ask the athlete to hold this position while you attempt to force the forearm into pronation (figure 13.32). Without the assistance of the biceps brachii, the remaining supinator muscles will not be able to resist this motion. A positive test is the inability to resist movement into pronation (Sallis et al. 2001).

Epicondylitis Tests

Use the following tests when you suspect acute or chronic tendinopathies of the flexor–pronator or extensor muscle groups.

Lateral Epicondylitis Test

You actively and passively test for lateral epicondylitis or tendinitis. The active test elicits pain during resisted wrist extension with the elbow flexed and forearm pronated (figure 13.33a). Adding radial deviation to the resisted motion increases the pain. Pain also occurs with passive flexion of the wrist with the elbow extended (figure 13.33b). Pain will increase when combined with ulnar deviation.

Medial Epicondylitis Test

You can use both passive and active tests to examine medial epicondylitis. For the active test, resist wrist flexion with the elbow flexed and forearm supinated (figure 13.34a). For the passive test, extend the wrist with the elbow extended and forearm pronated (figure 13.34b). In severe cases of epicondylitis, the athlete will complain of pain if he simply shakes hands or pulls open a door.

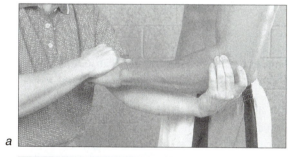

a

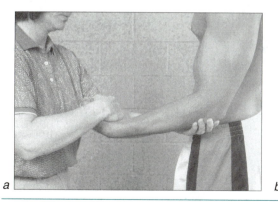

b

Figure 13.33   Lateral epicondylitis tests: *(a)* active and *(b)* passive.

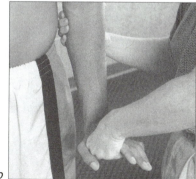

a   b

Figure 13.34   Medial epicondylitis tests: *(a)* active and *(b)* passive.

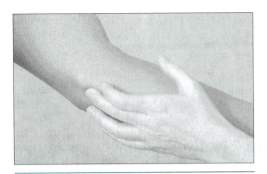

Figure 13.35 Tinel's test over the ulnar groove.

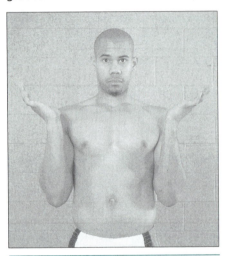

Figure 13.36 Elbow flexion test for ulnar nerve entrapment.

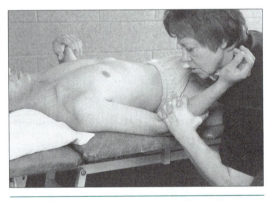

Figure 13.37 Humeroulnar joint mobility test.

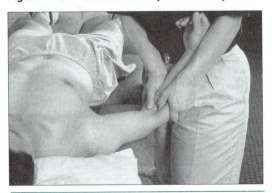

Figure 13.38 Radioulnar joint mobility test.

Nerve Compression and Neuropathy Tests

As previously discussed, nerve compression is common at the elbow and can occur in multiple locations. The following tests apply to the various entrapment locations.

Tinel's Sign

Tinel's sign identifies ulnar nerve compression or transmission interference at the elbow. Tap the ulnar nerve where it passes through the ulnar groove (figure 13.35) between the olecranon process and the medial epicondyle. The test is positive if it elicits a tingling or shooting sensation in the lateral forearm, hand, and fifth finger.

Elbow Flexion Test

You can examine ulnar nerve compression or entrapment in the cubital tunnel with the elbow flexion test. For this test, have the athlete maximally flex the elbow with the forearm neutral and wrist fully extended. The test position is held for 3 to 5 minutes and is positive if you find paresthesia along the medial border of the forearm and hand (figure 13.36).

Pronator Teres Test

To check for median nerve compression due to muscle hypertrophy of the pronator teres, apply sustained resistance against forearm pronation as the athlete extends the elbow from a starting position of 90° of flexion. A positive test reproduces symptoms of pain and paresthesia (hypesthesia) along the median nerve distribution in the hand.

Joint Mobility Examination

You should have already tested physiological joint motion during ROM examination. If the athlete lacks full joint motion, it may be due in part to joint capsule restriction. You can determine this in two ways: observing a capsular pattern of movement and examining joint accessory motion. An elbow capsular pattern is more limited with flexion than with extension and is equally limited in supination and pronation. In other words, a capsular restriction exists if the joint has lost more of its flexion than extension. If supination and pronation are restricted, they will be restricted equally. Examine joint accessory motion on the humeroulnar and radioulnar joints.

Humeroulnar Joint Mobility Test

With the athlete sitting or lying comfortably, stabilize the humerus and distract the ulna in a longitudinal caudal motion to examine the humeroulnar joint (figure 13.37).

Radioulnar Joint Mobility Test

To examine the proximal radioulnar joint, grasp the ulna with your stabilizing hand and the radial head with your mobilizing hand. Apply an anterior–posterior force to the radius, similar to the movement for testing joint stress (figure 13.38).

INJURY EXAMINATION STRATEGIES

As you have likely noted, multiple conditions involving a variety of structures can result from similar mechanisms. A thorough history, careful observation, and the appropriate use of the objective examination techniques just covered will help you identify and differentiate among the potentially involved structures.

On-Site Examination

A wrestler is thrown and lands awkwardly on an outstretched hand. He yells out in pain and grabs his arm. As you approach, you immediately note obvious deformity at the elbow joint.

The need for on-site examination of an elbow injury most often arises from direct contact, a fall on an outstretched hand, hyperextension, or a severe valgus or varus mechanism. As always, your goal is to quickly determine the nature and severity of the injury and check for any conditions indicating a medical emergency. As you approach the athlete, observe his response to the injury, his willingness to move the injured limb, and the position of the limb. As usual, conduct a primary survey immediately upon arrival.

History and Observation

As you reach the athlete, ask him or any bystanders what happened if you did not witness the injury. Observe closely for signs of immediate swelling, discoloration, and deformity. A gunstock deformity or varus angulation of the joint in a young athlete may indicate an epiphyseal fracture (refer to figure 13.25). Check if the olecranon process is more pronounced posteriorly, indicating a possible posterior humeroulnar dislocation.

Palpation and Neurovascular Status

If you observe an obvious deformity, immediately palpate for a distal pulse at the radial or ulnar artery as indicated. Also at this time, examine the sensory distribution of the peripheral nerves in the hand. If neurovascular findings are positive, immediately refer the athlete and stabilize the elbow in the position in which it was found for emergency transport. If neurovascular structures are intact, proceed with a cursory palpation of the bone and joint structures to check for bony tenderness, crepitus, or subtle deformities that would indicate a fracture or subluxation. Fractures and dislocations are usually easy to detect because of the superficial nature of joint structures. However, tenderness over the superficial bony structures will also occur with severe contusions due to direct contact, which also may result in considerable acute pain.

Range of Motion

If no obvious signs of fracture or dislocation and no severe bony tenderness are present, and all neurovascular signs are negative, have the athlete slowly flex and extend the elbow. If pain does not increase or become severe with movement, assist the athlete off the field for continued examination on the sideline. Since any muscle spasm will have little effect on stress testing at the elbow, you can defer ligament stress tests until the acute examination. If for any reason the athlete has difficulty standing, is in enough pain to hinder ambulation, or shows signs of shock, provide assisted transportation.

Acute Examination

In the opening scenario, Randy noticed that the inside of his elbow was sorer than usual. But he was facing the toughest batter on the other team, so he decided to throw a hard fastball for a strikeout that would end the inning. As Randy wound up and threw the ball, he felt a snap and tremendous pain in his elbow. After a quick consultation with the athletic trainer, he walked off the mound on his own power.

Checklist for On-Site Examination of the Elbow and Forearm

▷ **Primary Survey**

- ☐ Consciousness
- ☐ Airway, breathing, and circulation
- ☐ Severe bleeding
- ☐ Check for unusual positioning of the limb
- ☐ Examine for shock

▷ **Secondary Survey**

  ▷ **History**

- ☐ Chief complaint
- ☐ Mechanism of injury
- ☐ Location and severity of pain
- ☐ Information from bystanders

  ▷ **Observation**

- ☐ Note deformity, swelling, discoloration, pallor

  ▷ **Palpation**

- ☐ Bony tenderness, crepitus, and deformity along the medial supracondylar ridge, medial epicondyle, olecranon process and proximal ulna, lateral supracondylar ridge, lateral epicondyle, radial head, and proximal radius

  ▷ **Neurovascular examination**

- ☐ Sensory (C5, C6, C8, T1; ulnar, median, radial, musculocutaneous)
- ☐ Motor (C6, C7, C8, T1; ulnar, median, radial)
- ☐ Distal pulse (radial pulse; capillary refill)

  ▷ **Gentle, active range of motion**

- ☐ Elbow flexion, extension
- ☐ Pronation, supination

If all tests are negative, remove athlete from field for continued examination off-site.

A female basket ball player comes off the court holding her elbow in a flexed position. She states she used her outstretched arm to stop a pass and felt her elbow bend back.

Once the athlete has been removed to the sideline, you will perform a more detailed examination than on-site.

History

Begin with a detailed but focused history of the injury. Determining the injury's mechanism will help identify the injury's nature. Try to determine the patient's activity and the elbow's position at the time of pain or injury. Refer to the Acute Examination Checklist (see page 301) for appropriate questions. As always, a more thorough history will provide more information on which to base your objective examination.

Observation

As the athlete comes to the sideline, observe how she holds her elbow and look for any guarding or obvious expressions of pain. Note the location and degree of swelling and discoloration by comparing to the uninvolved side. If you conducted an on-site examination, has there been any change in appearance since that time? Diffuse and rapid swelling of the elbow or forearm can occur with elbow injuries and lead to a compartment syndrome, so you need to monitor closely for signs of excessive swelling and impending neurovascular compromise. If the athlete fell hard or received a direct blow to the posterior elbow, check for localized swelling of the olecranon bursa.

Next, check for alignment and the position of structures relative to one another, noting any differences between the right and left sides. Alignment includes the carrying angle and the relationship between the olecranon process and the epicondyles. Normal carrying angle is about 5° in males and 10 to15° in females, so the valgus angle of the elbow in extension is 175° in men and 165° to 170° in women (figure 13.23a on page 288). When the elbow is flexed, the carrying angle disappears (figure 13.23b). An abnormal carrying angle can be the result of a fracture or epiphyseal separation.

With the elbow flexed to 90°, the olecranon process and the medial and lateral epicondyles should form an isosceles triangle (figure 13.39a). When the elbow is in full extension, these same structures should form a straight line (figure 13.39b). Absence of this alignment may be due to fracture, subluxation, or dislocation.

Palpation

After your observation, palpate before performing special tests. Gently palpate around the injured area to detect temperature variations and soft tissue tightness or texture differences that may occur with the advent and progression of edema. Temperature changes occur naturally over different areas such as bony prominences compared to muscle bellies, but you can identify abnormal changes by comparing to the uninjured side. Check distal pulses again to ensure continued circulatory integrity. Depending on the injury mechanism, you may note tenderness on opposite sides of the joint. Diffuse tenderness anteriorly along with pain within the olecranon fossa posteriorly is common with hyperextension mechanisms. With valgus forces, you will note tenderness over the stressed medial structures as well as lateral tenderness due to compression. When patients experience pain on both sides of the joint with these mechanisms, the injury is typically more severe than if only one side of the joint is tender.

> Always test the uninvolved side first to examine quantity and quality of motion and to familiarize the athlete with the test.

Special Tests

Special tests for the elbow typically used in the acute examination are those that examine joint stability and muscle integrity:

- Medial and lateral stress tests (figure 13.30, a-b)
- Radioulnar joint test (figure 13.31)
- Distal biceps tendon rupture test (fiure 13.32)

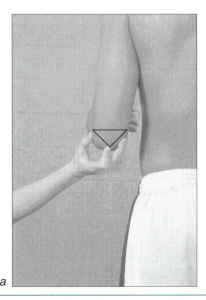
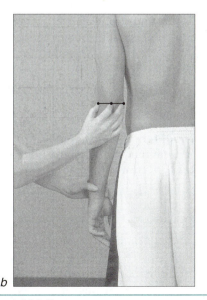

a   *b*

Figure 13.39   Normal elbow alignment at *(a)* 90° and *(b)* full extension.

Range of Motion

Examine active ROM through a full range for elbow extension and flexion, as well as for forearm supination and pronation. You may also wish to have the athlete perform active wrist flexion and extension, since the origin of the extrinsic muscles responsible for these motions crosses the elbow joint. If pain arises during any active motion, note where in the motion and over what range it occurs. As a rule of thumb, the earlier in the motion the pain occurs and the greater the pain is, the more serious the injury. Incomplete motion can be due to pain, weakness, spasm, or a bony block.

Next, perform passive ROM tests to examine the end feel of the joint and to determine the cause for any limitations in active ROM. Full passive motion without full active motion indicates weakness that can result from either muscle or nerve injury or pain. Incomplete passive motion is the result of a blockage that restricts motion.

Strength

Elbow musculature strength is commonly tested in midposition. Also perform manual resistance tests for wrist flexion and extension as well as shoulder flexion and extension, depending on the pathology. These tests are discussed in chapters 14 and 12, respectively. It is important to examine the shoulder to eliminate any possible referred pain from the shoulder into the elbow, and to examine the wrist because an elbow injury may affect wrist function and strength due to the many elbow muscles that function at the wrist.

Neurological Tests

If at any time the athlete complains of numbness, tingling, or referred pain into the elbow or forearm as a result of an elbow injury, follow with a complete neurological examination to test the integrity of both the primary nerve trunks and the peripheral nerves of the elbow and forearm (median, radial, musculocutaneous, and ulnar).

To examine motor function, perform isometric tests for each peripheral nerve. The musculocutaneous nerve has no innervation beyond the elbow, so you can only subject it to sensory testing. If you need to rule out shoulder or cervical involvement, also examine nerve root myotomes (see chapter 8).

Functional Tests

If your examination demonstrates no positive findings that indicate cessation of activity and pain has sufficiently subsided, perform functional tests to determine the athlete's readiness to return to activity. Functional tests are specific to sport and position. Examples of functional tests include gripping, swinging a bat, throwing, swimming with strokes specific to the athlete's competitive events, performing a tennis serve, performing a handstand or walkover, and throwing a discus. Execution of the activity should be painless and exhibit normal flow and joint excursion without hesitation, deficiency, or any unusual outcome. If you are ever uncertain whether the athlete is ready to return to activity, it is better to err on the side of caution for the sake of the athlete's health.

Clinical Examination

A high school tennis player comes into the athletic training facility at the beginning of the school year complaining of lateral elbow pain. You know this athlete well, and remember that she planned to attend an intensive tennis training camp over the summer to work on her game.

A 12-year-old Little League athlete presents with an achy feeling in his elbow that has persisted for over a month. His pain worsens with throwing and seems to be localized to the anterior lateral elbow. You note while talking with him that he does not fully extend his elbow.

Checklist for Acute Examination of the Elbow and Forearm

▷ **History**

Ask questions pertaining to the following:
- ☐ Chief complaint
- ☐ Mechanism of injury
- ☐ Unusual sounds or sensations
- ☐ Type and location of pain or symptoms
- ☐ Previous injury
- ☐ Previous injury to opposite extremity for bilateral comparison

▷ **Observation**
- ☐ Visible facial expressions of pain
- ☐ Swelling, deformity, skin coloration, abnormal contours, or discoloration
- ☐ Does athlete let arm hang and swing or does athlete hold or splint the arm?
- ☐ Overall position, posture, and alignment
- ☐ Carrying angle
- ☐ Alignment of the medial and lateral epicondyle and olecranon process (extended and flexed elbow)
- ☐ Flexed elbow posture
- ☐ Muscle development—are there areas of muscular atrophy?
- ☐ Bilateral comparison

▷ **Palpation**

Bilaterally palpate for pain, tenderness, and deformity over the following:
- ☐ Medial epicondyle and supracondylar ridge
- ☐ Olecranon process, olecranon fossa, and proximal ulna
- ☐ Lateral epicondyle and supracondylar ridge, radial head
- ☐ Flexor-pronator group, ulnar nerve, medial collateral ligament
- ☐ Olecranon bursa, distal triceps
- ☐ Extensor-supinator muscle group, brachioradialis, lateral collateral ligament, annular ligament
- ☐ Biceps tendon, brachial artery, median nerve

▷ **Special Tests**
- ☐ Collateral stress tests
- ☐ Radioulnar joint stress test
- ☐ Biceps tendon test

▷ **Range of Motion**
- ☐ Active ROM for elbow flexion and extension, forearm pronation and supination
- ☐ Active ROM for shoulder flexion and extension and wrist flexion and extension as appropriate
- ☐ Passive ROM for same motions as for active ROM
- ☐ Bilateral comparison

▷ **Strength Tests**
- ☐ Perform manual resistance against same motions as in active ROM
- ☐ Check bilateral comparison, note any pain or weakness
- ☐ Perform manual resistance for wrist flexion and extension and shoulder flexion and extension as appropriate

▷ **Neurovascular Tests**
- ☐ Sensory, motor, and reflex of nerve roots C5, C6, C7, C8, and T1
- ☐ Sensory and motor for median, ulnar, musculocutaneous, and radial peripheral nerves
- ☐ Distal pulse (radial pulse; capillary refill)

▷ **Functional Tests**

The clinical examination is similar to the acute examination, but includes additional examination techniques for chronic and postacute conditions.

History

Questions regarding the onset of symptoms, duration, aggravating and easing factors, past history of both involved and uninvolved sides, and previous rehabilitative care are as important as the questions you asked in the acute examination. Refer to chapter 3 as well as the history portion of the Clinical Examination Checklist (page 303) for specific questions you should ask. In particular, ask about sport- or work-related activities that may indicate excessive valgus overload or repetitive wrist flexion–extension or pronation–supination movements. Changes in training and equipment may equally influence task demands for the industrial athlete. For instance, if you are examining a factory worker, ask her if she has recently changed job tasks. All these questions, in addition to those asked in the acute examination, will give you a good idea of the injury's **SINS** (**S**everity, **I**rritability, **N**ature, **S**tage) and your examination objectives.

Observation

Observe how the patient holds her elbow. Does it hang freely when she walks, or is she guarding and supporting it with the other hand? If she maintains the joint in a flexed position, she may be experiencing joint swelling or pain in either the anterior capsule or olecranon fossa with full extension. This elbow posture is common with hyperextension injuries. Also notice whether the athlete uses the arm to open doors or carry heavy objects such as books. Upon direct observation, look for signs of swelling, redness or ecchymosis, changes in skin coloration, or any structures that appear abnormal in size or contour.

To test the quadrant position, place the neck in end range extension, rotation, and lateral flexion to the same side as the symptoms before applying overpressure to the head.

Differential Diagnosis

Elbow pain can also be referred from the shoulder and cervical regions. You must differentially rule out these areas as possible sources of the patient's complaints before focusing on the elbow. Active ROM with overpressure at the end ranges for cervical and shoulder motions eliminates these areas as possible referral sites. If straight-plane motions with overpressures for the cervical spine are negative, use the quadrant position discussed in chapter 11. If any of these cervical or shoulder motions reproduce the patient's complaints, you should further investigate them before moving on to the elbow.

Range of Motion

Perform active and passive ROM tests as discussed in the objective tests section. As with the acute examination, you can either perform each passive test immediately after each active motion or can perform all the active motions before all the passive tests. You can also record quantitative measurement of joint ROM at this time. If you find a capsular pattern of motion, include joint mobility tests in the examination.

Strength Tests

Manual strength tests are the same as those used for the acute examination. In addition, you should pay special attention to resisted wrist flexion and extension tests, as many chronic injuries involve the wrist flexor–pronator or extensor muscle groups that attach at the elbow. Elbow pain, especially subacute and chronic, can emanate from either the medial or the lateral epicondyle. Since these sites originate the common wrist flexor and extensor tendons, the athlete with epicondylitis experiences pain at the elbow with resisted movements of the wrist. The treatment facility may also provide you with tools to better quantify your strength examination.

Neurological Tests

If the athlete complains of burning, tingling, numbness, radiating pain, or weakness into the elbow, wrist, or hand, you should include a neurological examination to test sensory, motor, and reflex response as described for the acute examination (see page 300). With chronic conditions, sensory or motor deficits are likely due to a nerve compression syndrome, so you should follow with special tests.

Special Tests

Stress tests for the elbow's collateral ligaments and the proximal radioulnar joint are consistent with those outlined in the acute examination. Check for presence of pain and instability with stress application and compare bilaterally. Chronic injuries frequently require tests to identify nerve and tendon pathologies.

Palpation

Palpation in the clinical examination is similar to that for the acute examination. As you begin palpation, position the athlete comfortably, usually either supine or sitting. If the athlete or worker presents with tenderness over the medial or lateral epicondyle, pay special attention to tenderness and crepitus in the common flexor or extensor tendon, since the problem may be epicondylitis. Soft tissue examination into the bellies of these muscles can also elicit pain, especially if the athlete's injury has become chronic. Tendon palpation should begin lightly and then move deeper. Tendinitis can be very isolated, so start in a small area and progress outward from the initial palpation site. Once you locate the source of pain, continue palpating distally along the tendon and into the muscle for evidence of pain and soft tissue restriction. Comparison with the other elbow is crucial for accurate examination of soft tissue restriction.

Checklist for Clinical Examination of the Elbow and Forearm

▷ History

Ask questions pertaining to the following:
- ☐ Chief complaint
- ☐ Mechanism of injury
- ☐ Unusual sounds or sensations
- ☐ Type, location, onset, and duration of pain or symptoms
- ☐ Previous injury
- ☐ Previous injury to opposite extremity for bilateral comparison

If chronic, ascertain:
- ☐ Aggravating and easing activities
- ☐ Training history (changes in training or equipment)
- ☐ Activity restrictions
- ☐ Treatment if any

▷ Observation

- ☐ Visible facial expressions of pain
- ☐ Swelling, deformity, abnormal contours, or discoloration
- ☐ Does athlete let arm hang and swing, or does the athlete hold or splint the arm?
- ☐ Observe overall position, posture, and alignment
- ☐ Carrying angle
- ☐ Alignment of the medial and lateral epicondyle and olecranon process (elbow flexed and extended)
- ☐ Flexed elbow posture
- ☐ Muscle development—are there areas of muscular atrophy or hypertrophy?
- ☐ Bilateral comparison

▷ Differential Diagnosis

- ☐ Clear cervical region with overpressure tests in straight planes and quadrant position
- ☐ Clear shoulder region with passive overpressures in all ranges

(continued)

▷ *Range of Motion*

- ☐ Active ROM for elbow flexion and extension, forearm pronation and supination
- ☐ Passive ROM for same motions
- ☐ Active ROM for shoulder flexion and extension, wrist flexion and extension as appropriate
- ☐ Passive ROM for same motions
- ☐ Bilateral comparison

▷ *Strength Tests*

- ☐ Perform manual resistance against same motions as in active ROM
- ☐ Check bilaterally and note any pain or weakness
- ☐ Perform instrumented strength tests

▷ *Neurovascular Tests*

- ☐ Sensory, motor, reflex of nerve roots C5, C6, C7, C8, and T1
- ☐ Sensory and motor of median, ulnar, radial, and musculocutaneous peripheral nerves
- ☐ Distal pulse (radial)

▷ *Special Tests*

- ☐ Collateral stress tests
- ☐ Radioulnar joint stress test
- ☐ Epicondylitis tests (active, passive)
- ☐ Nerve compression tests

▷ *Joint Mobility Examination (as appropriate)*

Note capsular restriction and end feel:

- ☐ Humeroulnar
- ☐ Radioulnar
- ☐ Bilateral comparison

▷ *Palpation*

Bilaterally palpate for pain, tenderness, and deformity over the following:

- ☐ Medial epicondyle and supracondylar ridge
- ☐ Olecranon process, olecranon fossa, and proximal ulna
- ☐ Lateral eipcondyle and supracondylar ridge, radial head
- ☐ Flexor-pronator group, ulnar nerve, medial collateral ligament
- ☐ Olecranon bursa, distal triceps
- ☐ Extensor-supinator muscle group, brachioradialis, lateral collateral ligament, annular ligament
- ☐ Biceps tendon, brachial artery, median nerve

▷ *Functional Tests*

SUMMARY

1. Describe the etiology, signs and symptoms, and potential complications associated with acute and chronic injuries of the elbow and forearm commonly encountered in physically active people.

   Both acute and chronic injuries commonly occur at the elbow as a result of physical activity. Acute muscle strains and tendon ruptures of the biceps, triceps, and wrist flexor and extensor groups can result from violent muscle contractions. Traumatic injuries such as sprains, fractures, and dislocations most often occur as a result of extreme valgus, varus, and hyperextension forces; falls on an outstretched hand; and direct contact. Because of the close proximity of the major nerves and vessels to the elbow joint, neurovascular compromise can result as a complication of these traumatic injuries. Chronic overuse injuries are also prevalent, particularly in athletes engaged in overhead throwing sports and in sports such as tennis and golf that involve repetitive wrist motions. A variety of medial stress injuries can occur in both younger and older athletes due to valgus overload forces associated with overhead throwing activities. A careful examination is required to identify and differentiate the involved structure.

2. Identify the common pathologies associated with repetitive valgus overload stresses in the throwing athlete.

The late cocking phase of throwing places tremendous valgus forces on the elbow, resulting in traction injuries on the medial aspect and compression injuries on the lateral aspect of the joint. In the adult athlete, injury is usually to the ligament or tendon, resulting in medial epicondylitis and valgus instability. In the young athlete, injury more often involves the medial humeral apophysis and can result in apophysitis and eventually a traction apophyseal fracture if the stress is allowed to continue. Osteochondritis dissecans of the radial head as a result of medial compression with valgus overload can also occur in the young athlete who often performs throwing activities.

3. Identify causes of forearm compartment syndrome and the 5 Ps of neurovascular compromise.

Forearm compartment syndrome can result from any injury that compromises the vascular structures. Laceration or occlusion of the brachial artery secondary to fracture or dislocation or any trauma that causes rapid, excessive swelling in the elbow and forearm compromise blood flow to the forearm, ultimately resulting in venous collapse and tissue necrosis. Signs and symptoms of compartment syndrome include the 5 Ps: pain, pallor, pulselessness, paresthesia, and eventual paralysis. With traumatic injuries, you must examine neurovascular status immediately and monitor it often.

4. Identify the anatomical sites and signs and symptoms associated with nerve compression syndromes.

The peripheral nerves of the forearm and hand travel across the elbow through anatomical spaces created by bone, fascia, and muscle. Nerve compression can occur if these spaces are compromised due to excessive muscle hypertrophy, scar formation, fascial restriction, and swelling. Signs and symptoms are common and include pain, paresthesia, and possible muscle weakness along the involved nerve's distribution. Special tests that reproduce these signs and symptoms are positive for nerve compression syndromes.

5. Describe the normal anatomical alignment, carrying angle, and range of motion of the elbow joint.

To accurately examine joint position and motion, you need to understand the normal anatomical alignment of the elbow. In the anatomical extended position of 0°, the carrying angle of the elbow is slightly valgus, with females having a slightly greater angulation than males, and the medial and lateral epicondyle and olecranon process form a straight line. The elbow is capable of flexing about 145° actively and about 155° to 160° passively. In the flexed position, the valgus angulation disappears, and an isosceles triangle is formed by the olecranon process and the medial and lateral epicondyles.

6. Explain the purpose of and demonstrate the appropriate use of objective tests for the elbow and forearm.

As with all joints, your observation of the injury and the athlete's history dictate your objective test selection. It is best to palpate regionally with the elbow slightly flexed. Perform ROM tests first actively and then passively for flexion, extension, supination, and pronation. Follow with manual muscle testing for each motion to assess neuromuscular integrity and identify any motor weakness. Because of the close proximity of the neurovascular structures to the bone and joint surfaces of the distal humerus and elbow joint, you should perform neurological and vascular examinations with any significant trauma or suspected fracture or dislocation. Special tests for the elbow include tests for joint stability, tendon pathologies, and neuropathies.

7. Perform an on-site examination for the elbow and forearm, and determine criteria for immediate medical referral and mode of transportation from the field.

The immediate aims in an on-site examination of an elbow injury are to examine the joint for possible dislocation, fracture, and compromised vascular supply, as well as the athlete's overall condition. When you find obvious deformities, immediately examine neurovascular status; if the findings are positive, make a medical referral without delay because of the potential complications. If gross deformities are not present, palpate for any bony tenderness, crepitus, or subtle deformities that may indicate less serious fractures. If the injury is not serious, remove the athlete from the field for a more thorough examination on the sideline.

8. Perform an acute examination of the elbow and forearm, noting criteria for referral and return to activity.

During the acute examination, determine whether the athlete is able to return to sport participation by more thoroughly examining the severity of the injury, the structure involved, and the athlete's functional ability. This includes a more detailed history, observation, and palpation examination. Because of the superficial nature of many of the soft tissue and bony structures of the elbow, careful palpation is an important tool for identifying the specific structures involved. In addition, the acute examination includes active, passive, and resistive ROM tests in elbow flexion, extension, pronation, and supination. Also perform joint stability tests to determine medial and lateral collateral ligament integrity, and perform neurovascular tests as appropriate. If the examination reveals no significant injuries, use functional tests mimicking the forces and movements required of the upper extremity to determine the patient's readiness to return to activity.

9. Perform a clinical examination of the elbow and forearm, noting considerations for differential diagnosis.

Many conditions at the elbow are chronic and are often first reported in the athletic treatment facility. The clinical examination for the elbow is similar to the acute examination, with the addition of special tests to investigate more chronic conditions such as epicondylitis, tendinitis, and nerve compression syndromes. You should perform differential tests to rule out cervical and shoulder pathologies, as these pathologies may refer symptoms to the elbow. The clinical examination may also incorporate joint mobility tests to identify any joint or capsular restriction and to examine joint end feel.

REVIEW QUESTIONS

1. What is the normal carrying angle of the elbow? What is a gunstock deformity, and what are some of its potential causes?

2. What causes olecranon bursitis? What are the signs and symptoms associated with this condition?

3. Define the terms tendinitis, epicondylitis, and tendinosis. How do these conditions and their signs and symptoms differ?

4. Identify the injuries that cause a compartment syndrome. Describe the continuum of this pathology and the characteristic deformity that results without immediate care.

5. Discuss the causative factors, signs and symptoms, and structures involved in cubital tunnel syndrome. What special tests might you use to confirm this condition?

6. What are some secondary conditions that can result from chronic valgus overload in an athlete with valgus instability? Think about other structures that could be tractioned or compressed as a consequence of increased ligament laxity. What signs and symptoms would you expect if these structures were involved, and what special tests would you use to confirm their involvement?

7. How do you test the integrity of the medial (ulnar) collateral ligament? How would you determine the severity of the ligament injury?

8. Identify the peripheral nerve pathology that causes the following symptoms:
   - Weakness in pinch strength
   - Paresthesia over the dorsal web space
   - Deep ache in the extensor muscle mass with repetitive gripping
   - Paresthesia over the distal, radial aspect of the second digit
   - Intrinsic muscle weakness

CRITICAL THINKING QUESTIONS

1. You are asked to examine an 18-year-old pitcher who has had medial elbow pain for 6 weeks. His history reveals that he has been a pitcher for 6 years and has no previous injury. He complains of pain with hard throwing. Upon palpation, it is difficult for you to tell whether his tenderness is over the medial collateral ligament, medial condyle, or the musculotendinous origin of the flexor–pronator group. You also note that he has mild lateral joint pain. Given his age and sport, which condition or conditions might you suspect and why? What special tests would you use to differentiate the potential structures involved?

2. Identify the type of end feel you might find with the following pathologies and passive motions:
   - Posterior lateral osteophyte of the olecranon process with elbow extension
   - Valgus instability with valgus stress test
   - Biceps rupture with elbow extension
   - Acute anterior capsular strain with elbow extension
   - Lateral epicondylitis with pronation

3. You are at a wrestling match when you see an athlete fall onto his outstretched hand. You arrive at his side to find that he is in considerable pain, and you observe an obvious deformity. You immediately check distal pulse and find it absent. You know this is a medical emergency, and the coach's car is parked right next to the gym. The coach offers to take the athlete immediately to the emergency room. Do you accept his offer to get the athlete medical attention sooner, or do you wait for emergency medical services? Discuss what decision you would make and give your reasons.

4. Consider the scenario of the high school tennis player returning to school with lateral elbow pain after attending an intensive summer tennis camp. Her chief complaints include pain when initially waking and moving the wrist in the morning, and weakness and pain during her backhand stroke. Before beginning your objective examination, what important questions would you ask while taking a thorough history?

CITED REFERENCES

Alley, R.M., and A.M. Pappas. 1995. Acute and chronic performance related injuries of the elbow. In *Upper extremity injuries in the athlete*, ed. A.M. Pappas, 339-364. New York: Churchill Livingstone.

Andrews, J.R., and J.A. Whiteside. 1993. Common elbow problems in the athlete. *J Orthop Sports Phys Ther* 17(6): 289-295.

Behr, C.T., and D.W. Altchek. 1997. The elbow. *Clin Sports Med* 16(4): 681-704.

Bennett, J.B. 1993. Articular injuries in the athlete. In *The elbow and its disorders*, ed. B.F. Morrey, 581-595. Philadelphia: Saunders.

Cabanela, M.E., and B.F. Morrey. 1993. Fractures of the proximal ulna and olecranon. In *The elbow and its disorders*, ed. B.F. Morrey, 405-428. Philadelphia: Saunders.

Caldwell, G.L., and M.R. Safran. 1995. Elbow problems in the athlete. *Orthop Clin N Am* 26(3): 465-485.

Griggs, S.M., and A.P. Weiss. 1996. Bony injuries of the wrist, forearm, and elbow. *Clin Sports Med* 15: 373-400.

Grossfield, S.L., A.V. Heest, E. Arendt, and J. House. 1998. Pitcher's periostitis. *Am J Sports Med* 26(2): 303-307.

Jobe, F.W., H. Stark, and S.J. Lombardo. 1986. Reconstruction of the ulnar collateral ligament in athletes. *J Bone Joint Surg* 68A:1158-1163.

Larson, R.L., and L.R.Osternig. 1974. Traumatic bursitis and artificial turf. *J Sports Med* 2:183.

Lowery, W.D., P.R. Kurzweil, S.K. Forman, and D.S. Morrison. 1995. Persistence of the olecranon physis: A cause of "Little League Elbow." *J Elbow Shoulder Surg* 4(2): 143-147.

Morrey, B.F. 1993. Radial head fracture. In *The elbow and its disorders*, ed. B.F. Morrey, 383-404. Philadelphia: Saunders.

Nirschl, R.P. 1993. Muscle and tendon trauma: Tennis elbow. In *The elbow and its disorders*, ed. B.F. Morrey, 537-552. Philadelphia: Saunders.

Sallis R.E., D.A. Zillmer, B.A. Russell, and S.T. Doberstein. 2001. Confirming a biceps brachii tendon rupture. *Phys Sportmed* 29(2): 21.

Slowik, G.M., M. Fitzimmons, and J.M. Rayhack. 1993. Closed elbow dislocation and brachial artery damage. *J Orthop Trauma* 7(6): 558-561.

Takahara, M., M. Shundo, M. Kondo, K. Suzuki, T. Nambu, and T. Ogino. 1998. Early detection of osteochondritis dissecans of the capitellum in young baseball players. *J Bone Jt Surg* 80A(6): 892-897.

Takami, H., S. Takahashi, and M. Ando. 1997. Irreducible isolated dislocation of the radial head. *Clin Orthop Rel Res* 345:168-170.

Timmerman, L.A., and J.R. Andrews. 1994. Undersurface tear of the ulnar collateral ligament in baseball players: A newly recognized lesion. *Am J Sports Med* 22(1): 33-36.

Tyrdal, S., and B.S. Olsen. 1998. Combined hyperextension and supination of the elbow joint induces lateral ligament lesions: An experimental study of the pathoanatomy and kinematics in elbow ligament injuries. *Knee Surg, Sports Traum, Arthro* 6(1): 36-43.

Wadhwa, S.S., R. Mansberg, V.B. Fernandes, and S. Qasim. 1997. Forearm splints seen on bone scan in a weight lifter. *Clin Nuclear Med* 22(10): 711-712.

Weiker, G.G. 1995. Upper extremity gymnastic injuries. In *The upper extremity in sports medicine*, eds. J.A. Nicholas and E.B. Hershman, 840. St. Louis: Mosby.

Wilson, F.D., J.R. Andrews, T.A. Blackburn, and G. McCluskey. 1983. Valgus extension overload in the pitching elbow. *Am J Sports Med* 11(2): 83-87.

ADDITIONAL RESOURCES

Clarkson, H.M. 2000. *Musculoskeletal assessment: Joint range of motion and manual muscle strength.* 2nd ed. Philadelphia: Lippincott Williams & Wilkins.

Magee, D.J. 1992. *Orthopedic physical assessment.* 2nd ed. Philadelphia: W.B. Saunders.

Moore, K.L. 1992. *Clinically oriented anatomy.* 3rd ed. Baltimore: Williams & Wilkins.

CHAPTER 14

Wrist and Hand

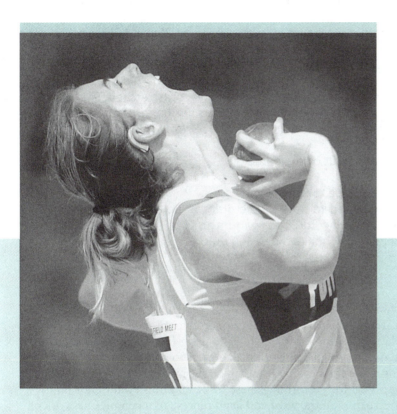

Objectives

After completing this chapter, the reader will be able to do the following:

1. Describe the types and mechanisms of acute and chronic injuries of the wrist and hand that physically active people commonly experience

2. Describe the potential complications and deformities that can result from seemingly simple sprains and strains

3. Identify the common sites and signs and symptoms of nerve compression injuries

4. Discuss the common fractures that occur in the wrist and hand and their characteristic deformities and signs and symptoms

5. Describe and perform the objective tests for wrist and hand examination

6. Perform an on-site examination of the wrist and hand, identifying the conditions that warrant immediate referral

7. Perform an acute examination of the wrist and hand, including special tests used to examine acute conditions

8. Perform a clinical examination of the wrist and hand, including examination techniques for chronic injuries

John was in his first year as an assistant athletic trainer at California State University and was excited to be accompanying the women's softball team to Oklahoma City for the NCAA national championships. Before the game, the coach from UCLA, the reigning national champions, approached John and informed him that their athletic trainer was back at the hotel with the flu.

She then asked, "Would you mind helping us out by coming onto the field if one of my players gets hurt during the game?"

John didn't see this as a problem, and injuries were rare in softball anyway. "Sure, I'd be glad to help. Just let me know if you need me."

It was the top of the seventh inning and CSU was behind by one run. UCLA was up to bat with one out, and their All-American pitcher (and fastest runner) was on first. On the next pitch, she made an attempt to steal second, sliding into the bag headfirst with hands outstretched. She was safe, but she was also obviously in a great deal of pain and was holding her hand. John realized he was needed and ran out to the injured player. It took only a moment to recognize that her fifth proximal interphalangeal joint was dislocated.

"Put it back in," she cried. "I've already come out of the game once and I have to pitch this last inning."

The coach also chimed in, "We need her—please take care of it for us."

John really wasn't sure what to do. It appeared to be a simple dislocation, and he knew how important this player was to the team. He certainly didn't want to be accused of not helping her because she was the opponent. He knew he had to make a decision quickly.

Since the purpose of the shoulder and elbow is to position the hand for a variety of tasks, the hand and its functions are the ultimate reason for upper-extremity design. The hand is a complex tool used for a large assortment of activities, ranging from fine motor activities such as writing, threading a needle, and picking up small objects to gross motor tasks such as throwing a baseball, gripping a tennis racket, or swinging on the uneven parallel bars. Proper wrist and hand functioning is vital for performing these tasks, and thus even minor injuries can be quite disabling. The structure of the wrist and hand represents a complex network of multiple bones, joints, ligaments, and intrinsic and extrinsic muscles that function together to provide the precision, coordination, mobility, and strength required to perform various tasks.

Because of the anatomical complexity of the wrist and hand, you are encouraged to review the structures and functions of this body region before continuing with the examination procedures in this chapter. As with any body region, a thorough knowledge of anatomy is essential for accurate examination and interpretation of your findings.

FUNCTIONAL ANATOMY

The wrist and hand are composed of 27 bones and more than 20 joints. The bones include 8 carpal bones (two rows of 4), 5 metacarpal bones, and 14 phalanges (figure 14.1). From proximal to distal, the articulations are the radiocarpal, intercarpal, carpometacarpal, metacarpophalangeal, and interphalangeal joints. The radiocarpal joint permits wrist flexion, extension, abduction, adduction, and circumduction. The intercarpal and carpometacarpal joints permit gliding movements. The metacarpophalangeal joints permit flexion, extension, abduction, and adduction, and the interphalangeal joints permit flexion and extension. The first carpometacarpal joint of the thumb is a saddle joint and as such allows

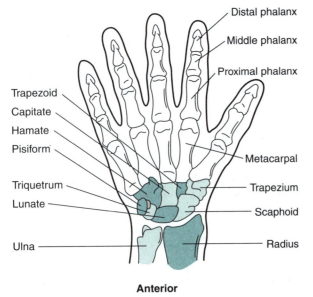

Figure 14.1 Skeletal anatomy of the wrist and hand.

Reprinted, by permission, from J.E. Donnelly, 1999, *Living anatomy* (Philadelphia: Lippincott, Williams & Wilkins), 60

more movement than the other four carpometacarpal joints. These motions include flexion, extension, abduction, adduction, opposition, and reposition.

The superficial nature of the bones and joints of the wrist and hand combined with their use for many activities renders them highly susceptible to sprains, dislocations, fractures, and tendon ruptures. A sound understanding of the surface anatomy of the wrist and hand can be invaluable. For example, you can palpate the carpal navicular (scaphoid) bone within a region known as the **anatomical snuffbox**, which is found between the extensor pollicis longus and extensor pollicis brevis muscle tendons (figure 14.2). The scaphoid is the most frequently injured carpal bone, and your ability to find and palpate the bone within the snuffbox can help you identify the point tenderness symptomatic of a possible fracture.

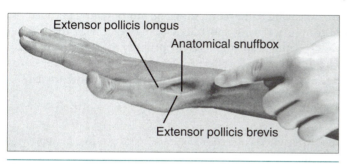

Figure 14.2   Anatomical snuffbox.

Five muscles act on the wrist joint. The flexor carpi radialis, palmaris longus, and flexor carpi ulnaris produce flexion, and the extensor carpi radialis longus and extensor carpi ulnaris produce extension. The flexor carpi radialis and extensor carpi radialis longus contract together to produce abduction, and the flexor carpi ulnaris and extensor carpi ulnaris work together to produce wrist adduction. Interestingly, approximately 12% of the population does not have a palmaris longus muscle, which works to tighten the palmar fascia. If you pinch the tips of your thumb and fingers together and simultaneously flex your wrist, the palmaris longus tendon, if you have one, becomes prominent at the wrist (figure 14.3).

Three extrinsic muscles in the forearm act on all four fingers. They include two flexor muscles (flexor digitorum superficialis and flexor digitorum profundus) and one extensor (extensor digitorum). Two smaller extrinsic muscles, the extensor indicis and extensor digiti minimi, assist with extension of the index and fifth finger, respectively. Eleven intrinsic muscles in the hand flex the proximal phalanges and extend the middle and distal phalanges. These muscles include four lumbricales in the palm and four dorsal and three palmar interossei muscles that lie between the metacarpal bones. Eight muscles produce the specialized movements of the thumb. Four are extrinsic because they originate from the forearm, including the extensor pollicis longus, extensor pollicis brevis, abductor pollicis longus, and flexor pollicis longus. Four intrinsic muscles that form the thenar eminence are the flexor pollicis brevis, opponens pollicis, abductor pollicis brevis, and adductor pollicis. Three intrinsic muscles on the medial aspect of the palmar surface of the hand form the hypothenar eminence, which acts on the little finger. These muscles include the abductor digiti minimi, flexor digiti minimi brevis, and opponens digiti minimi.

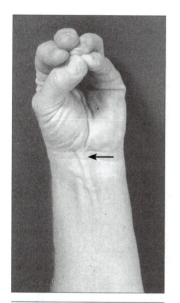

Figure 14.3   Prominence of palmaris longus with opposition of the thumb and finger.

Ruptures and avulsions of the muscle tendons acting on the fingers can produce characteristic deformities and dysfunctions and are described in detail later in this chapter. Accurate examination for these injuries necessitates thorough understanding of the tendon attachments to the bones of the hand and fingers and to the joints that they help move. For example, the extensor digitorum has a complex attachment to the finger that includes a central tendon insertion to the middle phalanx of the finger and two lateral bands that reconverge to form a common tendinous attachment to the distal phalanx (figure 14.4). A rupture of the central slip of the extensor tendon

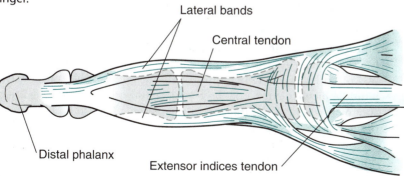

Figure 14.4   Extensor hood and tendons.

can result in a boutonniere deformity. A rupture of the distal extensor attachment to the distal phalanx can produce a deformity known as a mallet finger. On the palmar aspect of the hand, the flexor digitorum superficialis tendon inserts into the middle phalanx and the flexor digitorum profundus tendon inserts into the distal phalanx. As such, the superficialis flexes the metacarpophalangeal and proximal interphalangeal joints, while the profundus flexes these joints as well as the distal interphalangeal joint. A rupture of the profundus tendon from the distal phalanx produces a deformity known as a jersey finger.

WRIST AND HAND INJURIES

The dexterity and precision that the wrist and hand require for fine motor control often leave them unprotected and vulnerable to injury during sport activity. Contact with the ground (falls), opponents, and balls and other sporting implements is the primary mechanism for acute injury of the wrist and hand. The hand and wrist are also prone to repetitive stress injuries as well as other chronic conditions that may result from ignored or untreated acute injuries.

Acute Soft Tissue Injuries

Physically active people commonly experience contusions, sprains, and strains, primarily as a result of direct contact, falls, and other forces that either compress or place tension on the soft tissue structures.

Contusions

Because of the many bony prominences and superficial tendons exposed in the wrist and hand, contusions resulting from direct contact may be bothersome. Pain and swelling from contusions to the tendons and ligaments can decrease ROM and impair function. Rarely are these injuries serious, and pain and dysfunction usually dissipate quickly. Pain and loss of motion that continue for more than a few days should alert you to bony contusion, fracture, or both.

Sprains

Because of the multiple bones and joints in the wrist and hand, ligament injuries are quite common. Sprains to the wrist (distal radial ulnar joint and carpal bones) often result from extending or flexing the wrist beyond its normal range of motion. Mechanisms include falling on an outstretched hand (hyperflexion and hyperextension), jamming the wrist during blocking or vaulting activities, and twisting maneuvers. Excessive radial or ulnar deviation may also injure the wrist ligaments. Signs and symptoms associated with wrist sprain include pain, swelling, and point tenderness over the injured joint consistent with the degree of injury. The athlete will experience pain with both active and passive ROM. Muscular weakness may result secondary to pain with resisted motions. In cases of third-degree sprains, there may be joint instability and deformity.

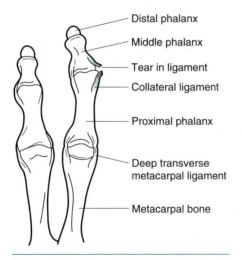

Distal phalanx

Middle phalanx

Tear in ligament

Collateral ligament

Proximal phalanx

Deep transverse metacarpal ligament

Metacarpal bone

Figure 14.5 Injury to the collateral ligament of the finger.

Collateral Ligament Sprain

Collateral ligament sprains of the fingers are among the most common injuries resulting from physical activity. Collateral ligament injuries can occur at either the metacarpophalangeal (MCP) joint, the proximal interphalangeal (PIP) joint, or the distal interphalangeal (DIP) joint. A mechanism frequently associated with collateral ligament sprains is jamming the finger while catching a ball, sliding into base, or tackling, among other activities, which can force the joints beyond their normal ROM and stretch the collateral ligaments (figure 14.5). Signs and symptoms associated with collateral ligament sprains include pain, swelling, point tenderness over the injured joint and ligament, increased pain with valgus or varus stress, and instability consistent with first-, second-, and third-degree classifications. Pain and swelling commonly persist for a significant amount of time. However, in some cases, chronic inflammation within the joint capsule (**capsulitis**) can ultimately result in adhesions and scarring that can deform the joint and permanently restrict its ROM. Therefore, even though collateral ligament injuries are often considered relatively minor, proper treatment and splinting are necessary to avoid permanent joint complications, particularly for the proximal interphalangeal joints.

Gamekeeper's or Skier's Thumb

A collateral ligament injury that can be particularly troublesome is known as **gamekeeper's** or **skier's thumb** and involves the ulnar (medial) collateral ligament (UCL) of the MCP joint of the thumb. The injury results from forced abduction and hyperextension of the thumb away from the hand that stretch and tear the UCL (figure 14.6). It has been termed

skier's thumb because the mechanism often occurs when skiers fall on an outstretched hand while holding onto a ski pole. However, it is equally common in sports in which the thumb is vulnerable to direct contact with a ball, person, or other object. Signs and symptoms include pain, point tenderness over the medial aspect of the MCP joint of the thumb, swelling, and varying degrees of instability consistent with the degree of ligament injury. In cases of second- and third-degree sprains, pain and weakness during grasping activities of the thumb and index finger will also result from the lack of stability at the joint.

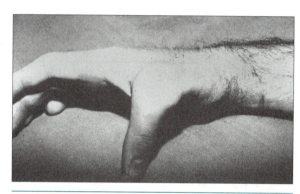

Figure 14.6   Gamekeeper's thumb.
Courtesy of Dr. Frank C. McCue, III.

A potential complication of UCL injury of the thumb is called a **Stener lesion**, in which the adductor aponeurosis comes between the ruptured ends of the ligament and prevents healing. Avulsion fractures may also result when the ligament tears at the bony attachment.

Volar Plate Rupture

Hyperextension of the PIP joint can rupture the volar plate. Signs and symptoms of volar plate injury include pain, tenderness over the palmar aspect of the joint, swelling, and loss of function. If unrecognized or untreated, volar instability can lead to a flexion or extension deformity at the joint. When the volar plate is disrupted from its distal attachment, subluxation and permanent hyperextension of the joint can occur. This hyperextension deformity may subsequently cause hyperflexion at the DIP joint caused by tensioning of the flexor tendons, resulting in a **swan-neck deformity** (figure 14.7a). Conversely, when the volar plate is disrupted from its proximal attachment, a flexion contracture or pseudoboutonniere deformity may result (figure 14.7b). Needless to say, proper management and treatment are imperative to prevent permanent joint deformity following a volar plate injury.

Volar refers to the palmar aspect of the wrist or hand. Although palmar is the most widely accepted term for this surface, volar continues to be used to describe some injury conditions.

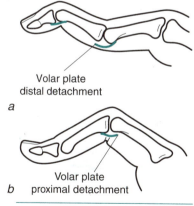

Figure 14.7   *(a)* Swan-neck deformity and *(b)* pseudoboutonniere deformity.

Strains and Tendon Avulsions

Finger tendon injuries are quite common in the physically active. Tendon injuries can result from a direct blow but more often result from abrupt forces applied in the direction opposite to that in which a joint is contracting. This mechanism can create considerable tensioning of the tendon, causing it to tear away from its distal attachment.

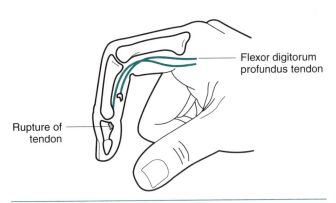

Figure 14.8   Jersey finger.

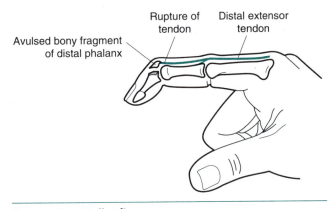

Figure 14.9   Mallet finger.

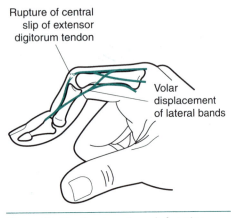

Figure 14.10   Boutonniere deformity.

Flexor Tendon Avulsion (Jersey Finger)

Flexor tendon avulsion injuries involve the flexor digitorum profundus tendon; they occur when the distal phalanx is forcefully extended while the finger is flexing. This injury is often called a **jersey finger** because it is frequently seen in athletes such as football players who get a finger caught while trying to grab and pull at an opponent's jersey. Signs and symptoms include immediate pain, swelling, and point tenderness at the attachment of the flexor tendon on the distal phalanx. With complete rupture (figure 14.8), the athlete will be unable to flex the distal phalanx while the proximal joint is held in extension. If the rupture is incomplete, you will note pain and weakness with flexion.

Extensor Tendon Avulsion (Mallet Finger)

Mallet finger, or **baseball finger**, occurs when the extended distal phalanx is suddenly and forcefully flexed. A common example is seen when an athlete attempts to catch a ball and the ball hits the tip of the extended finger. Rupture of the distal extensor tendon may or may not include avulsion of a bony fragment (figure 14.9). Signs and symptoms include pain, point tenderness over the distal attachment, flexion deformity of the distal phalanx, and an inability to actively extend the distal phalanx. Ruptures involving a bony avulsion have a greater chance of healing without surgical intervention if recognized early and appropriately splinted.

Extensor Tendon Rupture (Boutonniere Deformity)

A **boutonniere deformity** is characterized by flexion of the PIP joint and hyperextension of the DIP joint. This deformity most often results from injury to the central slip of the extensor digitorum tendon at its insertion at the base of the middle phalanx. Rupture of the extensor tendon at this location most often results from forced flexion of the PIP joint. Signs and symptoms include pain localized to the PIP joint, point tenderness near the tendon's insertion, swelling, and weakness when extending the PIP joint. As a consequence of this injury, the surrounding retinacular tissues are also disrupted and the intact lateral bands of the extensor tendon, which extend to the distal joint, begin to migrate toward the volar surface of the finger (figure 14.10). This migration changes the lateral bands' line of pull from PIP joint extensors to PIP flexors. Additionally, the flexed PIP joint will protrude through the lateral bands like a buttonhole, hyperextending both the MCP and DIP joints.

Chronic or Overuse Soft Tissue Injuries

Because of the repetitive nature of many hand movements, as well as the excessive use of the hands in many sport and occupational activities, chronic inflammatory conditions of the wrist, hand, and fingers are common. In addition, complications from unrecognized or untreated acute injuries can result in chronic and potentially disfiguring conditions.

Dupuytren's Contracture

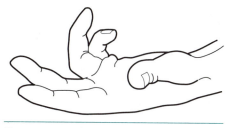

Figure 14.11 Dupuytren's contracture deformity with thickening of palmar fascia.

A flexion deformity more commonly seen in the older adult population is **Dupuytren's contracture**. This condition of unknown etiology is characterized by a flexion contracture of the MCP and PIP joints, usually of the fourth or fifth digits, as a result of thickness and contracture of the palmar fascia and its eventual adherence to overlying skin (Harris 1983) (figure 14.11). In addition to the obvious deformity, you may palpate thickening or nodules in the palmar fascia. The tight palmar fascia will also appear as rigid bands underneath the skin when the fingers are extended.

Wrist Ganglion

A wrist **ganglion**, or synovial cyst, is characterized by herniation of **synovial fluid** through the joint capsule or synovial sheath of a tendon. Minor sprains and strains often precipitate a wrist ganglion and are thought to weaken the capsule or synovial sheath, allowing fluid to escape and accumulate. Overuse mechanisms may also be an underlying cause of ganglion cysts. Wrist ganglions may form on either the dorsal or volar aspect of the wrist but are more common on the dorsal surface. Signs and symptoms include an observable and palpable localized mass over the wrist (figure 14.12). The mass may or may not be painful and may or may not restrict ROM or impede function. However, there is typically some tenderness, and the patient experiences mild to moderate pain and discomfort with wrist extension (dorsal ganglion). While some ganglion cysts can be small and others large, symptoms do not necessarily depend on size. Symptoms may be more related to the location of the cyst and the motions it may restrict.

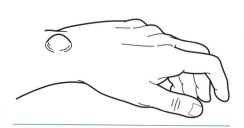

Figure 14.12 Wrist ganglion.

Tendinitis and Tenosynovitis

Tenosynovitis is an inflammatory condition of the tendon and its synovial sheath that causes pain, crepitus with palpation and movement, and decreased ROM.

Inflammation of the tendon or its surrounding synovial sheath is common in physically active people. Overuse or repetitive motion, direct trauma, and continual use following tendon injury are all common mechanisms of tendinitis and tenosynovitis. Signs and symptoms include point tenderness over the involved tendon, swelling, palpable crepitus, pain with active and resistive motion, and pain with passive stretching of the tendon. With tenosynovitis, the tendon, the synovial sheath, or both can become inflamed. This inflammation limits the tendon's ability to glide smoothly through the sheath, creating friction and discomfort. If the condition becomes chronic, the tissues can permanently thicken and limit motion. In severe chronic cases, tissue contracture may result.

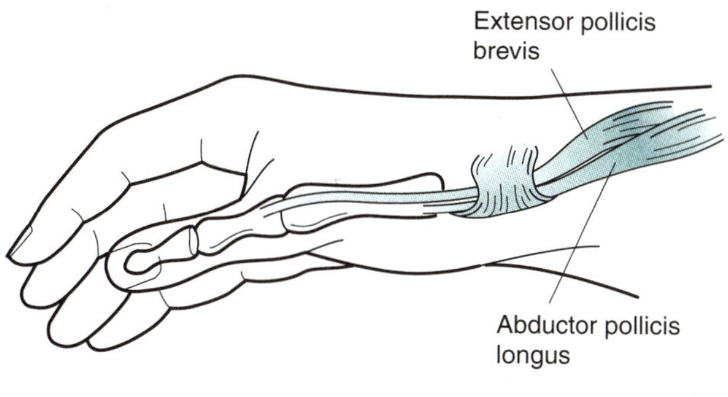

De Quervain's Disease

De Quervain's disease is a tenosynovitis of the abductor pollicis longus and extensor pollicis brevis tendons and their sheaths on the radial side of the thumb (figure 14.13). Repetitive motions that combine gripping with the hand and ulnar deviation of the wrist can inflame these tendons as they pass through their osseofibrous tunnel deep to the extensor retinaculum.

Extensor pollicis brevis

Abductor pollicis longus

Figure 14.13 Tenosynovitis of abductor pollicus longus and extensor pollicis brevis tendons (De Quervain's disease).

Signs and symptoms are consistent with typical tenosynovitis. The athlete complains of pain and crepitus at the base of the thumb, pain and weakness with active and resisted thumb extension or abduction, and increased pain when making a fist and deviating the wrist to the ulnar side (see the Finkelstein test later in this chapter).

Trigger Finger

Trigger finger is a condition associated with tenosynovitis of the flexor tendons, resulting from repetitive trauma to the flexor tendon sheath. Most commonly seen in the third and fourth digits, it results from thickening or nodules in the synovial sheath. This thickening decreases the space through which the tendon glides (stenosis) and causes the tendon to catch and then let go as it moves through the sheath during finger flexion. As the condition worsens and the synovial tunnel becomes more **stenotic** (narrow), the finger may stick in a flexed position, requiring passive assistance to return to an extended position. The hallmark sign of a trigger finger is an observable snapping of the finger as it actively flexes that mimics pulling a trigger. You may also hear a snap or click when this occurs. Depending on the state of the inflammatory response at the time of examination, you may also note signs and symptoms of tenosynovitis.

Stenosis is a stricture of any canal.

Bony Pathology

Fractures and dislocations of the wrist and hand are among the most common injuries in sport. The use of the hands for reaching, blocking, catching, and grabbing increases their vulnerability to injury during sport activities.

Traumatic Fractures

Traumatic fractures of the wrist and hand most often occur due to axial loading forces and falls on an outstretched hand.

Colles' Fracture

A Colles' fracture of the distal radius and ulna is typically caused by a fall on an outstretched

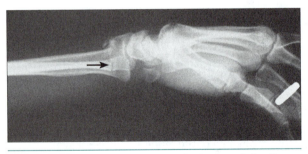

Figure 14.14 Colles' fracture with characteristic silver fork deformity.

hand with the wrist extended. It is characterized by **silver fork deformity** or dorsal displacement of the distal fragments of the radius and ulna in relation to their proximal shafts (figure 14.14). Signs and symptoms include immediate wrist pain, rapid swelling, tenderness, and deformity. Loss of wrist and hand function may result both from an unwillingness to move the extremity because of pain and from restrictions caused by the displacement. You may also note bony crepitus over the fracture. The displaced proximal fragments may injure the median nerve; when this happens, the patient may experience diminished sensation and motor function over the median nerve distribution.

Smith's Fracture

A Smith's fracture is the opposite of a Colles' fracture, displacing the distal radius and ulna volar to the proximal fragment. The mechanism of injury is most often a fall onto the back of the hand, causing hyperflexion of the wrist joint. Signs and symptoms are similar to those for Colles' fracture with the exception of their characteristic deformities.

Bennett's Fracture

A Bennett's fracture, involving the base of the first metacarpal bone (thumb), is most often caused by striking an object with a closed fist, making contact specifically with the thumb. This axial loading of the metacarpal bone causes a shear fracture at its base. While the proximal fragment maintains its position with the carpal bones, the metacarpal will be displaced

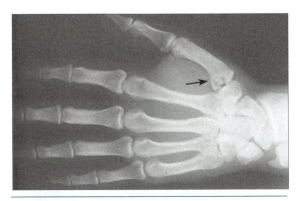

Figure 14.15   Bennett's fracture with metacarpal displacement.

Courtesy of Theodore E. Keats.

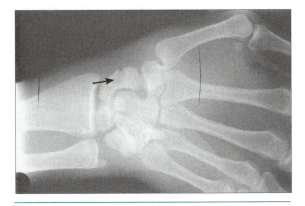

Figure 14.16   Navicular fracture.

Courtesy of Theodore E. Keats.

> A hallmark of a navicular fracture is point tenderness specifically over the navicular when you palpate the anatomical snuffbox.

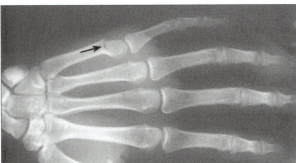

Figure 14.17   Boxer's fracture.

Courtesy of Theodore E. Keats.

because of the pull of the abductor pollicis longus muscle (figure 14.15). Signs and symptoms include immediate pain, rapid swelling, tenderness, and crepitus at the MCP joint of the thumb, as well as function loss. You may observe deformity depending on the extent of metacarpal displacement. Because this fracture occurs so near the joint, there may be false joint motion with movement.

Carpal Bones

Among the eight carpal bones, the navicular or scaphoid bone is the one most commonly fractured (figure 14.16). It can also be the most troublesome and slowest to heal. Navicular fractures typically occur when the bone is compressed against the radius during direct contact with the palm of the hand—for example, during blocking with the hands or in a fall in which the thumb and wrist are extended and the wrist is abducted. The patient complains of pain, swelling, and tenderness over the radial side of the wrist. A hallmark of a navicular fracture is point tenderness specifically over the navicular when you palpate in the anatomical snuffbox. You may also note crepitus and pain with wrist motion. Symptoms are commonly vague and this injury is often missed on initial X ray. Because of the poor vascular supply to the proximal portion of the bone, healing fractures in the region may be difficult; adequately immobilizing the fracture early optimizes the healing process. Therefore, suspect and rule out fracture any time there is pain in the anatomical snuffbox.

Metacarpal Bones

Fractures to the neck, shaft, and base of the metacarpal bones often result from axial loading of the metacarpal bone secondary to an indirect force such as striking an object with a closed fist. Other common causes are direct trauma or crushing injuries to the hand, such as when the hand is stepped on or landed on during sport activity. Signs and symptoms include pain, diffuse swelling over the dorsum of the hand, and tenderness over the metacarpal. Pain will likely increase with both longitudinal stress and axial compression or percussion of the metacarpal. You may note bony crepitus and also deformity if the bone is displaced. When the fracture specifically involves the neck of the fifth metatarsal, the injury is commonly referred to as **boxer's fracture** (figure 14.17).

Phalanges

Fractures of the phalanges can be caused by a variety of mechanisms, including direct contact, axial loading to the tip of the finger, torsion, and other indirect trauma. Fractures may also occur with sprains and dislocations. Signs and symptoms include pain, swelling, and point tenderness over the fracture site, as well as loss of function, deformity, and crepitus. If a displaced fracture occurs near a joint, there may be a false appearance of joint motion or dislocation. Fractures of the fingers are often missed or dismissed as sprains without careful examination and X ray. Because fractures through the joint have the potential for complications and permanent joint dysfunction, traumatic injuries to the phalangeal joints should be carefully examined by an orthopedist to rule out possible fracture.

Dislocation or Subluxation

The same forces and mechanisms responsible for wrist and hand fractures may also result in joint dislocation or subluxation.

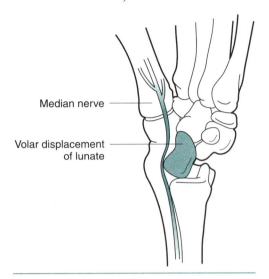

Median nerve

Volar displacement of lunate

Figure 14.18 Lunate dislocation.

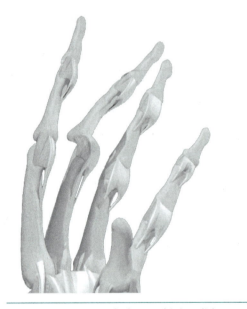

Figure 14.19 Interphalangeal joint dislocation.

Image courtesy of Primal Pictures.

Lunate Dislocation

In the wrist, the most commonly dislocated carpal bone is the lunate. Lunate dislocations can be caused by a fall on an outstretched hand or with hyperextension of the wrist. This mechanism displaces the lunate in a volar direction (figure 14.18). Volar displacement sometimes compresses the median nerve. Signs and symptoms include pain, swelling, and localized tenderness in the wrist. You may observe deformity and loss of function and find the lunate distinctly palpable on the volar aspect of the wrist. Numbness and tingling in the lateral palm and into the second and third fingers may also result from median nerve compression.

Metacarpophalangeal and Interphalangeal Joint Dislocations

Dislocation of the MCP and interphalangeal (IP) joints is consistent with third-degree sprains in which the ligaments and joint capsule are stretched or torn sufficiently to allow joint displacement. Unless the joint spontaneously reduces following injury, these injuries are quite obvious (figure 14.19); the distal bone can be displaced in any direction, depending on the offending force. Signs and symptoms of dislocation include obvious deformity, pain, rapid swelling, and loss of function. Often, the athlete or coach will reduce the dislocation and not seek medical attention. However, a physician should examine all first-time dislocations to rule out any associated articular fractures or volar plate disruptions.

Nerve and Vascular Injuries

Most cases of neurovascular compromise at the wrist and hand are attributable to chronic inflammatory conditions that compress these structures. On occasion, severe fractures or dislocations can also result in secondary injury or compression of the nearby nerve or vascular structure.

Carpal Tunnel Syndrome (Median Nerve Compression)

Carpal tunnel syndrome is a common wrist and hand condition characterized by compression of the median nerve as it passes through the carpal tunnel (figure 14.20). Compression of the median nerve within the tunnel can be caused by multiple factors, including overuse, bony protrusion into the tunnel, and fluid retention. Overuse resulting from repetitive use of the wrist and finger flexors can cause tenosynovitis and inflammation within the tunnel. Fractures and dislocations at the wrist may also compress the nerve in the tunnel secondary to protrusion of bony fragments and resultant swelling. Finally, fluid retention, which can result from a number of medical conditions, can cause swelling of the tissues within the carpal tunnel.

Carpal tunnel syndrome occurs more often in mature adults than in other age groups and more often in women than in men. It is less common in young adults but can occur in any sport involving repetitive wrist and finger flexion. Carpal tunnel syndrome may be unrelated to sport activity, as occupational and student activities such as excessive typing on

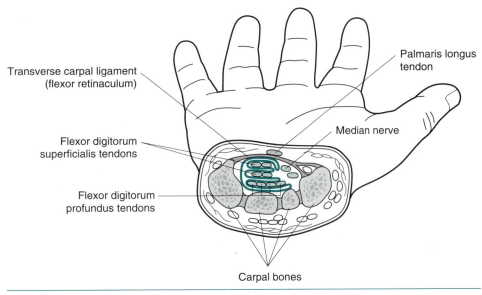

Transverse carpal ligament
(flexor retinaculum)

Palmaris longus
tendon

Flexor digitorum
superficialis tendons

Median nerve

Flexor digitorum
profundus tendons

Carpal bones

Figure 14.20   Median nerve through the carpal tunnel.

a computer keyboard are a causative factor. Signs and symptoms include pain, tenderness over the palmar aspect of the wrist, sensory changes, and motor weakness. Sensory changes may include tingling, numbness, and paresthesia over the median nerve distribution in the hand (palm and palmar aspect of the medial thumb and first and middle fingers). In severe or prolonged cases, muscle atrophy may occur in the thenar eminence; there may be weakness with flexion of the index and middle fingers and with flexion, abduction, and opposition of the thumb. Pain and sensory changes are usually exacerbated with the offending activity or when the wrist is held in a flexed position for a prolonged time, such as during sleep. Tapping or percussion over the flexor retinaculum at the wrist may also reproduce symptoms of pain and paresthesia (Tinel's sign). Other causes of median nerve compression include wrist fractures and dislocations as previously discussed. Median nerve palsy can also result from compression or injury at the elbow. In cases in which the thenar eminence muscles severely atrophy, thumb opposition and flexion are lost. Additionally, secondary to pull of the extensor muscles, an **ape hand deformity** may result, characterized by thumb extension and alignment in the same plane as the fingers (figure 14.21).

Palsy means partial to complete paralysis resulting from pressure on a nerve.

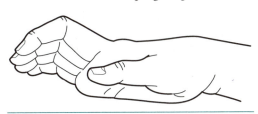

Figure 14.21   Ape hand deformity.

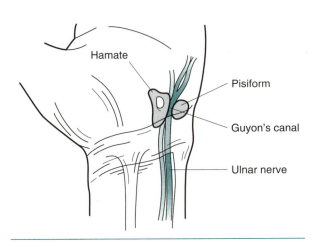

Hamate

Pisiform

Guyon's canal

Ulnar nerve

Figure 14.22   Ulnar nerve passing through the tunnel of Guyon.

Ulnar Nerve Compression

Compression injuries to the ulnar nerve can also occur at the wrist. Ulnar nerve **palsy** is commonly associated with cycling, as prolonged pressure of the handlebars over the hypothenar eminence irritates and compresses the ulnar nerve. Additionally, the nerve can be compressed in the tunnel of Guyon (figure 14.22) between the pisiform and hamate due to blunt trauma or fracture of the surrounding carpal bones. Signs and symptoms associated with ulnar nerve compression include pain, tingling, or numbness radiating into the ulnar distribution of the hand and fourth and fifth fingers. You may note motor weakness and atrophy in the hypothenar, dorsal interossei, and fourth and fifth lumbricale muscles. Wasting of these muscles resulting from ulnar nerve palsy is known as a **bishop's**, or **benediction**, **deformity**.

Radial Nerve Palsy

Wrist drop may be noted at the wrist with upper-extremity injuries resulting in radial nerve palsy. If the radial nerve is severely traumatized or injured, the wrist and finger extensors may be profoundly weakened or paralyzed so that the wrist "drops" into flexion. Because of the inability to extend the wrist, the patient will experience a flexion deformity. This condition points to the importance of differential diagnosis: Pathology seen in the hand can originate anywhere in the upper extremity.

Claw Hand Deformity

When both the median and ulnar nerves are injured, the consequent paralysis and wasting of the interossei and lumbricale hand muscles result in a claw hand deformity. A claw hand is characterized by hyperextension of the MCP joint and flexion of the PIP and DIP joints. When the hand loses intrinsic muscle function, it also loses the ability to flex the MCP joint and the joint hyperextends due to overpowering by the extrinsic finger extensors. This tenses the finger flexors, resulting in IP joint flexion. Claw hand deformity is often associated with a Volkmann's contracture (see figure 13.18).

Structural and Functional Abnormalities

The wrist and hand may show structural abnormalities of the joints, bones, and fingernails that indicate other medical conditions. Enlargement of the DIP joints (**Heberden's nodes**) and PIP joints (**Bouchard's nodes**) is often associated with arthritic conditions and disease. Severely concave, or **spoon-shaped, nails** may indicate fungal infections. Nails that are **clubbed**, or large and convexed, can result from hypertrophy of the underlying soft tissue and may also be associated with respiratory and congenital heart disorders.

OBJECTIVE TESTS

You will choose from the following special tests after considering your findings from the subjective history and objective observation. Because of the essential wrist and hand functions and their required fine motor coordination, you must appropriately select objective tests to delineate the involved structures and injury severity. While many finger injuries appear minor at first, they can lead to long-term dysfunction (e.g., joint contracture) if not properly examined and treated. Strategies for specific injury procedures for on-site, acute, or clinical examination follow this section and will help guide your test selection.

Palpation

Palpate the wrist and hand with the athlete seated and the arm relaxed. Because of the many small structures of the wrist, hand, and fingers, you will need to understand the anatomy before proceeding. Developing a systematic approach to palpation will also ensure that you locate and palpate each relevant structure.

Dorsal Structures

To palpate the dorsal hand, start at the radial styloid process and move just distal to the anatomical snuffbox. Palpate the scaphoid at the base of the snuffbox and the triquetrum at the top of the snuffbox. Tenderness here may indicate scaphoid fracture. The radial border of the snuffbox includes the abductor pollicis longus and extensor pollicis brevis, and the ulnar border is formed by the extensor pollicis longus. These tendons can be seen when the thumb is extended.

Moving medially on the dorsal aspect, palpate Lister's tubercle; this should be in line with the lunate, capitate, and third metacarpal (figure 14.23). Directly adjacent and distal to Lister's tubercle is a slight depression in which the lunate lies. If the wrist is slightly flexed, you can palpate the lunate as it moves into your fingertip. Tenderness here may indicate lunate dislocation.

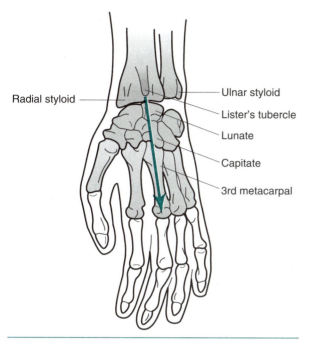

When the hand is held in a fist, you can see and palpate the carpi radialis longus and brevis as they insert on the base of the second and third metacarpals, respectively. You can palpate the extensor indicis and extensor digiti minimi if the index and little fingers are extended while the other fingers are flexed. Palpate the extensor digitorum communis with all the fingers extended.

Medial to the radius is the ulnar styloid process. Just distal to this process is the triquetrum. You can palpate the triquetrum when the wrist is radially deviated. The metacarpals are more superficial and easily palpated on the dorsal aspect and can be palpated along their length. The metacarpal heads are located at the level of the distal palmar crease. The dorsal aspect has a palpable groove through which the extensor tendons course. You can easily palpate the phalanges and IP joints for incongruity and tenderness.

Palmar Structures

Rotating the hand so you can palpate its palmar aspect, locate the pisiform on top of the anterior surface of the triquetrum. Palpate the flexor carpi ulnaris at the pisiform where it first inserts. Moving distally at a 45° angle from the pisiform in a line lateral to the index finger, palpate the hook of the hamate. The pisiform and hook of the hamate form the medial and lateral borders, respectively, of Guyon's tunnel. You can palpate the ulnar nerve in Guyon's tunnel. Tenderness here because of nerve palpation is common, so be sure to compare tenderness bilaterally. The palmaris longus becomes prominent in the central palmar wrist area when the patient opposes (touches) the thumb and little finger. The flexor carpi radialis is just lateral to the palmaris longus and can be palpated in the wrist and distal forearm when the patient flexes and radially deviates the wrist. It is also easy to palpate the thenar and hypothenar eminences, which you should investigate for muscle spasm, tenderness, atrophy, or other contour abnormalities. Palpate the radial pulse and pinch the nail beds to ensure that circulation is intact. Palpate the palmar surface of each phalange and IP joint for tenderness, swelling, and incongruity.

Figure 14.23   Lister's tubercle and surrounding bony anatomy.

Range of Motion

Wrist and hand ROM includes active, passive, and goniometric examinations. In addition, you can have the patient make a fist and then open it as wide as possible to quickly identify any gross deficiencies.

Perform passive motion either after each active motion has been tested or after all active motions have been tested.

Active ROM

Isolated joint motions include forearm supination and pronation (figure 14.24a); wrist flexion and extension (figure 14.24b), radial deviation and ulnar deviation (figure 14.24c); MCP flexion, extension, abduction, and adduction (figure 14.24, d-e); and interphalangeal flexion and extension (figure 14.24f). Thumb motions include flexion, extension, abduction, adduction, and circumduction (figure 14.24, g-i). The thumb and little finger also move in opposition to each other, and the thumb is able to oppose, or touch, all the fingers (figure 14.24j).

Passive ROM

Perform passive motion to examine joint end feel and help determine possible causes for any decreased range found during active motion testing. Most normal end feel sensations for the wrist and hand are tissue stretch. The exceptions include a bony end feel in radial and ulnar deviation and, of course, tissue approximation with thumb and finger adduction. Apply passive overpressure to each active motion. If overpressure reproduces the patient's pain, investigate

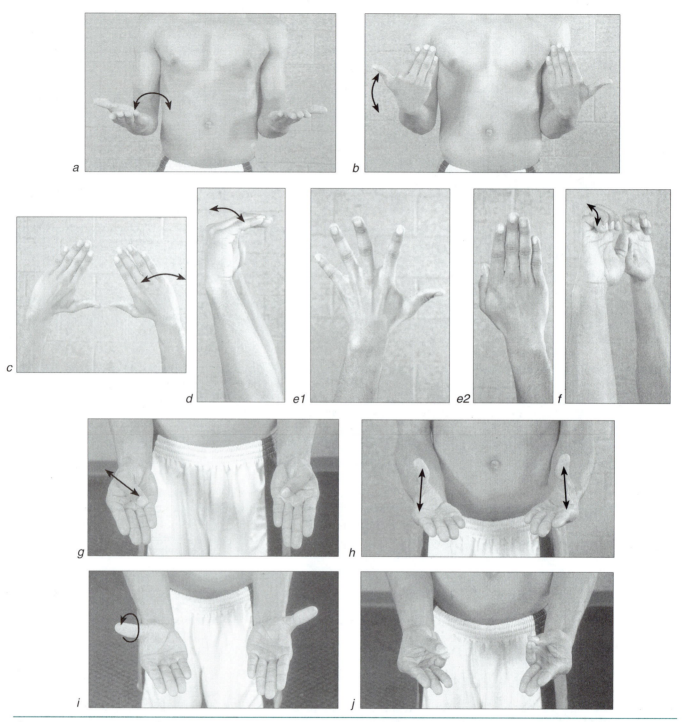

Figure 14.24 Active ROM for (a) forearm supination and pronation; (b) wrist flexion and extension; (c) radial and ulnar deviations; (d) MCP flexion and extension; (e) finger abduction and adduction; (f) interphalangeal flexion and extension; and thumb motions of (g) flexion and extension; (h) abduction and adduction; (i) circumduction; and (j) opposition.

further for possible ligamentous or capsular injury. Always conduct ligament stress tests and capsular mobility tests when pain occurs with overpressure.

Goniometric ROM Examination

You can apply goniometric wrist and hand examination to the majority of the active motions (table 14.1; figure 14.25). To accurately measure these motions, you must have access to the correct instruments. In particular, you will need smaller goniometers made specifically for finger examinations.

Table 14.1

Goniometric Examination of Wrist and Hand Motions

Motion	Location of goniometer	Movement	Normal range
Forearm supination	P: Seated, arm at side and elbow flexed to 90° holding a pencil with a closed fist A: Head of 3rd MC S: Perpendicular to floor M: Parallel with pencil	From neutral (pencil perpendicular to the floor), forearm is rotated laterally, with palm facing upward	0° to 90°
Forearm pronation	P: Seated, arm at side and elbow flexed to 90° holding a pencil with a closed fist A: Head of 3rd MC S: Perpendicular to floor M: Parallel with pencil	From neutral (pencil perpendicular to the floor), forearm is rotated medially, with palm facing downward	0° to 80-85°
Wrist flexion	P: Seated, forearm pronated, hand extended off table A: Ulnar styloid process S: Long axis of ulna M: Long axis of 5th MC	With fingers extended and relaxed, move palm toward volar aspect of wrist	0° to 90°
Wrist extension	P: Seated, forearm pronated, hand extended off table A: Ulnar styloid process S: Long axis of ulna M: Long axis of 5th MC	With fingers extended and relaxed, extend wrist by moving dorsum of hand toward dorsal aspect of wrist	0° to 70°
Radial deviation	P: Seated, forearm pronated and hand resting on table A: Over capitate on dorsal wrist S: Midline of forearm M: Long axis of 3rd MC	From neutral, move hand to the radial side, leading with thumb side of hand	0° to 20°
Ulnar deviation	P: Seated, forearm pronated and hand resting on table A: Over capitate on dorsal wrist S: Midline of forearm M: Long axis of 3rd MC	From neutral, move hand toward the ulnar side, leading with 5th finger side of hand	0° to 30°
MCP flexion*	P: Seated, arm resting on table A: MCP joint S: Long axis of metacarpal M: Long axis of proximal phalanx	With the PIP and DIP joints of the finger relaxed, move finger(s) to palm of hand	0° to 90°
MCP extension*	P: Seated, arm resting on table A: MCP joint S: Long axis of metacarpal M: Long axis of proximal phalanx	With the PIP and DIP joints of the finger relaxed, move finger(s) toward back of hand	0° to 30-45°
IP flexion*	P: Seated, arm resting on table A: DIP or PIP joint S: Long axis of most proximal phalanx M: Long axis of immediate distal phalanx	With distal and proximal joints relaxed, move test joint into full flexion	0° to 100° (PIP) 0° to 90° (DIP)
IP extension*	P: Seated, arm resting on table A: DIP or PIP joint S: Long axis of most proximal phalanx M: Long axis of immediate distal phalanx	With distal and proximal joints relaxed, move test joint into full extension	0° (PIP) 0-20° (DIP)
Thumb extension	P: Seated, arm and hand resting on table A: Carpometacarpal joint S: Long axis of radius M: Long axis of 1st MC	With wrist and fingers in extension, extend thumb fully	0° (MCP) 0-20° (IP)
Thumb flexion	P: Seated, arm and hand resting on table A: Carpometacarpal joint S: Long axis of radius M: Long axis of 1st MC	With wrist and fingers in extension, flex thumb by moving it across the palm	0° to 45° (MCP) 0° to 90° (IP)
Thumb abduction	P: Seated, arm and hand resting on table A: Midpoint, base of 1st and 2nd MC S: Long axis 2nd MC M: Long axis 1st MC	With wrist and hand in anatomical position, and thumb in contact with the MC of the 2nd finger (0° position), move thumb away from palm	0° to 70°

*A finger goniometer is preferred for these motions.

P = patient position; A = goniometer axis; S = stationary arm; M = movable arm; MC = metacarpal; PIP = proximal interphalangeal joint; DIP = distal interphalangeal joint; MCP = metacarpophalangeal joint.

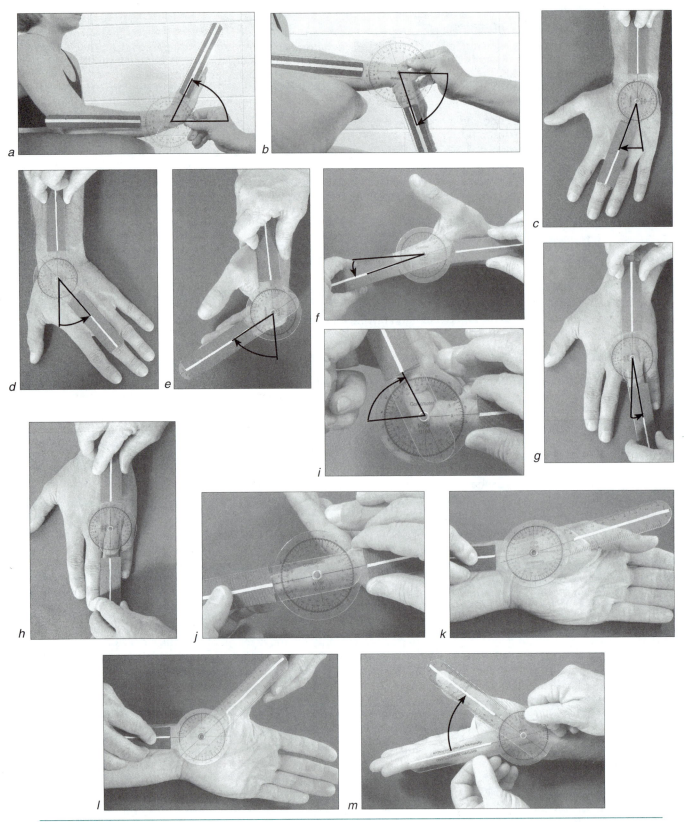

Figure 14.25 Goniometric measurement of *(a)* wrist extension, *(b)* flexion; *(c)* radial and *(d)* ulnar deviations; *(e)* MCP flexion and *(f)* extension; *(g)* finger abduction and *(h)* adduction; *(i)* interphalangeal flexion and *(j)* extension; and thumb motions of *(k)* carpometacarpal (CMC) flexion, *(l)* CMC extension, and *(m)* CMC abduction. (Measurement of pronation and supination is illustrated in chapter 13, figure 13.27.)

Strength

You can determine wrist and hand strength by manual muscle tests and instrumented strength examination.

Manual Muscle Tests

Manual muscle tests for the wrist and hand are described in table 14.2 and shown in figure 14.26. (See chapter 13, figure 13.28 for forearm pronation and supination.) To perform these

Table 14.2
Manual Muscle Tests for the Wrist and Hand

Motion	Athlete position	Stabilizing hand placement	Resistance hand placement	Instruction to athlete	Primary muscles tested
Forearm supination	Seated, elbow flexed to 90°	Elbow held at athlete's side	Grasp distal forearm, resistance on dorsal aspect	From neutral position, supinate forearm (laterally rotate) while you try to move forearm into pronation	Biceps brachii, supinator
Forearm pronation	Seated, elbow flexed to 90°	Elbow held at athlete's side	Grasp distal forearm, resistance on ventral aspect	From neutral position, pronate forearm (medially rotate) while you try to move forearm into supination	Pronator teres, pronator quadratus
Wrist flexion	Seated, forearm supinated	Distal forearm, just proximal to wrist	Palm	Move fingers and palm toward wrist	Flexor carpi radialis and ulnaris
Wrist extension	Seated, forearm pronated	Distal forearm, just proximal to wrist	Dorsal surface of hand over MCs	Move back of hand toward wrist	Extensor carpi radialis longus and brevis, extensor carpi ulnaris
Radial deviation	Seated, forearm neutral	Distal radius, just proximal to wrist	Radial side of palm	Deviate hand toward radial side (thumb) of forearm	Extensor carpi radialis longus and brevis, flexor carpi radialis
Ulnar deviation	Prone, forearm neutral	Distal ulna, just proximal to wrist	Ulnar side of palm	Deviate hand toward ulnar side (5th finger) of forearm	Flexor carpi ulnaris, extensor carpi ulnaris
MCP flexion	Seated, forearm supinated and hand resting on table	Over metacarpals	Over dorsal aspect of proximal phalanx of finger(s)	While maintaining DIP and PIP extension, move fingers toward palm	Lumbricales (2nd-4th), flexor digiti minimi (5th)
MCP extension	Seated, forearm pronated and hand extended off the table	Over metacarpals	Over dorsal aspect of proximal phalanx of finger(s)	Starting in slight flexion, extend MCP joints against your resistance	Extensor digitorum (2nd-5th), and extensor indices (2nd) or extensor digiti minimi (5th)

(continued)

Table 14.2
(continued)

Motion	Athlete position	Stabilizing hand placement	Resistance hand placement	Instruction to athlete	Primary muscles tested
MCP abduction	Seated, forearm pronated and hand resting on table	Over metacarpals	Radial (2nd & 3rd digits) or ulnar (3rd-5th digits) aspect of proximal phalanx	Move finger away from midline	Dorsal interossei (2nd-4th), abductor digiti minimi (5th)
MCP adduction	Seated, forearm supinated and hand resting on table	Over metacarpals	Ulnar (2nd digits) or radial (4th & 5th digits) aspect of proximal phalanx	Move finger toward 3rd finger	Palmar interossei
IP flexion (PIP, DIP)	Seated, forearm supinated and hand resting on table	Proximal phalanx (PIP) or midphalanx (DIP)	Midphalanx (PIP) or distal phalanx (DIP)	PIP: Flex PIP while maintaining DIP extension DIP: Flex DIP	Flexor digitorum superficialis (PIP) and profundus (DIP)
IP extension (PIP, DIP)	Seated, forearm pronated and hand off end of table	Same as IP flexion	Same as IP flexion	PIP: Extend PIP while maintaining DIP extension DIP: extend DIP	Extensor (2nd-5th) digitorum, and extensor indices (2nd) or extensor digiti minimi (5th)
Thumb flexion (MCP and IP)	Seated, forearm supinated and hand resting on table	Metacarpal (MCP) or proximal phalanx (IP)	Palmar surface proximal phalanx (MCP) or distal phalanx (IP)	MCP: Flex MCP while maintaining IP extension IP: Flex distal segment	Flexor pollicus longus (IP) and brevis (MCP)
Thumb extension (MCP and IP)	Seated, forearm pronated and hand resting on table	Metacarpal (MCP) or proximal phalanx (IP)	Dorsal surface proximal phalanx (MCP) or distal phalanx (IP)	MCP: Extend MCP while maintaining slight IP flexion IP: Extend distal segment	Extensor pollicus longus (IP) and brevis (MCP)
Thumb abduction	Seated, forearm supinated and hand resting on table	Proximal forearm and wrist	Lateral proximal metacarpal (APL) or phalanx (APB)	Move thumb away from palm	Abductor pollicis longus (APL) and brevis (APB)
Thumb adduction	Seated, forearm supinated and hand resting on table	Palmar aspect of hand	Medial aspect of thumb	Move thumb toward palm	Adductor pollicis
Opposition	Seated, forearm supinated and hand resting on table	Proximal wrist	Between the thumb and opposing 5th finger	Maintain contact between distal pads of thumb and 5th finger while you attempt to pull them apart	Opponens pollicis and digiti minimi

MCP = metacarpophalangeal joint; MC = metacarpal; IP = interphalangeal joint; DIP = distal interphalangeal joint; PIP = proximal interphalangeal joint.

tests, position the segment either neutrally or slightly into the motion, with the motion occurring against gravity. You can test the fingers either as a unit or individually. As an example, figures 14.26i-j demonstrate finger flexion isolating one finger and finger extension with resistance applied over all digits. Use individual finger strength tests if a finger is the injury site. Perform manual muscle tests for all the motions of the wrist and fingers.

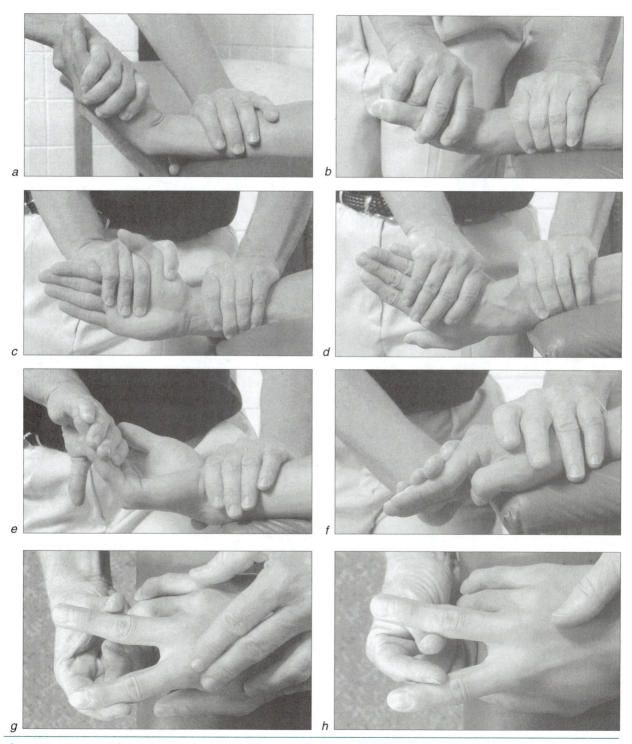

Figure 14.26 Manual muscle tests for *(a)* wrist flexion, *(b)* wrist extension, *(c)* radial deviation, and *(d)* ulnar deviation; MCP *(e)* flexion, *(f)* extension, *(g)* abduction, and *(h)* adduction.

(continued)

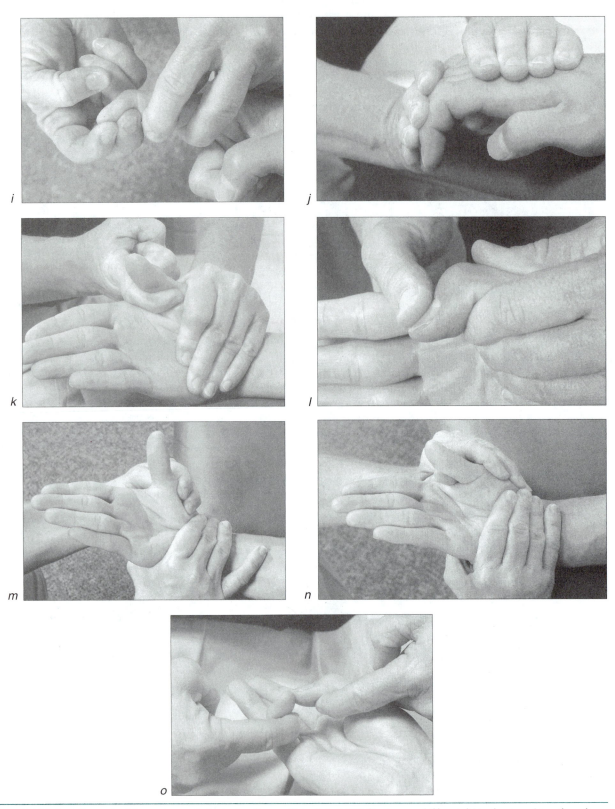

Figure 14.26 *(continued)* Manual muscle tests for finger *(i)* isolated DIP flexion and *(j)* combined extension; thumb *(k)* MCP flexion and *(l)* DIP extension; thumb *(m)* abduction, *(n)* adduction, and *(o)* opposition.

Instrumented Strength Examination

You can use dynamometers to examine grip and pinch strength (see figures 7.5 and 7.6). The pinch dynamometer examines chuck, tip, and lateral pinch grips. Have the patient perform the strength test with the uninvolved hand before attempting it with the involved hand. These tests were discussed in detail in chapter 7.

Neurovascular Examination

Neurovascular compromise to the wrist and hand can result from traumatic injury or compressive syndromes. Also perform neurovascular examination with any deep cut or laceration. Neurological examination for the wrist and hand is limited to sensory and motor testing of peripheral nerves; there are no reflex tests for this region. Additional tests for neurovascular compromise associated with specific conditions are included under special tests.

Sensory Tests

Use both light touch and pinprick methods to examine sensation over the sensory distributions of the hand. The hand is divided into median, ulnar, and radial nerve distributions (see chapter 8, figure 8.8). Dermatomal distributions include C6, C7, and C8. C6 provides sensation to the thumb, index finger, and half of the middle finger and hand area; C7 supplies sensation to the middle finger and corresponding hand area; and C8 supplies sensation to the ring and little fingers and corresponding hand area (see chapter 8, figure 8.7). The most sensitive and pure locations for examining each peripheral nerve are the dorsal web space (radial, C6); the distal, radial aspect of the second finger (median, C7); and the distal, ulnar aspect of the fifth finger (ulnar, C8).

Two-Point Discrimination Test

Although you can perform this test on any aspect of the hand and wrist, it is used most commonly to examine two-point discrimination sensation in the fingertips. Use a paper clip, calipers, or a specifically designed two-point discriminator device to examine the patient's ability to distinguish between one and two points. Normally, the fingertips can discriminate to a 4 mm (0.2 in.) distance between the two points. Place the ends of the device on the patient's fingertips and ask the patient—who keeps her eyes closed during the examination—if she feels one or two points (figure 14.27). The pressure should be light enough that it does not blanch the skin. If blanching occurs, the patient will rely on deep pressure sensation rather than light touch, and the test will not accurately examine the intended receptors. If the patient is unable to detect two points, widen the distance between the points by 1 mm (0.04 in.) and retest until she can feel two points.

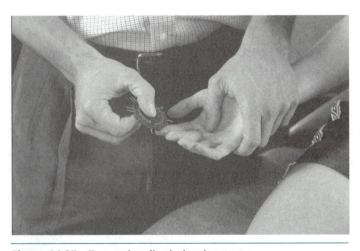

Figure 14.27 Two-point discrimination test.

Motor Tests

Use manual muscle tests for each peripheral nerve emanating from the brachial plexus. Test the radial nerve (C6-C7) with wrist extension and thumb extension, the ulnar nerve (C8) with finger abduction, and the median nerve (C6-T1) with thumb opposition (see chapter 8, figure 8.10). If you find it difficult to examine whether the patient's weak response is due to a neurological or other soft tissue injury to these muscle groups, you should test other muscles innervated by the nerve that are located away from the injured site. For example, if the patient responds weakly to a wrist extensor strength test, try testing thumb extension, which is also innervated by the radial nerve. If you find no deficit in thumb extension upon comparison to the uninvolved side, the injury is likely not nerve related. If you are not sure whether the neurological deficit is localized to the wrist and hand, testing strength more proximally strength may also be appropriate to check the integrity of the nerve root.

Vascular Tests

Vascular compromise to the wrist and hand is primarily examined via capillary refill testing and skin color and temperature (see chapter 9, figure 9.10).

Special Tests

Specials tests for the wrist and hand examine neurovascular compromise, presence of subtle fractures, ligament stability, tendon and muscle injury, chronic inflammatory conditions, and joint restrictions.

Neurovascular Compromise

In addition to or as follow-up to the standard on-site neurovascular examination, you can use special tests to examine further for neurovascular compromise. Hand and wrist injuries can compress or compromise both nerves and vessels, so examine for these problems if the hand is cold, discolored, or tingling, or if a radial pulse is diminished or absent.

Tinel's Sign

This test locates pathology of the median, ulnar, or radial nerve. To test for the median nerve, tap the surface over the carpal tunnel (figure 14.28a). Tap the radial nerve proximal to the radial styloid process (figure 14.28b). To test for the ulnar nerve, administer the tap over Guyon's tunnel (figure 14.28c). A positive test elicits pain with the tap.

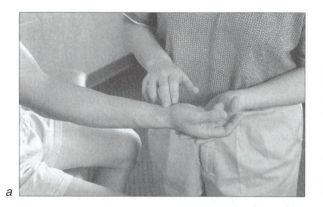

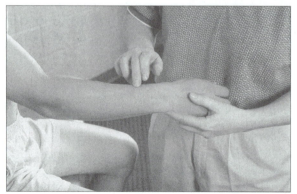

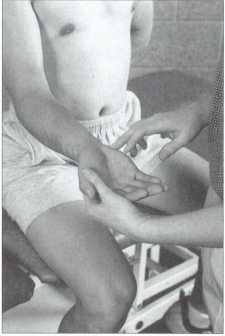

Figure 14.28 Tinel's location for the (a) median, (b) radial, and (c) ulnar nerve.

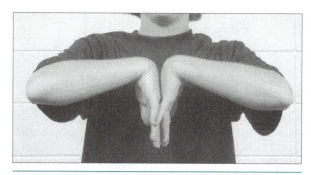

Figure 14.29   Phalen's test.

Phalen's Test

Phalen's test examines for carpal tunnel syndrome. The patient places the backs of the hands together with the wrists in full flexion. She then drops the elbows below the wrists and holds the position for about 1 minute or until the symptoms are reproduced (figure 14.29). Wrist pain is not a positive sign, but numbness or tingling in the thumb, index, or middle finger is.

Allen Test

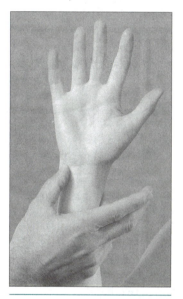

The Allen test determines the circulatory integrity of the hand. Instruct the patient to open and close the hand rapidly several times and then form a tightly closed fist. Apply pressure to the radial and ulnar arteries to compress them. While maintaining pressure, instruct the patient to relax the hand. Then release the pressure on one artery and observe the filling response (figure 14.30). Repeat the process bilaterally and compare between the two hands. If the filling response is uneven, the test is positive and indicates restricted circulation flow into the hand.

Fractures

Since the wrist and hand bones lie relatively close to the surface, most fractures in these areas are obvious. However, a fracture that is not displaced can be more difficult to identify without radiographic examination. Wrist fractures such as Colles' fracture and Smith's fracture usually present with deformity so that the examination is obvious. Phalangeal fractures are also often obvious because the force of the tendons displaces the bone fragments. However, fractures within the joint may be difficult to differentiate from joint sprains, and both may in fact be present. Fractures of the

Figure 14.30   Allen test.

carpals and metacarpals are sometimes less obvious. The following tests can be used to identify these fractures.

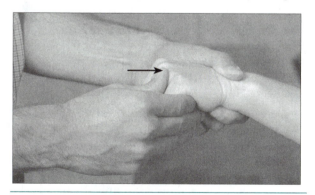

Figure 14.31   Compression test for metacarpal fracture.

Carpal and Metacarpal Fractures

Isolated soft tissue swelling around the site of the fracture is common. To easily confirm metacarpal fracture, have the patient relax the fingers so the MCP joints are flexed to 90°. Then apply compressive force to the end of the metacarpal (figure 14.31). If the patient reports pain with this maneuver in either the metacarpal or its corresponding carpal bone, a fracture is likely present.

Phalangeal Fractures

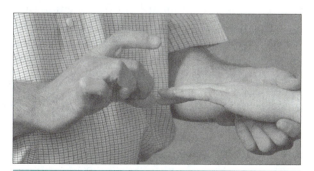

Figure 14.32   Vibration test for phalangeal fracture.

You can test phalangeal fractures either by an axial compressive force as described for the carpal and metacarpal fractures or by a **vibration test**. Apply the axial compressive force with the finger in full extension rather than flexed at the MCP joint as described earlier. Perform the vibration test with the patient's hand supported and the fingers relaxed. Flick the end of the suspected finger to cause a vibration along the digit (figure 14.32). If the patient reports significant pain, suspect a fracture.

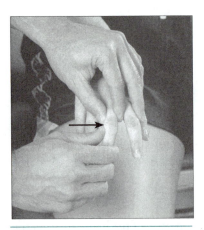

Figure 14.33   Collateral stress tests for the phalangeal joints.

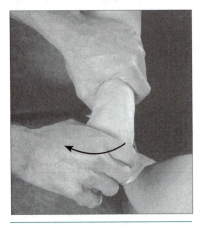

Figure 14.34   Radial collateral stress test for the wrist.

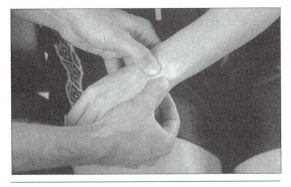

Figure 14.35   Lunatotriquetral ballottement (Reagan's) test.

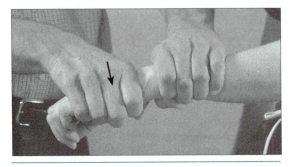

Figure 14.36   Anterior–posterior glide test of radiocarpal joints.

Ligament Stability Tests

You can examine joint integrity and instability caused by ligament injury using various stress tests, depending on the injury's location.

Valgus and Varus Stress Tests

The valgus stress test determines the integrity of the medial or ulnar collateral ligaments of the MCP and IP joints. The varus stress test determines the integrity of the lateral or radial collateral ligaments of the MCP and IP joints. Examine each joint individually. Stabilize the proximal segment of the joint and grasp the distal segment with your mobilizing hand. Then apply an ulnar (valgus) or radial (varus) force to the joint to stress the collateral ligaments (figure 14.33). Pain or laxity compared to what occurs in the opposite hand is a positive sign. You can also apply a collateral stress test to the wrist.

The radial collateral stress test examines radial collateral ligament (RCL) integrity, and the ulnar collateral stress test examines UCL integrity. Use one hand to stabilize the distal forearm and place your other hand over the patient's metacarpals to apply the collateral stress. Move your hand toward the little finger side to stress the RCL and toward the thumb side to stress the UCL (figure 14.34).

Lunatotriquetral Ballottement Test

This test, also called **Reagan's test**, determines the instability of the joint between the lunate and triquetrum. The lunate is the most commonly dislocated carpal bone. Stabilize the triquetrum by placing your index finger on one side and your thumb on the other. With your free hand, grasp the lunate on the anterior and posterior surfaces as you did for the triquetrum. Keeping the triquetrum stable, move the lunate in an anterior–posterior direction to examine for pain, laxity, and crepitus, which are positive signs for this test (figure 14.35). Compare between the patient's two hands.

Glide Tests

The glide tests are stress tests that determine ligamentous integrity and stability at various wrist joints and are used if the patient reports pain or reduced active motion. They examine joint laxity within the wrist in the carpal joints, the radiocarpal joint, the radioulnar joint, or a combination of these. The mobility of these joints depends on the specific movement. Thus, injury to a specific joint may cause more restriction in one movement than in another, depending on how much mobility the joint requires for the movement to occur. If the patient has pain and limited wrist extension, the injury may be in the radiocarpal joints. Pain and restricted wrist flexion may be secondary to injury at the midcarpals. Look to the distal radioulnar joint if supination or pronation is restricted or painful. Test the radiocarpal joints in an anterior–posterior glide test. Place your stabilizing hand around the patient's distal forearm so that it lies adjacent to the proximal carpal row. Place your mobilizing hand around the patient's hand so that it touches your stabilizing hand. Perform an anterior–posterior glide with your mobilizing hand as you examine for joint mobility and pain (figure 14.36). Then, with your hands in the same position, perform a posterior–anterior glide. Compare between the patient's two hands. A positive sign occurs if the patient

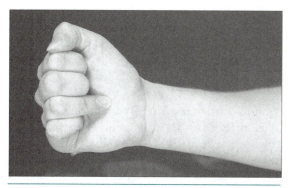

Figure 14.37   Jersey finger sign.

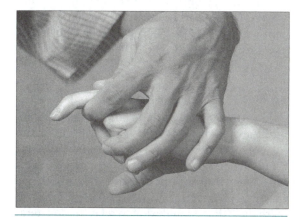

Figure 14.38   Mallet finger test.

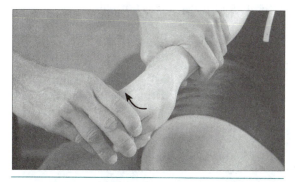

Figure 14.39   Finkelstein test.

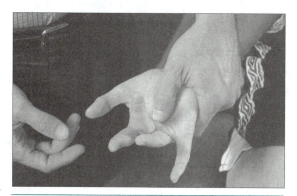

Figure 14.40   Trigger finger test.

reports pain, crepitus is present, or the area is either more or less mobile than its counterpart. These glide movements are called anterior and posterior glides, respectively. You can perform a side glide test with your hands in the same position by applying the force side to side rather than anterior to posterior.

Tendon and Muscle Pathology

The following are special tests for traumatic tendon injuries.

Flexor Tendon Avulsion Test

This avulsion test is also called the jersey finger sign because the injury occurs when an athlete attempts to make a tackle by grabbing onto an opponent's jersey. Instruct the athlete to make a fist. The sign is positive if the finger with the ruptured flexor digitorum longus tendon does not fully flex into the palm (figure 14.37).

Extensor Tendon Avulsion Test

This test is also called the **mallet finger test** because the mechanism often involves an impact compression force with sudden flexion of the distal phalanx. Instruct the athlete to fully extend all the fingers. The distal phalanx of the injured finger will remain in partial flexion if an extensor tendon avulsion is present (figure 14.38).

Inflammatory Conditions

The following tests can confirm the presence of tendinitis or tenosynovitis in the wrist and hand.

Finkelstein Test

Use the Finkelstein test to examine for De Quervain's disease, a tenosynovitis of the extensor pollicis brevis and abductor pollicis longus tendons. The patient places the thumb within the fist. Stabilize the forearm and move the wrist into ulnar deviation (figure 14.39). A variation of this test is to have the patient actively perform this movement. A positive sign is pain with the movement.

Trigger Finger Test

Use the trigger finger test, which identifies flexor tenosynovitis, if the patient complains that a finger locks in flexion when she attempts to extend it. The locking occurs because of the irregularity of the tendon's sheath that occurs with tendosynovitis and causes the tendon to catch in the retinaculum in the metacarpal area. Palpate the location along the tendon where the patient reports the locking, and have the patient then flex and extend the finger (figure 14.40). You can sometimes palpate a nodule, but the most common positive signs are pain with pressure over the area and a palpable clicking or snapping.

Ligamentous Tests for Joint Contractures

The following tests distinguish between tightness in the IP capsule and the collateral ligaments or intrinsic muscles.

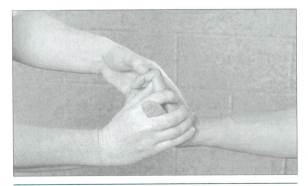

Figure 14.41 Bunnel-Littler test.

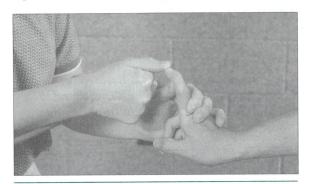

Figure 14.42 Retinacular test.

Bunnel-Littler Test

Use the Bunnel-Littler test if the patient demonstrates reduced flexion ROM of the PIP joints. A passive test, it distinguishes between tightness of the joint capsule and tightness of the intrinsic muscles. Passively place the patient's MCP joint in slight extension and then flex the PIP joint (figure 14.41). If the PIP joint cannot be flexed in this position, maintain the PIP joint position and slightly flex the MCP joint. If the joint capsule is tight, the PIP joint will not fully flex with MCP joint flexion. If the intrinsic muscles are tight, the PIP joint will fully flex with MCP joint flexion.

Retinacular Test

The passive retinacular test determines whether the cause of tightness in the PIP joint is the capsule or the retinacular (collateral) ligaments. Stabilize the PIP joint in neutral and then flex the DIP joint. If DIP movement is restricted, tightness may be present in either the capsule or collateral ligaments (figure 14.42). Then perform the test passively with the PIP joint in flexion to relax the collateral ligaments. If DIP movement is normal, the collateral ligaments are tight and the capsule is normal.

Joint Mobility Examination

When the patient presents with a capsular pattern of movement for any joint, joint mobility tests help you ascertain where the capsule is restricted and provide a basis for treatment. These tests are also used as treatment techniques.

For more information about joint mobility examination tests, refer to *Therapeutic Exercise for Musculoskeletal Injuries, Second Edition,* (Houglum 2005), chapter 6.

Wrist (Radiocarpal Joint)

You can examine radiocarpal joint mobility with the following mobilization techniques.

Distraction

The distraction test examines general joint mobility. Comparison to the uninvolved wrist joint shows whether laxity or restriction is present. With the patient seated, the involved forearm resting in pronation, and the wrist over the end of a table, stabilize the forearm with your hand on the distal forearm adjacent to the wrist joint. Place your mobilizing hand around the distal carpal row. With the mobilizing hand, apply a longitudinal distracting force to the wrist (figure 14.43).

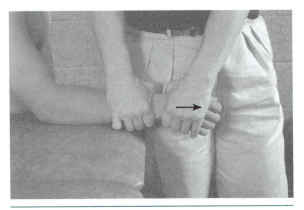

Figure 14.43 Radiocarpal joint distraction test.

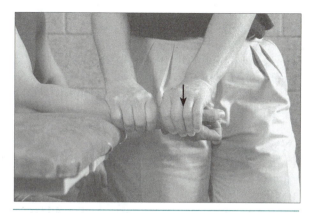

Figure 14.44 Dorsal glide test.

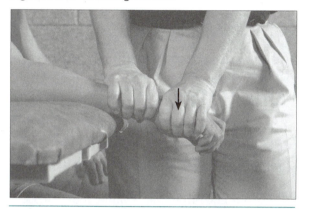

Figure 14.45 Ventral glide test.

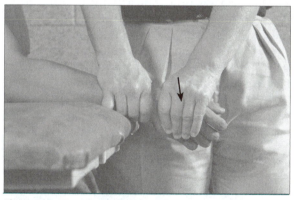

Figure 14.46 Ulnar glide test.

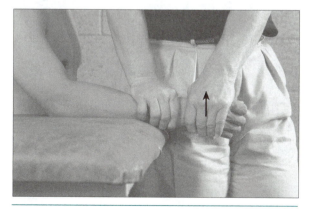

Figure 14.47 Radial glide test.

Glide Movements

The four glide tests for the radiocarpal joint are the dorsal (anterior–posterior) glide to examine wrist flexion; the ventral (posterior–anterior) glide to examine wrist extension; the radial glide to examine ulnar deviation; and the ulnar glide to examine radial deviation. Perform each movement individually. Since hand placement is the same for all tests, you can perform them in sequence; that is, you can complete one test and then move to the next one. It is best to perform the tests on the uninvolved side first as a means of comparison. As with the distraction test, the patient sits with the forearm on a table and the wrist and hand off the end of the table. Place your stabilizing hand on the distal forearm adjacent to the wrist joint and your mobilizing hand over the proximal carpal row. Perform the dorsal glide with the patient's forearm supinated. Provide an anterior–posterior glide to the wrist joint (figure 14.44). For the ventral glide, performed with the patient's forearm pronated, perform a downward glide in a posterior–anterior direction (figure 14.45). For the radial and ulnar glide tests, place the forearm in neutral with the thumb positioned up. For the ulnar glide, provide a downward force to move the wrist in an ulnar direction (figure 14.46); apply the radial glide force in an upward direction to move the wrist toward the radial aspect (figure 14.47).

Carpometacarpal Joints

#2-5 Carpometacarpal Ventral Glide

The #2-5 carpometacarpal ventral glide test examines general mobility of the second to fifth metacarpal and intermetacarpal joints. The patient sits with the forearm pronated and supported on a table and with the hand and wrist off the table. Place the thumb of your stabilizing hand along the metacarpal you wish to stabilize and your mobilizing thumb on the metacarpal you wish to mobilize. Apply a downward mobilizing force to the metacarpal to examine its mobility (figure 14.48).

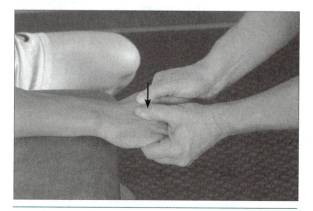

Figure 14.48 #2-5 carpometacarpal ventral glide.

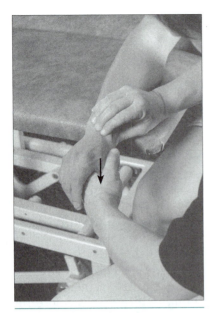

Figure 14.49 #1 carpometacarpal distraction.

#1 Carpometacarpal Distraction

This test examines general mobility of the thumb CMC joint. Seat the patient as you did for the other mobility tests. Using the thumb and index finger of your stabilizing hand, stabilize the scaphoid and trapezium bones; place the index finger and thumb of your mobilizing hand around the first metacarpal. Apply a longitudinal distraction force to the CMC joint (figure 14.49).

#1 Carpometacarpal Dorsal Glide

The #1 carpometacarpal dorsal glide examines thumb abduction. With the patient's forearm in supination and supported on a table as before, stabilize the proximal portion of the CMC joint with the thumb and index finger of your stabilizing hand. To examine joint mobility, place your thumb on top of the patient's anterior first metacarpal and apply a downward dorsal force to the joint (figure 14.50).

Metacarpophalangeal and Interphalangeal Joints

The MCP and IP joints are all tested in a similar fashion; use the same stabilizing and mobilizing hand positions and apply the same test forces.

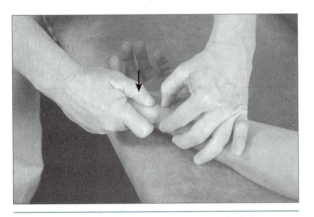

Figure 14.50 #1 carpometacarpal dorsal glide.

Metacarpophalangeal and Interphalangeal Joint Mobility Tests

The three test maneuvers are distraction to examine general mobility, dorsal glide to examine limited joint extension, and ventral glide to examine limited joint flexion. Position the patient as for other wrist and hand mobility tests. The forearm is in pronation with the wrist and hand over the end of a table. Stabilize the proximal arm of the joint you are testing with the index finger and thumb of one of your hands and apply the mobilizing force after placing the index finger and thumb of your opposite hand just distal to the joint (figure 14.51).

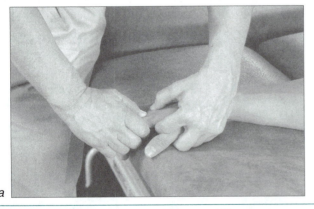 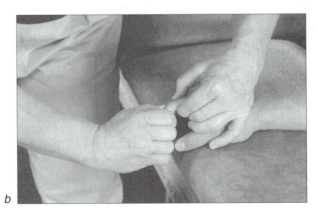

a   b

Figure 14.51 *(a)* MCP and *(b)* IP joint mobility tests.

INJURY EXAMINATION STRATEGIES

Because of its vital function in sport, the hand is a frequent injury site. Fortunately, most hand and wrist injuries sustained in sport are not serious. However, because the hand is so vital to upper-extremity function, even relatively minor injuries can severely hamper performance. Moreover, seemingly insignificant injuries are often left untreated, and as you learned from previous sections, ignoring injury can lead to inadequate bone healing, capsulitis, contractures, and deformities. Accurate and prompt examination is essential for successfully treating and restoring the injury site to full function.

On-Site Examination

It is the finals match of the NCAA women's volleyball championships. As Casey goes up for a solo block, her timing is a bit off and she is not able to completely square herself to the ball. The opposing player hits the ball hard off Casey's left hand. She immediately goes down on the court in pain, holding her left ring finger.

Daniel is a 14-year-old trying out for the high school soccer team. During the scrimmage, he trips and instinctively extends his right hand to break his fall. Upon contact with the ground, he hears a snap and feels immediate pain in his right wrist.

On-site examination of wrist and hand injuries should be relatively brief in most cases, with the majority of the examination being deferred to the sidelines. However, a short examination is necessary to determine the extent and severity of the injury and the need for medical referral, as well as to ascertain whether immobilization is necessary before moving the athlete.

As you approach the athlete, do a primary survey and check the surroundings as well as his position and immediate response. Ask him to describe the mechanism, the injury location, and any unusual sensations he heard or felt. Understanding the mechanism narrows down the potential structures involved. Observe bilaterally for obvious signs of severe bleeding, immediate swelling, discoloration, and deformity that indicate a fracture or dislocation. If you note deformity, immediately examine for any neurovascular deficits. Because many wrist and hand injuries are distal to the palpation site of the radial or ulnar pulse, you can check circulation by squeezing the nail bed, watching for blanching and capillary return. If you see any signs of serious injury, immobilize and refer the athlete for appropriate medical care. Because finger injuries can be quite painful, always remember to observe for signs and symptoms of shock, even if the injury appears relatively minor.

If there are no signs of serious injury, continue the on-site examination by palpating the musculoskeletal structures. As you palpate, check for point tenderness, crepitus, swelling, deformity, or irregularities over the distal radius, ulnar, carpal bones, metacarpals, and phalanges. If you do not identify a potential fracture and the athlete's pain has subsided sufficiently to allow ambulation, the athlete can leave the field for further examination on the sideline.

Acute Examination

As Casey heads off the volleyball court, she is still holding her ring finger. On the court, you saw no signs of obvious deformity or trauma. Now that she is on the sidelines, you note immediate and significant swelling.

Checklist for On-Site Examination of the Wrist and Hand

▷ **Primary Survey**

☐ Consciousness

☐ Airway, breathing, and circulation

☐ Severe bleeding

☐ Check for unusual positioning of the limb

☐ Examine for signs and symptoms of shock

▷ **Secondary Survey**

  ▷ **History**

    ☐ Mechanism of injury

    ☐ Location and severity of pain

    ☐ Unusual sensations heard or felt

    ☐ Information from bystanders

  ▷ **Observation**

    ☐ Deformity, swelling, discoloration, pallor, check for unusual limb positioning

  ▷ **Palpation**

    ☐ Bony tenderness, crepitus, and deformity along the distal radius and ulna, radiocarpal joint, carpal bones, and carpometacarpal joints

    ☐ Metacarpals, metacarpophalanageal joints, phalanges, proximal and distal interphalangeal joints

  ▷ **Neurovascular examination**

    ☐ Sensory (radial (C6), median (C7), ulnar (C8))

    ☐ Motor (radial, median, ulnar)

    ☐ Radial pulse or nail bed check

  ▷ **Gentle, active range of motion**

    ☐ Finger extension and flexion

    ☐ Wrist flexion, extension, and radial and ulnar deviation

If all tests are negative, remove from field for continued examination off-site.

PJ is a freshman linebacker for the local high school team and is playing in his first game. As the running back heads toward him, PJ misses the tackle but attempts to slow the player by grabbing his jersey. As the player pulls away, PJ tries to hold on, but then releases when he feels an intense burning pain in his middle finger. He walks over to you on the sideline, shaking his hand.

After the athlete has been assisted to the sideline, you can perform a more detailed examination to achieve a precise impression of the injury.

History

With the athlete in a comfortable position and the distal upper extremity supported, ask her to provide a more detailed history of the injury and if pertinent, any prior injuries to the area. Ask about the position of the hand and wrist at impact and about the direction the force came from. This is the time you ask the usual questions regarding intensity, quality, and specific location of the pain (refer to chapter 3 and the checklist for acute examination later in this section). Repeat questions regarding location and pain, because in many cases the athlete's symptoms will become more focused once the immediate pain of the injury subsides. Be sure to check for any previous injuries to both the involved and uninvolved sides, as bony or soft tissue irregularities may have resulted from previous injuries that are not consistent with the present injury.

Observation

Observe the athlete's facial expressions for signs of discomfort or pain. Also watch how he supports and moves the wrist, hand, and fingers. Is his movement guarded, or does he use the hand freely to gesture as he speaks? Observe the injured area for signs of discoloration, skin interruptions and scars, deformity, finger alignment, nail appearance and color, and abnormal contours; compare bilaterally. Check for skin creases in comparison to those on the other hand: Are creases on the injured hand normal, or have they been diminished by swelling? Also check for equal skin coloration.

Palpation

Start palpation proximally and proceed distally, moving to the area of injury last. Also palpate the distal forearm for any musculotendinous or bony tenderness, crepitus, or irregularity.

Special Tests

Special tests for traumatic wrist and hand injuries include those for neurovascular compromise, subtle fracture discovery, tendon and muscle injury, and ligament instability.

Range of Motion

Examine active ROM before passive motion. For a combined movement examination, have the patient make a fist and then open it as wide as possible. This allows you to quickly identify any gross deficiencies. Observe for quality and quantity of movement of isolated and multiple joints.

Strength

Perform manual muscle tests on the sideline to examine muscle strength. For each test, position the athlete's hand so that the muscle being tested works against gravity, unless this position is too inconvenient or difficult. Always perform strength tests on the uninvolved side and the structures surrounding the injury first, leaving the probable site of injury for last. You can perform a manual grip test in the acute examination to test general strength. Instruct the athlete to squeeze two or three fingers of your hand as hard as possible. Compare the involved and uninvolved sides by having the athlete perform the grip test on both your hands simultaneously.

Neurological Tests

If you suspect a nerve injury on the basis of deficits or weakness found thus far in your exam, perform a complete neurological examination for peripheral nerve integrity.

Functional Tests

Because the hand serves so many functions, you can use several different functional tests in addition to sport-related functional tasks.

To test motion and coordination, have the athlete perform a rapid thumb-to-finger touch test. The athlete moves the thumb tip from the index finger to the middle, ring, and little finger, then back again to the starting position as rapidly as possible. In another coordination test, the athlete supinates and pronates the injured segment as rapidly as possible while moving the opposite hand in opposing positions. For example, if the right wrist is injured, have the athlete supinate the right and pronate the left and then move the hands in opposite directions as rapidly as possible.

You can use more aggressive functional tests to examine strength and joint integrity. Weight bearing on the wrist in a push-up position with the palm flat on the floor, and then on the fingertips, examines overall hand strength and integrity of the wrist and finger joints. Grip activities can also represent a variety of functional tests, since the hand normally uses a number of different grips. Examples of power grips are grasping an object such as a bat, tennis racket, hockey stick, or lacrosse stick and grasping, catching, and throwing a ball. Examples of precision grips, used for more precise activities, are the chuck grip as in picking up a golf tee, the lateral pinch grip as in grasping a scorecard, and the pinch grip for fingertip prehension (i.e., tip to tip). Although the pinch grip is not often used in sport, it is vital for picking up very small objects such as a needle or coin.

Checklist for Acute Examination of the Wrist and Hand

▶ *History*

Ask questions pertaining to the following:

- ☐ Chief complaint
- ☐ Mechanism of injury
- ☐ Unusual sounds or sensations
- ☐ Type and location of pain or symptoms
- ☐ Previous injury
- ☐ Previous injury to opposite extremity for bilateral comparison

▶ *Observation*

- ☐ Visible facial expressions of pain
- ☐ Swelling, deformity, abnormal contours, or discoloration
- ☐ Skin creases, interruption, coloration, and scars
- ☐ Finger alignment, nail appearance and coloration
- ☐ Guarding of the wrist and hand
- ☐ Muscle development—are there areas of muscular atrophy?
- ☐ Bilateral comparison

▶ *Palpation*

Bilaterally palpate for pain, tenderness, and deformity from proximal to distal over the following:

- ☐ Distal radius and ulna, Lister's tubercle, extensor tendons
- ☐ Carpal bones, anatomical snuffbox, and tendon borders
- ☐ Flexor tendons, tunnel of Guyon
- ☐ Carpometacarpal joints, metacarpals (base, shaft, head), metacarpophalangeal joints
- ☐ Phalanges, proximal and distal interphalangeal joints
- ☐ Check radial pulse and look for nail bed blanching

▶ *Special Tests*

- ☐ Neurovascular compromise (Tinel's sign, Allen test)
- ☐ Fractures (compression, vibration)
- ☐ Tendon and muscle (flexor and extensor tendon avulsion)
- ☐ Ligament stress tests (collateral, Reagan's, glide tests)

▶ *Range of Motion*

- ☐ Active ROM for forearm pronation and supination
- ☐ Active ROM for wrist flexion, extension, radial and ulnar deviation
- ☐ Active ROM for MP flexion, extension, abduction, and adduction
- ☐ Active ROM for IP flexion, extension
- ☐ Active ROM for thumb flexion, extension, abduction, adduction, and circumduction
- ☐ Passive ROM for same motions as for active ROM
- ☐ Bilateral comparison

▶ *Strength Tests*

- ☐ Grip strength
- ☐ Perform manual resistance against same motions as in active ROM
- ☐ Check bilaterally and note any pain or weakness

▶ *Neurological Tests*

- ☐ Sensory and motor for radial, ulnar, and median nerve distributions

▶ *Functional Tests*

Clinical Examination

Beth returns to campus after working at basketball camps all summer. She comes to you complaining of continued pain and swelling in her index finger. She states she sprained it about 6 weeks ago, but it just doesn't seem to get any better. Her only treatment has been occasional icing and taping the finger to her middle finger whenever she plays.

Jeremy is a cycling enthusiast who recently started competing in long-distance road races. He comes to you complaining of pain and tingling in his right hand along the border of his fifth finger. He says it worsens as the ride progresses.

Frances is a 60-year-old-secretary who faithfully plays tennis on the weekends. She comes to you complaining of pain and numbness in her left hand. Although it bothers her somewhat when she plays tennis, she states the pain is worse at night and when she works on her computer. She has also noticed that her grip on the racket does not feel as strong.

Athletes commonly delay reporting wrist and hand injuries, so you may not have the opportunity to examine the injury until several days after it has occurred. Chronic or overuse injuries are typically not reported until they begin to interfere with work or performance.

History

When obtaining a history from a patient at some delay from the injury onset, get as much detailed information as possible regarding the incident. Ask the same questions you would ask during an acute examination, but in addition, ask about the time of onset and the duration of symptoms for more chronic conditions. Determine whether the injury has worsened or improved over time and what activities tend to aggravate or ease symptoms and to what extent. For chronic injuries, pay close attention to occupational or academic activities in addition to sport activities that may contribute to a repetitive stress injury. Ask the patient if she experiences any pain, weakness, or loss of motion with daily activities such as gripping, typing, and opening doors. If so, find out which motions are most bothersome.

Observation

As with all injuries, begin your observation when the patient enters the treatment facility. Observe for guarding versus free movement of the wrist and hand. Check for signs of swelling, discoloration, deformity, and muscle atrophy, and compare bilaterally. Check carefully for any areas of localized swelling or any nodules (such as on the dorsum of the wrist, which may indicate a wrist ganglion). Check for equal and bilateral skin creases and finger angulation.

Differential Diagnosis

Because the cervical or upper thoracic spine, shoulder, and elbow can refer symptoms into the wrist and hand, you should examine these areas to eliminate them as possible sources of the patient complaints. Use ROM movements with overpressure tests for each joint and include the quadrant position for the cervical spine. At the end of each active motion of each joint, apply an overpressure to move the joint to its maximum end range. If any of these movements reproduces the patient's symptoms, you should examine that joint more closely before continuing.

Myofascial restriction can also refer pain and symptoms into the wrist and hand. Travell and Simon (1983) showed that the most common sources of myofascial pain referral into

For more information on identifying particular pain patterns and their treatment, refer to *Therapeutic Exercise for Musculoskeletal Injuries, Second Edition,* (Houglum 2005), chapter 6.

the hand are the scalenes, infraspinatus, subscapularis, latissimus dorsi, coracobrachialis, brachialis, triceps, and forearm muscles. If pain is generalized and difficult to pinpoint, follows an atypical injury pattern, or radiates, you should perform soft tissue examination for possible myofascial-related referrals.

If the patient's pain follows a nerve pathway pattern or if she complains of tingling, burning, or shooting pain, suspect neural pathology and include a complete upper-extremity neurological examination for motor and sensory integrity and specific special tests for this pathology (see chapter 8).

Range of Motion

ROM examination in the clinic is consistent with that performed at the sideline. You can make a gross examination of ROM by having the patient perform full active motions in all planes for the forearm, wrist, and fingers while you observe for smoothness and fullness of motion. If there is any discrepancy or deficits in motion, make a more detailed examination of the area using goniometric techniques. Forearm supination and pronation occur primarily in the forearm with about 15° of movement taking place at the wrist, so if full supination or pronation is not possible, examine the forearm and wrist as possible sources of deficient motion. Wrist flexion occurs primarily at the intercarpal joint margin between the proximal and distal carpal rows, while wrist extension occurs primarily at the radiocarpal joint. Radial deviation occurs mostly between the proximal and distal carpal rows, and ulnar deviation occurs primarily at the radiocarpal joint (Kapandji 1970). In the fingers, the greatest degrees of motion occur in the PIP joints, with about equal motion occurring in the MCP and DIP joints.

The MCP joints have two degrees of freedom, whereas the IP joints have one. This allows for abduction or adduction and flexion or extension of the fingers at the MCP joints and only flexion and extension at the IP joints. Slight abduction and rotation are possible at the IP joints and rotation at the MCP joints. These movements are necessary for full function of the digits, but they occur only passively. Since the thumb plays the most vital role in hand function, it has the greatest degree of freedom of movement and is the only digit of the hand innervated by all three nerves.

During active ROM examination, check for capsular patterns in the wrist. The capsular pattern of the wrist is equal limitation of flexion and extension with mild limitation of supination and pronation at the distal radioulnar joint. The thumb's carpometacarpal (CMC) joint capsular pattern is more limited in abduction than in adduction, and the finger's MCP and IP joints are more limited in flexion than in extension. If you note this proportion of motion loss during active ROM, it is likely that capsular tightness is at least contributing to the patient's limited motion.

Strength

Administer manual muscle tests in the same way as for the acute examination. In addition, you can perform more objective strength tests with various machines. In the clinic, you can isokinetically examine forearm supination and pronation and wrist flexion and extension. Use grip and pinch dynamometers to objectively measure hand and finger strength.

Neurological Tests

The neurological examination for the wrist and hand includes sensory and motor testing. In addition to standard sensory tests, you can use a two-point discrimination test for fine sensory perception.

Special Tests

Any of the special tests described for the acute examination may be used in the clinical examination. Also use tests that identify chronic inflammatory conditions. As always, base your test selection on the client's history, your observations, and your objective findings up to this point.

Joint Mobility

Perform joint mobility tests if there is reduced ROM in order to help you determine whether the limited range is caused by capsular restriction or other factors.

Palpation

As with the acute examination, perform a methodical palpation of the distal forearm, wrist, hand, and fingers, moving from proximal to distal and from anterior to posterior. Carefully observe for areas of tenderness, deformity, spasm, swelling, crepitus, atrophy, nodules, and other abnormal contours. The forearm, thenar, and hypothenar areas may contain myofascial restriction and should be inspected for pain that may cause referral to other regions. Palpate the area of the patient's complaint last.

Functional Tests

Simple coordination exercises and activities such as push-ups and other strength maneuvers can be used along with sport-specific or work-specific activities to determine the patient's function and readiness to return to activity. The patient is ready to return to full participation if he performs all the functional tests well and without hesitation; he demonstrates balanced performance between the right and left upper extremities; he shows no evidence of pain; and he uses good motion, strength, endurance, power, agility, and control.

Checklist for Clinical Examination of the Wrist and Hand

▷ History

Ask questions pertaining to the following:
- ☐ Chief complaint
- ☐ Mechanism of injury
- ☐ Unusual sounds or sensations
- ☐ Type, location, onset, and duration of pain or symptoms
- ☐ Previous injury
- ☐ Previous injury to opposite extremity for bilateral comparison

If chronic, ascertain:
- ☐ Aggravating and easing activities
- ☐ Training and daily activity history (repetitive stresses)
- ☐ Activity restrictions
- ☐ Treatment if any

▷ Observation

- ☐ Visible facial expressions of pain
- ☐ Swelling, deformity, abnormal contours, or discoloration
- ☐ Skin creases, interruption, coloration, and scars
- ☐ Finger alignment, nail appearance and coloration
- ☐ Guarding of the wrist and hand
- ☐ Muscle development—areas of muscular atrophy
- ☐ Presence of localized nodules
- ☐ Bilateral comparison

(continued)

(continued)

▷ *Differential Diagnosis*

☐ Clear cervical region with overpressure tests in straight planes and quadrant positions
☐ Clear shoulder region with passive overpressures in all ranges
☐ Clear elbow region with passive overpressures in all ranges
☐ Perform complete upper quarter neurological screen if referred pain is noted

▷ *Range of Motion*

☐ Active ROM for forearm pronation and supination
☐ Active ROM for wrist flexion, extension, radial and ulnar deviation
☐ Active ROM for MP flexion, extension, abduction, and adduction
☐ Active ROM for IP flexion, extension
☐ Active ROM for thumb flexion, extension, abduction, adduction, and circumduction
☐ Presence of capsular patterns
☐ Passive ROM for same motions as for active ROM
☐ Bilateral comparison

▷ *Strength Tests*

☐ Check grip strength and pinch strength
☐ Perform manual resistance against same motions as in active ROM
☐ Check bilaterally and note any pain or weakness
☐ Perform instrumented strength tests

▷ *Neurological Tests*

☐ Sensory and motor for ulnar, radial, and median nerves
☐ Two-point discrimination test

▷ *Special Tests*

☐ Neurovascular compromise (Tinel's, Allen, Phalen's)
☐ Fractures (compression, vibration)
☐ Tendon and muscle (flexor and extensor tendon avulsion)
☐ Ligament stress tests (collateral, Reagan's, glide tests, Bunnel-Littler, retinacular)
☐ Tenosynovitis (Finkelstein, trigger finger)

▷ *Joint Mobility Examination*

Note capsular restriction and end feel:
☐ Radiocarpal distraction and glide
☐ Carpometacarpal distraction and glide
☐ Metacarpophalangeal and interphalangeal distraction and glide

▷ *Palpation*

Bilaterally palpate for pain, tenderness, and deformity from proximal to distal over the following:
☐ Distal radius and ulna, Lister's tubercle, extensor tendons
☐ Carpal bones, anatomical snuffbox, and tendon borders
☐ Flexor tendons, tunnel of Guyon
☐ Carpometacarpal joints, metacarpals (base, shaft, head), metacarpophalangeal joints
☐ Phalanges, proximal and distal interphalangeal joints
☐ Check radial pulse and observe for nail bed blanching

▷ *Functional Tests*

SUMMARY

1. Describe the types and mechanisms of acute and chronic injuries of the wrist and hand that physically active people commonly experience.

   The dexterity and precision required for fine motor control often leave the wrist and hand unprotected and vulnerable to injury during sport activity. Contact with the ground, an opponent, or balls and other sporting implements is the primary mechanism by which acute fractures, dislocations, sprains, and strains in the wrist and hand occur. The hand and wrist are also prone to repetitive stress injuries such as tendinitis, tenosynovitis, nerve compression syndromes, and capsulitis, as well as other chronic joint restrictions resulting from previous injury.

2. Describe the potential complications and deformities that can result from seemingly simple sprains and strains.

   Many times an athlete sustains a painful finger injury but dismisses it as a simple sprain. However, these injuries may also represent fractures or damage to the soft tissue structures that, if left unrecognized or untreated, will result in inadequate healing or permanent restriction. These injuries include intra-articular fractures, volar plate ruptures, extensor tendon ruptures, and capsulitis. To avoid these conditions, thoroughly examine all finger injuries and refer the patient if there is any question about the severity.

3. Identify the common sites and signs and symptoms of nerve compression injuries.

   Nerve compression in the wrist and hand occurs primarily in the carpal tunnel (median) or the tunnel of Guyon (ulnar). Carpal tunnel syndrome can result from a variety of factors including repetitive stress and carpal fractures. Ulnar nerve compression is commonly seen in cyclists as a result of prolonged pressure that occurs as the heel of the hand rests on the handlebars. Signs and symptoms, which are consistent with other nerve compression injuries, include pain, paresthesia along the nerve distribution, and, in chronic cases, muscle weakness and atrophy.

4. Discuss the common fractures that occur in the wrist and hand and their characteristic deformities and signs and symptoms.

   The small, fine bones of the wrist and hand are prone to fractures. Falling on an outstretched hand is a common mechanism for Colles' fracture and scaphoid fractures, whereas falling on the back of the hand may cause a Smith's fracture. While scaphoid fractures are often difficult to detect, Colles' and Smith's fractures each have a characteristic deformity. Both axial and longitudinal forces fracture the metacarpals and phalanges, and displacement is obvious because of the superficial nature of these bones. If you note any bony tenderness, refer the athlete to a physician for X ray.

5. Describe and perform the objective tests for wrist and hand examination.

   Palpate the wrist and hand with the patient seated and the arm relaxed. Because of the many small structures of the wrist, hand, and fingers, you will need to have a good grasp of the anatomy before proceeding. ROM and strength testing of the wrist and hand include active, passive, and manual resisted examinations of forearm supination and pronation; wrist flexion and extension, radial deviation and ulnar deviation; MCP flexion, extension, abduction, and adduction; and interphalangeal flexion and extension. The thumb has motions of flexion, extension, abduction, adduction, circumduction, and opposition. Sensory and motor testing are for the median, ulnar, and radial peripheral nerve distributions, and the C6, C7, and C8 dermatomes. Special tests exist for neurovascular compromise, fracture, ligament instability, musculotendon pathology, and joint contracture.

6. Perform an on-site examination of the wrist and hand, identifying the conditions that warrant immediate referral.

   Most wrist and hand injuries are not severe enough to require immediate medical referral. When dealing with an on-site injury, direct your attention to any evidence of severe bleeding, potential fractures and dislocations, or neurovascular compromise. If you identify any of these injuries, immediate medical care and referral are required. If these conditions are not present, the athlete can be moved to the sideline for further examination.

7. Perform an acute examination of the wrist and hand, including special tests used to examine acute conditions.

Except in the case of serious injury, you will examine most hand and wrist injuries on the sideline once the athlete has left the field. At the sideline, thoroughly palpate all structures and perform a more detailed examination for active and passive ROM, strength, ligamentous stability, musculotendinous injury, and neurovascular integrity. Perform vibration and compression tests to detect less obvious fractures.

8. Perform a clinical examination of the wrist and hand, including examination techniques for chronic injuries.

The clinical examination is similar to the acute examination for the wrist but includes tests to examine more chronic conditions such as nerve compression, tenosynovitis, and joint restrictions. With chronic conditions, it is important to gain a history of both sport and daily living activities, as these may equally expose the wrist and hand to repetitive stress injuries.

REVIEW QUESTIONS

1. What characteristic joint postures and structural pathology are associated with the following deformities?
   - Boutonniere
   - Pseudoboutonniere
   - Silver fork
   - Ape hand
   - Benediction
   - Claw hand

2. What are the signs and symptoms of a volar plate rupture? How would you distinguish this injury from a collateral ligament sprain?

3. Name the sensory distributions and motor tests for each of the peripheral nerves. When would you include a neurological examination in your examination of a wrist or hand injury?

4. Describe the etiology and signs and symptoms of carpal tunnel syndrome. If you suspect that a patient has carpal tunnel syndrome, what special tests would you use to rule out or confirm your impressions? What questions about activity may you ask?

5. Now that you have studied the complete upper extremity, identify the joints and associated conditions that can refer pain to the wrist and hand. What differential tests would you use to rule out pathology in these other joints?

6. What is the purpose of Phalen's test? How do you perform it, and what constitutes a positive result?

7. How do you determine whether tightness in a PIP joint is caused by capsular, ligamentous, or muscle restrictions?

CRITICAL THINKING QUESTIONS

1. Think back to the scenario at the beginning of the chapter. Considering what you have learned, what would you do in this situation? Explain your rationale and discuss any examination procedures you would perform before making your decision.

2. A 20-year-old soccer player comes into the athletic training room holding her wrist. While playing soccer she lost her balance and put out her hand to break the fall.

She complains of pain in her wrist, primarily on the palmar side. She reports no previous injury. On exam, you find some mild swelling on the palmar aspect of her wrist but no immediate discoloration or deformity. On palpation, she is point tender over the same area but does not appear to have any bony crepitus, palpable deformity, or mass. You check for tenderness in the anatomical snuffbox, and it is mildly tender but similar bilaterally. On active motion, the athlete's pain intensifies with full wrist extension and lessens considerably with flexion. On passive testing, the pain is considerable with wrist extension and nonexistent with wrist flexion, except at the extreme end range. The patient denies any referred pain into her hand. Given this history, what condition would you most likely suspect, and what specific tests would you use to confirm your suspicions and to rule out other potential injuries?

3. An industrial worker who plays on his company's baseball team comes to you complaining of pain in the radial aspect of his wrist. He states that the pain has come on gradually over time, and he notices it primarily during batting, especially when he breaks the wrists at the end of his swing. He has had no previous injury to either hand. When you ask about his occupation, you find that he works on the assembly line in an automobile factory and that his job requires him to place about 100 radiator caps on radiators each day. Upon palpation, you notice tenderness and crepitus at the base of the thumb. You note pain and weakness with resisted thumb extension. On the basis of this history and symptoms, what condition might you suspect, and how would you confirm your findings?

4. Consider the three scenarios presented at the opening of the clinical examination section (see page 341). What types of history questions would you ask in each of these cases?

5. Consider the case of PJ, the linebacker who attempted to slow another player by grabbing his jersey. He complains of pain and a burning sensation on the palmar aspect of his middle finger. Upon observation, you find no deformity, but there is some mild swelling on the palmer aspect of his middle phalanx. You ask PJ to open his fist as wide as possible and tightly close it again so you can quickly examine gross movement. You note he has full extension in all digits, but as he makes a fist, he is unable to flex the injured finger into his palm. Given the injury mechanism, the pain location, and these findings, what injury might you suspect? What objective tests would you use to confirm your suspicions?

CITED REFERENCES

Harris, R.B. 1983. *Textbook of disorders and injuries of the musculoskeletal system.* 2nd ed. Baltimore: Williams & Wilkins.

Houglum, P.A. 2005. *Therapeutic exercise for musculoskeletal injuries.* 2nd ed. Champaign, IL: Human Kinetics.

Kapandji, I.A. 1970. *The physiology of the joints: Upper limb.* Vol. 1. New York: Churchill Livingstone.

Travell, J.G., and D.G. Simon. 1983. *Myofascial pain and dysfunction, the trigger point manual: The upper extremities.* Vol. 1. Baltimore: Williams & Wilkins.

ADDITIONAL RESOURCES

Clarkson, H.M. 2000. *Musculoskeletal assessment: Joint range of motion and manual muscle strength.* 2nd ed. Philadelphia: Lippincott Williams & Wilkins.

Hoppenfeld, S. 1976. *Physical examination of the spine and extremities.* Norwalk: Appleton and Lange.

Houglum, P.A. 2005. *Therapeutic exercise for musculoskeletal injuries.* 2nd ed. Champaign, IL: Human Kinetics.

Kendall, F.P., E.K. McCreary, and P.G. Provance. 1993. *Muscles: Testing and function.* 4th ed. Philadelphia: Lippincott Williams & Wilkins.

Moore, K.L. 1992. *Clinically oriented anatomy.* 3rd ed. Baltimore: Williams & Wilkins.

Lower Thoracic and Lumbar Spine

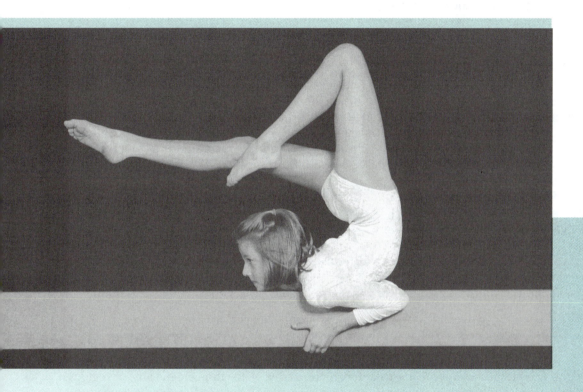

Objectives

After completing this chapter, the reader will be able to do the following:

1. Describe the etiology, signs and symptoms, and potential complications associated with acute and chronic injuries of the thoracic and lumbar spine commonly encountered in the physically active

2. Describe the congenital and degenerative conditions of the thoracic and lumbar spine

3. Describe the common causes, signs and symptoms, and indicative tests for nerve root compression in the lumbar spine

4. Identify the characteristics of and potential contributing factors to functional and structural deformities in the thoracic and lumbar spine

5. Describe and demonstrate the objective tests for examining the lower thoracic and lumbar spine

6. Perform an on-site examination of the lumbar spine, identifying criteria for immediate medical referral and transportation from the field

7. Perform an acute examination of the lumbar spine

8. Perform a clinical examination of the lumbar and thoracic spine, noting considerations for differential diagnosis

Max had been working at a shipping company during the summers and holidays for the past three years to help put himself through school. He enjoyed his job, except for the fact that his supervisor was constantly on him about lifting properly when loading his truck. Max considered himself a strong specimen and a good athlete—he certainly didn't think lifting a few boxes was any big deal.

It was the Christmas holidays, and work was nuts! Max was tired and cranky. He bent over and reached for a box at his side, but it was heavier than he had expected. Instead of turning around to get a better angle, he took a deep breath and lifted it hard and fast. At once, a searing pain shot through his back, and he dropped the box with a gasp. He could barely stand and needed assistance to get to the industrial clinic. There he encountered Ruth, a certified athletic trainer, who had recently been hired to head up the company's recreational sport program and work in the clinic.

When taking his history, Ruth asked, "Can you tell me what happened and where your pain is?"

"All I did was pick up a box. It was heavy, but no heavier than a lot of the packages I lift."

"Can you tell me how you picked it up? What position were you in?" Ruth asked. When Max explained the mechanisms, Ruth had a pretty good idea why the injury had occurred. She continued with a thorough examination, including a neurological examination to check for nerve root compression. Max showed no signs of neurological deficits but appeared to have a significant lumbar strain or sprain. However, because of his pain, she referred him to his physician for a follow-up examination and possible medication.

After a couple of weeks of treatment in the clinic, Max was as good as new. "Hey, thanks for all your help, Ruth. I feel great!"

"I'm glad to hear it, Max. You know, you were lucky. Lifting like that, your injury could have been a lot worse, and it may be worse next time. You really need to work on your lifting mechanics if you want to stay active in sports and not have a 70-year-old back by the time you're 30. Before you leave, let's work on it, okay?"

Max had a new appreciation for his supervisor's concern. "Yeah, I think that would be a good idea."

Considerable mechanical and muscular forces are exerted on the thoracic and lumbar regions of the spine during jumping, twisting, bending, and lifting activities. The lumbar spine provides both mobility and stability for upper-extremity and torso movements and effectively absorbs and transmits forces between the upper and lower extremities. Because of its greater mobility and load-bearing function compared to the thoracic and sacral spines, the lumbar spine is particularly susceptible to pain and injury. This chapter explores both the acute and chronic injuries that often occur in the lumbar spine and provides the essential examination techniques for examining these conditions and appropriately treating and referring them. While the primary focus is on the lumbar spine, lower thoracic spine pathologies that may also affect the lumbar spine region are covered as necessary.

FUNCTIONAL ANATOMY

The lumbar spine consists of the strongest and thickest spinal vertebrae, providing both stability and mobility for the upper torso. The lumbar spine achieves its stability through large anterior vertebral bodies, strong anterior and posterior longitudinal ligaments, intervertebral discs, and broad musculature. Two adjacent vertebrae separated by a vertebral disc constitute the basic functional unit of the lumbar spine (figure 15.1). The anterior segment (one vertebral body and the intervertebral disc) bears weight and absorbs shock. Each intervertebral disc is composed of a nucleus pulposus surrounded by a thick annulus fibrosis (figure 15.2). The fibers of the annulus fibrosis run obliquely to strongly attach one vertebra to the next. This oblique fiber arrangement puts the disc under greatest tension in rotation; thus it is most often

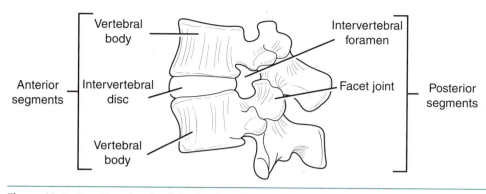

Figure 15.1   Functional unit of the lumbar spine.

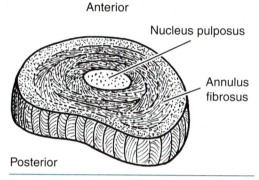

Figure 15.2   Each intervertebral disc is composed of a nucleus pulposus surrounded by the thick annulus fibrosis.

injured as a result of torsional movement. The posterior segment, which does not bear weight except in extreme extension, serves as a protective structure for the spinal cord (figure 15.3). The paired facet joints (see figure 15.1) direct and limit movement of the functional unit and prevent forward slipping of one vertebra on another. These joints are often the site of inflammation and overstress injuries. Between the anterior body and the posterior facet joints lies the intervertebral foramen that serves as the nerve root exit from the lumbar plexus into the lower extremity (see figures 15.1 and 15.3). Degenerative change or disc herniation can compromise this space, causing nerve compression and neurological symptoms in the lower extremity.

The muscles that move the lumbar region include the abdominal flexors and the back extensors. The abdominal muscles are the rectus abdominis, external oblique, internal oblique, and transversus abdominis (figure 15.4). The rectus abdominis includes three tendinous intersections that can clearly be seen in lean people with good muscular development. These intersections are found at the

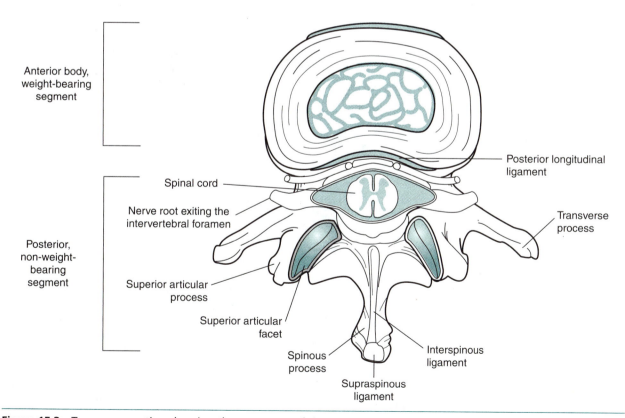

Figure 15.3   Transverse section showing the structures of the posterior segment, and the relationship of the spinal cord and nerve roots.

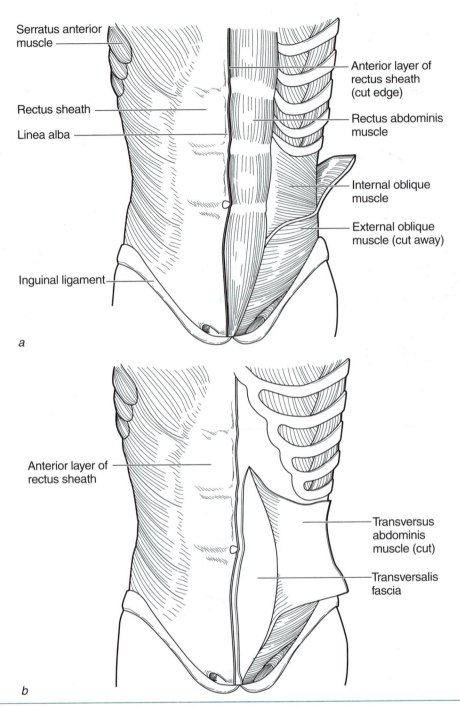

Serratus anterior muscle

Rectus sheath

Linea alba

Inguinal ligament

Anterior layer of rectus sheath (cut edge)

Rectus abdominis muscle

Internal oblique muscle

External oblique muscle (cut away)

a

Anterior layer of rectus sheath

Transversus abdominis muscle (cut)

Transversalis fascia

b

Figure 15.4   Abdominal musculature: *(a)* intermediate dissection and *(b)* deep dissection.

top of the xyphoid process, the umbilicus, and halfway between these two landmarks. The rectus abdominis is the prime flexor of the trunk. The external and internal obliques assist with flexion and also produce rotation and lateral flexion. The transversus abdominis is largely responsible for increasing intra-abdominal pressure through the Valsalva maneuver. The back extensor muscles include the erector spinae (spinalis, longissimus, and iliocostalis), lattisimus dorsi, transversospinalis, interspinales, and quadratus lumborum (figure 15.5). These muscles also contribute to trunk rotation and lateral flexion. The abdominal flexors and back extensor muscles are important for maintaining good posture and moving the trunk.

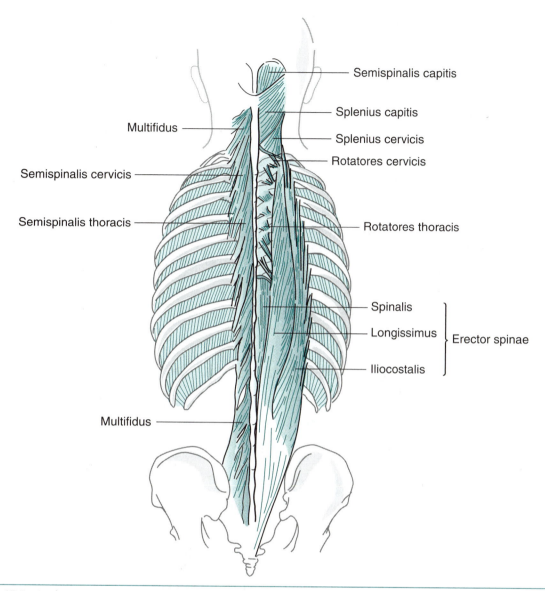

Figure 15.5 Back extensor musculature.

LOWER THORACIC AND LUMBAR SPINE INJURIES

Lumbar and thoracic pain is most often due to acute and chronic strains of the postural muscles supporting the lumbar region. Chronic strain may result from poor posture, poor mechanics, weakness, stiffness, and muscle restrictions. Occasionally congenital defects or degenerative changes cause low back pain. Traumatic injuries such as fractures may also occur, and you must always consider the potential for spinal cord injury and potential paralysis with severe injuries.

Acute and Chronic Soft Tissue Injuries

Soft tissue injuries make up the majority of injuries encountered in the lumbar spine. The soft tissue injuries that physically active people most commonly experience include contusions, sprains, and strains.

Contusions

The spinal structures vulnerable to direct contact and contusions are the spinous processes and their overlying superficial ligaments. Contusions to these structures may result in point tenderness, localized swelling, and pain with flexion and extension. The surrounding musculature is also vulnerable to contusions resulting from direct contact with an opponent (football), a sport implement (baseball, lacrosse stick), or the ground. Contusions to the musculature may cause considerable muscle swelling, stiffness, and spasm resulting in loss of range of motion and function. Although these contusions are rarely serious or debilitating, patients who have received significant direct trauma to the lower trunk and complain of severe or unrelenting low back pain should be thoroughly examined for possible kidney or other visceral trauma.

Sprains

Sprains in the lumbar and thoracic region typically result from sudden loading or torsional movements. They can also result from direct or indirect trauma that forces the spinal segments beyond their normal ranges of motion, as well as from compressive loading forces. The more common injury mechanism in the lumbar region is sudden extension with rotation. The lumbar spine depends heavily on the surrounding musculature to increase its stability during mechanical loading. Suddenly loading the spine when the muscles are unprepared places greater demands on the ligament and capsular structures. Therefore, weak or poorly conditioned trunk and abdominal muscles may make an athlete more susceptible to lumbar sprains. Sprains at the lumbosacral junction can result from this mechanism but may also result from a jamming mechanism, such as landing off balance on a straight leg, in which the spine absorbs most of the load.

Signs and symptoms of lumbar sprain include pain, swelling, muscle spasm, and decreased ROM. If the spasm is severe, you may see a lateral shift of the spinal column toward the spasm. Because of muscular involvement, sprains are painful with both active movement and passive stretching; consequently it is often difficult to distinguish a sprain from a strain.

Strains

The mechanisms for muscular strains are similar to those for sprains, causing sudden contraction or stretching of the involved musculature. Sudden eccentric loading of an already contracting muscle is also a common cause of muscular strain. Strains can result from a single episode of muscle overload but also frequently result from cumulative stress. Factors such as poor posture; muscular imbalance; poor conditioning; weak abdominal muscles; and inflexibility of the hamstrings, hip flexors, or back extensors can increase susceptibility to muscular strains. Signs and symptoms include pain, point tenderness, muscle spasm, and possible swelling in and around the involved musculature. You may note a lateral deviation in the spine with severe spasm. You will also see decreased ROM and increased pain with active contraction and passive stretching of the involved muscle.

Bone and Joint Pathologies

Bone and joint pathologies are less common than soft tissue injuries. While traumatic fractures may occur in the lumbar and thoracic spine, the vast majority of bone and joint pathologies result from congenital weakening, degenerative processes, or both.

Traumatic Fractures of the Thoracic Spine

Because of the stability of the thoracic spine, fractures and dislocations are rare in athletes. Thoracic spine fractures typically involve compression of the vertebral body resulting from violent forward flexion or axial loading in a forward flexed position. Axial loading forces originate superiorly as a result of contact or of forces exerted through the head and shoulders, including heavy lifting techniques. Axial forces can also be transmitted inferiorly through the thoracic spine in a hard fall on the buttocks. Dislocation or instability is uncommon

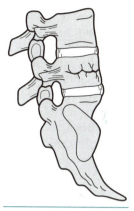

Figure 15.6 Compression of the vertebral body.

with these injuries and neurological injury rarely results. Signs and symptoms include localized pain and discomfort, tenderness with palpation over the spinous process of the involved vertebra, muscle spasm and guarding, and increased pain with forward flexion and other movements of the thoracic spine. It is not uncommon for athletes with thoracic spine fractures to get up and walk off the field following injury, so you must carefully examine localized, central thoracic spine pain after a traumatic injury before allowing the athlete to return to activity.

Traumatic Fractures of the Lumbar Spine

Traumatic fractures are relatively uncommon with sport activities, with the possible exception of high-speed impact sports. The structures most likely to be fractured secondary to acute trauma are the vertebral body, transverse processes, spinous processes, and pars articularis. Compression of the vertebral body typically results from high compressive or axial loading forces to a partially flexed lumbar spine (figure 15.6). Because of the larger vertebral body size, designed to better withstand axial loading forces, compression fractures in the lumbar spine are considerably less common than in the thoracic spine. However, skeletally immature athletes and athletes with diminished bone density secondary to aging, eating disorders, and amenorrhea may be more at risk for compression fractures in this area. Fractures of the transverse processes can result from direct trauma, violent torsional movements, or an avulsion of the psoas major muscle following a violent contraction (figure 15.7). Avulsion fractures of the transverse process can cause considerable pain and bleeding. Fractures of the relatively unprotected spinous processes are typically attributable to blunt trauma but may also result from forced hyperflexion of the lumbar spine. Pars interarticularis fractures are more commonly the result of stress reactions, but may also occur acutely with forced hyperextension or landing with the spine in hyperextension, particularly in athletes with underlying bony abnormalities or defects (figure 15.8).

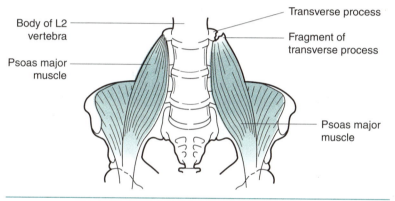

Body of L2 vertebra

Psoas major muscle

Transverse process

Fragment of transverse process

Psoas major muscle

Figure 15.7 Transverse process with psoas avulsion.

Signs and symptoms associated with fracture include immediate pain, direct or indirect tenderness over the vertebral segment, crepitus, decreased ROM, and an unwillingness to move. If the fracture encroaches on the spinal cord or nerve root, signs and symptoms of sensory or motor deficits associated with nerve compression or injury may also be present. Although unstable fractures with nerve involvement are rare in the lumbar spine, you should conduct a thorough neurological examination whenever you suspect spinal fracture following acute trauma.

Spondylolysis and Spondylolisthesis

A condition that is often attributed to a congenital abnormality but may not manifest itself until the patient is physically active is spondylolysis. **Spondylolysis** involves a fracture of **pars interarticularis**, located between the inferior and superior facets (see figure 15.8). It is typically thought to be a stress fracture secondary to a congenital weakening. Spina bifida occulta may also be a contributing factor in some athletes.

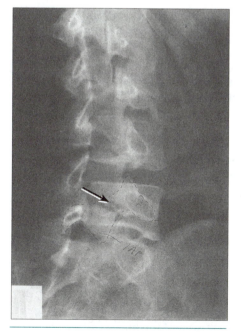

Figure 15.8 Pars fracture of the lumbar spine.

Courtesy of Theodore E. Keats

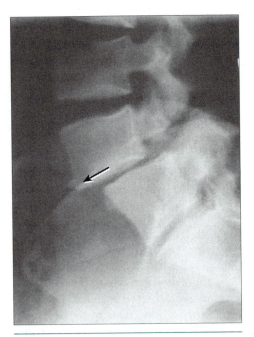

Figure 15.9 Spondylolisthesis with forward slippage.

Courtesy of Theodore E. Keats.

These injuries occur most often in young, skeletally immature athletes and do not necessarily preclude physical activity except when the fracture is acute. When spondylolysis occurs bilaterally, a secondary condition known as spondylolisthesis may result.

Spondylolisthesis is characterized by a forward subluxation of the involved vertebra (figure 15.9). Because of the orientation of the facet joints, the spondylolytic vertebra displaces anteriorly in relation to the vertebra directly below. Spondylolisthesis is frequently found in gymnasts, weight lifters, and football linemen secondary to the repetitive flexion and hyperextension loading forces inherent in their activities. Progression of forward slippage appears to be a concern only during athletes' preadolescent and adolescent growth years; rarely does forward subluxation progress in adults. In young athletes with this condition, the extent of forward subluxation should be examined regularly. The extent of subluxation of the vertebral body in relation to the inferior vertebral body is typically graded from stage I to stage IV. Athletes with stage I (<25% subluxation) and even stage II (25-50%) may continue activity provided that pain and symptoms allow. Progression to stage III (51-75%) often requires removal from activity and surgical management for stabilization.

Signs and symptoms associated with spondylolysis and spondylolisthesis are centralized low back pain (possibly radiating into the buttocks and posterior thighs), swelling, muscle spasm, and a straightening of the lordotic curve. Patients with these conditions may exhibit decreased ROM and increased pain with hyperextension. Standing on only the leg of the affected side and extending the spine also increases pain. A step deformity, when palpating the spinous processes, may be noted with spondylolisthesis. Symptoms may mimic those of lumbar sprains and strains and spondylolisthesis usually requires an X ray for definitive identification.

Facet Syndrome

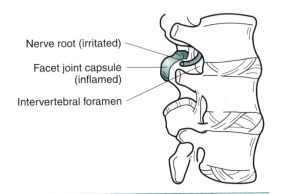

Figure 15.10 Facet joint syndrome with nerve root irritation.

Nerve root (irritated)

Facet joint capsule (inflamed)

Intervertebral foramen

Facet syndrome refers to an inflammation (**spondylitis**) of the facet joint and its surrounding capsule. Facet syndrome can result from acute trauma or chronic repetitive insult. Extension overload of the facet joint, particularly when combined with rotation, can compress and irritate the joint. Consequently, patients with scoliosis are more susceptible than others to facet joint pain and dysfunction. Inflammation of the facet joint may also irritate the nearby nerve root as it exits through the intervertebral foramen (figure 15.10). Because the facet joint is richly innervated, facet syndrome may be associated with considerable pain. Other signs and symptoms include localized swelling, paraspinal muscle spasm, tenderness upon palpation and movement of the facet joint, and increased pain with extension, compression, and rotation to the involved side. Pain may also be referred down the leg. There may also be a deviated posture (functional scoliosis) secondary to muscle spasm or in an attempt to avoid pain due to joint compression.

SI Joint Dysfunction

Low back pain can also be referred from a sprain or dysfunction of the sacroiliac (SI) joint. While these conditions and tests are covered in the discussion of the hip and pelvis, they are mentioned here simply to alert you of potential injuries affecting the lumbar spine region. See chapter 18 for more information about these conditions.

Degenerative Pathologies

Whereas spondylolysis and spondylolisthesis may be the more common causes of bony pathology in the adolescent athlete, spondylitis and **spondylosis** (degenerative changes) of the vertebrae and disc are more frequently the cause of back pain in the physically active adult. The water content in the intervertebral disc decreases with age. This often results in microtears and degeneration of the richly innervated annulus fibrosis, leading to low back pain and discomfort. Chronic joint inflammatory conditions resulting from cumulative and repetitive stress (e.g., spondylitis, facet syndrome) may also bring about degenerative changes such as osteophytes and capsular fibrosis. The L4/L5 and L5/S1 levels are particularly vulnerable to pain and degeneration because these segments are the most mobile, accounting for 80 to 90% of lumbar flexion. Moreover, the transition from the very mobile L5 vertebrae to the relatively stable S1 vertebrae makes this joint prone to shear forces that cause pain and injury. Poor posture, weak abdominal and back musculature, and inflexibility may contribute to the cumulative stresses placed on the spine and may hasten degenerative changes.

Patients with degenerative disc and joint disease report decreased pain in the morning and increased pain throughout the day as prolonged standing and sitting compress the disc and joints. Other signs and symptoms include pain across the lower lumbar region and into the buttocks and decreased ROM into flexion, extension, or rotation. As degenerative changes progress, nerve compression syndromes may result from narrowing of the intervertebral foramen (stenosis) secondary to encroachment by osteophytes or disc herniation. Although degenerative joint disease may be a normal process of aging, symptoms can often be reduced and severe degeneration avoided through identifying and correcting faulty posture and through training geared toward increasing flexibility, muscular strength, and spinal stability.

Intervertebral Disc Herniation

Intervertebral disc **prolapse** (bulge) or herniation can be caused by both acute trauma and cumulative stress mechanisms. Faulty posture, faulty movement mechanics, weak musculature, and inflexibility can all contribute to repetitive microtrauma that weakens the annulus fibrosis and allows **protrusion** and possible **extrusion** or **sequestration** of the disc material (figure 15.11). Twisting and holding a heavy object away from the body while lifting is a frequent mechanism for acute lumbar disc herniation.

While the inner part of the disc is aneural and early protrusion does not cause pain, once the nucleus pulposus herniates through a tear in the annulus fibrosis, the extruded or sequestered portion of the disc exerts pressure on adjacent structures that are richly innervated and compresses the nearby spinal cord (posterior herniation) or nerve root (posterior-lateral herniation) (see chapter 11, figures 11.10 and 11.11). Disc herniation can occur at any level but most frequently occurs at L4/L5 and L5/S1 levels. Posterolateral lesions are more common because of the strong posterior longitudinal ligament that stabilizes the spine and disc. However, central herniations do occur and pressure the **cauda equina**, which can result in **cauda equina syndrome** with loss of bowel or bladder function.

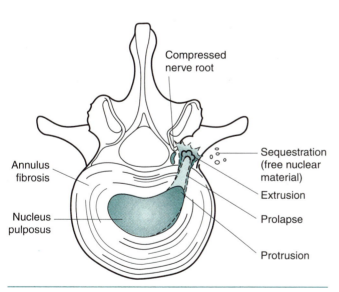

Figure 15.11   Four stages of disc herniation.

Signs and symptoms of disc herniation include centralized back pain, point tenderness over the spinal level, muscle spasm, and **sciatica**, or referred pain along the nerve distribution. Signs and symptoms associated with nerve compression will also be present; these are covered in the next section.

Nerve Compression

Nerve compression injuries of the thoracic and lumbar spine most often involve the nerve roots of the sciatic nerve as they exit the intervertebral foramen of the lumbar vertebrae.

Nerve Compression Injuries of the Lumbar Spine

Nerve compression can result from an encroaching prolapsed or herniated intervertebral disc (see figure 15.11) or from degenerative osteophytes causing stenosis of the intervertebral foramen (figure 15.12). In rare cases, nerve compression may result from excessive forward subluxation of the vertebral body in stage III or IV spondylolisthesis.

When injuries are associated with nerve compression, the patient typically complains of sciatica, or radiating pain down the thigh, lower leg, and foot along the distribution of the sciatic nerve. The specific pain location and pattern depends on the lumbar level at which the nerve is compressed (figure 15.13). Coughing, sneezing, or straining (Valsalva maneuver) significantly increase intrathecal pressure and pain. The patient will list to one side, typically away from the side of nerve root compression. Side-bending and extension with rotation toward the involved side will close down the foraminal space and increase nerve compression and pain. Pain and increased symptoms with special tests, including the straight-leg raise, well straight-leg raise, Hoover, and Kernig tests, indicate nerve compression. You may also note paresthesia or numbness over the specific dermatome, motor weakness of the inner-vated muscles, and a diminished reflex. Patients exhibiting positive neurological signs require immediate referral. If the patient complains of bowel or bladder dysfunction, a cauda equina syndrome may be present, which constitutes a medical emergency.

> ⚠ If a patient complains of changes in bowel or bladder function as a result of a back injury, consider the condition a medical emergency and immediately refer the patient to prevent permanent dysfunction.

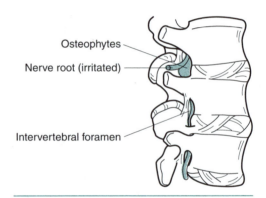

Figure 15.12 Osteophytes and stenosis of intervertebral foramen causing nerve root compression.

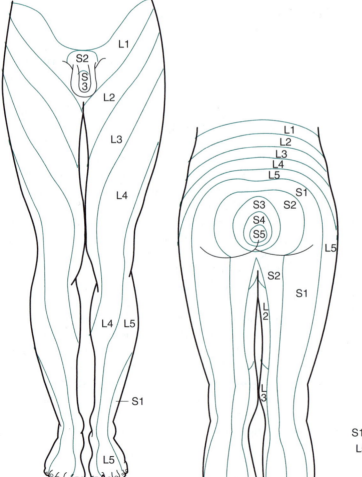

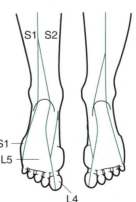

Figure 15.13 Sensory nerve distribution for the lumbar plexus.

Structural and Functional Abnormalities

Other structural and functional abnormalities of the thoracic and lumbar spine are not necessarily symptomatic or associated with trauma. However, you should recognize these abnormalities, as they may contribute to cases of occasional or chronic low back pain. Although some of these abnormalities can be identified only through X ray, others offer visible signs that are easily noted with careful observation.

Café au Lait Spots

Note abnormalities in skin appearance, as they may indicate underlying pathologies. **Café au lait spots**, or darkened patches of skin, indicate collagen disease is affecting the connective tissue.

Spina Bifida Occulta

Spina bifida occulta, a congenital malformation of the lumbar spine, is characterized by incomplete closure of the posterior lamina at birth. The athletic population will include only those with mild cases, as more severe cases would likely preclude activity. Superficial signs indicating this underlying condition include a hairy patch (**faun's beard**), dimpling, and fatty deposits of the skin overlying the lumbar spine. Unless it has been problematic prior to athletic involvement, this condition is not likely to exhibit symptoms except for occasional low back pain. However, those with spina bifida occulta are thought to be more prone than others to have pars interarticularis defects (see the discussion of spondylolysis on pages 355-356).

Scoliosis

Scoliosis, a deformity in which the spinal column has a lateral "C" or "S" curvature (figure 15.14), may be either structural or functional. **Structural deformities** are characterized by permanent structural changes in the bone and are usually congenital. Structural or permanent changes may also result from mechanical dysfunction, ultimately leading to permanent degenerative changes that disrupt the normal contours and motions of the spine over time. With structural scoliosis, the vertebrae are rotated with the anterior body toward the convex side. This rotation causes the posterior ribs and posterior chest wall to be more prominent on the convex side and less prominent, or sunken in, on the concave side.

Functional deformities do not involve permanent bony changes and typically result from mechanical dysfunction due to poor posture, leg length discrepancy, joint inflammation, nerve root irritation, muscular imbalance, soft tissue shortening, or a combination of these. These conditions are marked by observable postural deformity and loss of spinal ROM. A distinguishing factor of functional versus structural curvatures is that functional curvature disappears with forward flexion of the spine. Because of the muscular imbalances and compensatory changes created by these spinal curvatures, patients with scoliosis often complain of pain, muscular fatigue, and spasm in the postural muscles.

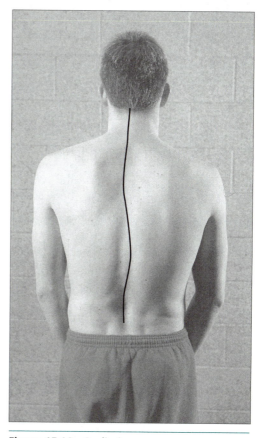

Figure 15.14   Scoliosis.

It is important to recognize functional scoliosis in the physically active and to correct the mechanical dysfunction in order to prevent irreversible structural changes over time.

Kyphosis and Scheuermann's Disease

As discussed in chapter 11, **kyphosis** is an excessive posterior curvature of the upper and midthoracic spine (figure 15.15). The rounded contour of the upper thoracic spine is accentuated secondarily to congenital factors, compensatory changes, muscular imbalance, joint disease, compression fractures, osteoporosis in older adults, and Scheuermann's disease in young persons (see chapter 11, page 203). These conditions are mentioned here as they may cause compensatory pain and dysfunction in the lumbar spine region.

Lordosis

Lordosis, the opposite of kyphosis, is an excessive anterior (forward) curvature of the lumbar spine (figure 15.16). An increased lordotic curve may be congenital, but may also be acquired secondary to muscle imbalances such as weak abdominals, tight hip flexors, and tight back extensors that rotate the pelvis anteriorly. Increased lumbar lordosis can result in low back pain because it increases musculature stress as well as placing stress on the posterior, non-weight-bearing elements of the spine (facet joints).

Ankylosing Spondylitis

Ankylosing spondylitis (AS) is a rheumatic disease that causes arthritis of the spine and sacroiliac joints. According to the American College of Rheumatology (2000), the disease may afflict as many as 129 out of 100,000 people in the United States, mostly affecting adolescents and young adult males. Symptoms can vary from intermittent episodes of back pain to a severe chronic disease that attacks the spine, peripheral joints, and other body organs, resulting in joint and back stiffness, loss of motion, and deformity.

Delayed diagnosis is common because symptoms often mimic more common back problems. Early warning signs include gradual onset of back pain during adolescence or early adulthood (<35 years of age), morning stiffness that improves with physical activity and worsens with inactivity, and symptoms that persist for more than 3 months. Signs and symptoms include a marked decrease in flexibility in the lumbar spine and pain in the lumbar and sacroiliac areas. The patient may also complain of pain in the neck and upper back. Related rheumatic symptoms may include fever, fatigue, weight loss, anemia, and inflammation of the eyes, lungs, and heart valves. You may note arthritic changes on X rays and bone scans.

Lumbarization and Sacralization

Two other structural abnormalities that may contribute to low back pain are lumbarization and sacralization. In **lumbarization**, the S1 vertebral segment remains mobile and separate from the sacrum and appears as a sixth lumbar vertebra on X ray. Conversely, **sacralization** is a congenital fusion of the L5 and S1 vertebrae. On X ray there will appear to be only four lumbar vertebrae. These abnormalities are often asymptomatic but may occasionally contribute to lower back pain in the physically active.

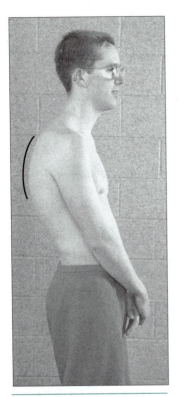

Figure 15.15   Kyphosis.

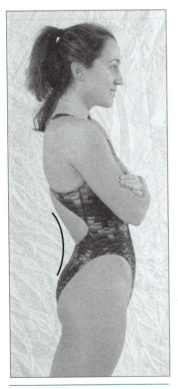

Figure 15.16   Lordosis.

OBJECTIVE TESTS

Because the lumbar spine both mobilizes and stabilizes the upper extremity and torso, it requires adequate motion and strength to perform everyday activities. While lumbar and thoracic pain is most often due to acute and chronic strains of the postural muscles supporting the lumbar region, pain and dysfunction can also result from bone and joint pathology. Objective tests aim to isolate the underlying cause for the pain and dysfunction, and differentiate structural from functional abnormalities.

Palpation

Palpation of the lumbar spine proceeds from superficial to deep layers.

Check first for temperature variations with the back of your hand, moving your hand from the left to right sides of the thoracic, lumbar, and sacral regions. Then palpate the spinal column and pelvis for tenderness, crepitus, or subtle deformity. Palpate the spinous processes, interspaces, transverse processes, ribs and their interspaces, ilium, sacrum, sacroiliac joints, sacrotuberous ligament, and ischial tuberosities for tenderness or abnormal structures. Next examine superficial soft tissue mobility from the thoracic region downward, followed by deeper soft tissue palpation of the muscles. Palpate spinal muscles first, then move to lateral muscles. Routinely include the paraspinals, quadratus lumborum, lateral abdominals, latissimus dorsi, lower trapezius, hip rotators (especially the piriformis), and gluteals. Examine the muscles bilaterally for spasm, tenderness, and any restricted mobility.

Range of Motion

Thoracolumbar ROM includes forward flexion, back extension, lateral flexion, and trunk rotation. Examine active ROM first; if the movement is free of pain, apply an overpressure force to examine passive motion and end feel. Since spine movement is a composite of motions of several vertebral levels, overpressure provides only a gross estimate of end feel. Specific end feel of individual vertebral joints is most appropriately examined through individual joint examination (see the section on joint mobility examination later in this chapter).

Active ROM

It is easiest to observe forward **flexion** by having the patient bend over to touch his toes. You should observe two factors: how far he can reach to the floor and the curvature of the thoracic and lumbar spines as he bends forward. Normal excursion allows the patient to touch the fingers to the floor; if the motion is more limited, measure and document the distance between the fingertips and the floor. A normal curve is smooth and continually rounded from the upper thoracic spine to the sacrum, with movement progressing from one vertebral level to the next as the patient moves into full trunk flexion (figure 15.17). An abnormal curve is apparent when you observe flat sections or sharp angulations (figure 15.18). Remember, you cannot assume that forward flexion motion is normal solely because the patient touches the floor. For example, a straight spine with little segmental movement between the vertebrae can be compensated for by greater hip flexibility. This is why you should note the spine curvature and the way the spine moves in addition to observing how far the patient is able to reach.

The majority of **extension** occurs in the lumbar spine with minimal extension in the thoracic spine. The patient should place both hands in the small of the back to provide stability during extension motion (figure 15.19). As the patient moves into extension, the thoracic curve should become straight and the lumbar curve more lordotic. Normal extension is approximately 30°.

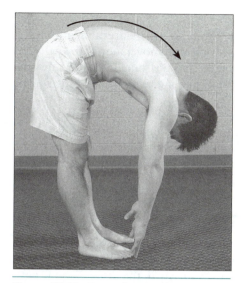

Figure 15.17 Normal active forward flexion.

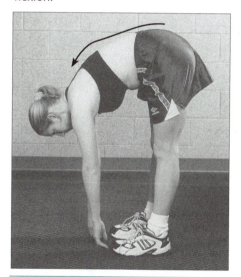

Figure 15.18 Abnormal active forward flexion.

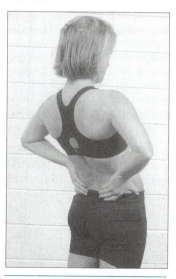

Figure 15.19 Active back extension.

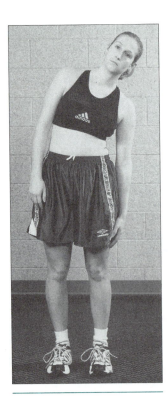

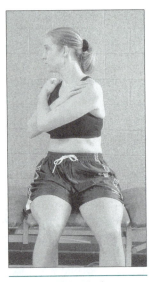

Figure 15.21 Active trunk rotation.

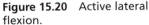

Figure 15.20 Active lateral flexion.

The patient should perform **lateral flexion** without compensatory lateral movement of the pelvis to the opposite side. To limit spinal rotation substitution, instruct the patient to keep her hips square and to run her hand down the lateral thigh as she laterally flexes. As you observe lateral flexion, the thoracolumbar spine should move sequentially as it did during flexion and extension and should produce a smooth curve (figure 15.20). Normal lateral flexion should be equal on both sides and 30 to 40° in each direction.

The patient should perform **rotation** while sitting to eliminate hip and thigh movement. With the arms crossed and hands on opposite shoulders, she rotates to the left and right as far as possible (figure 15.21). Rotation occurs primarily in the thoracic spine with minimal contribution from the lumbar spine and is 50 to 70°.

Passive ROM

If the patient reports pain with any active motion, defer passive motion examination. If no pain is reported, carefully apply passive overpressure to the end of active movement. All motions should produce a soft tissue stretch sensation without a bony or hard end feel. Normally, overpressure is pain free.

Goniometric Examination of ROM

Various measurement techniques (goniometry, inclinometry, and a standard tape measure) are used to examine thoracolumbar ROM. Motions most commonly tested with a tape measure are presented in table 15.1 and demonstrated in figure 15.22 (Clarkson 2000).

Strength

Strength is best examined with the trunk moving against gravity (table 15.2).

Manual Strength Testing

Test abdominals with the patient supine (figure 15.23a-b), lateral flexors in a side-lying position (figure 15.23b), and extensors while prone (figure 15.23c). Strength is usually examined without resistance, as trunk weight alone provides considerable resistance and makes the movement quite challenging.

Instrumented Strength Examination

In some cases you may wish to quantify trunk strength. Dynamometers and other equipment are commercially available for examining trunk strength, but they are rather costly and not available in most athletic treatment facilities. You are more likely to find and use these instruments in industrial health care settings. Less costly alternatives are free and machine weights designed to strengthen the trunk. For examining trunk strength, a 10 repetition maximum (RM) or higher is recommended over a 1RM. The patient should be familiarized and proficient with the desired strength movement before beginning testing.

Neurological Examination

Neurological tests include motor, sensory, and reflex examination of the lumbar plexus. Perform both sensory and motor tests bilaterally, simultaneously whenever possible, so that you can immediately compare sides and identify subtle differences. Neurological examina-

Table 15.1

Tape Measure Examination of Thoracolumbar (TL) and Lumbar (L) ROM

Motion	Location of tape measure	Movement	Measurement	Normal range
TL flexion	Spanning C7 to S2 spinous processes	Begin neutral, bilateral stance (feet shoulder-width apart); trunk moves into forward flexion to limit of motion	Increase in measured distance (cm) between C7 and S2 from neutral stance to full flexion	10 cm
TL extension	Suprasternal notch to surface of table	Begin prone, with pelvis stabilized; trunk raises into a push-up (hands at shoulder level) to limit of motion, without lifting pelvis from the table	Measured distance (cm) between table and suprasternal notch	Will vary with stature
L flexion	Spanning distance from S2 to a mark 10 cm superiorly	Begin neutral, bilateral stance (feet shoulder-width apart); trunk moves into forward flexion to limit of motion	Increase in measured distance (cm) between mark and S2 from neutral stance to full flexion	5 cm
L extension	Spanning distance from S2 to a mark 10 cm superiorly	Begin neutral, bilateral stance (feet shoulder-width apart) and hands on the iliac crests; trunk moves into hyperextension to limit of motion	Decrease in measured distance (cm) between mark and S2 from neutral stance to full hyperextension	2 cm
Lateral flexion	Spanning fingertip to floor surface	Begin neutral, bilateral stance (feet shoulder-width apart); side bend to limit of motion (watch for trunk rotation, hip hike, and lateral deviation of pelvis)	Distance (cm) between 3rd fingertip to floor	Will vary with stature—should be equal bilaterally
Trunk rotation	None—observation only			
Muscle length (toe touch)	Spanning fingertip to floor surface	Begin neutral, bilateral stance (feet shoulder-width apart); trunk moves into forward flexion to limit of motion— attempts to reach toes	Distance (cm) between 3rd finger tip to floor	Able to touch floor. For hypermobility, have athlete stand on box and record distance beyond box surface
Costo-vertebral motion	Place the tape measure circumferentially around the athlete's chest just below the axilla (T4)	Maximal expiration followed by maximal inspiration	Difference (cm) between end inspiration and expiration	3 to 7.5 cm

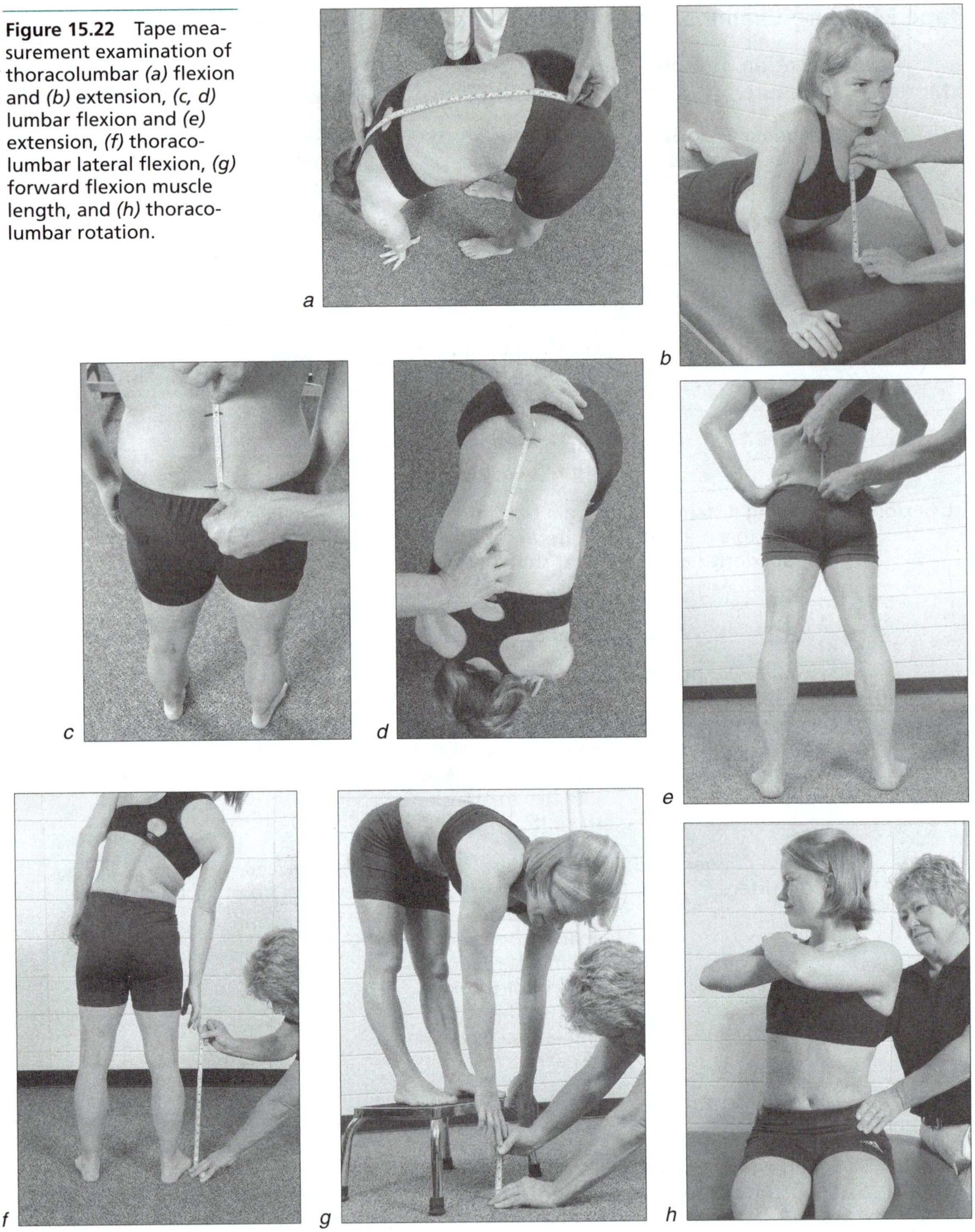

Figure 15.22 Tape measurement examination of thoracolumbar *(a)* flexion and *(b)* extension, *(c, d)* lumbar flexion and *(e)* extension, *(f)* thoracolumbar lateral flexion, *(g)* forward flexion muscle length, and *(h)* thoracolumbar rotation.

tion procedures and examination checklists for the lumbar plexus are detailed in chapter 8 and briefly reviewed here.

Sensory Testing

Perform sensory testing for the lumbar plexus with light touch or pinprick methods over the anterior thigh (L2), the medial aspect of the knee (L3), the medial lower leg (L4), the lateral lower leg and dorsum of the foot (L5), the lateral plantar foot (S1), and the posterior thigh (popliteal fossa) and posterior lateral heel (S2) (see table 8.7 and figure 8.13).

Table 15.2
Manual Muscle Tests for the Thoracolumbar Spine

Motion	Athlete position	Stabilizing hand placement	Resistance hand placement	Instruction to athlete	Primary muscles tested
Trunk flexion	Supine, hook-lying position	None required	None required	With hands at ear level, perform an abdominal curl; if unable to complete full motion (grade 5), move hands to chest (grade 4), then to sides (grade 3)	Rectus abdominis
Trunk rotation	Supine, hook-lying position	None required	None required	With hands at ear level, perform an abdominal curl toward the right and then toward the left knee; if unable to complete full motion (grade 5), move hands to chest (grade 4), then to sides (grade 3)	Internal and external abdominal obliques
Lateral flexion	Side-lying	Lower extremities	None required	Lift shoulders and trunk off table with hands at ear level (grade 5), across chest (grade 4), or at sides (grade 3)	Abdominal obliques and erector spinae working unilaterally
Trunk extension	Prone, pelvis stabilized	Lower extremities	None required	Lift head and shoulders off the table with hands behind head (grade 5), behind back (grade 4), or at sides (grade 3)	Erector spinae

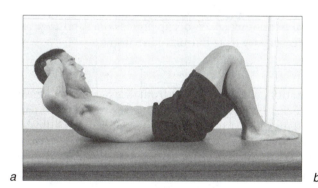

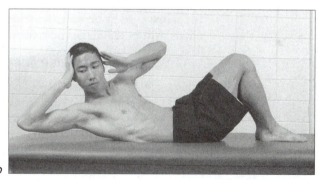

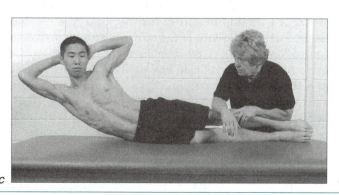

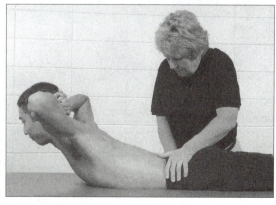

Figure 15.23 Strength testing for (a) trunk flexion, (b) trunk rotation, (c) side-lying lateral trunk flexion, and (d) prone trunk extension.

Motor Testing

Motor tests include manual resistance to hip flexion (L1-L2), knee extension (L3-L4), ankle dorsiflexion (L4), great toe extension (L5), ankle eversion or hip extension (S1), and knee flexion (S2). These tests are also described in table 8.7 and demonstrated in figure 8.15 of chapter 8.

Reflex Testing

To examine deep tendon reflex and to differentiate between an upper and lower motor neuron lesion, perform brisk tendon taps over the patellar tendon (L3-L4), Achilles tendon (S1-S2), and medial hamstring tendon (L5-S1) with a reflex hammer. An involved nerve root or peripheral nerve will diminish the reflex, whereas a central cord lesion may exhibit a hyperreflexivity. Refer to chapter 8, table 8.4 and figure 8.17, for the description of these tests. The reflex grading scale is provided on page 123 (table 8.3).

Special Tests

Special tests for the lumbar spine examine neuropathies, spinal cord lesions, and joint dysfunction.

Neuropathy Tests

Neuropathy tests identify neurological dysfunctions such as disc herniation or nerve irritation caused by nerve compression, inflammation of the nerve or its sheath, or restricted tissue mobility.

Valsalva Maneuver

Intrathecal describes a location within the spinal canal.

The **Valsalva maneuver** examines for a herniated disc or other space occupying lesion within the spinal canal. To perform the test, have the patient take a deep breath and hold it while bearing down as if moving the bowels, or blow into a closed fist (see chapter 11, figure 11.26). This technique increases intrathecal pressure and pain if pressure is being applied to the spinal cord by herniated disc material or another space-occupying lesion. A positive sign elicits pain in the nerve root and along its sensory distribution (dermatome).

Straight-Leg Raise Test

This test identifies sciatic nerve root irritation, which can result from disc herniation, muscle spasm (especially in the piriformis), facet pathology, or sciatic nerve restriction or inflammation. When the test includes dorsiflexion and neck flexion, it is known as **Lasegue's test**. Perform it passively with the patient supine. Position the patient's hip in internal rotation and adduction with the knee in full extension. Then, slowly flex the hip until the patient reports pain in the back or leg or until you perceive tightness in the posterior thigh. Then reposition the leg in slightly less hip flexion so that the pain resolves. Next, passively dorsiflex the foot either with or without active neck flexion (figure 15.24). A positive result occurs if the patient reports a return of the leg pain first noted with the straight-leg raise. Normal ROM for a straight-leg raise should be 80 to 90°. Disc involvement limits the straight-leg raise to about 30°. Pain in the 50° to 70° range can indicate nerve irritation without disc herniation.

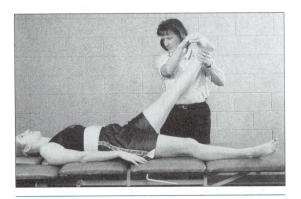

Figure 15.24 Straight-leg raise.

Well Straight-Leg Test

This test identifies a large disc lesion that protrudes medially to the nerve root. Perform the straight-leg test already described on the uninvolved side. A positive sign occurs if the patient reports pain on the involved side with the straight-leg raise of the uninvolved leg.

Kernig-Brudzinski Test

This active test determines nerve root, meningeal, or dural irritation and is actually a combination of two separate tests, the **Kernig test** and the **Brudzinski test**. In the Kernig test, only the neck is flexed (figure 15.25); in the Brudzinski test, only the hip motion is performed to tension neural structures and elicit symptoms.

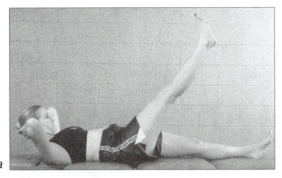

Figure 15.25 Kernig test.

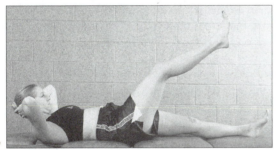

a

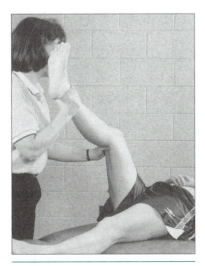

In the Kernig-Brudzinski test, the patient lies supine with both hands clasped behind the head and both legs extended. She flexes the neck to bring the chin to the chest; then actively flexes the hip with the knee extended until she feels pain in the back or leg (figure 15.26a). Keeping the hip in the position where pain is first felt, flex the patient's knee (figure 15.26b). The test is positive if the pain disappears.

Bowstring Test

The bowstring, a modification of the straight-leg test, is also called the **cram test**, or **popliteal pressure test**. It identifies compression or tension on the sciatic nerve. With the patient supine, move the leg into a straight-leg raise until you produce radicular pain. Then flex the knee slightly (about 20°) to relieve the pain and apply pressure to the popliteal fossa with your thumbs or fingers (figure 15.27). The test is positive if the patient reports a return of the pain with popliteal pressure.

Hoover Test

Use the Hoover test only when you feel it necessary to find out whether the patient is **malingering** (pretending to be injured) or is truly unable to lift the leg. With the patient supine, place one hand under each heel and lift both heels slightly off the table. Then instruct the patient to try to lift one of the legs. If the patient is truly trying, you should feel a downward or counterpressure of the oppositive heel against your other hand (figure 15.28). If you do not feel any pressure on the other hand, the patient is most likely not giving a full effort.

b

Figure 15.26 Kernig-Brudzinski test: *(a)* extension and *(b)* flexion of the knee.

Radicular describes pain referred into the extremity.

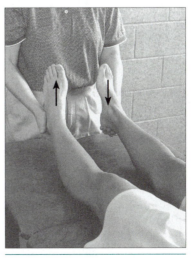

Figure 15.27 Bowstring test.

Figure 15.28 Hoover test.

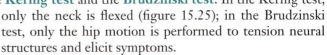

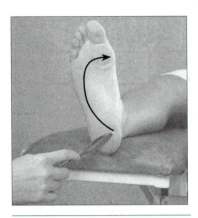

Figure 15.29 Babinski test.

Tests for Spinal Cord Lesions

Tests for upper motor neuron (spinal cord) lesions include the

- Babinski (figure 15.29),
- Chaddock,
- clonus,
- Gordon, and
- Oppenheim tests.

These pathological reflex tests are described in detail in chapter 8 (see table 8.4).

Joint Dysfunction Tests

The joint dysfunction tests determine joint integrity of the lumbar spine or sacroilium. You should rule out pathology in these areas when patients complain of lower lumbar pain.

Stork Standing Test

This active test is also known as the **spondylolisthesis test** or the **single leg stance test**. While balancing on one leg, the patient extends the spine backward (figure 15.30) and then repeats the test on the opposite side. If the test produces back pain, the patient may have a pars fracture. If the pain occurs while the patient stands on one leg but not the other, the pars fracture may be unilateral. In the case of unilateral pain, pathology is typically present on the same side as the support leg.

Spring Test

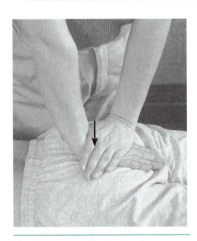

The passive spring test determines whether or not the sacroiliac joint is the source of the patient's pain. The patient is prone with a rolled towel under the anterior superior iliac spine (ASIS) bilaterally. Place the base of one of your hands over the apex of the patient's sacrum and place your other hand on top of the first hand. A shear stress between the sacrum and ilium occurs when you apply downward pressure over the apex of the sacrum (figure 15.31). Pain is the positive sign. If you find pain or dysfunction in the sacroiliac region, perform other special tests for the sacroiliac joint as described in chapter 18.

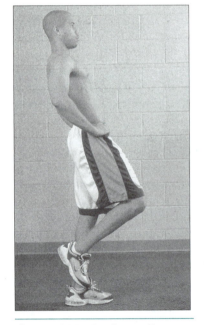

Figure 15.30 Stork standing test.

Figure 15.31 Spring test.

Joint Mobility

Abnormal end feel is the primary reason to examine joint mobility of the thoracolumbar spine. Examine pain and joint play along with joint mobility. For all the procedures described here, the patient is prone. It may be necessary to position a pillow under the abdomen for comfort.

Caudal means away from the head.

Cephalad means toward the head.

Before joint mobility examination, palpate the spinous processes of the middle and lower thoracic and lumbar vertebrae for alignment and tenderness. T7 is at the level of the inferior angle of the scapula, and the L4 and L5 interspace is at the level of the crest of the ilium. To begin joint mobility assessment, palpate each spinous process either from caudal to cephalad or cephalad to caudal. Posterior–anterior (PA) vertebral pressure can be applied centrally and unilaterally. Apply a central PA pressure over each spinous process, directing pressure from your shoulders through your thumbs (figure 15.32). Apply the force slowly and precisely in order to determine end feel movement, excursion, and quality. Also apply unilateral PA force with the thumbs through a vertical force from the shoulders, but apply it lateral to the spinous process over the transverse process of each vertebra. Compare the left and right sides of each level. The degree of movement and end feel should be the same and should be pain free bilaterally.

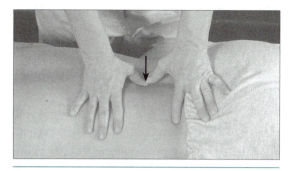

Figure 15.32 Examination of central posterior–anterior (PA) mobility over the spinous process.

INJURY EXAMINATION STRATEGIES

Back pain, a frequent complaint in the physically active, commonly results from acute traumatic episodes as well as cumulative stress. Although not usual in sport, the most severe consequence of a back injury is paralysis. You must be able to quickly and effectively recognize the signs and symptoms of a serious back injury and manage it accordingly to prevent further injury and neurological insult. However, the majority of examinations will take place in the clinic or treatment facility on athletes with postacute or chronic low back complaints. Even then there is potential for nerve root compression and neurological deficits, and you must recognize these symptoms early to ensure appropriate care and complete restoration. Whenever examining back pain, remember that pain experienced in the thoracic and lumbar spine can also be referred from the viscera or can be a result of lower-extremity dysfunction. Conversely, pain in the lower extremity can be caused by back pathology. It is vital to consider these relationships when examining the low back.

On-Site Examination

It was nearing the end of the third quarter with less than 2 minutes on the clock. Ryan knew he needed to make this reception if his team was to stay in the game. The ball was a little off target, coming high and to the inside of the field. As Ryan leapt to catch the ball, he was hit off balance and landed hard on his buttocks. He felt immediate pain in his lower back and a dull ache radiating into both legs. After landing, he lay on his side, afraid to move.

When approaching a downed athlete with a back injury on the field, observing his response and movement provides immediate and important clues to the extent of the injury. If the athlete is rolling around and trying to move, even though in pain, a spinal cord injury is of little concern. But if the athlete is lying very still, you must consider the potential for a serious back and spinal cord injury.

Primary Survey

Once at the athlete's side, perform a primary survey: Examine the level of consciousness; airway, breathing, and circulation; severe bleeding; obvious signs of deformity or trauma; and look for signs of shock. If the athlete is unconscious, assume a serious spine injury and stabilize the head and neck. If the athlete is conscious and not moving, determine why. If the reason is that the athlete can't or won't move because of pain or fear, you must consider a serious spine injury until you have proven otherwise.

Secondary Survey

Once you have confirmed that the athlete's vital signs are stable, begin your secondary survey by obtaining a brief history of what happened, whether or not you observed the injury. Knowing whether the injury was caused by a helmet directed at the small of the back, a tackle through the shoulder resulting in axial loading of the thoracic and lumbar spine, or a noncontact twisting motion will help you determine the nature of the injury. Gain a clear picture of the type and location of the athlete's pain and symptoms before moving or allowing the athlete to move. Find out whether the pain is centralized over the spine or lateral over the musculature; also determine if the athlete felt any unusual sensations of numbness, burning, or tingling at the time of injury and whether he feels them now. Is the athlete able to wiggle the toes? If there is radiating pain, numbness, or inability to move the lower extremities, suspect a serious spine injury.

If these symptoms are negative except for centralized back pain, perform a cursory sensory and motor neurological examination before moving the athlete. Examine for sensation bilaterally with light touch on the upper thigh (L2), medial knee (L3), medial lower leg (L4), dorsum of the foot (L5), and lateral foot (S1). Since a spinal injury can affect both extremities equally, compare the sensation of light touch in the lower extremity to that in the upper extremity. For motor tests, have the athlete dorsiflex the foot and big toe and plantar flex the foot against your resistance, noting any change in symptoms or muscle weakness.

Checklist for On-Site Examination of the Lumbar and Thoracic Spine

▷ *Primary Survey*

- ☐ Check surroundings and environment
- ☐ Gain history from bystanders if you did not witness
- ☐ Note position of body
- ☐ Consciousness
- ☐ Airway, breathing, and circulation
- ☐ Check for severe bleeding
- ☐ Check for movement of the extremities

▷ *Secondary Survey (Examine in the Position Found)*

- ☐ If athlete is unconscious, manage as a serious spinal injury

If conscious, examine the following:

- ☐ Presence and location of back pain
- ☐ Sensations of numbness, tingling, or burning
- ☐ Difficulty in moving extremities

If any of these are positive, assume serious spine injury. If back pain only:

- ☐ Sensory testing over L2-S1 dermatomes
- ☐ Motor testing for dorsiflexion, big toe dorsiflexion, plantar flexion
- ☐ Palpation for tenderness and deformity

If signs are positive, assume serious spine injury. If signs are negative:

- ☐ Perform active ROM of lower extremities
- ☐ Examine for sensory changes with motion

If signs are positive, assume serious spine injury. If negative:

- ☐ Allow athlete to sit, then stand, then move off-site for further examination
- ☐ Continue to monitor vitals
- ☐ Continue to check sensory and motor function in extremities

If you find no neurological deficits, palpate the lumbar spine for any tenderness along the spinous processes. Although this may be difficult if the athlete is lying supine, you can typically reach your hand under the small of the back without moving the athlete. If pain is present over the spine, assume a serious spine injury. If there is no central spine pain and the pain is primarily in the surrounding musculature, ask the athlete to actively move the legs and examine for any changes in sensation. If your examination has shown that the athlete does not have a serious lumbar or lower thoracic spine injury, and the pain is not so severe that the athlete is unable to ambulate, you can slowly move the athlete to sitting and then standing. If her condition remains unchanged during standing, assist the athlete off the field to a location where you can perform an acute examination.

If at any time you suspect a serious spinal injury, notify emergency medical services and take every precaution to transport the athlete according to the correct procedures. Fortunately, most lumbar injuries are not this extreme and include only temporarily painful but not life-changing signs and symptoms. The most immediate symptom with a back injury is often muscle spasm. If severe enough, this can cause immediate pain and disability that prevents the athlete from ambulating unaided. When performing an on-site examination, you must determine the injury severity and whether the athlete needs passive transport off the field.

For a discussion of procedures for transporting an athlete with a suspected spinal injury, refer to *Introduction to Athletic Training, Second Edition,* (Hillman 2005), chapter 8.

Acute Examination

Recall Max from the opening scenario. Max was fatigued when he bent over and reached for a heavy box at his side. Instead of turning around to get a better angle, he took a deep breath and lifted it hard and fast. At once, a searing pain shot through his back and left lower leg and he dropped the box with a gasp. He could barely stand and needed assistance to get to the industrial clinic.

You will perform an acute examination in the event that an athlete walks off the field with a low back injury or as a follow-up to any on-site examination. Since the postural muscles of the back and trunk are active in any position except lying down, the patient may be most comfortable in a reclined position as you conduct the history portion of the examination. If a table is not available at the sideline, it may be best to move the patient into the treatment facility if feasible, since getting up and down from the ground may be difficult for an athlete in acute pain and spasm. If a table is not available and a facility is not close by, use your best judgment as to whether the patient can remain standing for early portions of the examination. Here is a summary of the acute examination procedures for the lower thoracic and lumbar spine.

History

Once on the sideline, reexamine the patient's perception of the location, quality, and severity of the pain. Ask again about the injury mechanism and any unusual sensations the athlete may be experiencing. This is also the time to obtain a history regarding any past injuries to the lumbar or thoracic spine. If the patient has a history of back pain, determine the number, severity, and duration of previous injury episodes and find out about their treatment or examination.

Observation

As usual, your observation should begin when the patient comes off the field. Observe for freedom versus guarding of movement. When the patient left the field, was he able to easily straighten, or were his movements slow and painful? Patients with acute low back injuries are often quite guarded, which can make examination difficult. Observe the patient's posture—is it different than normal? If you have the patient recline on a table, note any difficulty or hesitancy as the patient gets onto the table, and observe how well he moves from side-lying to supine. As you prepare for the objective examination, make the same observations as the

Checklist for Acute Examination of the Lumbar and Thoracic Spine

▷ History

Ask questions pertaining to the following:

- ☐ Chief complaint
- ☐ Mechanism of injury
- ☐ Unusual sensations of numbness, tingling, burning pain into the lower extremities
- ☐ Type and location of pain or symptoms
- ☐ Previous injury (number of prior episodes and comparison with current episode)

▷ Observation

- ☐ Visible facial expressions of pain
- ☐ Swelling, deformity, abnormal contours, or discoloration
- ☐ Freedom of movement and ability to get on and off the table
- ☐ Overall position, posture, and alignment
- ☐ Muscle development—are there areas of muscular spasm or atrophy?

▷ Palpation

Bilaterally palpate for pain, temperature, tenderness, spasm, and restricted mobility:

- ☐ Bony: spinous processes, interspaces and interspinous ligament, ilium, sacrum, sacroiliac joint, sacrotuberous ligament, ischial tuberosities
- ☐ Soft tissue (superficial to deep): paraspinals, quadratus lumborum, abdominals, latissimus dorsi, lower trapezius, hip rotators (piriformis), gluteals

▷ Special Tests

- ☐ Neuropathy tests (Valsalva, straight and well leg raise, Kernig-Brudzinski, bowstring)
- ☐ Joint dysfunction tests (stork, spring)

▷ Range of Motion

- ☐ Active ROM for forward flexion, extension, lateral flexion, and rotation
- ☐ Passive ROM for the same motions if nonpainful in active ROM
- ☐ Costovertebral motion

▷ Strength Tests

- ☐ Active ROM against gravity and weight of trunk for abdominals, lateral flexion, and extension

▷ Neurological Tests

- ☐ Sensory for L2-S2
- ☐ Motor for L2-S2
- ☐ Reflex (patellar, hamstring, and Achilles tendons)

▷ Functional Tests

patient gets off the table and returns to standing. Once the patient is standing, note any immediate signs of swelling, discoloration, deformities, unusual markings, obvious muscle spasm, or irregularities. Observe the lumbar spine for symmetry and correct alignment. From the side, check for a normal lumbar curve; when standing behind the patient, check for soft tissue balance and straightness versus lateral curvature of the spine.

Palpation

As with the acute examination of other body areas, palpation follows your observations and moves from superficial to deep structures. The patient should be prone during your examination to allow the back musculature to relax, facilitating palpation. When you begin palpating, move systematically throughout the thoracic and lumbar spine regions.

Special Tests

Use special tests in the acute examination to rule out or investigate neurological pathology or joint dysfunction.

Range of Motion

If the patient is able to stand, attempt active ROM testing of the trunk and lumbar spine and examine for quality and quantity of movement in all planes. If the patient reports pain with any active motion, defer passive motion examination. If no pain is reported, you can cautiously apply overpressure at the end of the movement.

Strength

Perform AROM against gravity to examine muscle function and dynamic trunk stability. Although a treatment table will likely not be available, these tests can be performed with more limited motion on the ground or floor.

Neurological Tests

Perform neurological testing when the patient reports weakness, referred pain, numbness, or tingling into the lower extremities. Be sure to examine sensory, motor, and reflex responses bilaterally.

Functional Tests

Since functional tests are usually part of clinical examination rather than acute examination, they are discussed under that section (see page 376).

Clinical Examination

Kim was in her third year of competitive NCAA Division I gymnastics. The pain she was experiencing in her back was getting to be too much to bear. It was no longer restricted to hard landings and dismounts, and she was having difficulty just bending forward. Her pain and stiffness upon waking in the morning was nearing a severity of 7 out of 10. Although she knew the coach wouldn't like it, she decided it was time to visit a professional about her pain.

It is common for patients to report back injuries or back pain some time after their onset. Because the back is complex and has many structures that can be the source of pain, and because many of those structures can refer pain to the lower extremities, examination of back injuries is a challenging task. It can be difficult to narrow down potential causes of the pain and identify the source of the problem. A systematic approach that uses a thorough history to limit the possibilities along with a complete objective examination that pinpoints and confirms your suspicions is invaluable. Many elements of the acute examination are used in the clinical examination. The primary distinguishing factors are the breadth of the history, observation, and differential diagnosis examinations. Quantitative techniques for ROM and strength are also especially valuable in the clinical examination.

History

In addition to taking the history as outlined for the acute examination, make further inquiries when examining a patient in the clinic. Since the injury is postacute or chronic at this point, other questions will help you obtain a better history of the nature, duration, and irritability of the patient's symptoms.

- **Nature.** When asking about unusual sensations such as numbness, tingling, or burning pain into the leg, include questions regarding any changes in or difficulty with coordination (e.g., tripping), urination, or bowel movements. If the patient complains of urinary or bowel dysfunction, immediately refer him to a physician. Try to get a sense of the quality and nature of the pain—whether it is superficial or deep, localized or radiating, central over the spine or lateral in the musculature. Ask about aggravating symptoms, such as increased pain with coughing, sneezing, or laughing, that may indicate a disc lesion. Determine whether the pain changes with activity or during the course of the day. Pain with activity may be related to disc pathology, whereas arthritic pain will be worse in the morning and ease with some activity. If pain is activity related, ask what motions cause the most pain, and if the pain increases or decreases with sitting, standing, walking, or getting up from a chair. Standing and walking are extension activities, while sitting is a flexion activity; mechanical dysfunctions can be related to both.
- **Duration.** To determine the duration of symptoms, ask the patient when and where his pain initially occurred. Determine whether the pain has been intermittent or constant and whether it has improved or intensified over time. Most pain is intermittent and normally changes over time. Rarely is it constant or consistent over time, and patients with this type of pain may have psychological overlay.
- **Irritability.** To get a sense of the condition's irritability, ask how intense the pain is when it occurs and how long it lasts. Very irritable injuries become painful easily and persist, while less irritable conditions may exhibit delayed pain into or after an activity and have shorter durations. Disruption of sleep patterns also suggests increased irritability.
- **Previous injury history.** Obtain a history of any previous injury to the back, including information about the number and frequency of earlier episodes and a specific account of the most recent episode, treatments and their success or failure, medications received, examinations performed, and prior identification of the injury. If the patient is taking medications, find out what they are, as some medications may mask the pain or aid in relieving inflammation, clouding the picture.

Observation

Your observation begins from the moment you see the patient and continues through the history portion of the examination. Does the patient sit and move comfortably or hesitate with movement? Does the patient maintain a position without difficulty or change positions frequently? Does the patient avoid certain positions, such as standing or sitting? Is the gait normal? You should perform a posture examination as outlined in chapter 4 before conducting any other portion of the objective examination. Consider posture from anterior, lateral, and posterior views. A postural checklist is provided on pages 53-54.

For further discussion on posture examination, refer to *Therapeutic Exercise for Musculoskeletal Injuries, Second Edition,* (Houglum 2005), chapter 11.

Differential Diagnosis

Differential diagnosis is the component that differs between the acute and clinical examination. Since the spine can refer into the lower extremities and present symptoms similar to those of many other injuries, conduct a differential diagnosis to rule out injuries within the extremities and sacroiliac region is necessary.

Full Squat Test

A quick test for the lower extremities is a full squat test. Ask the patient to go into a full squat while you observe quality and quantity of motion. The patient should be able to fully flex the hips and knees while keeping both heels on the floor, and she should be able to maneuver easily into full flexion and then into full standing. If the patient hesitates or is unable to complete the exercise, further examine the lower extremities.

Sacroiliac Dysfunction

Sacroiliac dysfunction is quickly identified with the patient standing. Stand behind the patient and place one thumb on a posterior superior iliac spine (PSIS) and the other thumb on the sacral spinous process. The patient then flexes the hip of the palpated PSIS (figure 15.33a). The thumb on the PSIS should move caudally; the test is abnormal if the PSIS moves upward. Repeat the test on the other side with one thumb on the opposite PSIS and the other on the sacral spinous process. Next, place one thumb on an ischial tuberosity and the other on the central apex. When the patient flexes the ipsilateral hip, the ischial tuberosity should move laterally; the result is abnormal if it moves upward (figure 15.33b). Repeat this test on the opposite side. If these tests are positive, the sacroiliac joint requires further investigation.

Range of Motion

Active and passive movements are consistent with those previously described for the acute examination. In addition, you perform a more quantitative examination, recording ROM with a tape measure (measure reach distance from ground), goniometer, or inclinometer as described in the objective tests section of this chapter.

Strength

Manual resistance strength tests are consistent with those described previously. Additionally, if you are fortunate to have isokinetic or other back strength testing equipment available, use it to identify specific weaknesses. The trunk flexors are generally not as strong as the trunk extensors. If the patient reports any possible nerve root or referred pain symptoms, avoid rotation tests and perform machine testing with caution to avoid aggravating the injury.

Neurological Tests

In addition to the standard neurological testing, a variety of sensory tests, such as temperature, deep pressure, or vibration, can further identify sensory deficiencies; use the same dermatome, myotome, and reflex distribution patterns as previously described to identify levels of involvement (see chapter 8, tables 8.4 and 8.7 and figures 8.13, 8.15, and 8.17). If no neurological deficiencies with symptoms distal to the gluteal fold are evident, you can defer the neurological examination. In the absence of symptoms, the examination would be negative.

Special Tests

The same tests that were described for the acute examination can be used in the athletic training clinic. Although many other special tests are

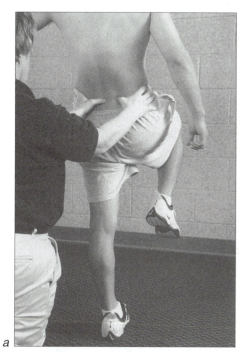
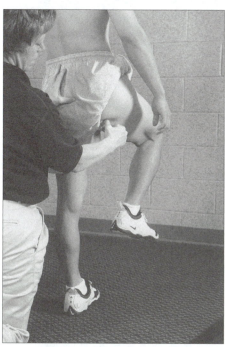

Figure 15.33 Sacroiliac dysfunction tests: (a) Upward movement of PSIS and (b) upward movement of the ischial tuberosity when flexing the ipsilateral hip are considered abnormal.

available to examine the low back for neuropathology and joint dysfunction, those presented in this chapter are most commonly used for athletic injuries.

Palpation

Palpation should be an integral part of the clinical examination. Soft tissue with areas of tenderness and limited mobility can be a common source of pain in patients with a history of previous injuries and in older patients. Note any evidence of active trigger points and areas of myofascial restriction.

Functional Tests

Perform functional tests only if the patient has minimal symptoms and has full, unrestricted mobility. While the patient is performing these tests, observe closely for any hesitation; lack of normal movement, power, and flexibility; inability to bend, cut, turn, twist, or make contact with opponents; reduced quality in stride, throw, or stroke; diminished effort; or lack of confidence. You should examine the patient's condition after the functional tests, since postactivity pain or spasm commonly occurs if a back injury is not completely resolved. If the patient executes all tests well, has no pain or muscle spasm, displays confidence in skill execution, and has normal ROM, strength, agility, and performance, she is able to return to full sport participation.

Checklist for Clinical Examination of the Lumbar and Thoracic Spine

▷ History

Ask questions pertaining to the following:
- ☐ Chief complaint
- ☐ Mechanism of injury
- ☐ Unusual sensations of numbness, tingling, burning pain into the lower extremities
- ☐ Bowel or bladder dysfunction
- ☐ Type, quality, and location of pain or symptoms
- ☐ Previous injury (number of prior episodes and comparison with current episode)

If chronic, ascertain:
- ☐ Onset and duration of symptoms and pain patterns over time
- ☐ Aggravating and easing factors
- ☐ Irritability of symptoms

▷ Observation

- ☐ Visible facial expressions of pain
- ☐ Swelling, deformity, abnormal contours, or discoloration
- ☐ Ability to sit, stand comfortably; freedom of movement versus guarding
- ☐ Overall position, posture, and alignment
- ☐ Muscle development—are there areas of muscular spasm or atrophy (compare bilaterally)?

▷ Differential Diagnosis

- ☐ Squat test
- ☐ Sacroiliac dysfunction

▷ *Range of Motion*

- ☐ Active ROM for forward flexion, extension, lateral flexion, and rotation
- ☐ Passive ROM for same motions if nonpainful in active ROM
- ☐ Costovertebral motion

▷ *Strength Tests*

- ☐ Active ROM against gravity and weight of trunk for trunk flexion (abdominals), lateral flexion, and extension

▷ *Neurological Tests (If Pain or Symptoms Below the Gluteal Fold)*

- ☐ Sensory for L2-S1
- ☐ Motor for L2-S2
- ☐ Reflex (patellar and Achilles tendons)

▷ *Special Tests*

- ☐ Neuropathy tests (Valsalva, straight and well leg raise, Kernig-Brudzinski, bowstring)
- ☐ Joint dysfunction tests (stork, spring)
- ☐ Spinal cord lesion tests (as indicated)

▷ *Joint Mobility Examination*

- ☐ Central PAs over spinous processes
- ☐ Unilateral PAs over transverse processes

▷ *Palpation*

Palpate for increased temperature, pain, tenderness, spasm, and restricted mobility:

- ☐ Bony: spinous processes, interspaces and interspinous ligament, ilium, sacrum, sacroiliac joint, sacrotuberous ligament, ischial tuberosities
- ☐ Soft tissue (superficial to deep): paraspinals, quadratus lumborum, abdominals, latissimus dorsi, lower trapezius, hip rotators (piriformis), gluteals

▷ *Functional Tests*

- ☐ Check for normal and unrestricted movement
- ☐ Check ability to bend, turn out, cut, twist, run, stride
- ☐ Check for postactivity pain and spasm

SUMMARY

1. Describe the etiology, signs and symptoms, and potential complications associated with acute and chronic injuries of the thoracic and lumbar spine commonly encountered in the physically active.

   Physical activity places tremendous mechanical loads on the lumbar spine, making it susceptible to injury. Lumbar and thoracic pain is most often due to acute and chronic strains of the postural muscles supporting the lumbar region. Chronic strain may result from poor posture, poor mechanics, weakness, stiffness, and muscle restrictions. Occasionally congenital defects or degenerative changes cause low back pain. Traumatic injuries such as fractures may also occur, and you must always consider the potential for a spinal cord injury and paralysis with severe injuries.

2. Describe the congenital and degenerative conditions of the thoracic and lumbar spine.

> On occasion, low back pain results from a congenital weakness or degenerative changes with repetitive stress over time. Spondylolysis is thought to result from congenital weakness of the pars interarticularis. This condition is most often seen in young, skeletally immature athletes. If the defect is bilateral, spondylolisthesis, or forward slippage of the vertebrae, may result. In older adults, degenerative changes may be the culprit, causing back pain and ranging from chronic inflammatory conditions to degenerative disc changes to osteophyte formation. Poor posture, weak abdominals and back musculature, and poor mechanics often mechanically stress the spine.

3. Describe the common causes, signs and symptoms, and indicative tests for nerve root compression in the lumbar spine.

> Nerve root compression can be caused by any space-occupying lesion that impinges on the spinal cord or nerve root. Lumbar disc lesions often cause nerve root compression due to disc herniation into the central or intervertebral foramen. Osteophytes resulting from degenerative changes may also narrow the intervertebral foramen and pressure the nerve. The signs and symptoms of a nerve root compression include pain into the lower extremity along the distribution of the involved nerve root, paresthesia along the dermatome, motor weakness, and diminished reflex. Special tests that tension the nerve root and increase intrathecal pressure elicit pain and increase symptoms. Signs and symptoms of bladder and bowel dysfunction can occur with compression of the cauda equine, which constitutes a medical emergency.

4. Identify the characteristics of and potential contributing factors to functional and structural deformities in the thoracic and lumbar spine.

> Structural and functional deformities of the lumbar spine are not uncommon; they include lumbarization of the spine, spina bifida occulta, scoliosis, and excessive thoracic kyphosis and lumbar lordosis. Whereas structural deformities are characterized by a permanent structural change that is often congenital, functional deformities are usually caused by mechanical stress, muscle imbalance, and dysfunction. However, a functional deformity can ultimately become a structural deformity if it leads to degenerative and permanent changes in the spine.

5. Describe and demonstrate the objective tests for examining the lower thoracic and lumbar spine.

> While lumbar and thoracic pain most often result from acute and chronic strains of the postural muscles supporting the lumbar region, it can also result from bone and joint pathology. Objective tests aim to isolate the underlying cause of the pain and dysfunction and to differentiate structural from functional abnormalities. Palpation is best performed with the patient relaxed and supine. ROM testing for the thoracolumbar region includes passive and active motions for forward flexion, back extension, lateral flexion, and trunk rotation. Strength testing for these motions is best examined with the trunk working against gravity. Neurological tests include motor, sensory, and reflex examination of the lumbar plexus (L1-S2) and are performed bilaterally. Special tests identify the presence and location of neuropathies, joint dysfunction, and spinal cord lesions.

6. Perform an on-site examination of the lumbar spine, identifying criteria for immediate medical referral and transportation from the field.

> Although severe, life-changing injuries to the lumbar spine are uncommon in sport, you must be constantly aware that they are a possibility and must rule them out before removing the athlete from the playing field. If you find any evidence of sensory or motor deficits or centralized spine pain, immobilize the athlete and transport her on a spine board for further medical examination. In addition to ruling out catastrophic spinal cord injury, the immediate examination must accurately determine the athlete's

alertness and respiratory and cardiovascular status; you must be aware of any signs of bleeding, fractures, dislocations, or shock. Only then should you determine the appropriate method of transportation.

7. Perform an acute examination of the lumbar spine.

   Once the athlete is on the sideline, you can examine the injury more thoroughly. Obtain a more detailed history and perform an objective examination that includes observation, palpation, special tests, active and passive ROM, and strength. Perform neurological tests if the athlete reports any symptoms below the gluteal fold. Although many special tests for spine injuries are available, only the most common were presented in this chapter, including the Valsalva maneuver, straight-leg raise test, well straight-leg raise test, Babinski test, Oppenheim test, Kernig-Brudzinski test, bowstring test, Hoover test, stork standing test, and spring test.

8. Perform a clinical examination of the lumbar and thoracic spine, noting considerations for differential diagnosis.

   If the patient does not report the injury immediately, you will first see the spine injury in the treatment facility at some interval after it occurred. In this case you must obtain a more detailed history and pain profile and must perform tests that will provide a differential diagnosis, eliminating other potential causes of the patient's complaints. Most of the tests used in the acute examination are also used in the clinical examination. In addition, joint mobility tests further define the injury, and functional tests determine if the patient is able to return to work or sport participation.

REVIEW QUESTIONS

1. What are the common mechanisms of sprains and strains? What are some of the causative factors of these injuries, and what preventive measures can be taken to avoid these injuries?

2. Discuss some of the locations where spinal fracture can occur and the potential complications that may be associated with each.

3. What is the difference between spondylolysis, spondylolisthesis, spondylosis, and spondylitis? What, if any, are the differential signs and symptoms of each, and what implications do these conditions have for physical activity?

4. Discuss the causes, pathology, and signs and symptoms associated with a lumbar intervertebral disc herniation. What are some of the special tests you would use to confirm a lesion?

5. What is the difference between the straight-leg and well straight-leg raise tests?

6. What tests examine for low back pain caused by sacroiliac dysfunction?

7. Review the sensory and motor neurological examination for the lumbar plexus.

CRITICAL THINKING QUESTIONS

1. A basketball player comes to you complaining of pain in his lower lumbar region that travels down the left buttock and into the lateral lower leg. Upon examination, you note some spasm and guarding. During your objective examination, you find increased pain with active extension and with lateral flexion and rotation to the left side. On neurological testing, you note paresthesia on the lateral leg and dorsum of the foot and mild weakness with extension of the great toe. The athlete denies pain with coughing, sneezing, or laughing, and the Valsalva maneuver is negative. Straight-leg raise is positive. On the basis of these findings, what injury or condition do you suspect, and at what level?

2. A young gymnast comes to you complaining of central lower back pain. She describes a strip of pain that runs across her back at the level of the iliac crests. She describes

the pain as a deep ache that travels into both buttocks, but she denies any pain down her leg. On observation, you note an increased lordotic curve. Although she does not complain of pain in forward flexion, you note that the spinous process at L4 does not seem to be as apparent as at L3 and L5. Her pain increases on active extension. What conditions and level might you suspect, and what tests would you use to confirm your suspicions?

3. You are invited to speak at an educational workshop for industrial workers on the prevention of back pain and injury. Based on the knowledge you have gained in this chapter, what information do you think would be important to share with the audience, and what prevention strategies could you offer?

4. Consider the scenario presented at the beginning of the on-site examination section. The receiver lands hard on his buttocks and feels immediate pain in his back and in both lower extremities. As you approach, you notice he is talking to his teammates but is lying very still. What are you most concerned about and how would your examination proceed?

5. Gerald is a 12-year-old swimmer who specializes in the fly and breaststroke. He goes to see Charlie, the club's part-time athletic trainer, because of increasing pain and discomfort in his midback. He tells Charlie it doesn't so much bother him while he is swimming, but it bothers him quite a bit during prolonged study periods. As the boy approaches, Charlie thinks to himself how poor Gerald's posture is. Given his chief complaint, sport, and competitive events, what possible muscle imbalance and postural deviations might you suspect in this young athlete? Recalling what you learned in chapter 4, how would you go about performing a postural examination on Gerald?

CITED REFERENCES

American College of Rheumatology. 2000. www.rheumatology.org (accessed August 13, 2004).

Clarkson, H.M. 2000. *Musculoskeletal assessment: Joint range of motion and manual muscle strength.* 2nd ed. Philadelphia: Lippincott Williams & Wilkins.

ADDITIONAL RESOURCES

Hillman, S.K. 2004. *Introduction to athletic injuries.* 2nd ed. Champaign, IL: Human Kinetics.

Houglum, P.A. 2005. *Therapeutic exercise for musculoskeletal injuries.* 2nd ed. Champaign, IL: Human Kinetics.

Kendall, F.P, E.K. McCreary, and P.G. Provance. 1993. *Muscles: Testing and function.* 4th ed. Philadelphia: Lippincott Williams & Wilkins.

Magee, D.J. 1992. *Orthopedic physical assessment.* 2nd ed. Philadelphia: W.B. Saunders.

Leg, Ankle, and Foot

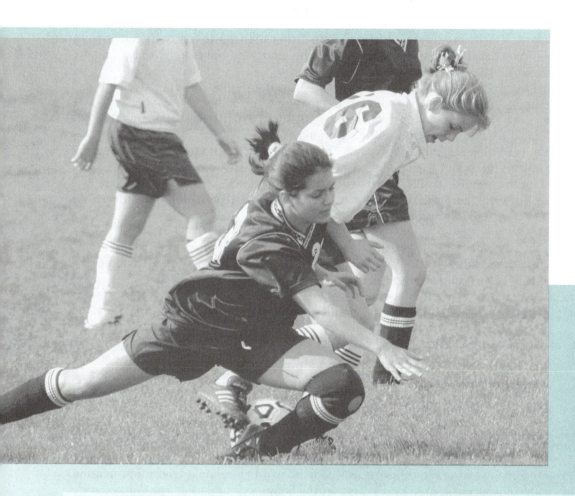

Objectives

After completing this chapter, the reader will be able to do the following:

1. Describe the etiology, signs and symptoms, and potential complications associated with acute injuries of the foot, ankle, and leg commonly encountered in the physically active

2. Describe the etiology, signs and symptoms, and potential complications associated with chronic or overuse injuries of the foot, ankle, and leg commonly encountered in the physically active

3. Identify the signs and symptoms of neurovascular injury at the foot and ankle and identify which ones indicate a medical emergency

4. Identify the common functional and structural abnormalities of the foot and their potential effects on lower-extremity mechanics and injury

5. Describe and demonstrate the objective tests for the leg, ankle, and foot

6. Perform an on-site examination of the leg, ankle, and foot, noting criteria for medical referral and mode of transportation from the field

7. Perform an acute examination of the leg, ankle, and foot

8. Perform a clinical examination of the leg, ankle, and foot, including differential diagnosis of referring lumbar, hip, knee pathologies, and functional tests for return to activity

Bill was covering baseball practice at Monrovia University when Eddie got hit in the shin with a line drive while pitching batting practice.

"Hey, Eddie, looks like you took a pretty good shot! Where did it hit you?" Bill asked as he approached.

"It hit me right in the muscle," Eddie said, in a great deal of pain.

As Bill looked, he could see swelling and discoloration already forming over the belly of Eddie's anterior tibialis. It was pretty obvious what had happened, so rather than waste any time, Bill got an ice bag and wrapped it on Eddie's shin to try to control the bleeding and the pain. Twenty minutes later, Eddie was still restless.

"Man, Bill, this really hurts. I've been hit in the shin before, but this pain is out of control. I'm also getting some numbness in my foot. Do you think this bandage is too tight?"

"Maybe. Let's loosen it up a bit and see if that relieves the pressure," Bill offered. As he took off the wrap, he noticed that the leg was even more swollen than before.

After another 20 minutes, Eddie called Bill over again. "Hey, Bill, you gotta do something about this—this isn't feeling any better. I can't even move my foot, it hurts so bad."

Bill came and looked at the leg. The whole anterior compartment was now swollen and the skin was taking on a whitish, glossy appearance. "Eddie, can you feel when I touch you here?" Bill asked as he did a sensory check over the dorsum of the foot.

"No, I can't!"

"How about trying to bring your toes up toward your shin—can you try that for me?" Bill was getting concerned at this point. Eddie tried to lift his foot, but he couldn't. Bill palpated for a pedal pulse and felt one, but it felt faint compared to the one in the other leg.

"Eddie, I think you have a little more than a contusion here—I think we better get you to the emergency room right away." Bill called emergency medical services and within 5 minutes they arrived.

About an hour later, Bill saw Doc Rogers, Monrovia's team physician. "Hi, Doc, how's Eddie?"

"Hi, Bill. Eddie's on his way to surgery. He developed an acute anterior tibial compartment syndrome from the hemorrhage resulting from the contusion. He was lucky that you were there and recognized the signs and symptoms."

Actually, Bill was wishing he had recognized the signs a little sooner.

The primary functions of the leg, ankle, and foot are to provide a rigid lever for propulsion and a stable but adaptable structure to support the body's weight during gait. Appreciating the balance between mobility and stability at the foot and ankle is essential, as changes in joint function resulting from injury and functional and structural abnormalities can tremendously influence this balance and thus influence lower-extremity mechanics, stress, and future injury.

FUNCTIONAL ANATOMY

The lower leg, ankle, and foot form a complex relationship of 28 bones (tibia, fibula, 7 tarsals, 5 metatarsals, and 14 phalanges), multiple ligaments, and intrinsic and extrinsic muscles that function together to provide stability, adaptability, and shock absorption for optimal support and locomotion of the entire body. The lower-leg complex is often referred to in three segments: the hindfoot, midfoot, and forefoot (figure 16.1). Although movement at any one joint may be minimal, in combination the joints of the foot and ankle offer a great deal of flexibility and adaptability.

The majority of physiological movement occurs in the hindfoot, at the talocrural and subtalar joints. Two motions of the subtalar joint that you will read about throughout this chapter are pronation and supination. These are not true motions but rather a composite of three motions occurring at the joint. In the open chain (foot is free to move), **pronation**

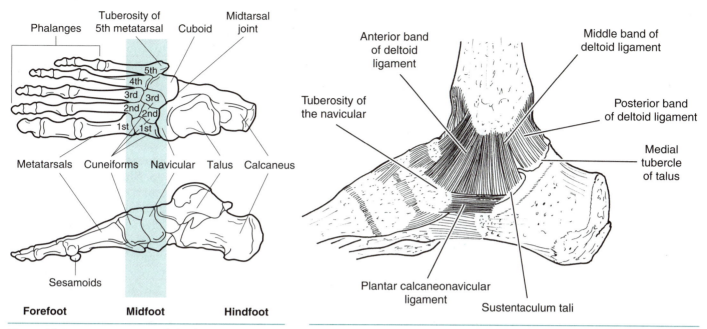

Figure 16.1 Bony anatomy of the foot, including the hindfoot, midfoot, and forefoot.

Figure 16.2 Medial ligaments of the ankle.

results from eversion, dorsiflexion, and abduction of the foot; **supination** results from inversion, plantar flexion, and adduction of the foot. In the closed chain (weight bearing), however, pronation is a result of eversion, plantar flexion, and abduction, whereas supination is a result of inversion, dorsiflexion, and adduction. It is important to understand these composite motions, as they play a major role in lower-extremity function and mechanics. As you will note throughout this chapter, excessive or reduced subtalar motion can substantially affect foot and ankle mechanics, abnormally stressing the joints and soft tissue structures.

Refer to chapter 4 for a more complete discussion on the role of supination in gait and posture.

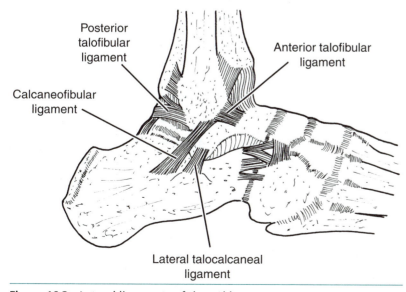

Figure 16.3 Lateral ligaments of the ankle.

The majority of the ankle's plantar flexion and dorsiflexion occurs at the talocrural joint. Inversion and eversion occur at the subtalar and transverse tarsal joints. The broad deltoid ligament supports the medial aspect of the ankle (figure 16.2), and the anterior talofibular, calcaneofibular, and posterior talofibular ligaments support the lateral aspect of the ankle (figure 16.3). Two anatomical features of the ankle likely account for the much higher incidence of inversion versus eversion sprains. First, the four components of the deltoid ligament create a much broader and stronger ligament in comparison to the three lateral stabilizing ligaments. Second, the fibula extends more distally than the tibia, preventing excessive ankle eversion.

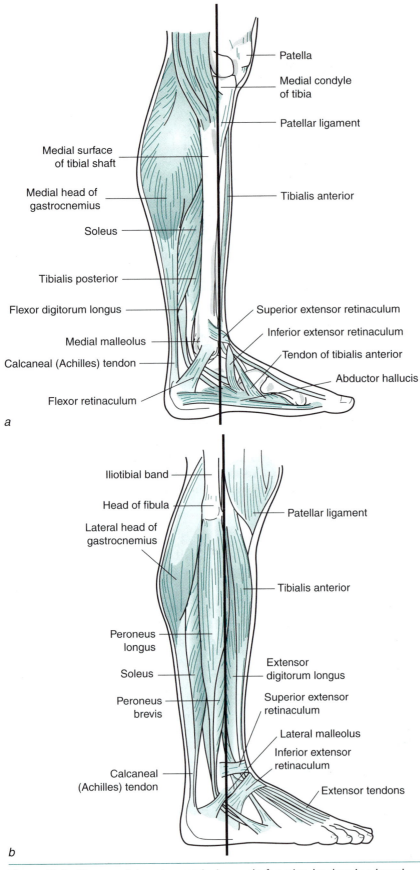

Patella

Medial condyle of tibia

Patellar ligament

Medial surface of tibial shaft

Medial head of gastrocnemius

Tibialis anterior

Soleus

Tibialis posterior

Flexor digitorum longus

Superior extensor retinaculum

Inferior extensor retinaculum

Medial malleolus

Tendon of tibialis anterior

Calcaneal (Achilles) tendon

Abductor hallucis

Flexor retinaculum

a

Iliotibial band

Head of fibula

Lateral head of gastrocnemius

Patellar ligament

Tibialis anterior

Peroneus longus

Soleus

Extensor digitorum longus

Peroneus brevis

Superior extensor retinaculum

Lateral malleolus

Inferior extensor retinaculum

Calcaneal (Achilles) tendon

Extensor tendons

b

Figure 16.4   You can determine extrinsic muscle function by drawing imaginary lines that divide the ankle into (a) medial and (b) lateral and anterior and posterior components.

The ankle is most stable in 90° of dorsiflexion and becomes less stable as the talorcrural joint moves into plantar flexion. In 90° of dorsiflexion, inversion stress is restricted largely by the calcaneofibular ligament and the articulation of the bones creating the ankle mortis. As the ankle moves into plantar flexion, the anterior talofibular ligament helps prevent excess inversion. Since the joint is far more stable in dorsiflexion, most inversion ankle sprains occur with the ankle slightly plantar flexed. Minor inversion ankle sprains almost always involve the anterior talofibular ligament, while more severe inversion sprains typically injure both the anterior talofibular and calcaneofibular ligaments.

The muscles acting on the foot and ankle are described as either intrinsic or extrinsic. **Intrinsic** muscles both originate and insert within the foot and move the toes. **Extrinsic** muscles originate from the leg (and in one case the posterior thigh) and insert in the foot. They act on the ankle and in some cases the toes, depending on their point of insertion. The extrinsic muscles are classified as dorsiflexors, plantar flexors, invertors, or evertors. Two imaginary lines will help you remember the role each muscle plays (figure 16.4). One line splits the foot into medial and lateral components, and the other passes through the axis of rotation created by the malleoli. Any muscles passing anterior to the malleolar axis of rotation must produce dorsiflexion, and any muscles passing posterior must produce plantar flexion. The muscles traversing into the foot medial to the midline must contribute to inversion, and those passing lateral to the midline must contribute to eversion.

The triceps surae muscle group, the primary plantar flexors of the ankle, consists of the gastrocnemius and soleus muscles and the Achilles tendon. The gastrocnemius is a biarticulate muscle, meaning that as it originates from the posterior femur and inserts into the calcaneus, and it crosses two joints, the knee and ankle.

The soleus is a uniarticulate muscle, originating from the tibia and fibula and inserting into the calcaneus. When the knee is extended, the gastronemius is the primary plantar flexor, and when this muscle becomes shortened by knee flexion, the soleus becomes the primary plantar flexor. These length–tension principles are important to remember as you examine muscle function and teach patients how to stretch the muscles of the calf. In addition, although the gastrocnemius and soleus are the primary plantar flexors, the other muscles passing posterior to the malleolar axis of rotation also contribute to plantar flexion. As such, a patient can completely rupture the Achilles tendon and still be able to plantar flex the ankle (albeit not very powerfully) by contracting the peroneal muscles and the tibialis posterior, flexor digitorum longus, and flexor hallicus longus.

The leg fascia give rise to intermuscular septa and retinacula that create several compartments and tunnels through which muscles, nerves, arteries, and veins traverse. The anterior compartment of the leg and the tarsal tunnel of the ankle have special clinical relevance. The structures within the leg's anterior compartment include the tibialis anterior, extensor digitorum longus, and extensor hallucis muscles, the anterior tibial artery and vein, and the deep peroneal nerve (figure 16.5). Trauma to the anterior aspect of the leg can swell the muscles and increase pressure within the anterior compartment in a condition known as anterior compartment syndrome. The deep peroneal nerve innervates the dorsiflexor muscles and provides sensation to the first web space of the foot. Excessive pressure on the nerve can prevent the muscles from producing dorsiflexion (dropfoot) on a temporary or permanent basis. The flexor retinaculum of the ankle sends three septa to the tibia and creates four compartments for the tibialis posterior muscle, flexor digitorum longus muscle, tibial nerve and posterior tibial vessels, and flexor hallicus longus muscle (figure 16.6). Increased pressure within the tunnel, known as tarsal tunnel syndrome, can compress the tibial nerve and numb and weaken the skin and muscles it innervates. These examples illustrate the importance of knowing the muscle and sensory innervations of the nerves that lie within the compartments and tunnels of the leg and ankle.

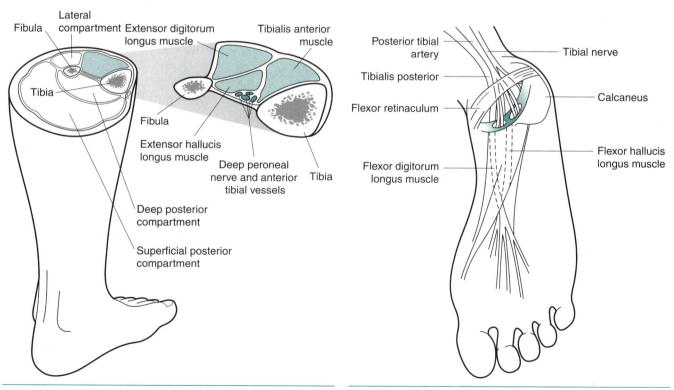

Figure 16.5   Contents of the anterior compartment of the leg.

Figure 16.6   Structures passing through the tarsal tunnel.

LEG, ANKLE, AND FOOT INJURIES

The majority of the active population experiences leg and foot problems sometime in their life. Tremendous forces, both compressive and rotational, are transmitted through the weight-bearing structures of the foot, ankle, and leg. Consequently, both traumatic and chronic injuries frequent this region. Even seemingly minor injuries can be debilitating given the foot and ankle's need for strength and stability in daily weight-bearing activities, let alone sport activities. Additionally, leg and foot problems can alter gait or lower-body mechanics, increasing stress and compensatory problems up the kinetic chain in the knee, hip, or low back.

Acute Soft Tissue Injuries

The leg complex relies on the integrity of active and passive soft tissue structures for both stability and propulsion. Dynamic sport activity places tremendous loads and demands on the foot and ankle. Soft tissue injuries commonly occur as a result of direct contact and intrinsic or extrinsic forces acting on the foot, ankle, and leg.

Contusions

> ⚠ You should closely monitor severe contusions to a muscular compartment for excessive swelling and neurovascular compromise.

The leg, ankle, and foot are vulnerable to direct trauma in sport activity. Making contact with the ground or an opponent, kicking an unyielding object, being hit in the shin by a baseball, and being stepped on or kicked by another player are all common injury mechanisms for soft tissue and periosteal contusions. Signs and symptoms include pain, swelling, and discoloration. Direct contact to the superficial and unprotected anterior medial border of the tibia can result in localized inflammation (**periostitis**) and hematoma formation under the periosteum, which can take considerable time for the body to absorb. Disability and function loss are usually more severe with muscle contusions due to tenderness, swelling, and spasm within the muscle tissue. Decreased range of motion and strength also occurs and varies according to the degree of tissue injury. Although muscle contusions rarely result in serious injury, complications can arise from severe contusions and excessive bleeding within the enclosed anterior tibial compartment of the leg (see the discussion of anterior compartment syndrome later in this chapter). You should closely monitor severe contusions to a muscular compartment for neurovascular compromise.

A heel contusion, or **stone bruise**, can be particularly problematic. A heel bruise can result from landing hard on the heel during jumping activities or stepping on an uneven surface or a stone at heel strike with little or no footwear protection. A contusion to the fat pad of the heel can cause considerable pain and point tenderness, making it difficult to bear weight or walk with a normal gait. Discoloration and swelling may or may not be evident, depending on severity.

Sprains

The foot and ankle include multiple joints and ligaments that stabilize the body during weight-bearing activities. Given the tremendous forces exerted on these structures with landing, cutting, and running, the ligaments are prone to injury when activity forces the joint beyond its normal ROM. Sprains occur most often at the **hindfoot**, which is composed of the inferior tibiofibular (syndesmosis), talocrural (tibia, fibula, and talus), and subtalar (talus, calcaneus, navicular) joints. Ligamentous support is essential for stabilizing the hindfoot, particularly when the ankle plantar flexes. Stability is provided laterally by the anterior talofibular, calcaneofibular, and posterior talofibular ligaments (refer to figure 16.3) and medially by the deltoid ligament complex (refer to figure 16.2). The distal tibiofibular joint is stabilized by the interosseous membrane and the anterior and posterior tibiofibular ligaments. Although sprains occur most often at the hindfoot, sprains in the **midfoot** (talocalcaneonavicular, cuneonavicular, intercuneiform, and calcaneocuboid joints) and **forefoot** (tarsometatarsal, intermetatarsal, metatarsophalangeal, and interphalangeal joints) are not uncommon. The injury mechanism determines which joint structures are involved.

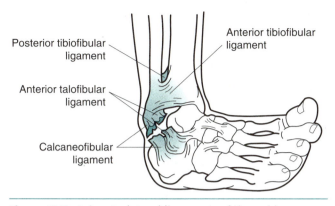

Figure 16.7   Injury to lateral ligaments of the ankle.

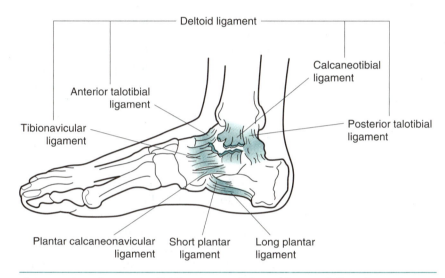

Figure 16.8 Injury to medial ligaments of the ankle. Carefully palpate the distal fibula for possible fracture with all serious eversion injuries.

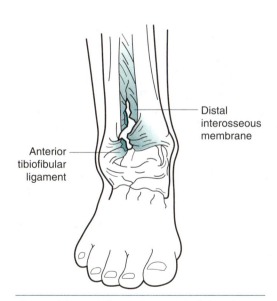

Figure 16.9 Syndesmotic sprain of the tibiofibular joint.

Lateral Ankle Sprains

The most common mechanism of ankle injury involving the lateral ligament complex is inversion with or without plantar flexion. In typical scenarios, a basketball player comes down on an opponent's foot or lands awkwardly on the outside of his own foot, causing the ankle to turn in (inversion mechanism). The athlete complains of immediate pain upon injury and may hear a "pop." Injury almost always involves the anterior talofibular ligament (figure 16.7). The calcaneofibular and, less often, the posterior talofibular ligaments are also involved. Signs and symptoms are consistent with first- through third-degree ligament sprains. With second- and third-degree sprains, there may also be injury to the medial structures of the ankle due to compression from the inversion force. Dislocation of the ankle mortise rarely results with third-degree ligament injuries, but associated avulsion or push-off fractures of the lateral and medial malleolus, respectively, are not uncommon with more severe ankle sprains.

Medial Ankle Sprains

Medial ankle sprains resulting from eversion forces are considerably less common, primarily due to the greater stability of the medial ankle, a consequence of the thickness and strength of the deltoid ligament complex as well as the longer lateral malleolus, which prevents excessive eversion (figure 16.8). Palpate the distal fibula for possible fracture with severe eversion injuries. Signs and symptoms are consistent with first-, second-, and third-degree sprains. However, disability and recovery may be prolonged with medial ankle sprains, given the support the deltoid ligament provides to the medial longitudinal arch of the foot so that even simple weight-bearing stresses the injured structures. Furthermore, pes planus and excessive pronation may result from chronic medial instability.

Syndesmotic Sprains

Syndesmotic, or **high-ankle sprains**, disrupt the tibiofibular ligaments and distal interosseous membrane, causing instability of the tibiofibular joint and widening of the ankle mortise (figure 16.9). Although less frequent than lateral ankle sprains, this injury can result in prolonged disability and recovery when not identified and managed properly. Syndesmotic ankle sprains are typically caused by forced hyperdorsiflexion or lateral rotation of the foot, which forcibly separate the distal tibiofibular joint. These injuries are most often seen in contact sports such as football, in which the foot is planted and laterally rotated as contact is made to the lateral aspect of the leg. Signs and symptoms include pain and swelling anterior to the ankle joint. Pain in the anterolateral aspect of the ankle with weight bearing, passive lateral rotation of the foot, or forced dorsiflexion also indicates injury to the syndesmosis.

Foot Sprains

Given the number of bony articulations and ligaments in the foot, myriad sprains can result from both direct and indirect forces. Because of the foot's stability, sprains to the mid- and forefoot are less common than sprains to the ankle joint. Sprains to the metatarsal and long arch can result from both chronic overuse and acute traumatic forces that stretch the supporting ligamentous structures, causing midfoot hypermobility and a fallen arch. Signs and symptoms of foot and arch sprains include pain, point tenderness over the involved structure, swelling, discoloration, and difficulty with weight bearing. A rupture of the Lisfranc's ligament between the first and second tarsometatarsal joints has been described as a subtle injury that can occur when the foot is laterally rotated and pronated, with all of the body weight applied to the first metatarsal head (Shapiro, Wascher, and Finerman 1994). Signs and symptoms include feeling a "pop" in the midfoot, immediate pain that increases with weight bearing, and joint instability with stress testing. Radiographic examination shows widening (diastasis) between the first and second metatarsal bases during weight bearing. Because it is often difficult to distinguish bony from ligamentous injury in the foot given the smaller structures, physician examination and radiographic examination are often necessary to rule out fracture.

Toe Sprains

Toe sprains most often result from direct contact at the end of the toe, such as stubbing or jamming the toe while kicking an unyielding object. However, any direct or indirect mechanism that forces the joint beyond its normal range can result in sprains. Most problematic are sprains to the great toe, also known as **turf toe**. Turf toe can result from extreme dorsiflexion of the first metatarsophalangeal joint during push-off, extreme plantar flexion or axial compression while kicking an unyielding object, or quick stops that slide the foot forward in the shoe. Signs and symptoms of toe sprains include pain, swelling, and ecchymosis. You will also note decreased ROM and pain with passive and active movements. There may be joint instability with second- and third-degree classifications. Pain is particularly apparent with push-off, hindering normal gait and running.

Strains

Numerous muscles originating from the leg and terminating in the foot and toes are responsible for a variety of ankle and foot motions. Given the strong mechanical forces associated with running, jumping, and cutting, muscle strains commonly result from overstretch and muscular overload. Strains of the lateral peroneal muscles can result from forced and rapid eversion forces or overstretching with excessive inversion motions. Strains of the triceps surae muscles and common Achilles (calcaneal) tendon typically result from forceful and rapid plantar flexion during sport activities. Acute strains to the posterior tibial and toe flexor muscle and tendons can also occur with forceful plantar flexion and inversion, although repetitive stress and chronic tractioning with a valgus foot are more frequent causes.

Signs and symptoms of muscle and tendon strains include pain with active and resistive movement, pain with passive stretch, muscle spasm, swelling, and point tenderness over the injured area. You may note a palpable defect with second- and third-degree muscle injuries. While the degree of symptoms and disability vary according to the severity, even first-degree (mild) strains can be debilitating given the constant demands placed on these structures during walking and weight bearing. Muscle spasms are also common, particularly in the calf muscles. Muscular fatigue, dehydration and electrolyte imbalance, and direct blows are typical predisposing factors. Signs and symptoms of muscle spasm include immediate pain,

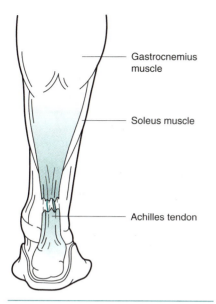

Figure 16.10 Achilles tendon rupture.

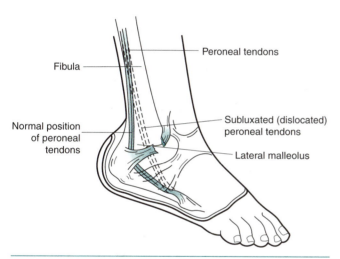

Figure 16.11 Ruptured peroneal retinaculum, allowing the peroneal tendons to dislocate.

💡 **Fibular** and **fibularis** are synonymous with *peroneal* and *peroneus*. Although some of the newer anatomical texts use *fibular* and *fibularis* with reference to specific muscles and nerves of the lower extremity, this text uses the more familiar terms *peroneal* and *peroneus*.

observable spasm, and loss of function. If spasm is severe and prolonged, signs and symptoms consistent with a first-degree strain may be present the following day.

Rupture of the Achilles (Calcaneal) Tendon

Rupture of the Achilles tendon (figure 16.10) can result from sudden, violent plantar flexion during eccentric loading in full weight-bearing activity. A rapid punch in gymnastics and the push-off in tennis are common mechanisms. The athlete complains of immediate pain and disability and often reports a feeling of being kicked or shot in the calf. Considerable swelling and discoloration also occurs, accompanied by an observable defect in the contour of the Achilles tendon. The athlete will be unable to actively plantar flex the foot and a Thompson test will be positive.

Rupture of the Plantaris Muscle

The plantaris muscle can also rupture with forceful contraction or stretch at its musculotendinous unit during running, jumping, and rapid change of direction. The patient complains of a sudden, sharp pain deep in the posterior leg with push-off that may also resemble a feeling of being kicked or shot in the back of the leg. Pain, spasm, and possible loss of function may occur, and you may observe swelling and discoloration around the ankle the next day. You may note tenderness deep to the belly of the gastrocnemius, and pain may increase with passive dorsiflexion. Given the relatively insignificant function of the plantaris muscle, pain and disability after the initial acute stages of injury are usually minimal.

Rupture of Peroneal Retinaculum

The peroneal (fibular) retinaculum, which tethers the peroneus longus and brevis tendons behind the lateral malleolus, can be strained or ruptured by direct blow, forceful eversion or plantar flexion, or inversion ankle injury (figure 16.11). When the peroneal retinaculum is disrupted, the peroneal tendons sublux and snap over the lateral malleolus when the foot moves into eversion and plantar flexion. Other signs and symptoms include pain, swelling, and inflammation of the tendons with repetitive subluxation.

Chronic or Overuse Soft Tissue Injuries

Chronic soft tissue injuries are a frequent complaint in physically active people as a consequence of repetitive microtrauma resulting from abnormal friction, traction, structural mechanics, or some combination of these. As you will note, excessive pronation is associated with a number of chronic overuse conditions. In the stance phase of gait, the foot begins to pronate immediately after heel strike, unlocking the midtarsal joints, and **flexibility** increases in the forefoot and rearfoot to absorb the shock of heel strike and to adapt to the ground surface. During midstance, the foot begins to supinate, which acts to lock the midtarsal joints to provide maximum **stability** to the forefoot, making the foot rigid for maximal propulsion during push-off. When pronation is excessive and continues past midstance, it increases stress on the medial long arch and soft tissue structures that can transmit abnormal stresses further up the lower-extremity chain.

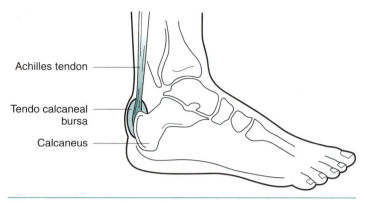

Achilles tendon —

Tendo calcaneal bursa —

Calcaneus —

Figure 16.12 Retrocalcaneal bursitis.

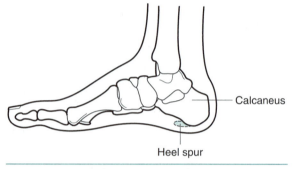

— Calcaneus

Heel spur

Figure 16.13 Heel spur resulting from chronic tractioning of a tight plantar fascia.

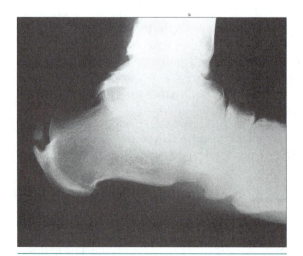

Figure 16.14 Calcaneal apophysitis (Sever's disease).

Courtesy of Theodore E. Keats

Retrocalcaneal Bursitis

The tendo calcaneal bursa lies between the calcaneus and the distal insertion of the Achilles tendon (figure 16.12). Inflammation and swelling of this bursa can result from repetitive overuse with running, direct pressure, or friction from poorly fitting footwear. Signs and symptoms include localized swelling, redness, and point tenderness near and around the calcaneal attachment of the Achilles tendon. You may also note pain with active or resistive plantar flexion. Bursa thickening and eventual calcium formation may occur in chronic cases.

Plantar Fasciitis

Inflammation of the plantar fascia is seen most often in athletes with abnormal foot alignment and is precipitated by overuse, poor footwear or playing surface, or improper conditioning. The patient's history is your primary evaluative tool. The patient typically complains of a gradual onset of pain and stiffness on the plantar surface of the foot, extending from the heel to the metatarsal heads. If the condition is prolonged, a **heel spur** may develop at the proximal calcaneal attachment (figure 16.13). Note that the heel spur is not the cause of plantar fasciitis, but a result.

Tendinitis and Tenosynovitis

Tendinitis and chronic strain of the peroneal, posterior tibial, and Achilles tendons are common in the athletic population. In all cases, injury results from repetitive overuse, friction, or tendon traction. Improper mechanics and abnormal foot alignment are often predisposing factors. Tendinitis may also occur in the toe extensor tendons where they cross superficially on the dorsum of the foot. Typically, inflammation of these tendons results from shoe pressure or friction or from shoelaces that are too tight. Signs and symptoms associated with tendinitis include pain, point tenderness, and crepitus over the inflamed tendon, decreased ROM, and swelling. Pain with passive stretch or active or resistive movement of the involved muscle or tendon occurs as well. Inflammation and irritation of the Achilles tendon may also involve the synovial sheath (tenosynovitis), with swelling and snowball crepitus that are more pronounced than with simple tendinitis. Chronic thickening of the tendon may occur with prolonged inflammation.

Calcaneal Apophysitis (Sever's Disease)

In young, skeletally immature athletes, the calcaneal apophysis can become inflamed secondary to repetitive traction stress of the Achilles tendon (figure 16.14). Common signs and symptoms include posterior inferior heel pain, point tenderness, and increased pain with weight bearing, running, or jumping. Decreased dorsiflexion range secondary to tightness of the Achilles tendon during rapid growth phases is likely a predisposing factor.

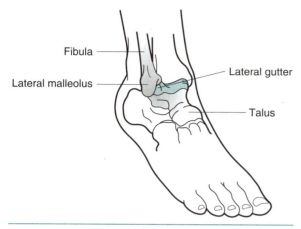

Figure 16.15 Anatomical location of the sinus tarsi (lateral gutter) and impingement.

Pes cavus is an abnormally high or excessive arch.

Pes planus is a flat foot that has lost normal concavity on its plantar surface.

⚠ If medial shin pain becomes localized or if bone percussion causes pain, suspect a tibial stress fracture and refer the patient to a physician.

Anterolateral Impingement

Chronic anterolateral ankle pain can result from synovitis and scar tissue thickening following lateral ankle injuries (Ferkel et al. 1991). Specifically, anterolateral impingement is caused by chronic inflammation and impingement of hypertrophic scar tissue between the talus and fibula in the sinus tarsi (lateral gutter) (figure 16.15). Signs and symptoms include persistent pain over the anterolateral aspect of the ankle for weeks and even months following a lateral ankle sprain. Refer patients with persistent anterior lateral ankle pain that does not respond to conservative treatment and rest to a physician for further examination.

Medial Tibial Stress Syndrome (MTSS)

Medial tibial stress syndrome (MTSS), commonly referred to as **shin splints**, is usually an inflammation of the periosteum (periostitis) along the posterior medial tibial border at or near the insertion of the long toe or ankle flexors. There are a number of predisposing factors. Excessive pronation; inflexibility of the calf muscle, Achilles tendon, posterior tibialis, or long toe flexors (i.e., flexor hallucis longus); dorsiflexor weakness or fatigue; and foot conditions such as pes cavus and pes planus can alter the shock-absorbing or decelerating capabilities of the leg and transmit increased stress to the shin and leg muscles. The condition is typically brought on by abrupt changes in footwear, running surfaces, or training regime. Medial tibial stress syndrome is characterized by diffuse pain, point tenderness, and inflammation along the medial border of the tibia. The pain is usually diffuse along a broad area of the medial tibial surface.

You should differentiate shin pain due to MTSS from other sources of shin pain, including stress fractures, compartment syndrome, and bone tumors. Compartment syndrome (especially that of the deep posterior compartment) causes diffuse pain along the posterior medial border of the tibia, but the pain also extends into the involved compartment, which is also palpably taut and tender. Pain that dramatically increases with stretching the compartment and neurovascular compromise are also signs of compartment syndrome (see the section on compartment syndrome for more information). If pain becomes localized or if bone percussion causes pain, suspect a tibial stress fracture and refer the patient to a physician for diagnostic imaging (bone scan, MRI). Deep, nagging pain at night with radiating symptoms may indicate bone pathology such as a tumor. You must differentiate and rule out these conditions through careful examination.

Traumatic Fractures

Traumatic fractures can result from the same mechanisms that cause ankle and foot sprains. In fact, it is not uncommon for both fracture and ligament injury to result from traumatic ankle injury.

Tibia and Fibula

Traumatic fractures of the tibia and fibula can result from a direct blow or indirect torsional stress in association with inversion and eversion ankle injuries. Fractures to the fibula shaft can result from a direct blow to the lateral aspect of the leg or from severe eversion or lateral rotation stress. Fractures to the tibial shaft, which are less common, require much greater forces; they can occur in contact sports such as football with a direct blow to the shin, or in skiing with a severe torsional stress. Fractures involving the epiphyseal plate of the distal tibial typically result from either compressive or torsional forces in skeletally immature athletes. Avulsion fractures of the distal fibula (lateral malleolus) occur secondary to an inversion stress (figure 16.16), while push-off fractures are caused by eversion when the everted calcaneus butts

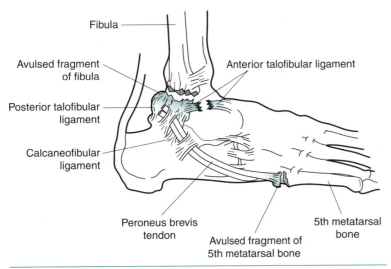

Figure 16.16   Avulsion fractures of both the distal fibula and proximal fifth metatarsal.

up against the distal fibula. Fractures to the medial malleolus of the tibia similarly result from severe eversion (avulsion) or inversion (push-off secondary to contact with the talus) forces. **Bimalleolar fractures** can also result from these mechanisms. A **Pott's fracture** occurs when forcibly everting the foot causes an avulsion fraction of the medial malleolus and a shear fracture of the lateral malleolus or distal fibula. Fractures through the articulating surface of the tibia (chondral and osteochondral fractures) may also occur when the ankle joint is forcibly compressed into excessive inversion and plantar flexion or eversion and dorsiflexion.

Signs and symptoms of fracture include immediate pain, swelling, and possible deformity if the fragments are displaced. You will note tenderness over and around the fracture site. Muscle splinting and spasm may also occur. Other signs of fracture include pain with bony percussion or with transverse stress such as that produced when the tibia and fibula are squeezed together. You may also note false joint motion or crepitus when manipulating the bone. While a fracture of the tibia results in an inability or unwillingness to bear weight, this may not be the case in the non-weight-bearing fibula. However, you will observe pain with active or resisted eversion.

> ⚠ The ability of a patient to bear weight on an injured ankle does not rule out the possibility of a fracture.

Foot

Traumatic fractures in the foot typically involve the metatarsals and phalanges. The mechanisms associated with toe sprains also apply here. Traumatic fractures of the metatarsal shafts most often result from direct trauma, such as when an athlete is stepped on by another player or when a weight is dropped on the foot. Pain with longitudinal stress applied to the plantar surface of the foot, axial stress to the bone, or torsional stress applied through twisting the toe often indicates metatarsal fractures. A dislocated fracture of the midfoot characterized by one or more displaced proximal metatarsals is known as a **Lisfranc's fracture**. This fracture is caused in athletics by a direct blow to the Lisfranc joint (between the midfoot and forefoot) or by axial loading along the metatarsals, coupled with either a medially or laterally directed rotational force (figure 16.17). Fracture at the base of the fifth metatarsal (**Jones' fracture**) is usually caused by indirectly loading the bone with plantar flexion and eversion stress. Avulsion fractures of the proximal fifth metatarsal may also occur at the insertion of the peroneus brevis tendon with inversion stress injuries (see figure 16.16). Suspect fracture whenever there is point tenderness over the base of the fifth metatarsal or pain with resisted eversion.

Although less common, fractures of the calcaneus and talus can also occur secondary to athletic activity. The most frequent cause of calcaneus fracture is direct trauma from falling or landing on the heel from a height. Talar dome fractures are typically associated

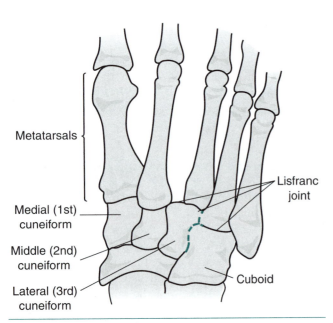

Figure 16.17   Lisfranc's fracture.

with compressive ankle injuries. General signs and symptoms of foot fractures are consistent with those previously mentioned.

Bony Defects Secondary to Repetitive Stress

The bone is also susceptible to chronic stress injuries secondary to repetitive traction or compression. Stress injuries to the bone include stress fractures, bone spurs, and degenerative changes.

Stress Fractures

Amenorrhea is the absence or cessation of menses.

The tibia and metatarsals are the most common sites of stress fractures in the leg, ankle, and foot, which result from repetitive stress associated with running and jumping activities. Stress fractures of the fifth metatarsal and fibula are also common secondary to repetitive tractioning of the peroneal muscles with eversion and plantar flexion. Tibial stress fractures most often occur in the distal one-third of the tibia, and metatarsal stress fractures most often involve the second or third metatarsal shafts. Athletes with excessive pronation or impaired shock absorption due to an immobile pes cavus, a hypermobile pes planus, muscle weakness, or muscular fatigue are especially susceptible to tibial and metatarsal stress fractures. Female athletes with compromised bone density associated with secondary **amenorrhea** are also thought to be at increased risk.

Sequela refers to the progressive course of a pathological condition.

Typical **sequelae** of a developing stress fracture include an insidious onset of pain that initially occurs only during activity and subsides with rest. If the repetitive stress continues, the athlete will also complain of continued pain after activity and into the night. Eventually, if the stressful activity is not curtailed, the athlete experiences pain throughout the day. Typically the athlete reports no history of trauma, but his training history will likely indicate recent high-intensity training or an abrupt change in training practices, surface, or equipment (footwear). Other signs and symptoms may include localized tenderness over the bone, pain with axial and transverse stress, and swelling.

Exostosis

Excessive calcification, or **bone spurs**, is identified by radiographic examination and can develop at various locations of the foot and ankle secondary to repetitive stress and contact. Repetitive contact between the head of the talus and distal tibia with extreme dorsiflexion can result in an anterior **talotibial exostosis**. The athlete experiences anterior ankle pain, palpable tenderness over the anterior talar dome, pain and limited ROM into dorsiflexion, and pain with push-off. Similarly, repetitive extreme plantar flexion causes spurring of the posterior talus and calcaneus. Pain deep in the posterior aspect of the heel and pain with forced plantar flexion are hallmark symptoms. A posterior **calcaneal exostosis**, or **pump bump**, can result from chronic irritation at the Achilles tendon attachment. Athletes with an already prominent posterior calcaneal tuberosity are more susceptible to irritation, usually chronic friction and pressure from ill-fitting shoes. Signs and symptoms in addition to the bony prominence include pain, localized swelling, and redness. Inflammation and irritation associated with a calcaneal exostosis may also involve the retrocalcaneal bursa and distal Achilles tendon.

Osteochondritis Dissecans

Avascular necrosis (osteochondritis dissecans) is tissue death resulting from lack of blood supply (ischemia).

The talar dome is the most common site of osteochondritis dissecans in the leg and foot. Although rare, compression associated with inversion, eversion, and dorsiflexion can impinge on and injure the articular surface of the talus, resulting in avascular necrosis of the subchondral bone. Signs and symptoms may resemble those of an ankle sprain. The patient typically complains of nonspecific ankle joint pain and swelling that worsen with activity. You may notice locking, clicking, and decreased ROM if there is a loose fragment in the joint. Refer patients complaining of prolonged ankle pain that does not respond to conservative treatment to a physician for further examination.

As with any dislocation or fracture, perform distal pulse and neurological checks to rule out vascular or nerve injury.

Dislocation and Subluxation

Dislocations of the ankle, hindfoot, and midfoot joints are relatively uncommon. Such injuries require tremendous forces; thus when these dislocations occur, they are almost always associated with fracture. Dislocation of the phalanges commonly results from the same mechanisms that cause sprains and fractures. Dislocations are readily apparent secondary to obvious joint deformity. Immediate pain, swelling, and loss of function also occur.

Nerve and Vascular Injuries

Because of the compartments and tunnels that the nerves and vessels of the lower extremity pass through on their way to the foot, neurovascular compromise is not uncommon. Neurovascular compromise can result from both acute and chronic compression mechanisms; acute conditions usually represent more serious injury. You should be able to distinguish between these conditions and know which signs and symptoms represent a medical emergency.

Tarsal Tunnel Syndrome

Tarsal tunnel syndrome is characterized by compression of the tibial nerve in the tarsal tunnel. The tarsal tunnel is a fibroosseous, inelastic tunnel formed by the talus, calcaneus, tibialis posterior, flexor digitorum longus, and flexor hallucis longus (the floor) and flexor retinaculum (roof) (see figure 16.6) (Jackson and Haglund 1991). Because of the tunnel's inelasticity and fixed space, the tibial nerve can become entrapped by surrounding structures when normal spatial relationships are disrupted. Although the nerve within the tunnel can be compressed or tractioned as a consequence of direct trauma, acute fractures, or dislocation, you will most often see this condition in patients with abnormal foot and ankle mechanics that result in chronic eversion and excessive pronation.

Symptoms of tarsal tunnel syndrome include pain and numbness in the foot's longitudinal arch that can radiate upward into the medial ankle region. Running activities and ankle dorsiflexion often increase the discomfort. Pain may also worsen at night. You may find foot fatigue, numbness, and burning on the plantar surface and into the toes (Jackson and Haglund 1991). Weakness of the foot intrinsic muscles and toe flexors may also occur in prolonged conditions.

Medial Plantar Nerve Compression Syndrome

The medial plantar nerve is a distal branch of the posterior tibial nerve. It can become entrapped in the longitudinal arch as it passes under the spring ligament (figure 16.18). This occurs most often in runners who have rearfoot valgus. The athlete reports symptoms of burning in the arch that can extend in the sole from the heel to the great toe.

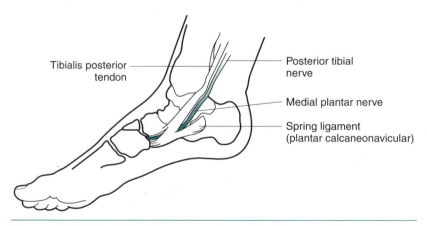

Figure 16.18   Medial plantar nerve passing under the spring ligament.

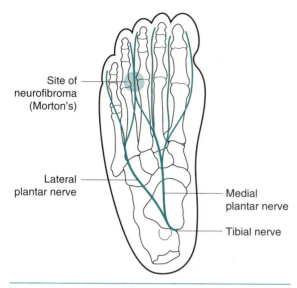

Site of
neurofibroma
(Morton's)

Lateral
plantar nerve

Medial
plantar nerve

Tibial nerve

Figure 16.19 Location of Morton's neuroma
between the third and fourth metatarsal heads.

Morton's Neuroma

Also referred to as **metatarsalgia**, Morton's neuroma usually occurs at the bifurcation of the lateral plantar nerve as it angles sharply and branches off between the third and fourth metatarsal heads (figure 16.19). This is a prime area of pressure and friction that can cause fibrous tumor formation or tissue buildup around the nerve. Common complaints include pain with weight bearing and tight shoes, burning, numbness, and shooting pain.

Peroneal Nerve Palsy

The peroneal nerve is susceptible to injury with inversion ankle injuries. Since this nerve has a significant sensory branch, the patient will complain of sensory changes in the dermatome along the lateral leg and dorsum of the foot. Eversion weakness thought to be due to lateral muscle weakness, as well as pain associated with the ankle sprain, may in fact be the result of superficial peroneal nerve injury. When weakness is prolonged or accompanied by sensory changes, suspect peroneal nerve injury. Plantar flexion and ankle inversion often exacerbate sensory disturbances.

Compartment Syndrome

In a **compartment syndrome**, pressure within a muscle compartment increases to the point that it causes neurovascular compromise. There are four muscular compartments in the leg: anterior, lateral, deep posterior, and superficial posterior (see figure 16.5). Each is bound by a thick, elastic fascial sheath that limits compartment expansion during significant swelling. Although any compartment can be affected, the most common site of compartment syndrome is the anterior tibial compartment, which houses the anterior tibialis, extensor hallucis longus and extensor digitorum longus muscles, the anterior tibial artery and vein, and the deep peroneal nerve. These structures are surrounded and enclosed by the fibula, tibia, intermuscular septum, and the crural fascia. A compartment syndrome can be classified as either chronic (exertional) or acute.

• **Chronic (Exertional) Compartment Syndrome.** Chronic or exertional compartment syndrome usually results from excessive muscle hypertrophy during exercise. During activity, tissue pressure remains high during contractions, impeding blood flow and causing muscle ischemia. This transient ischemia causes the athlete to stop or slow activity secondary to symptoms of pain, muscular fatigue, a feeling of heaviness within the compartment, and reduced dorsiflexion muscle function. Passive plantar flexion exacerbates the pain. Once activity ceases, interstitial volume and blood flow return to normal and symptoms subside. In exertional compartment syndromes, the pressure is usually not high enough to cause vascular collapse and rarely results in a medical emergency. It is common to see fascial defects and muscle herniation through the fascia resulting from increased intracompartmental pressure. Athletes who experience exertional compartment syndromes may in severe cases require a surgical fasciotomy to remove the fascial restriction and allow sufficient room for muscle hypertrophy during activity.

• **Acute Compartment Syndrome.** Acute compartment syndrome represents a medical emergency and typically results from acute trauma such as a fracture, a kick to the leg, or other direct trauma. Intensive exercise can be a causative factor, although this is rarely the case. As a result of the acute trauma, vasodilatation and bleeding within the compartment increase pressure and cause venous compromise and eventual collapse. Given the higher pressure of the anterior tibial artery as compared to the veins, blood continues to flow into the compartment even after venous collapse, further contributing to the rising pressure. If the condition is left untreated, muscle ischemia and tissue necrosis occur within 6 to 12 hours. Immediate recognition and medical referral are imperative.

Signs and symptoms of an impending acute compartment syndrome include pain out of proportion to the injury that greatly intensifies with plantar flexion of the ankle. The compartment will be warm to the touch, and the overlying skin will be tense, glossy, and pale. You will find sensory and motor loss over the distribution of the deep peroneal nerve, with motor deficits ranging from weakness of great toe extension and dorsiflexion to eventual foot drop. If any of these signs are apparent, refer the patient immediately for medical attention. In addition, do not compress the injury as this can create further pressure and vascular compromise. Elevation of the limb further reduces blood flow in an already compromised and ischemic limb.

Deep Vein Thrombophlebitis

Deep vein thrombophlebitis is the inflammation of a deep vein and may be associated with a **thrombus**, or blood clot. The leg, particularly the calf, is the most frequent site of these conditions. Venous inflammation or clotting in patients may result from direct trauma such as the impact of a batted ball or a hard kick to the calf, or it may follow a period of cast immobilization. Signs and symptoms include a vague, dull ache in the posterior calf, swelling, pallor, diminished or absent pedal pulse, and a positive Homan's sign (see the special tests section later in this chapter). A potential complication of a thrombus is a **pulmonary embolism**, which occurs if the clot breaks loose and travels to and obstructs the pulmonary artery or one of its branches.

Structural and Functional Abnormalities

Collectively, the joints of the midfoot and forefoot form structural arches that provide spring and shock absorption both lengthwise and crosswise. The four arches of the foot that contribute to its stability and its shock absorption are the medial longitudinal, lateral longitudinal, transverse, and metatarsal arches (figure 16.20). Structural or functional foot abnormalities may alter these supportive arches, leading to decreased stability or shock absorption or both. Changes resulting from these structural and functional abnormalities can tremendously influence gait, lower-extremity alignment, and mechanics, leading to a host of chronic stress and compensatory problems not only in the foot and ankle, but also up into the knee, hip, or low back.

> ⚠ If an acute compartment syndrome is left untreated, muscle ischemia and tissue necrosis will occur within 6 to 12 hours. Immediate recognition and medical referral are imperative.

> ⚠ Compression and elevation are contraindicated with a suspected compartment syndrome, as they can increase intercompartmental pressure and vascular compromise.

> ⚠ Watch for the 5 Ps of an impending compartment syndrome: *P*ain, *P*aresthesia, *P*allor, *P*ulselessness, and *P*aralysis.

> ⚠ A potential complication of a thrombus is a pulmonary embolism, which occurs when a clot breaks loose and travels to and obstructs a pulmonary artery.

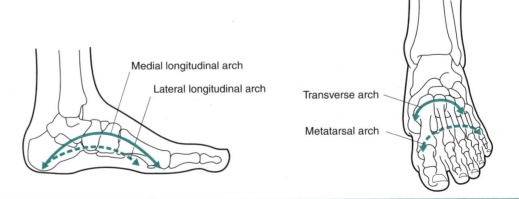

Figure 16.20   Arches of the foot.

Foot Alignment in Relaxed Weight-Bearing Position

Part of the leg, ankle, and foot examination includes identifying the foot's alignment when weight bearing and non-weight bearing. Because the foot is a mobile segment, joint positions and alignment can change between weight bearing and non-weight bearing; you should not assume the two positions reveal the same alignment. This section presents normal alignment, followed by possible pathological variations.

Anatomic Alignment When Standing

View the patient from anterior, lateral, and posterior views. Ask the patient to remove shoes and socks and stand comfortably. Observe the patient's alignment in a relaxed standing position and then compare to alignment when the talus is in a neutral position. Ideally, both positions should be the same, but more often, they differ. For normal talar neutral alignment, the following should occur:

- Metatarsal heads are in the same plane as the ground and in the same plane with each other.
- Calcaneus is centrally located below the leg and perpendicular to the floor, with both condyles flat on the ground.
- Talus is neutral.
- Medial border of the foot lies in a straight line from heel to big toe.
- Each toe is flexible and in straight alignment.
- Medial longitudinal arch is visible and forms a gentle, smooth curve.
- Normal ROM is available at the ankle ($-10°$-$65°$).
- Muscles have good tone and strength.
- Weight is distributed between heel and ball of foot with all metatarsal heads on the floor.
- Foot is asymptomatic.

Forefoot–Rearfoot Relationships

Clinicians commonly use the term *excessive pronation* to describe deviations of the subtalar joint relative to a neutral position. *Excessive* defines a pronation that is either greater than normal or occurs within the gait cycle for a prolonged period. In contrast, *excessive supination* is seen in rigid feet with little intertarsal or metatarsal mobility. As previously mentioned, however, these deviations are relatively complex, with pronation and supination representing a composite of three planes of motion. During weight bearing, excessive pronation results from excessive eversion, plantar flexion, and abduction of the foot and is characterized by a collapsed medial arch (pes planus) or a drop in the height of the navicular bone (see Feiss Line on page 411). Excessive foot pronation is associated with hypermobility in the subtalar joint, requiring greater effort by the foot and ankle stabilizers to maintain stability during weight-bearing activities. Excessive supination is characterized by a rigid, inverted, dorsiflexed, and adducted foot. The hypomobile subtalar joint adversely affects the foot's ability to absorb shock.

Given the interrelationship of the three planes of motions contributing to supination and pronation, a variety of anatomical alignment deviations between the forefoot and rearfoot can contribute to gross pathologies. In particular, the relationship between the forefoot and rearfoot, defined by the alignment of the metatarsal heads (forefoot) and plantar surface of the calcaneus (rearfoot), plays a significant role in these deviations. In a normal or neutral foot, the plane of the metatarsal heads is perpendicular to a line bisecting the calcaneus in the frontal plane. The more common structural deformities resulting in deviations from neutral alignment are described here.

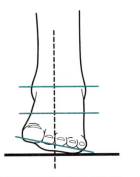
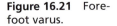
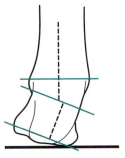

Figure 16.21 Fore-foot varus.

Figure 16.22 Rearfoot varus.

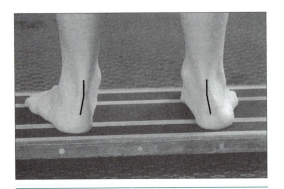

Figure 16.23 Rearfoot valgus.

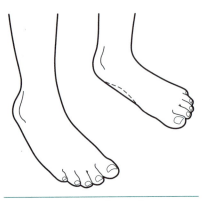

Figure 16.24 Pes planus foot.

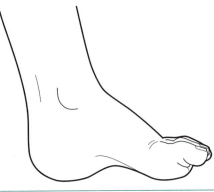

Figure 16.25 Pes cavus foot.

Forefoot Varus

Forefoot varus is characterized by inversion of the forefoot relative to the rearfoot secondary to inadequate rotation of the talus medially. Consequently, the medial side of the foot is raised (figure 16.21). In an effort to bring the first metatarsal into contact with the ground for push-off, the patient pronates the foot excessively; this adaptation resembles a pes planus foot. Excessive pronation can precipitate a host of lower-extremity complaints including posterior tibial and Achilles tendinitis, patellofemoral disorders, and hip or low back pain.

Forefoot Valgus

Forefoot valgus is an eversion of the forefoot relative to the rearfoot. Excessive medial rotation of the talus everts the plane of the metatarsals, with the lateral border of the forefoot riding higher than the medial side. To compensate, the patient supinates at the midfoot to bring the lateral border of the foot into contact with the ground. Common lower-extremity complaints associated with a forefoot valgus include increased susceptibility to inversion ankle sprains and lateral knee pain.

Rearfoot (Hindfoot) Varus

Rearfoot varus, the most common structural foot deformity (Tiberio 1988), is characterized by an inverted calcaneus that causes the medial condyle of the calcaneus to lose contact with the ground (figure 16.22). Either **tibial varum** or **genu varum** may also be present and contribute to a rearfoot varus. The result is that the lateral aspect of the foot makes initial contact, requiring compensatory plantar flexion of the first ray or subtalar pronation to bring the medial calcaneal condyle and forefoot into contact with the ground. Chronic injuries that may ensue include plantar fasciitis, metatarsalgia or stress fracture of the second ray, hallux valgus (see figure 16.26), posterior tibialis tendinitis, and medial tibial stress syndrome (Tiberio 1988).

Rearfoot (Hindfoot) Valgus

Hindfoot valgus is a calcaneus eversion (figure 16.23). This may result in a hypermobile foot and excessive subtalar pronation. Hindfoot valgus is typically less problematic than rearfoot varus.

Pes Planus

Pes planus, or **flatfoot,** is caused by hypermobility resulting from increased ligament laxity and muscle weakness on the plantar surface of the foot (figure 16.24). It can also result from trauma such as severe medial ankle and arch sprains. Patients with a pes planus foot may have greater and more prolonged subtalar pronation during gait secondary to the hypermobility, resulting in medial stress injuries at the ankle, lower leg, and knee. They may also complain of medial arch pain and fatigue with activity. However, many active athletes with a pes planus foot have no complaints of pain.

Pes Cavus

A **pes cavus** foot is characterized by an abnormally high and rigid arch, contracture of plantar soft tissue structures, prominent metatarsal heads, and elevation of toes off the ground (figure 16.25). The plane of the metatarsals is plantar flexed in relation to the calcaneus. The pes cavus foot is typically hypomobile and therefore has poor shock-absorbing capabilities. Callus formation, plantar fasciitis, Achilles tendon tightness, and stress injuries are frequent complaints in athletes with a pes cavus foot.

Plantar Flexed First Ray

Plantar flexion of the first ray relative to the rest of the metatarsal plane can be attributable to either a structural or functional deformity. As mentioned previously, plantar flexion of the first ray may occur as a compensatory motion for a rearfoot varus. A structural deformity is often present with a congenitally pes cavus foot. A rigid plantar flexed first ray compromises normal mechanics at the first metatarsophalangeal joint during gait and may result in joint rigidity (Tiberio 1988). Callus formation under the first metatarsal head will usually be more pronounced than normal.

Equinus Deformity

Equinus deformity refers to a limited dorsiflexion range at the ankle. It can be caused by a structural forefoot equinus, in which the forefoot is plantar flexed relative to the rearfoot, or by a rigid forefoot varus or abnormally tight calf or Achilles tendon. The consequence is midtarsal hypermobility and excessive pronation to compensate for the lack of dorsiflexion at push-off.

Toe Deformities

Toe deformities may be congenital or acquired as a consequence of other forefoot and rearfoot deformity or dysfunction.

Hallux Valgus and Bunions

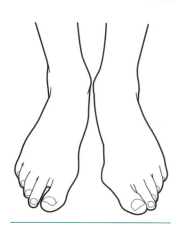

Hallux valgus is a valgus deformity at the first metatarsophalangeal joint characterized by a medial deviation of the joint and lateral angulation of the phalanx (figure 16.26). It may be congenital or result from trauma or ill-fitting shoes.

As a result of the angulation, the extensor and flexor hallucis longus tendons deviate laterally and compromise joint function. The prominent medially deviated metatarsophalangeal (MP) joint will be subject to increased pressure and friction from footwear. A bunion develops secondary to callus formation, bursal thickening, and excessive bone formation.

Figure 16.26 Hallux valgus.

Hallux Rigidus

Degenerative or arthritic changes resulting from joint dysfunction or pathomechanics may lead to fusion and rigidity at the first metatarsophalangeal joint. Signs and symptoms include decreased active and passive ROM and palpable joint tenderness. Because of his inability to fully extend the toe, the patient experiences pain with push-off and demonstrates an altered gait.

Claw Toes

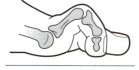

Figure 16.27 Claw toes.

Claw toes are often found in conjunction with a pes cavus foot and are characterized by hyperextension of the metatarsophalangeal joint and flexion of the distal and proximal interphalangeal joints (figure 16.27). They can also result from neurological problems, dysfunction of the lumbricals and interosseous muscles, or both.

Hammer Toes

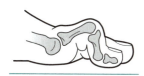

Figure 16.28 Hammer toes.

Similar to claw toes, hammer toes are characterized by hyperextension of the metatarsophalangeal joint and a flexion contracture of the proximal interphalangeal joint. However, the distal interphalangeal joint may be flexed, hyperextended, or neutral (figure 16.28). You will frequently find a callus over the flexed and prominent proximal interphalangeal joint due to contact and friction with the top of the shoe. This deformity may be congenital or may result from poorly fitting shoes or intrinsic muscle dysfunction. Intrinsic muscle insufficiency results in an inability to hold neutral or to flex the metatarsophalangeal joint, and consequently results in a hyperextension deformity due to the overpowering extrinsic toe extensors. This hyperextension in turn tenses the toe flexors, resulting in a flexion deformity of the proximal interphalangeal joint.

Mallet Toe

Mallet toe, which is similar to mallet finger, is a flexion of the distal IP of the toe. As a consequence of a mallet toe, a callus may form over the dorsal aspect of the distal joint. This deformity is fairly benign and causes little or no joint dysfunction or compensatory motion.

Morton's Toe

With Morton's toe, the second toe is longer the first; therefore, push-off subjects the second metatarsal to unusually large stress. This may alter the function and mobility of the first metatarsophalangeal joint and increase the risk of stress fracture in the second metatarsal.

OBJECTIVE TESTS

By now you should appreciate the variety of conditions, both acute and chronic, that you may encounter when examining the foot and ankle. To examine and differentiate among these injuries, you need a sound knowledge of injury pathology and a good understanding of normal foot alignment and mechanics. The following examination components provide the additional tools you will need to accurately determine the severity, irritability, nature, and stage of the injury. Some of these tools will also become important when you examine chronic conditions further up the chain (chapters 17 and 18), as these conditions may originate from, or be exacerbated by, structural or functional foot abnormalities. As always, the patient's past and present history and your observations will guide objective test selection.

Palpation

Because of the many and small structures that constitute the foot and ankle, it is particularly important to develop a systematic routine for palpation to help you avoid inadvertently omitting a structure. Palpate all structures bilaterally and focus on the area of pain last. This chapter describes the palpation sequence regionally (anterior and dorsal, medial, lateral, and posterior and plantar), moving from proximal to distal structures. (You may wish to refer to figures 16.1 through 16.6 at the beginning of this chapter or an anatomy text when reviewing this section.)

- **Anterior and dorsal structures.** Anterior structures of the leg and ankle include the tibial crest, anterior tibiofibular joint and ligament, anterior dome of the talus, anterior tibialis muscle and tendon, and extensor tendons as they cross the anterior ankle joint. Having the patient actively dorsiflex the ankle will aid palpation of these tendons; alternatively, having the patient relax the ankle joint facilitates palpation of the anterior tibiofibular and talotibial joints. Distal into the foot, the anterior (dorsal) structures include the bony contour of the cuneiforms, metatarsals, and toes and the soft tissue characteristics of the extensor hallucis longus, extensor digitorum longus, and brevis tendons. You will also palpate the dorsalis pedis pulse on the dorsum of the foot, between the tibialis anterior and extensor digitorum longus tendons over the tarsal area.

- **Medial structures.** Moving proximal to distal, the medial leg and foot structures consist of the tibial shaft; medial malleolus; deltoid ligament; three tendons (tibialis posterior, flexor digitorum longus, and flexor hallucis longus) as they pass posteriorly to the medial malleolus; posterior tibial artery; sustentaculum tali; navicular tuberosity; spring ligament; medial cuneiform; abductor hallucis; first metatarsal base, shaft, and head; and first toe. Also in this region is the posterior tibial nerve, which sits just posterior to the tibialis posterior, flexor digitorum tendons, and posterior tibial artery (ordered anterior to posterior as they pass behind the medial malleolus), and anterior to the flexor hallucis longus tendon.

- **Lateral structures.** Lateral structures of the leg, ankle, and foot include the fibula shaft, peroneal muscles and tendons, lateral malleolus, anterior and posterior talofibular ligaments, calcaneofibular ligament, sinus tarsus, cuboid, base of the fifth metatarsal, and fifth phalanx.

- **Posterior and plantar structures.** Posterior leg and ankle structures include the gastrocnemius and soleus muscles, Achilles tendon, and calcaneus. Be sure to palpate the skin over the calaneus for signs of bursal thickening or ectopic bone growth (exostosis). Plantar structures include the calcaneal fat pad, plantar aponeurosis (fascia) from its attachment on the medial tubercle of the calcaneus to its distal expanse, the metatarsal heads, and toes. As the flexor hallucis longus passes the first metatarsal head on its way to the great toe, it passes through two sesamoid bones in the tendon of the flexor hallucis brevis. If there is tenderness in this area, palpate the medial and lateral sesamoid bones for tenderness and crepitus.

Range of Motion

ROM examination includes motion at the talocrural (ankle), subtalar, and metatarsophalangeal joints. Examine bilaterally and note pain, motion quality, joint restriction, or excessive motion.

Active ROM

The patient can perform bilateral non-weight-bearing movements simultaneously for easy comparison of left and right. Ankle dorsiflexion (figure 16.29a), plantar flexion (figure 16.29b), inversion (figure 16.29c), and eversion (figure 16.29d), as well as toe extension (figure 16.29e), flexion (figure 16.29f), and abduction, are performed with the ankles over the end of the bench or table. In weight bearing, the movements can also be performed with the two feet simultaneously. The movements should include ankle plantar flexion (raising toes), dorsiflexion (lifting toes off the ground, standing on heel), inversion (lifting medial border and rolling onto lateral border of foot), and eversion (lifting lateral border, rolling onto medial border of the foot), as well as toe flexion (toe curl) and extension (toes lifted off ground). Observe for differences in total range for each motion and pain or hesitancy with any of the movements.

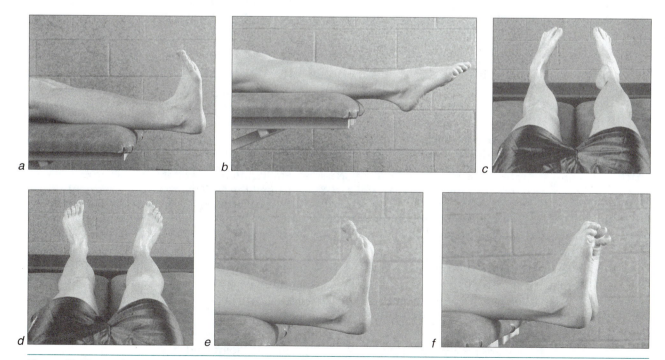

Figure 16.29 Active ROM movements for *(a)* ankle dorsiflexion, *(b)* plantar flexion, *(c)* inversion, *(d)* eversion and for *(e)* toe extension and *(f)* flexion.

Passive ROM

If active ROM is full, perform passive overpressures at the end of each motion. Overpressure response is normally pain free, and end feel for these motions should produce a soft tissue stretch sensation. If active movements were not full, passively move the ankle and foot into full dorsiflexion, plantar flexion, rearfoot inversion, rearfoot eversion, forefoot inversion, and forefoot eversion, and passively perform toe flexion and extension.

Goniometric Examination of ROM

Goniometric measurement of ankle and foot motions are described in table 16.1 and illustrated in figure 16.30.

Table 16.1
Goniometric Examination of Ankle and Foot ROM

Motion	Location of goniometer	Movement	Normal range
Ankle dorsiflexion	P: Supine, knee flexed to 30° and gastrocnemius relaxed A: Just inferior to lateral malleolus S: Long axis of fibula M: Lateral border of foot	From neutral position (goniometer reading 90°), dorsiflex the ankle to limit of motion	0° to 10-30°
Ankle plantar flexion	P: Supine, knee flexed to 30° and gastrocnemius relaxed A: Just inferior to lateral malleolus S: Long axis of fibula M: Lateral border of foot	From neutral position (goniometer reading 90°), plantar flex the ankle to limit of motion	0° to 45-65°
Subtalar inversion	P: Prone, foot off edge of table with marks bisecting the superior and inferior aspects of the posterior calcaneus A: Midpoint, superior aspect of calcaneus S: Long axis of leg M: Long axis, midline of calcaneus	Invert the calcaneus to the limit of motion	0° to 30-50°
Subtalar eversion	P: Prone, foot off edge of table with marks bisecting the superior and inferior aspects of the posterior calcaneus A: Midpoint, superior aspect of calcaneus S: Long axis of leg M: Long axis, midline of calcaneus	Evert the calcaneus to the limit of motion	0° to 15-30°
MTP flexion	P: Seated, foot relaxed and resting on table A: Dorsum (2nd-4th) or side (1st & 5th) of MTP joint S: Long axis metatarsal M: Long axis proximal phalanx	Stabilizing the metatarsal, flex the MTP joint to limit of motion	0° to 40°
MTP extension	P: Seated, foot relaxed and resting on table A: Plantar surface (2nd-4th) or side (1st & 5th) of MTP joint S: Long axis metatarsal M: Long axis proximal phalanx	Stabilizing the metatarsal, extend the MTP joint to limit of motion	0° to 50° (2nd-5th) 0° to 70-90° (1st)
1st MTP abduction and adduction	P: Seated, foot relaxed and resting on table A: Dorsum of 1st MTP joint S: Long axis of 1st MT M: Long axis of proximal phalanx	Passively abduct and adduct the great toe to the limit of motion	0° to 10-20°
1st IP flexion and extension	P: Seated, foot relaxed and resting on table A: 1st IP joint S: Long axis proximal phalanx M: Long axis distal phalanx	Extend and flex the IP to full limit of motion with the MTP joint held in extension	0° to 80-90°

P = patient positioning; A = goniometer axis; S = stabilizing arm; M = movable arm; MTP = metatarsal phalangeal joint; IP = interphalangeal joint; MT = metatarsal.

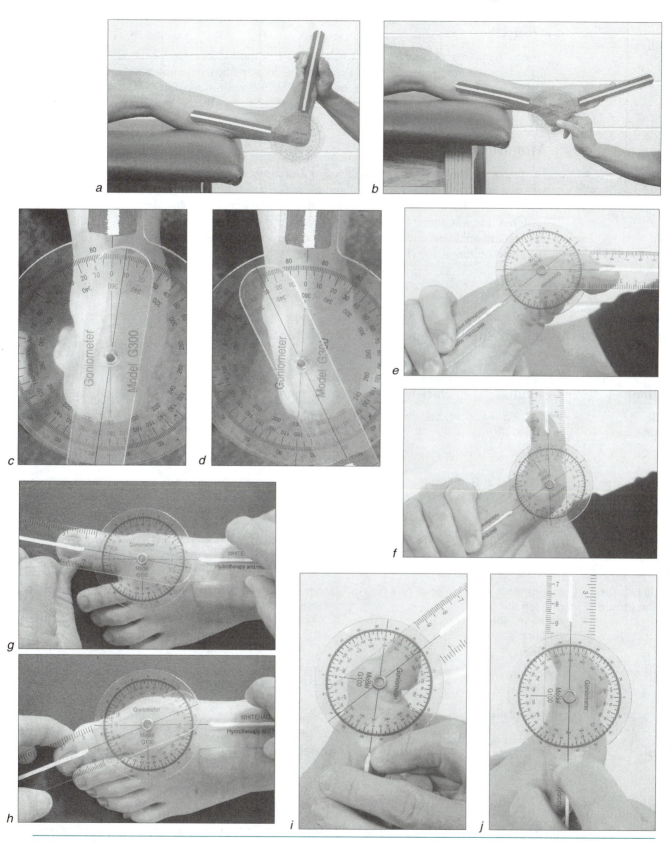

Figure 16.30 Goniometric examination of *(a)* ankle dorsiflexion; *(b)* ankle plantar flexion, *(c)* inversion, and *(d)* eversion; *(e)* MTP flexion and *(f)* extension; *(g)* great toe abduction and *(h)* adduction; *(i)* first interphalangeal flexion and *(j)* extension.

Strength

Due to the large mechanical forces associated with running, jumping, and cutting, muscles of the foot, ankle, and lower leg play a critical role in providing dynamic stability, adaptability, and shock absorption for the foot and ankle. When examining foot, ankle, and lower leg strength, consider both the adequacy of strength as well as the balance of strength between muscle groups.

Manual Muscle Testing

Manual muscle tests for the leg, ankle, and foot musculature include knee flexion; ankle dorsiflexion, plantar flexion, inversion, and eversion; and toe flexion and extension (table 16.2, figure 16.31). Because of the strength of the plantar flexor muscles, the grade 5 test is best performed as a standing heel raise. Knee flexion is covered in chapter 17, but is included in the leg and ankle examination because of the gastrocnemius muscle's origination proximal to the tibiofemoral joint.

Table 16.2

Manual Muscle Testing for the Leg, Ankle, and Foot Musculature

Motion	Athlete position	Stabilizing hand placement	Resistance hand placement	Instruction to athlete	Primary muscles tested
Ankle dorsiflexion	Seated, leg extended off table	Distal posterior tibia	Dorsomedial surface of the foot	Dorsiflex and invert the foot by bringing the big toe toward shin	Tibialis anterior
Ankle plantar flexion (grade < 5)	Seated, foot and leg extended off table	Distal anterior tibia	Plantar surface of foot	With knee extended (gastrocnemius) and flexed >45° (soleus), point foot against resistance	Gastrocnemius, soleus
Ankle plantar flexion (grade 5)	Standing on one leg using hand on table to balance	None	None—uses body weight	Raise heel 20 times, or until unable to complete full motion	Gastrocnemius, soleus
Inversion	Side-lying, lying on side to be tested, foot slightly plantar flexed	Distal medial tibia	Medial aspect of foot	Raise medial border of foot toward ceiling	Tibialis posterior
Eversion	Side-lying, on side not to be tested, foot slightly plantar flexed	Distal lateral tibia	Lateral aspect of foot	Raise lateral border of foot toward ceiling	Peroneal longus and brevis
2nd-5th MTP and IP toe flexion	Supine, foot resting on table	MTP: Metatarsal PIP: Proximal phalanx DIP: Middle phalanx	MTP: Proximal phalanx PIP: Middle phalanx DIP: Distal phalanx	Flex or curl toes	MTP: Lubricales PIP: Flexor digitorum brevis DIP: Flexor digitorum longus

Motion	Athlete position	Stabilizing hand placement	Resistance hand placement	Instruction to athlete	Primary muscles tested
2nd-5th MTP and IP toe extension	Supine, foot resting on table	Metatarsals	Distal phalanx	Extend toes	Extensor digitorum longus and brevis
Great toe flexion	Supine, foot resting on table	MTP: 1st metatarsal IP: MTP joint	MTP: Proximal phalanx IP: Distal phalanx	Flex great toe	MTP: Flexor hallucis brevis IP: Flexor hallucis longus
Great toe extension	Supine, foot resting on table	1st metatarsal	Proximal and distal phalanx	Extend great toe	Extensor hallucis brevis (PIP) and longus (DIP)
Great toe abduction	Supine, foot resting on table	1st metatarsal	Medial aspect of proximal phalanx	Abduct the toe against resistance or place in abduction and say, "don't let me move you"	Abductor hallucis

MTP = metatarsalphalangeal joint; PIP = proximal interphalangeal joint; DIP = distal interphalangeal joint; IP = interphalangeal joint.

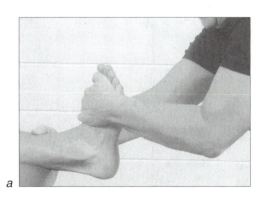

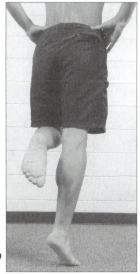

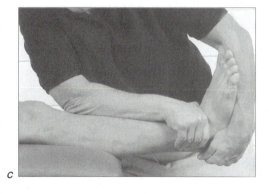

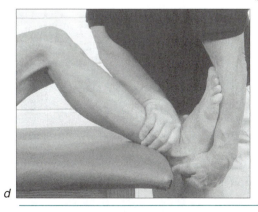

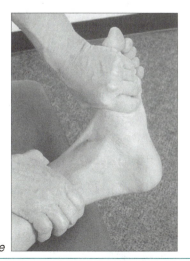

a

b

c

d

e

Figure 16.31   Manual muscle testing for (a) ankle dorsiflexion; (b) ankle plantar flexion in standing, and seated with (c) knee extended and (d) knee flexed; (e) inversion.

(continued)

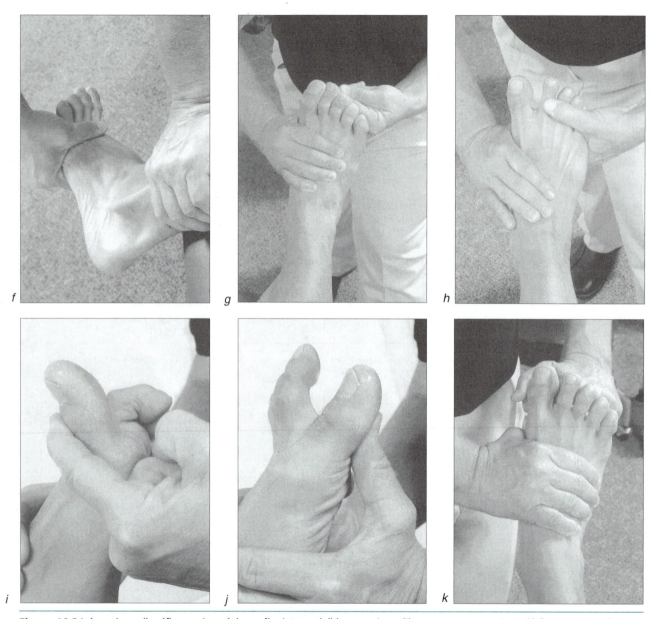

Figure 16.31 *(continued)* *(f)* eversion; *(g)* toe flexion and *(h)* extension; *(i)* great toe extension, *(j)* flexion, and *(k)* abduction.

Instrumented Strength Examination

Isokinetic dynamometers can quantify strength and endurance for ankle plantar flexion and dorsiflexion and inversion and eversion (figure 16.32). Less expensive methods of quantifying foot and ankle strength include the use of free weights (e.g., ankle weight boot), or machine weights (e.g., calf raise machine) to perform 1RM or 10RM tests.

Neurovascular Examination

Perform and compare all neurovascular tests bilaterally. Vascular examination includes comparing distal pulse, skin color and temperature, and capillary refill. A detailed review of these tests is covered in chapter 8.

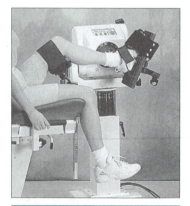

Figure 16.32 Isokinetic testing of ankle inversion and eversion.

Courtesy of Biodex Medical Systems.

Neurological Examination

Neurological examination includes sensory, motor, and reflex testing of the peripheral nerve branches of the lumbosacral plexus.

Sensory Testing

Peripheral sensory nerve examination should include the deep peroneal nerve in the first dorsal web space, the superficial peroneal nerve on the dorsum of the foot and lateral leg, the tibial nerve over the posteriomedial plantar heel, the medial plantar nerve over the medial three digits, and the lateral plantar over the fifth digit. Any abnormal result warrants a more detailed sensory examination (see chapter 8, table 8.7).

Motor Testing

For myotome examination, the posterior tibial nerve, which innervates the muscles in the posterior compartment, is examined with resistance to plantar flexion and toe flexion. The superficial peroneal nerve innervates the lateral compartment muscles and is tested with eversion. The deep peroneal nerve innervates the muscles in the anterior compartment and can be tested with dorsiflexion and great toe extension. Test the integrity of the medial plantar with great toe abduction (abductor hallucis) and the lateral plantar nerve with abduction of the fifth digit (abductor digiti minimi). See chapter 8, table 8.7 and figure 8.16, for illustrations of these tests.

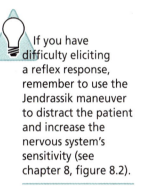

If you have difficulty eliciting a reflex response, remember to use the Jendrassik maneuver to distract the patient and increase the nervous system's sensitivity (see chapter 8, figure 8.2).

Reflex Testing

For symptoms below the knee, you can elicit a deep tendon reflex from the Achilles tendon (S1-S2) (chapter 8, figure 8.17). If you find the response diminished or absent, ensure that the patient is not inhibiting the response by having him perform the Jendrassik's maneuver (chapter 8, figure 8.2). You can also test the posterior tibialis tendon (L4-L5) on the medial aspect of the ankle for reflex response, but this site is not commonly used.

Vascular Compromise

If you suspect vascular compromise, palpate the dorsalis pedis over the dorsum of the foot in the space between the tibialis anterior and the extensor digitorum longus, and palpate the posterior tibial artery just posterior to the medial malleolus. Check for presence and strength of pulse (figure 16.33). Also look for changes in skin color and temperature, and normal capillary refill of the nail bed. Skin that is warm, glossy, and pale suggests increased compartmental pressure. You can also identify tissue ischemia by unusually intense pain when the muscle is stretched.

Special Tests

Special tests for the leg, ankle, and foot include tests to identify fractures, ligament instability, neurovascular compromise, and muscle and fascial injury, and tests to examine structural alignment.

Fracture Tests

A number of tests can be used to determine if a fracture is present. It is a misconception that an athlete is unable to

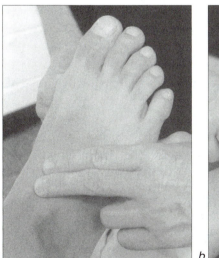
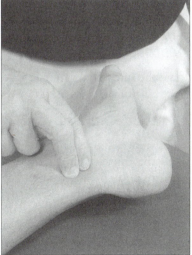

a   b

Figure 16.33 Palpation of the (a) dorsalis pedis and (b) posterior tibial pulses.

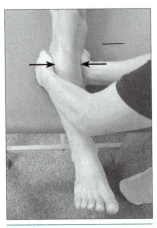

Figure 16.34   Pott's compression test.

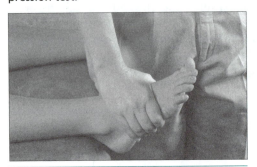

Figure 16.35   Morton's test for metatarsal stress fractures and Morton's neuroma.

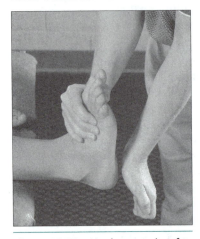

Figure 16.36   Heel percussion for tibial stress fracture.

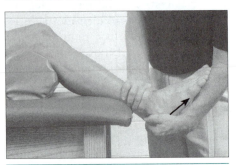

Figure 16.37   Anterior drawer test.

walk if a bone is fractured. Traumatic injury with torsion or impact forces can fracture the leg and foot bones. Although an X ray is the definitive means for diagnosing a fracture, you can tentatively identify a fracture with these commonly used tests.

Pott's Compression (Squeeze) Test

A Pott's fracture occurs in the distal leg, but if the bones are not displaced it may be difficult to detect. The following test will often enable you to identify a Pott's fracture. Place your hands on either side of the upper aspect of the leg with the pad of one hand just distal to the fibular head and the pad of the other hand at the same level on the medial tibia. Then push your hands together to squeeze the tibia and fibula (figure 16.34). A positive sign occurs if the athlete reports increased pain in the distal fibula or tibia.

Morton's Test

The metatarsals are the most frequent site of stress fractures in the lower quarter. To test for fracture, have the patient lie supine. Grasp the midfoot region and squeeze the metatarsal heads together (figure 16.35). If the test produces pain, there may be a stress fracture. You can also use this test in suspected cases of Morton's neuroma. If the result is positive, refer the patient to a physician for further examination.

Percussion Test (Tap or Bump Test)

Another way to identify fractures is with vibration or percussion. To differentiate a tibial stress fracture from medial tibial stress syndrome, apply a percussive force (tap or bump) to the plantar surface of the heel (figure 16.36). If localized pain occurs near the suspected fracture site, the test is considered positive. You can also apply a percussion test to the metatarsals by stabilizing the toe in the neutral position and tapping the end of the toe to create a vibration down the shaft of the metatarsal.

Hoffa's Test

This test rules out a calcaneal fracture. With the patient prone and the feet over the end of the table, instruct her to plantar flex and dorsiflex the ankle while you palpate the Achilles tendon. A positive sign occurs if the Achilles tendon on the injured side is less taut during movement than the uninjured side; in this case, refer the patient to a physician for further testing.

Ligamentous Stability Tests

To examine the integrity of the medial, lateral, and tibiofibular ligaments of the ankle, perform the following tests.

Anterior Drawer Test

This test examines the integrity of the anterior talofibular ligament and the calcaneofibular ligament. A positive sign can occur with a tear of only the talofibular ligament, but laxity is greater when both ligaments are injured. With the patient in either a sitting or a supine position and the knee slightly flexed to relax the gastrocnemius, passively position the ankle in about 20° plantar flexion and stabilize the leg. Grasp the calcaneus and pull the foot forward (figure 16.37). A positive result occurs if this produces pain and laxity. You will commonly see a dimple in the skin over the site of the anterior talofibular ligament during this test. In an alternate testing position, the patient is

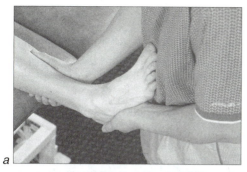

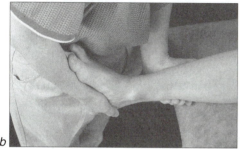

Figure 16.38 Talar tilt tests at *(a)* end range varus to stress lateral ligaments and *(b)* end range valgus to stress medial ligaments.

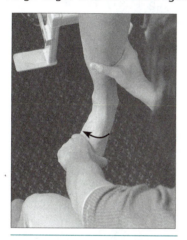

Figure 16.39 Kleiger test.

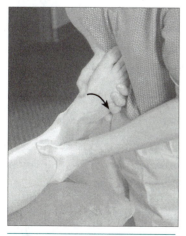

Figure 16.40 Stress test for the syndesmosis.

prone with the foot hanging off the edge of the table. Place one hand under the distal anterior surface of the tibia and apply an anteriorly directed force to the calcaneus.

Talar Tilt

This test determines the integrity of the calcaneofibular and deltoid ligaments. The patient can be positioned supine, sitting, or side-lying. Place the ankle in the anatomic position and stabilize the distal tibia and fibula. Then adduct and invert the calcaneus into a varus position to test the calcaneofibular ligament. Test the deltoid ligament with the calcaneus abducted and everted into a valgus position. Pain or laxity with end range varus (figure 16.38a) is positive for calcaneofibular ligament injury, and pain or laxity with end range valgus (figure 16.38b) is a positive sign for deltoid ligament injury.

Kleiger Test (Lateral Rotation Test)

This test examines the integrity of the deltoid ligament. With the patient sitting, her knee flexed to 90°, and her foot relaxed and not bearing weight, grasp the foot and rotate it laterally (figure 16.39). A positive test occurs with medial and lateral ankle pain with or without palpated talus displacement.

Syndesmotic Separation

This test examines the integrity of the anterior tibiofibular ligament and syndesmosis. To stress the syndesmosis, fully dorsiflex the ankle to end range, forcing the dome of the talus to stress the inferior tibiofibular joint. You can further stress the joint by laterally rotating the foot when it is in this dorsiflexed position (figure 16.40). Pain over the anterior distal tibiofibular joint demonstrates a positive test. The main differences between this and the Kleiger test are the specific ligaments that are stressed due to the degree of ankle dorsiflexion.

Neurovascular Tests

Use additional neurovascular testing to determine peripheral nerve injuries or circulatory problems in the leg and ankle. Whereas both nerve and vascular injuries can occasionally result from acute trauma, nerve compression injuries more often result from overuse and chronic inflammatory conditions. Examine any complaint of numbness, burning, or tingling along a specific nerve pathway for possible nerve compression or injury. In nontraumatic cases, look to structural malformations or malalignments as possible causes of nerve compression.

Homan's Sign

Homan's sign identifies deep vein thrombophlebitis. With the patient in a relaxed position, passively extend the knee while passively dorsiflexing the ankle. Pain in the calf is a positive sign. Palpating the calf can also elicit complaints of tenderness.

Deep Peroneal Nerve Compression Tests

The deep peroneal nerve runs through the anterior compartment and into the dorsum of the foot; both of these are sites for compression secondary to acute trauma or increased volume within the leg compartment after prolonged activity. (High arches or tight shoelaces can also help compress the anterior tibial branch of the deep peroneal nerve as it passes superficially along the dorsum of the foot.) The sensory loss is often less than the motor loss, since the deep peroneal nerve primarily supplies the anterior foot muscles. Loss of dorsiflexion, reduced ankle control, and pain or burning during plantar flexion are the primary complaints. Forceful passive plantar flexion reproduces the patient's pain, especially after activity. You may find reduced strength for toe extension or ankle dorsiflexion when compared to the strength in the uninvolved extremity. Refer patients who demonstrate positive test results to a physician for additional examination.

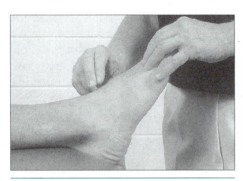

Figure 16.41 Tinel's sign for the anterior tibial branch of the deep peroneal nerve.

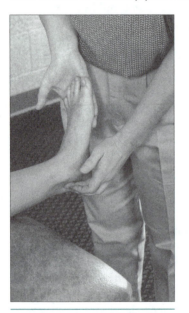

Figure 16.42 Tinel's sign for posterior tibial nerve pathology at the ankle.

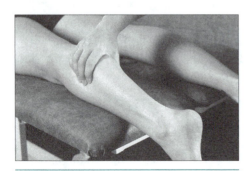

Figure 16.43 Thompson test.

Superficial Peroneal Nerve

The superficial peroneal nerve can be injured during ankle sprains. Since this nerve has a significant sensory branch, the patient complains of sensory changes along its dermatome in the lateral leg and dorsum of the foot. Eversion weakness that may be masked by weakness of the lateral muscles in an ankle sprain may be the result of superficial peroneal nerve injury, especially if the weakness is accompanied by sensory changes. Sensory disturbances will occur when the nerve is placed on stretch with plantar flexion and inversion of the ankle.

Tinel's Sign

This is also called the percussion test, and it identifies nerve pathology, usually compression or entrapment. There are two places in the ankle where you can use Tinel's sign to examine nerve compromise. One is on the dorsum of the proximal foot over the anterior ankle where the anterior tibial branch of the deep peroneal nerve emerges (figure 16.41). The other is just behind the medial malleolus where the posterior tibial nerve passes (figure 16.42). A tapping or percussion of the nerve should not normally produce any sign or symptom; paresthesia or tingling is a positive sign of nerve dysfunction.

Morton's Test

Morton's test confirms a Morton's neuroma. Passive extension of the toes with pressure over the neuroma site reproduces the patient's pain. The Morton's test for stress fracture previously mentioned (squeezing the metatarsal heads) may also compress the nerve and reproduce the patient's pain (see figure 16.35).

Muscle and Fascial Tests

Muscle and fascial tests examine injuries of the Achilles tendon and plantar fascia.

Thompson Test

The Thompson test examines the integrity of the Achilles tendon. The patient lies prone with the foot over the end of the table. With the patient relaxed, squeeze the calf. Normal response is foot movement into plantar flexion (figure 16.43). Lack of foot movement is a positive sign for an Achilles tendon rupture. When you do not have access to a table on the sidelines, you can also perform this test as the patient kneels with the foot unencumbered.

Plantar Fasciitis

The patient's history is the primary examination tool for plantar fasciitis. The patient will report a gradual onset of pain that occurs especially in the morning upon arising and also after prolonged sitting and that improves after taking a few steps. The hallmark of plantar fasciitis is significant pain with direct, point pressure to the medial calcaneal tubercle on the plantar surface of the anterior aspect of the heel.

Alignment Tests

If the results of one or more of the following tests are positive, malalignment may be causing the patient's injury and pain, particularly if the condition is either chronic or recurring. Correction of the malalignment is often necessary to completely resolve the injury. These alignment tests require considerable practice to produce reliable (consistent) measures. However, once mastered, they can be quite valuable in the examination of structural malalignments.

Calcaneal–Tibial Alignment

This alignment identifies a rearfoot valgus or varus and reliably determines rearfoot supination or pronation. The patient lies prone with the foot over the end of the table; the opposite leg is flexed, and the ankle on that leg is crossed over the knee of the leg being investigated (see figure 16.44a). This position stabilizes the pelvis and prevents unwanted movement of the lower extremity. Palpate the calcaneus and draw a line from the medial to the lateral calcaneal process. Then, palpate and mark the center of the calcaneus near the insertion of the Achilles tendon. Draw a perpendicular line from the midcalcaneal mark to the horizontal line. Mark the medial–lateral midpoint of the distal third of the tibial shaft, and draw a line to connect this point with the midcalcaneal point. After marking the leg, place the rearfoot in the neutral alignment by palpating the talus medially and laterally while moving the forefoot with your hand over the distal lateral fourth and fifth metatarsal heads (figure 16.44b). The rearfoot is neutral when you palpate the talus equally on its medial and lateral aspects. The patient must remain relaxed during this process so that you can obtain an accurate position and alignment. In this position, the alignment of the two vertical lines should be straight or in slight varus, no more than approximately 5° to 8°. If the inversion angle is greater than 8°, the rearfoot is in varus. If the heel is angled in eversion, the rearfoot is in valgus.

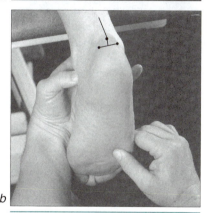

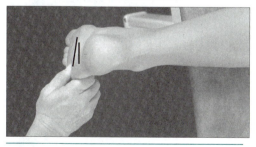

Figure 16.44 (a) Position for calcaneal–tibial alignment test and (b) patient's foot in neutral alignment and with reference lines marked.

Forefoot–Rearfoot Alignment

This test determines the alignment between the rearfoot and forefoot. Position the patient as you did in the calcaneal–tibial alignment examination (prone in a figure-4 position). Place the rearfoot in neutral alignment as described earlier, and then visually examine the relationship between the rearfoot angle and the forefoot angle. In the normal foot, the plantar surface of the heel and the metatarsal heads are parallel in the same plane. If the metatarsal head of the great toe is higher than that of the little toe, the forefoot is in varus (figure 16.45). If the first metatarsal head is lower than the fifth metatarsal head, the forefoot is in valgus.

Figure 16.45 Forefoot–rearfoot alignment test showing forefoot varus.

Feiss Line

The Feiss line examines navicular drop, and navicular drop in turn can determine rearfoot–forefoot alignment. Draw a line from the inferior aspect of the medial malleolus to the plantar aspect of the metatarsophalangeal joint of the great toe. With the patient standing normally and relaxed and the feet about 15 cm (6 in.) apart, determine the position of the navicular tuberosity. It should lie on the line. If the navicular tuberosity is below the line, the foot is considered pes planus with a low longitudinal arch (figure 16.46). If the navicular tuberosity lies above the line, the foot is considered an equinus foot with a high arch.

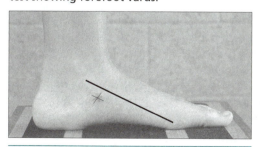

Figure 16.46 Feiss line. Note that the navicular tuberosity is below the line, indicating a pes planus foot.

Navicular Drop

The navicular drop is an alternative method for determining how much the subtalar joint deviates from neutral. The drop represents the change in navicular height between subtalar neutral and relaxed stances. You can perform the test with the patient seated or standing; however, measuring in full weight bearing may provide a more representative measure of functional joint motion.

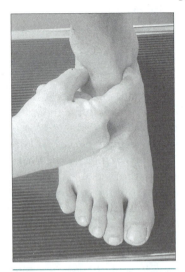

Figure 16.47 Measurement of navicular drop.

Before beginning the measurement, mark the most prominent lateral aspect of the navicular bone. Next, have the patient stand in a bilateral stance on the floor or on a raised platform with the feet shoulder-width apart. Determine the neutral position of the subtalar joint by placing your thumb and index finger over the anterior dome of the talus, with your fingers positioned just below the inferior border of the anterior tibia and anterior to the medial border of the distal fibula and the lateral border of the distal tibia (figure 16.47). While palpating the anterior talar dome, have the patient slowly invert and evert the hindfoot and ankle while using your thumb and index finger to sense when the prominence of the medial and lateral aspects of the talar dome equalize. With the foot held in the referenced subtalar neutral position, use a ruler to measure the distance from the mark on the navicular to the floor or platform. Report this measurement in millimeters (mm). Then instruct the patient to relax the foot into full weight bearing, and again use a ruler to measure the distance between the resulting navicular position and the floor. Record the difference in distance between the original height of the navicular and its final weight-bearing position as the patient's navicular drop. While the literature does not agree on how much navicular drop constitutes excessive pronation, values between 0 and 10 mm are generally considered in the normal range.

Joint Mobility Tests

Accessory movements of the leg, ankle, and foot are complex because of their numerous joints. A few of the commonly used joint mobility examination techniques are discussed here. These techniques determine hypomobility or hypermobility of the joints in this lower-extremity segment. They can also treat hypomobile areas.

For treatment techniques, refer to *Therapeutic Exercise for Musculoskeletal Injuries, Second Edition,* (Houglum 2005), chapter 6.

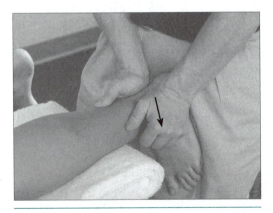

Figure 16.48 Distal tibiofibular ventral glide test.

Distal Tibiofibular Joint

Since the fibula moves with ankle motion, restriction of fibular movement can limit ankle dorsiflexion and plantar flexion. Examine tibiofibular joint mobility if ankle motion is limited in its last few degrees of motion.

Ventral Glide

Have the patient lie prone, with the foot over the end of the table and a padded wedge under the distal leg. Place your stabilizing hand over the distal tibia just above the medial malleolus and place the thenar eminence of your mobilizing hand over the posterior distal fibula just above the lateral malleolus. With the mobilizing hand, apply a posterior–anterior (PA) force to take up the joint slack, and then apply an additional force to examine the amount of movement available (figure 16.48).

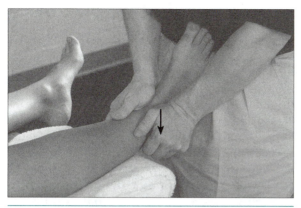

Figure 16.49   Distal tibiofibular dorsal glide test.

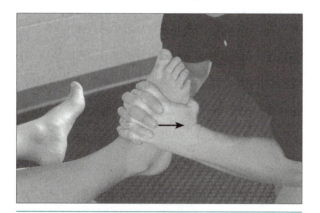

Figure 16.50   Talocrural joint distraction test.

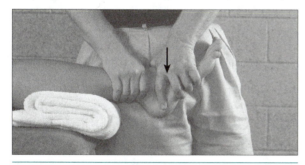

Figure 16.51   Dorsal talar glide test.

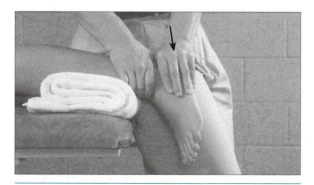

Figure 16.52   Ventral talar glide test.

Dorsal Glide

Have the patient lie supine with the heel off the end of the table. Apply your stabilizing hand to the distal tibia just above the malleolus and apply the thenar eminence of your mobilizing hand on the anterior distal fibula just above the lateral malleolus (figure 16.49). Apply an anterior–posterior (AP) force to the fibula to examine the amount of movement available.

Talocrural Joint

If you observe a capsular pattern of motion in the sagittal plane, examine joint mobility and compare bilaterally.

Distraction

Use distraction to examine general mobility of the talo-crural joint. Have the patient lie supine with the foot just off the table and the leg strapped to the table. With the ankle in about 10° of plantar flexion and in neutral inversion and eversion, place your hands around the patient's foot with your ulnar borders close to the talus and apply a distraction force to the foot, primarily from the medial aspects of your hands (figure 16.50).

Dorsal Talar Glide

This technique examines AP movement of the talus. If dorsiflexion is limited, this movement is likely to be restricted. Have the patient lie supine with the foot over the end of the table. Place your stabilizing hand on the distal leg while your mobilizing hand grasps the talus and midfoot to maintain the joint in a loose-packed position (figure 16.51). Apply an AP force to the talus perpendicular to the tibia's long axis as you examine the amount and quality of movement and end feel.

Ventral Talar Glide

This maneuver examines PA movement of the talus. If plantar flexion is limited, this movement will be restricted if the capsule is restricted. Have the patient lie prone, with the foot over the end of the table and a pad placed under the distal leg. Place your stabilizing hand over the distal leg and place your mobilizing hand around the calcaneus and talus (figure 16.52). Apply a downward PA force to examine the amount and quality of movement and end feel.

Midfoot Glide Tests

Just as the ankle joint can be restricted within its capsule, other joints in the foot can also demonstrate capsular restriction. This is particularly true if the joint has been immobilized. Examine joint mobility in these instances.

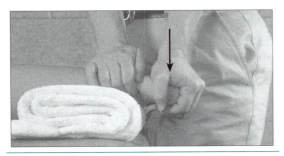

Figure 16.53   Medial–lateral glide of subtalar joint.

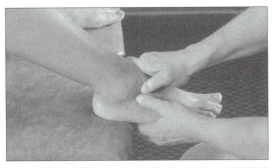

Figure 16.54   Midtarsal joint anterior–posterior and posterior–anterior glides.

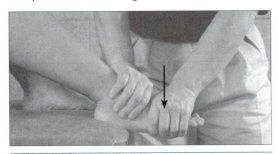

Figure 16.55   Tarsometatarsal joint anterior–posterior glide.

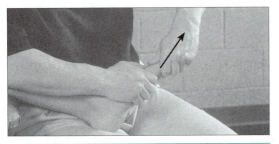

Figure 16.56   Metatarsophalangeal and interphalangeal joints distraction.

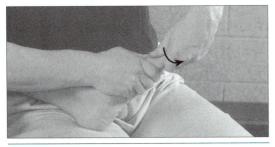

Figure 16.57   Metatarsophalangeal and interphalangeal joints rotation.

Subtalar Joint Medial–Lateral Glide

This is a test of lateral motion within the subtalar joint. Restriction of inversion or eversion limits medial–lateral glide in this movement. The patient is side-lying with the foot over the end of the table and a pad under the distal leg. Place your stabilizing hand on the distal leg and your mobilizing hand around the calcaneus. Use your thigh to maintain the patient's foot in neutral alignment (figure 16.53). Apply a downward force in the same plane as the subtalar joint. The opposite glide can be examined in two ways: either apply the force in an upward direction to the calcaneus with the patient in the same position or rotate the patient to the opposite side and apply a downward force to the joint in the opposite direction.

Midtarsal Joint Anterior–Posterior and Posterior–Anterior Glides

These movements will be restricted if capsular adhesions of the midtarsal joints limit foot abduction or adduction. With the patient supine and the foot supported either on the table or on your thigh, use the index finger and thumb of your stabilizing hand to secure one tarsal bone while placing the index finger and thumb of the mobilizing hand around the adjacent tarsal bone (figure 16.54). Apply an AP and a PA force parallel to the joint's surface.

Tarsometatarsal Joint Anterior–Posterior Glide

These movements examine the mobility between each distal tarsal and metatarsal. With the patient supine and the hip and knee flexed so that the heel is supported on the end of the table, grasp the distal tarsal row with your stabilizing hand and the metatarsal with your mobilizing hand (figure 16.55). Apply an AP glide to each tarsometatarsal joint to examine accessory movement excursion, quality, and end feel.

Metatarsophalangeal and Interphalangeal Joints

The following tests are used to examine mobility of the metatarsaphalangeal and interphalangeal joints.

Distraction

This movement examines general joint mobility. With the patient comfortably supine and the foot on your thigh, stabilize the proximal joint end with one hand and grasp the distal joint end with the mobilizing hand (figure 16.56). Apply a traction force to separate the joint as you examine it for mobility and end feel.

Rotation

Rotation examines general joint mobility and end feel. Position the patient's foot on your thigh as for the distraction movement. Grasp the proximal end of the joint with your stabilizing hand and the distal end with your mobilizing hand (figure 16.57). Apply a rotational force with the mobilizing hand in a clockwise and then counterclockwise direction.

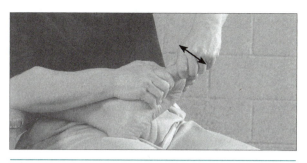

Figure 16.58 Dorsal and ventral glide tests of the metatarsophalangeal and interphalangeal joints.

Dorsal and Ventral Glides

Dorsal (PA) glides, used to examine extension mobility, are restricted if the capsule prevents full extension. Ventral or plantar (AP) glides, which examine flexion mobility, are restricted if the capsule prevents full joint flexion. With the patient's heel anchored on the table or your thigh, grasp the proximal segment of the joint with your stabilizing hand and the distal segment of the joint with the index finger and thumb of your mobilizing hand (figure 16.58). Apply PA and AP glides parallel to the joint surface.

INJURY EXAMINATION STRATEGIES

While injuries of the leg, foot, and ankle are rarely life threatening, they often result in significant disability due to the weight-bearing demands they fulfill. By now you have learned the objective examination tools for examination of acute and chronic conditions of the leg, ankle, and foot. In addition, you will use posture and gait examination to help you delineate specific structural and functional abnormalities. These next sections focus on the examination strategies you will use when encountering an acute (on-site and acute examinations) versus a postacute or chronic injury. As always, the injury environment, the patient's history, and your observations will guide the breadth and depth of your examination.

On-Site Examination

James, a running back, is down on the field. From your observation of the tackle from the sideline, it appears that James planted his foot to change direction and received a hard blow to the outside of his right leg. As you run onto the field, James is rolling around in pain, holding his ankle.

You are called to gymnastics practice where Stella is sitting on the floor exercise mat holding her right leg. When you ask what happened, she tells you that she was near the completion of her final tumbling run, and when she went to punch into her double backflip, she felt a pop and sharp pain in her calf. She describes the pain as feeling like someone had kicked her.

Although injuries to the leg, ankle, and foot are rarely life threatening, severe injuries to these areas demand accurate and rapid examination and efficient and effective transport and care. You should be aware of the signs and symptoms of acute injuries that occur in these areas and be ready to treat them appropriately.

When the athlete suffers an injury to this lower segment and is unable to stand, either the injury is significant or the athlete's tolerance is limited. In any case, you must be able to quickly examine the nature and severity of the injury and determine the method of transport off the playing surface. As you approach the downed athlete, complete a primary survey and observe her for movement and reaction to the injury. Check the position of the injured leg and observe whether the athlete is willing to move the injured area.

History

Injury to the foot and ankle can be very painful, and your first responsibility may be to calm the athlete. Once the athlete is calm, obtaining relevant injury history should help you quickly focus on the area of injury (see On-Site Examination Checklist on page 417 and chapter 3 for specific questions). Athletes with Achilles tendon rupture commonly report a sensation of having been kicked in the calf. For second- and third-degree ankle sprains, it is not unusual for athletes to state that they heard a pop at the time of injury. However, this sign may also indicate a fracture and you must carefully examine the injury before moving the athlete.

Observation

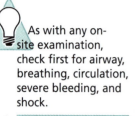

As with any on-site examination, check first for airway, breathing, circulation, severe bleeding, and shock.

Observe for immediate signs of swelling, deformity, or discoloration. Depending on the injury severity, this may require taking time on the field to carefully remove the shoe and sock. You should also remove the shoe and sock on the uninvolved side to allow bilateral comparison and observation of skin and nail coloration so you can monitor any circulatory impairment.

Palpation

Palpate the area to determine any tenderness, crepitus, or abnormalities that may not be obvious upon observation; to identify the structure involved; and to rule out any potential fracture or dislocation. Palpation of the injured area should be brief but thorough, including the distal tibia, tip of the medial malleolus, deltoid ligament, distal fibula, lateral malleolus, lateral ligament complex, anterior tibiofibular joint, Achilles tendon, tarsals, metatarsals (including the base of the fifth), and phalanges. If you suspect fracture or dislocation, palpate the pedal pulse and quickly check sensation along the lateral and medial borders of the foot to rule out neurovascular compromise.

Special Tests

Dislocations are usually obvious in the leg, foot, and ankle, but fractures may not be obvious, even after palpation. The Pott's compression test can quickly examine a potential distal leg fracture. If you suspect an ankle sprain, use an anterior drawer test to determine severity of the injury. If you find bony deformity, tenderness, or crepitus, immobilize the limb and remove the athlete from the field by passive transport. Passive transport is also necessary when the injury is painful or severe enough to prevent weight bearing. Even if the athlete is willing to stand and ambulate with assistance, two people should support the athlete to move her off the playing surface and avoid weight bearing on the injured segment pending a more detailed examination on the sideline.

For more details on passive transport and two-person support, refer to *Introduction to Athletic Training, Second Edition,* (Hillman 2005), chapter 8.

Acute Examination

Julie is a graduate assistant covering the women's basketball team. Amy, the team's center, came down from a rebound, landing on another player's foot and sustaining an inversion injury of the right ankle. While on the court, Julie performed a cursory examination, including palpation of the bony structures, and found no gross deformities or bony tenderness. She did, however, note point tenderness over the distal fibula and lateral ligament structures. With the help of two teammates, Amy was carried off the court to the bench where Julie continued her examination and observed moderate swelling around the anterolateral ankle. By the look on Amy's face, she was still in considerable pain.

When an athlete is removed from the field because of an ankle or foot injury, perform a thorough acute examination to determine more precisely the nature and severity of the injury and the athlete's playing status.

Checklist for On-Site Examination of the Leg, Ankle, and Foot

▷ *Primary Survey*

☐ Survey scene
☐ Level of consciousness
☐ Airway, breathing, and circulation

▷ *Secondary Survey*

▷ *History*

☐ Mechanism of injury and chief complaint
☐ Quality, location, and severity of pain
☐ Unusual sounds and sensations
☐ Information from bystanders

▷ *Observation*

☐ Athlete's response to injury
☐ Deformity, swelling, discoloration
☐ Unusual positioning of the limb
☐ Skin coloration

▷ *Palpation*

☐ Distal tibia, medial malleolus, deltoid ligament
☐ Distal fibula, lateral malleolus, lateral ligaments
☐ Anterior tibiofibular ligament, anterior talar dome
☐ Achilles tendon
☐ Tarsals, metatarsals, phalanges

▷ *Neurovascular Examination*

☐ Pedal pulse
☐ Sensory over dorsum of foot, lateral border of foot, posterior calcaneus

▷ *Special Tests*

☐ Pott's compression test
☐ Anterior drawer test

▷ *Active Range of Motion*

If all tests are negative, assist the athlete from the field and have athlete avoid weight bearing until complete examination is performed off-site.

History

Obtain a thorough history of the injury mechanism and location and the type and severity of symptoms. With ankle injuries, try to determine whether the mechanism resulted in inversion, eversion, or rotation. Determine whether the foot was planted and ascertain the direction of the applied force. Ask the athlete what he was doing at the time of the injury: Was he pushing off, jumping, landing, cutting, or pivoting? Knowledge of previous injuries to either the involved or uninvolved side may influence your findings. For example, a previous severe injury to the uninvolved ankle may have resulted in laxity from ligament damage or restricted mobility from scar tissue, leaving a poor comparison for the injured side.

Observation

If the athlete was able to walk off the field, observe for normal gait, equal weight bearing, stride, and swing-through side-to-side. Does the athlete exhibit full ROM when walking, or does she avoid toe-off or full dorsiflexion? If you did not do so on the field, remove both socks and shoes. Observe closely, comparing bilaterally, for signs of local or diffuse swelling, discoloration, and deformity. Note the "attitude" of the foot and observe whether the foot rests in a more inverted position compared to the uninvolved side; this may indicate second- or third-degree injury to the lateral ligament complex. Also check for any scars or indications of previous injury that the athlete may have forgotten to mention when giving the history.

Palpation

Palpate the bony prominences and joints for tenderness, swelling, crepitus, lack of conformity, and other signs of pathology. Palpate the muscles for areas of tenderness, swelling, myofascial restriction, herniation, and nodules, and incongruity compared left and right. Palpate the tendons for tenderness, nodules, and crepitus during both active and passive movement. For a complete list of structures to palpate, refer back to pages 400-401.

Special Tests

Special tests for on-site and acute examination of the leg, ankle, and foot are primarily stress tests for examining the integrity of a bone, ligament, or tendon. Always compare bilaterally, testing the uninvolved side first.

Range of Motion

Follow the standard guidelines for ROM testing: Test and compare bilaterally each movement of the legs, ankles, and feet, using the uninvolved side as a guide for what is normal for the athlete. Perform painful movements last, and follow active movements by passive overpressure if the athlete can tolerate it. Passive motion can immediately follow active motion in the non-weight-bearing position.

Strength

If you find adequate active ROM and strength examination is indicated, you can perform manual muscle tests in a non-weight-bearing position. Apply manual resistance to ankle dorsiflexion, inversion, and eversion and to toe flexors and extensors, with the joint positioned at midrange of the motion you are testing. If you find calf strength difficult to resist manually, examine plantar flexion in a weight-bearing position. Have the athlete stand on only the involved leg and raise the heel off the floor. If she is able to complete a full ROM, have her perform 10 to 20 repetitions and compare bilaterally. Observe for movement control throughout the ROM and for heel height. Test the uninvolved leg first for comparison.

Neurovascular Tests

Suspected fractures and dislocations and significant trauma (e.g., direct trauma to the anterior tibial compartment or over the peroneal nerve as it courses superficially around the fibular head) warrant a full neurovascular examination. Pay particular attention to the attitude of the ankle and any evidence of foot drop that would suggest direct or indirect trauma to the deep peroneal nerve. Because of the potential for increasing swelling in the muscular compartments of the leg, repeat neurovascular examination periodically if intercompartmental swelling is a concern.

Functional Tests

Some ankle sprains may be mild enough to allow immediate return to participation following the acute examination. Before allowing the athlete to return to full participation, you must first determine his readiness and the readiness of the ankle.

The functional tests for the ankle include general and specific tests for strength, power, flexibility, and agility. The general tests may or may not be sport specific but will determine the ankle's general functional mobility, strength, and response to mechanical stresses. The activities include change of direction with figure-8 runs; forward–backward running; side-to-side movements such as cariocas and side shuffles; forward and lateral jumps; and sudden stop–start maneuvers such as cutting, stop jumps, and zigzag running. The athlete should first perform these functional tests at half speed, using large sweeping arcs of movement, and progress to faster speeds, tighter circles, and sharper cuts.

Use the same progression for functional tests that mimic a particular sport activity. For example, you may have a basketball player run, jump, and land on one foot, as in a layup. A volleyball player may run and stop with a two-footed jump and land with immediate lateral movement or may perform jump squats and backward and lateral runs.

To pass these functional tests, the athlete must perform the movements without hesitation and without favoring the injured ankle; the athlete must also demonstrate adequate strength, flexibility, and agility without increasing or recurring pain and without compensatory movements. You should weigh any questionable performance with other determining factors before allowing the athlete to return to full participation.

Clinical Examination

Jane is a cross country runner who has come to you with a chief complaint of foot pain. She states she first noticed her pain about 3 weeks ago, but only occasionally during sprint training; then about a week ago, she began to feel pain with her distance runs, but it eased with rest. She is now having pain with walking. As she removes her shoes for you to examine her foot, you note her shoes are worn and show an unusual wear pattern.

Stanley is a 60-year-old male who has recently taken up tennis. He immediately fell in love with the sport, and is playing four or five times per week. About 4 weeks ago, he began having pain and cramping in his arch. For a while, he was able to work through the pain, as it improved after a few minutes of warm-up. However, the pain is now worse, especially with the first few steps out of bed in the morning. He is hoping you can tell him what the problem is so he can get back to playing tennis as soon as possible.

Most acute leg, ankle, and foot injuries that occur during practice or competition are first examined on the field or sideline. However, on occasion, lesser injuries will not be immediately reported as significant pain and swelling may not appear until the following day. These types of acute injury, as well as chronic and overuse injuries, are more commonly seen in the treatment facility. The foot and ankle are equally prone to overuse conditions, but the cause of the condition is not always obvious. The clinical examination uses a number of tools to help identify the nature and severity of the condition as well as predisposing factors that may have contributed to the injury.

History

In addition to asking the questions discussed in the acute examination, you must obtain a thorough history of the patient's training and activity. First establish the onset and duration of symptoms to determine the stage of the injury. Identify aggravating and easing factors to determine the level of irritability and also the potential structures involved. Whereas stress fractures are more painful with activity and ease with rest, tendon and muscle injuries may warm up with activity and be more painful at rest. Inflammatory conditions are usually stiff in the morning and loosen as the day progresses, with a return of pain from fatigue and overuse toward the end of the day. Further ascertain the nature of the injury through careful questioning about the patient's training practices, as sudden changes in workout intensity or terrain are frequent culprits in overstress injuries.

Checklist for Acute Examination of the Leg, Ankle, and Foot

▷ *History*

Ask questions pertaining to the following:

- ☐ Chief complaint
- ☐ Mechanism of injury and position of the limb when injured
- ☐ Unusual sounds or sensations
- ☐ Type and location of pain or symptoms
- ☐ Previous injury
- ☐ Previous injury to opposite extremity for bilateral comparison

▷ *Observation*

- ☐ Visible facial expressions of pain
- ☐ Swelling, deformity, abnormal contours, or discoloration
- ☐ Gait, willingness to bear weight, range of ankle motion
- ☐ Overall posture and alignment of lower leg, ankle, and foot
- ☐ Bilateral comparison

▷ *Palpation*

Bilaterally palpate for pain, tenderness, crepitus, defects, and deformity over the following:

- ☐ Tibial crest, anterior tibiofibular ligament, anterior dome of talus, anterior tibialis muscle and tendon, extensor digitorum and hallucis tendons, extensor digitorum brevis, dorsalis pedis pulse, cuneiforms, metatarsals, and phalanges
- ☐ Fibula, peroneal muscle and tendons, lateral malleolus, anterior and posterior talofibular ligaments, calcaneofibular ligament, sinus tarsus, cuboid, base of fifth metatarsal
- ☐ Gastrocnemius, soleus, Achilles tendon, calcaneus
- ☐ Plantar fascia, metatarsal heads
- ☐ Tibial shaft, medial malleolus, deltoid ligament, tibialis posterior tendon, flexor digitorum tendon, flexor hallucis longus tendon, tibial nerve and tibial artery, navicular tubercle, medial cuneiform, and first metatarsal (base, shaft, and head)

▷ *Special Tests*

- ☐ Fracture tests (Pott's compression, Morton's, Percussion, and Hoffa's)
- ☐ Thompson test
- ☐ Ligament laxity tests (anterior drawer, talar tilt, Kleiger, syndesmosis)
- ☐ Bilateral comparison

▷ *Range of Motion*

- ☐ Active ROM for plantar flexion, dorsiflexion, inversion, eversion, toe flexion and extension
- ☐ Passive ROM for plantar flexion, dorsiflexion, rearfoot inversion and eversion, forefoot inversion and eversion, toe flexion and extension
- ☐ Bilateral comparison

▷ *Strength Tests*

- ☐ Perform manual resistance against same motions as in active ROM
- ☐ Check bilaterally and note any pain or weakness

▷ *Neurovascular Tests*

- ☐ Sensory over dorsum of the foot (deep peroneal), lateral border of the foot (superficial peroneal), posterior heel (posterior tibial)
- ☐ Motor for dorsiflexion (deep peroneal), eversion (superficial peroneal), and plantar flexion (posterior tibial)
- ☐ Dorsalis pedis and posterior tibial pulses

▷ *Functional Tests*

Thoroughly investigate any previous injuries, the dates and number of the incidents, the method and effectiveness of the treatments, and the duration of disability for each occurrence, especially the most recent. If the current injury is a repeat of a previous overuse injury, the underlying cause may still exist, and you must account for this in the objective examination. If the patient has suffered prior ankle sprains, find out when the last episode occurred and compare the severity of the previous and present injuries. There may be scar tissue that either restricts mobility or is weaker than normal tissue, making the ankle susceptible to chronic inflammatory or impingement conditions. If the patient's leg was casted for a previous injury, there may be weakness or tightness within the calf muscle that reduces ankle dorsiflexion and makes the gastrocnemius vulnerable to strains. Also obtain information regarding injuries to other segments of the lower extremities, as these may affect the current injury. For example, immobilization of the knee may result in secondary weakness, reduced flexibility, and soft tissue restriction in the ankle and leg.

Observation

As the patient moves toward you, observe whether the gait is normal, whether a limb is favored, and whether the ankle exhibits reduced ROM. Note whether weight bearing is equal or whether the patient shifts weight to avoid putting pressure on the injured joint. Is the patient cautious when removing the shoe and sock? Observe for any deformity, ecchymosis, muscle atrophy, or swelling in the lower leg, ankle, or foot. Localized swelling and discoloration are common around the lateral malleolus with postacute inversion ankle sprains. Note any scars, calluses, blisters, or bony structural changes that indicate previous injury or areas of increased pressure or friction.

What are the structure and position of the leg, ankle, and foot when bearing weight and not bearing weight? Compare their structure and alignment to what you would expect for a healthy foot and lower extremity as outlined previously in this chapter and chapter 4. How does the relationship of these structures change when the patient moves from weight bearing to non-weight bearing? Does the height of the longitudinal arch or angle of the Achilles tendon change? Check the alignment of the toes and feet with the leg, as well as hip and knee alignment and any influence they might have on the leg, foot, and ankle. Your observation should also include inspecting the patient's footwear and a thorough gait examination. Note the type of shoes, excessive or abnormal wear patterns, differences in wear patterns left to right, and the amount of breakdown. Compare these findings to what you observe in your posture and gait examinations.

Differential Diagnosis

Since you did not witness the injury, you must eliminate potential injuries from other regions such as the back, hip, and knee that may refer pain to the leg, ankle, and foot before you proceed with the objective examination. You can quickly eliminate the back as a source of leg and foot pain by having the patient perform trunk ROM with overpressure. Eliminate the hip and knee as sources of pain using active ROM and overpressures for each joint motion. The hip and knee motions are best performed with the patient lying supine. If none of these joint motions reproduce the patient's pain, proceed to the specific objective examination for the leg, ankle, and foot. If, on the other hand, any motion does reproduce the patient's complaint, investigate that joint further before examining the leg and foot.

Range of Motion

Examine active and passive motions as previously described. You can use goniometric examination to better objectify your findings. Examine passive movement of the ankle into dorsiflexion and plantar flexion with the rearfoot in and out of neutral. Also examine movement of the rearfoot into supination and pronation and examine movement of the first ray for laxity or restriction. In particular, note if there are any restrictions into dorsiflexion. If sufficient dorsiflexion is not available, increased mobility or compensations in other segments in order to accommodate normal gait are likely. If you suspect inflammation of the extensor and flexor digitorum longus tendons, also perform toe flexion and extension with and without ankle plantar flexion and dorsiflexion.

Strength

Strength examination allows you to determine if any muscle weakness has resulted from the injury and to better delineate the muscles involved if the soft tissue is injured. You can also use isokinetic devices and other instrumental ankle-testing machines to obtain more precise objective measures. You can examine dorsiflexion, plantar flexion, inversion, and eversion for strength, endurance, and power on most isokinetic and instrumented ankle devices. Remember that the gastrocnemius muscle is biarticulate. Knee flexion strength may also need to be assessed, and remember to test plantar flexion with the knee both flexed and extended.

Neurological Tests

Perform neurological testing if you suspect that the patient's symptoms stem from a back or neurological injury, or if you observe symptoms of a nerve compression syndrome or exertional compartment syndrome. Routinely use neurological testing when the source of the patient's symptoms is unknown; when the patient reports numbness, burning, tingling, or weakness; or when objective findings indicate leg weakness. Neurological tests examine motor, sensory, and deep tendon reflexes. If you suspect the symptoms stem from a back injury, perform sensory and motor testing of the lumbar and sacral plexus nerve root (see chapter 8, table 8.7 and figures 8.13 and 8.15 for further detail). When you suspect injury at the knee or below, perform sensory and motor examination of the peripheral nerves as previously described in this chapter.

Special Tests

All the acute tests discussed earlier apply to the clinical examination. In addition, include tests for malalignment, chronic, and inflammatory conditions. If you have not done so, thoroughly examine static and dynamic lower-extremity function by examining posture and gait. To review a detailed discussion on examining posture, gait, and lower-extremity alignment, refer to chapter 4.

Palpation

Palpation should proceed systematically: Start at one location and gradually cover all tissue within the leg, ankle, and foot. Pay particular attention to any tenderness and restriction along the medial border of the tibia, which may indicate a medial tibial stress syndrome. Also be sure to palpate the medial calcaneal tubercle on the plantar aspect of the heel at the insertion of the plantar fascia if the patient is experiencing pain around the calcaneus and plantar surface of the foot. Because stress fractures are common in the foot, carefully palpate and differentiate between tenderness over soft tissue versus bone.

Functional Tests

Proprioception, agility, and balance are all important functional qualities of athletic performance; they are particularly important in the lower extremity to ensure safe participation and prevent secondary injury due to compensatory motions. As mentioned in relation to the acute examination, functional activities include running, jumping, lateral movements, rapid acceleration and deceleration movements, and combined upper- and lower-extremity movements. The activities you test depend on the athlete's specific sport and position within the sport.

Checklist for Clinical Examination
of the Leg, Ankle, and Foot

▷ *History*

Ask questions pertaining to the following:

- ☐ Chief complaint
- ☐ Mechanism of injury
- ☐ Unusual sounds or sensations
- ☐ Type and location of pain or symptoms
- ☐ Previous injury
- ☐ Previous injury to opposite extremity for bilateral comparison

If chronic, ascertain:

- ☐ Onset and duration of symptoms
- ☐ Aggravating and easing factors
- ☐ Training history (change in practice intensity, duration, frequency, training surface, footwear, orthotics)

▷ *Observation*

- ☐ Swelling, deformity, abnormal contours, discoloration, scars, calluses, blisters, exostosis
- ☐ Gait, weight bearing, ankle motion
- ☐ Overall position, posture, and alignment of foot, ankle, and lower extremity
- ☐ Muscle development—are there areas of muscular atrophy?
- ☐ Inspect shoes bilaterally for abnormal, uneven, or excessive wear
- ☐ Bilateral comparison

▷ *Differential Diagnosis*

- ☐ Clear low back, hip, and knee with active ROM and overpressure tests

▷ *Range of Motion*

- ☐ Active ROM for plantar flexion, dorsiflexion inversion, eversion, and toe flexion and extension
- ☐ Passive ROM for plantar flexion, dorsiflexion, rearfoot inversion and eversion, forefoot inversion and eversion, and toe flexion and extension
- ☐ Bilateral comparison

▷ *Strength Tests*

- ☐ Perform manual resistance against same motions as in active ROM
- ☐ Check bilaterally and note any pain or weakness

▷ *Neurovascular Tests*

- ☐ Sensory over anterior thigh (L2, L3), anteromedial leg (L3, L4), lateral leg and dorsum of foot (L5), lateral plantar foot (S1), medial plantar, and posterolateral plantar heel (S1, S2)
- ☐ Peripheral sensory examination over dorsal web space (deep peroneal), dorsum of foot and lateral leg (superficial peroneal), posteromedial plantar heel (posterior tibial)
- ☐ Examination of myotomes with ankle dorsiflexion (L4), great toe extension (L5), ankle plantar flexion and eversion (S1), great toe flexion (S2)
- ☐ Peripheral motor examination with ankle dorsiflexion (deep peroneal) and plantar flexion and toe flexion (posterior tibial) and eversion (superficial peroneal)
- ☐ Reflex with Achilles tendon (S1, S2)

(continued)

(continued)

▷ *Special Tests*

- ☐ Pott's compression test
- ☐ Thompson test
- ☐ Ligament laxity tests (anterior drawer, talar tilt, Kleiger, syndesmosis)
- ☐ Alignment tests (calcaneal–tibial, forefoot–rearfoot, Feiss' line)
- ☐ Stress fracture tests (Morton's, percussion, Hoffa's)
- ☐ Neurovascular (Homan's, deep and superficial peroneal nerve compression, Tinel's, Morton's)
- ☐ Bilateral comparison

▷ *Joint Mobility Examination*

- ☐ Distal tibiofibular (ventral and dorsal glides)
- ☐ Talocrural (distraction and glides)
- ☐ Subtalar (medial–lateral glides)
- ☐ Midtarsals (anterior–posterior (AP) and posterior–anterior (PA) glides)
- ☐ Tarsometatarsals (AP glides)
- ☐ Metatarsophalangeal and interphalangeal (distraction, rotation, and AP and PA glides)

▷ *Palpation*

Palpate for pain, tenderness, crepitus, defects, and deformity over the following:

- ☐ Tibial crest, anterior tibiofibular ligament, anterior dome of talus, anterior tibialis muscle and tendon, extensor digitorum and hallucis tendons, extensor digitorum brevis, dorsalis pedis pulse, cuneiforms, metatarsals, and phalanges
- ☐ Fibula, peroneal muscle and tendons, lateral malleolus, anterior and posterior talofibular ligaments, calcaneofibular ligament, sinus tarsus, cuboid, base of fifth metatarsal
- ☐ Gastrocnemius, soleus, Achilles tendon, calcaneus
- ☐ Calcaneal tubercle and insertion of the plantar fascia, plantar fascia, metatarsal heads
- ☐ Tibial shaft, medial border of the tibia, medial malleolus, deltoid ligament, tibialis posterior tendon, flexor digitorum tendon, flexor hallucis longus tendon, posterior tibial artery and nerve, navicular tubercle, medial cuneiform, and first metatarsal (base, shaft, and head)

▷ *Functional Tests*

SUMMARY

1. Describe the etiology, signs and symptoms, and potential complications associated with acute injuries of the foot, ankle, and leg commonly encountered in the physically active.

   The leg, ankle, and foot are the most frequently injured region of the body. The foot and ankle undergo tremendous stress during sporting activities because of their propulsive and weight-bearing functions. Acute injuries often result when the forces exerted on the ankle and foot exceed the tensile strength of the soft tissue or exceed the allowable ROM. Lateral ankle sprains, the most common injury in the leg, typically result from inversion mechanisms. Medial ankle sprains are less common because of the anatomical makeup of the joint and the strength of the deltoid ligaments. Dislocations are rare, but fractures are common, resulting from the same mechanisms that produce sprains. Contusions and muscle strains also occur frequently.

2. Describe the etiology, signs and symptoms, and potential complications associated with chronic or overuse injuries of the foot, ankle, and leg commonly encountered in the physically active.

Because of their weight-bearing and propulsive functions, the leg, ankle, and foot are also prone to chronic and overstress injuries as a result of repetitive stress. Many times, these injuries are precipitated by structural or functional abnormalities that compromise the stability and shock-absorption capabilities of the foot and ankle. Chronic stress injuries occurring commonly in the leg complex include retrocalcaneal bursitis, plantar fasciitis, tendinitis and tenosynovitis, anterolateral impingement, and tibial stress syndrome.

3. Identify the signs and symptoms of neurovascular injury at the foot and ankle and identify which ones indicate a medical emergency.

Neurovascular compromise can result from both acute and chronic conditions. An acute anterior compartment syndrome, which constitutes a medical emergency, occurs when pressure within one of the muscular compartments of the leg exceeds the vessel pressure, causing vascular collapse. If the syndrome is not recognized and treated immediately, avascular necrosis and irreversible nerve damage result. A more transient ischemia can occur with an exertional compartment syndrome, but it usually does not cause vascular collapse. Nerve compression syndromes can also result from chronic narrowing of a space or tunnel through which a nerve travels. Be able to differentiate the signs and symptoms of acute versus chronic neurovascular compromise and identify those that indicate a medical emergency.

4. Identify the common functional and structural abnormalities of the foot and their potential effects on lower-extremity mechanics and injury.

The ability to recognize foot malalignments is essential. Many deformities can sufficiently affect alignment and mechanics to cause abnormal stress and a host of lower-extremity injuries, including tendinitis, medial tibial stress syndrome, plantar fasciitis, and stress fractures. Depending on the structural abnormality, shock absorption or stability of the foot structures may be compromised.

5. Describe and demonstrate the objective tests for the leg, ankle, and foot.

To be able to examine and differentiate the variety of conditions that you may encounter at the foot and ankle, you will need sound knowledge of injury pathology and a good understanding of normal foot alignment and mechanics. Remember to palpate all structures bilaterally, and focus on the area of pain last. Because of the many and small structures that constitute the foot and ankle, it is particularly important to develop a systematic, methodical routine for palpation of these structures to help you avoid inadvertently omitting a structure. Range of motion and strength examination includes passive, active, and resisted motions at the ankle (plantar flexion, dorsiflexion), subtalar (inversion, eversion), and metatarsophalangeal (toe extension, flexion and abduction) joints. Neurological examination includes sensory, motor, and reflex testing of the peripheral nerve branches of the lumbosacral plexus. If vascular compromise is suspected, palpate the dorsalis pedis posterior tibial artery for presence and strength of pulse. Also note skin coloration and temperature. Special tests for the leg, ankle, and foot are primarily used to identify fractures, ligament instability, neurovascular compromise, and muscle and fascial injury, and to examine structural alignment.

6. Perform an on-site examination of the leg, ankle, and foot, noting criteria for medical referral and mode of transportation from the field.

The goal of the on-site examination is to quickly determine the presence of severe trauma, including any potential fracture or dislocation that warrants immobilization and medical referral before the athlete is transported from the field. The on-site examination should include a brief history to determine the mechanism and location of injury; careful observation for immediate signs of swelling, discoloration, or deformity; examination for neurovascular compromise if fracture or dislocation is suspected; a brief but thorough palpation of bony and soft tissue structures to identify any defects, deformities, or crepitus; and stress tests for bone and ligament integrity. Once it is clear that there are no signs of severe trauma, the athlete is assisted off the field and prevented from bearing weight pending a more thorough examination.

7. Perform an acute examination of the leg, ankle, and foot.

Acute examination includes a complete investigation of current and past injury history and a more thorough observation and palpation examination. A clear picture of the mechanism of injury will help greatly in defining the potential structures involved. Additional stress tests, as well as active, passive, and resistive ROM, are performed to examine ligamentous and muscle integrity. Before the athlete returns to activity, all tests should be negative and pain should be sufficiently controlled to allow full, unrestricted participation without hesitation or compensation.

8. Perform a clinical examination of the leg, ankle, and foot, including differential diagnosis of referring lumbar, hip, and knee pathologies and functional tests for return to activity.

If the first time the patient is seen is in the athletic injury treatment facility, the injury may be the result of an acute trauma that has worsened over the first 24 to 48 hours following injury or may be the result of overuse. Many of the examination procedures are the same as for the acute examination. Additional tests examine alignment and structural faults that may contribute to lower-extremity pain and dysfunction, stress fractures, nerve compression syndromes, and joint mobility.

REVIEW QUESTIONS

1. What are the two primary functions of the leg and foot? What roles do pronation and supination play in these functions?

2. Describe the mechanisms that result in lateral, medial, and syndesmosis ankle sprains. What tests would you use to determine ligament integrity?

3. What is Sever's disease? How is this condition different from retrocalcaneal bursitis and Achilles tendinitis?

4. Describe the mechanisms of injury associated with the following fractures:
   - Push-off fracture of the lateral malleolus
   - Avulsion fracture of the lateral malleolus
   - Jones' fracture
   - Stress fractures of the tibia and metatarsals

5. What is the difference between an acute and a chronic anterior tibial compartment syndrome? Describe the hallmark signs and symptoms of each and identify the symptoms that indicate a medical emergency.

6. Describe the normal alignment characteristics of the foot. How do the following structural abnormalities deviate from normal alignment?
   - Rearfoot varus
   - Rearfoot valgus
   - Equinus deformity
   - Hallux valgus

7. What is the purpose of the Thompson test? If the test is positive, what condition is indicated? What are the other signs and symptoms associated with this injury?

CRITICAL THINKING QUESTIONS

1. A 26-year-old female runner comes to you complaining of shin splints along the medial border of the tibia. Describe how you would differentiate in your examination among

medial tibial stress syndrome, posterior tibial tendinitis, and a tibial stress fracture. What questions would you ask in the history, and what clues could the athlete provide to help differentiate these conditions?

2. Syndesmotic and medial ankle sprains, less common in sport than lateral ankle sprains, often result in prolonged disability due to difficulty with bearing weight. On the basis of the structures involved, discuss why bearing weight would be difficult and why bearing weight too soon after injury may prolong healing.

3. A basketball player complains of occasional pain, numbness, and tingling along the posteromedial ankle and into the medial arch. She states that when she runs, her symptoms worsen and she gets an aching, burning sensation on the bottom of her foot. You have noted in the past when she runs down the court that she appears to pronate excessively. What nerve compression syndrome might you suspect, and what special tests might you use to identify this condition? What structural or functional abnormalities may contribute to this condition, and how would you examine for these?

4. Consider the scenario where Stella is sitting on the floor exercise mat holding her right leg. When you asked what happened, she told you that she was near the completion of her final tumbling run, and when she went to punch into her double back flip, she felt a pop and sharp pain in her calf. She describes the pain as having felt like someone had kicked her. Your initial observation reveals swelling and deformity around the Achilles tendon. Upon palpation, there is a palpable defect in the tendon. Based on this brief history and observation, what specific injury might you suspect? Describe what objective tests you would use to further confirm this injury, and their sequential order.

CITED REFERENCES

Ferkel, R.D., R.P. Karzel, W. Del Pizzo, M.J. Friedman, and S.P. Fischer. 1991. Arthroscopic treatment of anterolateral impingement of the ankle. *Am J Sports Med* 19(5): 440-470.

Jackson, D.L., and B. Haglund. 1991. Tarsal tunnel syndrome in athletes. *Am J Sports Med* 19(1): 61-65.

Shapiro, M.S., C. Wascher, and G.A.M. Finerman 1994. Rupture of Lisfranc's ligament in athletes. *Am J Sports Med* 22(5): 687.

Tiberio, D. 1988. Pathomechanics of structural foot deformities. *Phys Ther* 68(12): 1840-1849.

ADDITIONAL RESOURCES

Clarkson, H.M. 2000. *Musculoskeletal assessment: Joint range of motion and manual muscle strength.* 2nd ed. Philadelphia: Lippincott Williams & Wilkins.

Hillman, S.K. 2005. *Introduction to athletic training.* 2nd ed. Champaign, IL: Human Kinetics.

Houglum, P.A. 2005. *Therapeutic exercise for musculoskeletal injuries.* 2nd ed. Champaign, IL: Human Kinetics.

Magee, D.J. 1992. *Orthopedic physical assessment.* 2nd ed. Philadelphia: W.B. Saunders.

Moore, K.L. 1992. *Clinically oriented anatomy.* 3rd ed. Baltimore: Williams & Wilkins.

Mosby's medical, nursing, and allied health dictionary. 2002. 6th ed. St. Louis: Mosby.

Knee and Thigh

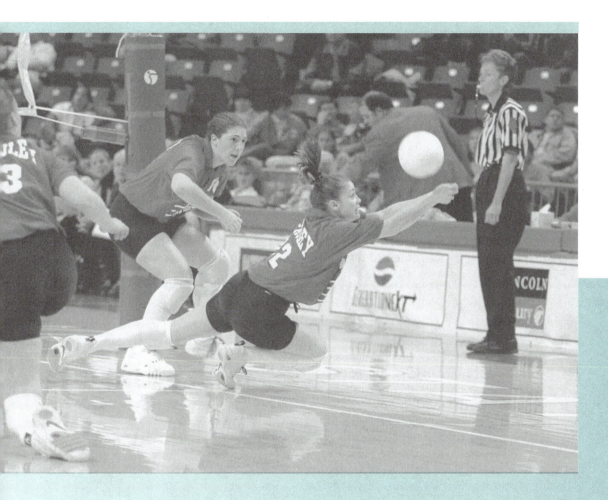

Objectives

After completing this chapter, the reader will be able to do the following:

1. Describe the etiology, signs and symptoms, and potential complications associated with acute and chronic injuries of the knee frequently encountered in the physically active

2. Describe the etiology and signs and symptoms, including predisposing structural and biomechanical factors, associated with chronic patellofemoral pathologies

3. Describe and perform the stress tests for examining internal derangement of the knee joint

4. Describe and perform the special tests for examining patellofemoral dysfunction

5. Describe and demonstrate the objective tests for examining the knee and thigh

6. Perform an on-site examination of the knee, indicating criteria for immediate medical referral and mode of transportation from the field

7. Perform an acute examination of the knee, including functional criteria for return to activity

8. Perform a clinical examination of the knee, including examination of lower-extremity alignment and considerations for differential diagnosis of referring pathologies from the back, hip, foot, and ankle

Connie was enjoying the break from the athletic training room while covering women's basketball practice at Virginia State University. About 30 minutes into practice, Molly, the point guard, ran down the court and quickly changed direction to go around a defender. Connie saw Molly's knee buckle, and Molly went down in a heap, holding her knee. Just from watching the injury occur, Connie already had a good sense of what had happened.

"I felt my knee give out and I heard a pop," Molly said, in obvious pain.

Connie did not observe any immediate swelling, deformity, or discoloration and found no palpable tenderness along the joint line, bony prominences, or surrounding soft tissue. Given the mechanism of injury, Connie performed a Lachman test to examine the integrity of Molly's anterior cruciate ligament, first on the uninjured leg and then on the injured leg. There was an obvious difference, and Connie could feel no end point on the injured leg.

"Let's help you off the court and get some ice on this right away. The doc will be in the athletic training room in a couple of hours and we'll have him take a look." Four hours later, as Connie was attending to another athlete, Dr. Steve came out of the exam room to talk to Connie about Molly. "Molly is very sore, swollen, and apprehensive. It was difficult to get a good examination. What did you find when you examined her immediately after injury, Connie?"

"She clearly had a positive Lachman and had no previous injury to either knee. Her joint swelling developed within about 2 hours. I saw her go down, and her mechanism was consistent with an ACL tear."

"That's what I suspected as well. The information from your initial examination immediately after the injury is very helpful. Let's get her scheduled for an MRI to confirm. Good call, Connie!"

The knee is a complex joint that absorbs and transmits forces through the lower extremity while weight bearing and that provides mobility for locomotion. Although the knee can easily withstand three to four times body weight in compressive loads, because of its bony configuration it has a much lower tolerance to shear and rotational loads. As the link between the femur and tibia, the knee experiences considerable torque through these long levers during physical activity. These factors make the knee vulnerable to injury. The knee joint injury pathologies, their effects on knee joint function, and the examination tools used to identify them are the focus of this chapter.

FUNCTIONAL ANATOMY

The knee comprises three joints: the tibiofemoral, patellofemoral, and proximal tibiofibular joint (figure 17.1). The tibiofemoral joint, the primary weight-bearing joint, is the largest joint in the body. It is a modified hinge joint that allows a large flexion and extension range, limited rotation, and minimal abduction and adduction. The congruency of the tibiofemoral articulation is improved by the medial and lateral menisci, which attach to the periphery of the tibial plateaus (figure 17.2). The menisci help to stabilize the joint by deepening the articular surface, improving weight

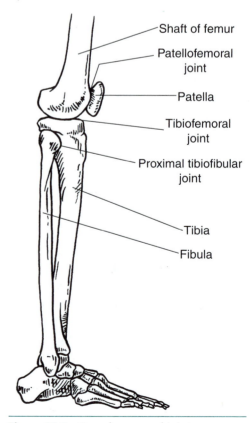

Figure 17.1 Knee bones and joints.

- Shaft of femur
- Patellofemoral joint
- Patella
- Tibiofemoral joint
- Proximal tibiofibular joint
- Tibia
- Fibula

Anterior

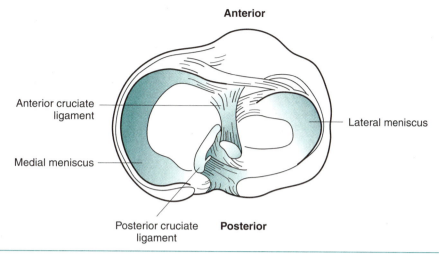

Anterior cruciate ligament

Lateral meniscus

Medial meniscus

Posterior cruciate ligament

Posterior

Figure 17.2 Medial and lateral menisci at their attachments on the tibial plateau.

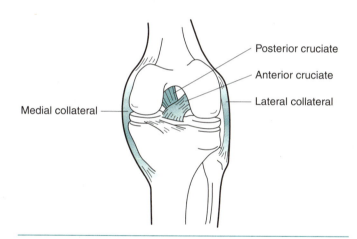

Posterior cruciate

Anterior cruciate

Medial collateral

Lateral collateral

Figure 17.3 Primary stabilizing ligaments of the knee.

distribution, and increasing contact area between the tibia and the femur. They also serve as shock absorbers to decrease the loading stress placed on the joint during weight-bearing activities. Injury to these structures affects joint stability and biomechanical function. The menisci tend to have a poor vascular supply, and for this reason injury to a meniscus often necessitates removing part or all of the meniscus. Orthopedic surgeons often attempt to repair a meniscus to avoid the loss of joint stability and articular degeneration that can occur with complete removal of the structure.

Except in the case of axial loading forces, the knee joint relies primarily on ligament, capsular, and muscular support, since there are no bony limitations in the transverse plane. The primary stabilizing knee ligaments (anterior cruciate, posterior cruciate, medial collateral, and lateral collateral) guide skeletal motion as the knee moves between flexion and extension and provide the principal support system to limit excessive motion between the tibia and the femur (figure 17.3). Secondary support is provided by the capsule and menisci and through dynamic muscular activation of thigh and lower leg muscles that cross the knee joint. When mechanical loads stress the joint, the primary stabilizing ligaments are most often injured.

The cruciate ligaments check excessive anterior and posterior translation of the tibia on the femur, and the collateral ligaments limit valgus and varus stress to the knee. The mechanisms of ligamentous injury usually involve stresses that exceed the ligament's ability to check these motions. These injuries can be either self-inflicted (noncontact) or caused by contact with other players. An especially debilitating injury is a rupture of the anterior cruciate ligament, which frequently occurs from a noncontact mechanism involving deceleration or a sudden change in the body's direction. Contact with another player that produces an excessive valgus force to the knee can injure the medial collateral ligament. Occasionally the same valgus force to the knee injures the anterior cruciate ligament (ACL), medial collateral ligament, and medical meniscus; this condition is known as the Unhappy Triad of O'Donohue. The medial meniscus is injured because the deep fibers of the medial collateral ligament attach to the periphery of the meniscus. In contrast, the lateral collateral ligament has no attachment to the lateral meniscus. In this chapter you will learn how to examine the integrity of

432 Examination of Musculoskeletal Injuries

the cruciate and collateral ligaments by applying controlled amounts of anterior, posterior, valgus, and varus stress to the knee joint.

Knee extension and flexion occur when the powerful quadriceps and hamstrings contract. The quadriceps' three vasti muscles (medialis, intermedius, lateralis) originate from the femur, while the rectus femoris originates from the anterior pelvis (figure 17.4). As such, the vasti muscles are uniarticulate, acting only as knee extensors, while the rectus femoris is biarticulate, acting both as a knee extensor and a hip flexor. All four muscles commonly insert into the tibia through the patellar tendon. The hamstring muscles consist of the semitendinosus, semimembranosus, and biceps femoris (figure 17.5). All except for the short head of the biceps femoris originate from the posterior pelvis and insert into the medial tibia (semitendinosus and semimembranosus) and lateral tibia and fibula (biceps femoris). Consequently, the hamstring muscle group is biarticulate and important not only as a knee flexor but also as a hip extensor. The insertion of the hamstrings also internally and externally rotates the tibia and counters anterior translation of the tibia on the femur. Closed-chain exercises, such as the squat, optimally contract the hamstrings by involving both the knee and hip and help counter anterior shearing (anterior tibial translation) in an ACL-deficient knee.

Biomechanical knee function relies on the coordination between muscular control and static constraints to guide skeletal motion through its full range of motion (ROM). This coordinative motion occurs at the joint surfaces and is a combination of roll, slide, and glide movements that allow unrestricted motion and optimal joint efficiency as the knee moves between full flexion

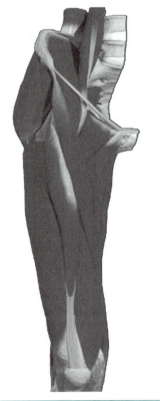

Figure 17.4 Anterior thigh musculature and quadriceps tendon.
Courtesty of Primal Pictures.

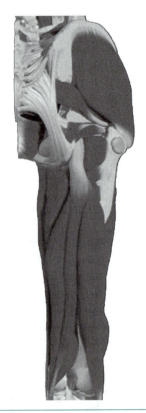

Figure 17.5 Posterior thigh musculature.
Courtesty of Primal Pictures.

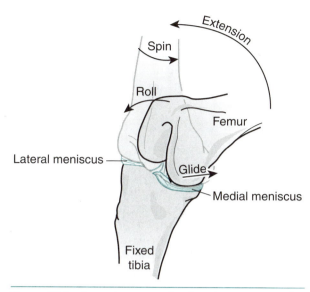

Figure 17.6 Screw home mechanism that occurs as the knee moves from flexion to extension, with the femur rolling on a fixed tibia.

and extension. Specifically, the **screw home mechanism** describes the biomechanical movement of the femur on the tibia as the knee extends and flexes. Starting in flexion with the distal segment stabilized (as in weight bearing), the femur rolls anteriorly on the tibia and menisci as the quadriceps contract and the knee extends (figure 17.6) until the posterior cruciate ligament (PCL) becomes taut and limits the forward roll. At this point, the femur then glides posteriorly on the tibia to allow continued forward roll and as knee extension continues, the ACL becomes taut and fits into the intercondylar groove. However, full extension is not yet achieved, as the lateral femoral condyle still has room to roll forward.

To achieve terminal knee extension, the femur must pivot around the taut ACL that is now positioned tightly in the intercondylar groove, spinning the medial femoral condyle on the medial tibial plateau as the lateral femoral condyle completes its forward roll. The end result is an observable internal rotation of the femur at terminal knee extension. During this knee extension movement, the menisci also move anteriorly with the femur through active and passive processes. As the quadriceps contract, the patellomeniscal fibers that attach to the anterior horns of the menisci pull the menisci forward while at the same time the forward roll of the femur mechanically pinches the menisci from a posterior to anterior position (this pinching mechanism is also know as the cherry pit mechanism).

Moving now from full extension into flexion, the popliteus muscle contracts to unlock the tibiofemoral joint by externally rotating the femur on the tibia. As the knee moves into flexion with contraction of the hamstring muscles, the femur rolls posteriorly until the ACL becomes taut, and then glides anteriorly to allow continued flexion. The menisci also move posteriorly during flexion, secondary to contraction of the politeus and the semimenbranosis muscles, which attach to the lateral and medial posterior horns of the menisci, respectively. As with anterior movement, the cherry pit mechanism passively aids the posterior translation of the menisci, as the posterior roll of the femur pinches the menisci from an anterior to posterior position. Understanding the screw home mechanism becomes important as you interpret positive findings of special tests for joint stability and internal derangement. If injury damages any of the structures contributing to joint control, the normal mechanics of the knee will be disrupted, resulting in either joint restriction or instability that can severely hamper physical activity and sport performance.

The patellofemoral joint, also susceptible to injury, is formed by the articulation of the patella with the anterior surface of the femur in the intracondylar groove. The patella, the largest sesamoid bone in the body, is completely contained within the quadriceps tendon (see figure 17.4); it functions to protect the anterior knee joint and improve the mechanical advantage of the quadriceps with knee extension. As the knee moves from flexion to extension, the surface and area of joint contact vary considerably, as do the compressive loads. This is a common area for overstress injuries, particularly when structural malalignments in the lower extremity (including ankle and hip) alter the position of the patella in the intracondylar groove, causing abnormal joint contact and compressive loads. Females tend to have a higher incidence of patellofemoral pathology, and the anatomical configuration of the pelvis, thigh, knee, and tibia (known as the quadriceps angle) contributes to this problem. Later in this chapter you will learn how to use three anatomical landmarks, the anterior superior iliac spine, patella, and tibial tubercle, to determine the quadriceps angle (Q-angle) of the lower extremity.

Quadriceps angle (Q-angle) is the angle created by a line from the anterior superior iliac spine through the midpoint of the patella and a line from the tibial tubercle through the midpoint of the patella. See table 17.1 and figure 17.39.

The relatively shallow patellofemoral articulation also occasionally exposes the patella to dislocation, usually in the lateral direction. This injury is distinguished from knee dislocation, which is a disarticulation of the femur and tibia. The latter injury is extremely serious as it extensively disrupts the knee ligaments and often damages the popliteal artery that passes through the knee joint and vascularizes the leg. Trauma to the popliteal artery creates the potential for loss of limb.

KNEE AND THIGH INJURIES

The knee joint is one of the most frequently injured joints in physically active people. It is particularly susceptible to injury because of its lack of bony stability, its reliance on soft tissue structures for stability, and the large mechanical forces it experiences with sport activity. Compressive, varus and valgus, anterior and posterior shear, and rotational forces are constantly applied to the knee joint during sport activities, particularly those that require running, jumping, cutting, and rapid change of direction. Injury results when intrinsic or extrinsic forces exceed the structural integrity of the supporting tissues.

Acute Soft Tissue Injuries

Because the knee relies so heavily on the soft tissue structures for stability, injuries to these structures are common. Acute soft tissue injuries can result from both contact and noncontact mechanisms, with or without the foot contacting the ground.

Contusions

To allow full, unrestricted motion, the knee and thigh are often unprotected during sport activity, leaving the area vulnerable to direct contact with a sport implement, another player, or the ground. Because of the mobility required at the knee, contusions around the joint can be particularly bothersome. Signs and symptoms include pain, swelling, point tenderness, and discoloration. Contusion may also limit ROM and function secondary to pain and swelling.

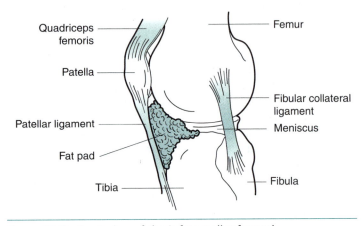

Figure 17.7   Contusion of the infrapatellar fat pad.

Contusion of the Infrapatellar Fat Pad

With knee hyperextension injuries, the tibia and femur can impinge the infrapatellar (IP) fat pad, resulting in a contusion (figure 17.7). Signs and symptoms of a fat pad contusion include pain, swelling, and point tenderness deep to and on either side of the patellar tendon. ROM is limited in knee extension, and the patient is apprehensive about fully extending the knee because of increased pain. The patient may also complain of the knee giving out with activity as a result of an unconsciously avoiding pain into extension.

Quadriceps Contusion

Muscle contusions in the thigh, particularly the quadriceps, can be quite troublesome and result in prolonged disability. Quadriceps contusions occur most often when the muscle sustains direct contact while contracted rather than relaxed. Significant pain, spasm, and loss of function immediately follow injury. ROM into flexion will be limited secondary to pain and spasm, but gentle stretching and ice with the knee flexed may afford relief. With severe contusions in the muscle belly, considerable hemorrhage and swelling can occur over the 24 to 48 hours following injury. You may also note discoloration and a palpable hematoma. An increase in leg circumference of 2.5 cm (1 in.) or more indicates significant hemorrhage. Depending on the injury severity, the patient may be unable to fully contract the quadriceps or achieve end range extension. Knee flexion may also be severely limited secondary to hemorrhage and spasm.

Myositis Ossificans

A potential consequence of a quadriceps muscle contusion is **myositis ossificans**, which occurs when the body's inflammatory response during hematoma absorption causes calcification or forms bony deposits in the muscle. Calcification most often occurs secondary to severe hemorrhage, repetitive insult, or a too aggressive or early return to activity following a severe contusion. The calcification may occur solely within the muscle belly or may appear as a bony stalk off the femur that extends into the muscle; the latter is typically more restrictive because it attaches the muscle to the bone (figure 17.8). Signs and symptoms of myositis ossificans include a history of severe or repetitive insult to the quadriceps, pain, a palpable mass within the muscle belly, decreased knee flexion range, decreased quadriceps strength, and radiograph evidence within 3 to 4 weeks after injury.

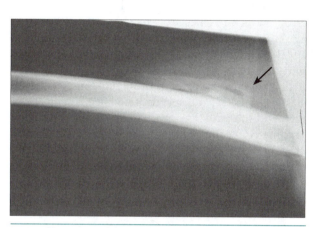

Figure 17.8 Myositis ossificans in the quadriceps.
Courtesy of Theodore E. Keats.

Traumatic Bursitis

Direct contact over one of the superficial knee bursae may cause traumatic bursitis. Falling on the knee and making knee-to-knee contact with another player are the most common mechanisms. The bursae most prone to traumatic injury include the prepatellar, suprapatellar, infrapatellar, and pes anserine (figure 17.9). Signs and symptoms include immediate observable bursal swelling, redness, and mild pain. The area is warm to the touch, and you can palpate a soft, fluid-filled pouch. Limited ROM with flexion results from the swelling and increased pressure in the bursa as the skin tightens over the knee during flexion.

Sprains

The cruciate (anterior, posterior) and collateral (medial, lateral) ligaments act as the primary stabilizers of the knee joint (see figure 17.3). Injury to these ligaments often occurs during athletic activities and may cause considerable instability and activity restriction. Although each ligament injury is discussed separately, injury commonly affects more than one structure, particularly with contact mechanisms. Injuries to more than one ligament, or associated injury of the capsule or meniscus, can result in rotatory or multiplanar instabilities at the knee.

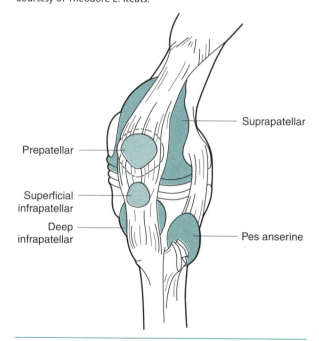

Prepatellar

Superficial infrapatellar

Deep infrapatellar

Suprapatellar

Pes anserine

Figure 17.9 Locations of the prepatellar, suprapatellar, infrapatellar, and pes anserine bursae.

Anterior Cruciate Ligament

The anterior cruciate ligament (ACL) originates from the intercondylar eminence of the tibia and runs in a posterior, lateral, and superior direction to attach on the posterior medial aspect of the lateral epicondyle of the femur. It consists of three bundles arranged such that some portion of the ligament is taut throughout the range. The ACL is tightest in extension and most lax in 45° of flexion. Its primary functions are to limit extension, forward translation (glide), medial rotation, and extreme lateral rotation of the tibia relative to the femur and to act as a guide for the femur as it rolls from flexion into extension. Anterior cruciate ligament sprains have become the most prevalent third-degree ligament injury at the knee (Johnson et al. 1992). Both contact and noncontact mechanisms can injure the ACL. In a contact mechanism, the foot is firmly planted and laterally rotated when a valgus force is applied to the lateral aspect of the knee (or lower extremity) with the knee slightly flexed. Noncontact mechanisms account for the majority of ACL injuries (Boden et al. 2000), particularly in females (Arendt and Dick 1995). In fact, females are 2 to 8 times more likely to injure their ACL than males, depending on the sport (Arendt et al. 1995, 1999; Biondino 1999; Ferretti et al. 1992; Malone et al. 1993; Myklebust et al. 1998; Oliphant and Drawbert 1996). With noncontact mechanisms, injury is usually associated with a sudden deceleration or change of direction, so it is not surprising that the majority of these noncontact injuries occur in sports such as basketball, gymnastics, lacrosse, and soccer. The knee is typically at or near full extension at the time of injury, and the athlete complains of the knee buckling or giving way during a sudden stop or landing from a jump, or cutting or pivoting. Landing off balance with the center of body mass lateral and posterior to the landing leg can also injure the ACL secondary to excessive valgus and rotary forces imparted at the knee upon ground contact.

Signs and symptoms include immediate pain and unwillingness to move the knee. The athlete may also hear a pop at the time of injury. Immediate symptoms usually subside sufficiently enough within a few minutes to allow a full knee examination. A large joint effusion and loss of motion usually result within 24 hours. You need to examine the knee shortly after injury because examination becomes much more difficult once pain, swelling, and muscle guarding set in. The athlete will initially be unwilling to bear weight or will have a sense of weakness or instability with weight bearing. You will note anterior and rotatory instability with stress tests on second- and third-degree sprains. Second-degree ACL sprains are rare.

Posterior Cruciate Ligament

The posterior cruciate ligament (PCL), which has a wide attachment on the anterior surface of the medial femoral condyle, expands posteriorly under the ACL to attach to the posterolateral tibial plateau. Much shorter than the ACL, it limits extension, posterior translation, and medial rotation of the tibia on the femur. It is most taut in flexion and most lax in 45° of flexion, but because of its short length, it is fairly taut throughout the full ROM. It also functions biomechanically to limit the forward roll of the femur and to cause the femur to pivot as the knee moves from flexion into extension.

The PCL is most often injured secondary to a direct blow to the anterior tibia that drives it posteriorly on the fixed femur. Common scenarios are making contact with the dashboard during a traffic collision and falling on the anterior tibia with the knee flexed and the foot and ankle plantar flexed. Additionally, any hyperflexion or hyperextension mechanism that forces the tibia posteriorly in relation to the femur can stretch or tear the PCL and posterior joint capsule. Signs and symptoms include pain, joint effusion, and limited ROM into full flexion and extension. With complete rupture there may be an audible pop at the time of injury. With more serious second-degree as well as third-degree injuries, you will observe a posterior sag of the tibia when the quadriceps are relaxed and will note posterior instability with posterior stress tests. Athletes who have good quadriceps and hamstrings strength may not complain of instability with weight bearing, so these injuries are sometimes missed. Athletes with PCL tears often do well following rehabilitation and return to full activity without surgical intervention.

Medial (Tibial) Collateral Ligament

The medial collateral ligament (MCL) is a broad, fan-shaped ligament that consists of superficial (extra-articular) and deep (intra-articular) fibers. The superficial fibers run outside the joint capsule, extending from the medial femoral epicondyle to the medial condyle and superior flare of the tibia. The deep fibers dive into the joint capsule, attaching firmly to the medial meniscus and the fibrous capsule of the knee joint. The MCL limits abduction of the tibia on the femur and also assists in limiting extension and lateral rotation of the tibia. In addition, the deep fibers stabilize the medial meniscus. A straight valgus stress can result in an isolated MCL injury. Typically the foot is planted in neutral or lateral rotation when contact is made to the lateral aspect of the abducted leg, resulting in a valgus stress to the medial joint structures. With severe valgus injuries, the ACL and medial meniscus are commonly injured also (i.e., the **unhappy triad**) if the valgus force continues once the MCL fails.

Signs and symptoms of MCL injury include pain, mild to moderate swelling, discoloration, and point tenderness in the middle portion of the MCL or near its femoral or tibial attachment. Pain may also occur at the medial joint line if the deep portion of the ligament or its attachment to the medial meniscus is torn. Since the ligament is primarily located outside of the joint capsule, there is usually no joint effusion with an isolated MCL sprain. The athlete experiences increased pain when the ligament is taut during full knee flexion and extension, as well as with an applied valgus stress. You will note instability during valgus stress with second- and third-degree injuries.

Lateral (Fibular) Collateral Ligament

The lateral collateral ligament (LCL) runs from the lateral epicondyle of the femur to its attachment on the fibular head. It is completely separate from the capsule and does not attach to the lateral meniscus. It limits knee extension and adduction of the tibia relative to the femur. It also assists in limiting lateral rotation of the tibia when the knee is extended. The LCL is injured less frequently than the other knee ligaments. The mechanism for LCL injury is a varus force applied to the medial aspect of the knee. The LCL is most vulnerable when the varus force occurs while the leg is adducted and the tibia medially rotated. Injuries to the LCL happen most often in contact sports such as football, soccer, and wrestling when one player falls into or makes contact against the medial side of another player's planted lower extremity. Signs and symptoms include pain, lateral knee swelling, ecchymosis, and point tenderness over the fibular collateral ligament. The athlete may hear or feel a pop with complete rupture and you will note varus instability with second- and third-degree injuries. The athlete experiences increased pain when the ligament is tensed during full knee flexion, extension, and during varus stress. Pain and swelling also limit ROM. Unlike the MCL, the LCL lies completely outside of the joint capsule, and a joint effusion associated with this injury typically indicates injury to the capsule or meniscus as well. Injury to the posterolateral capsule commonly accompanies an LCL sprain.

Rotary and Multiplanar Instabilities

The mechanisms just described commonly injure more than one structure. In addition to the primary ligament, injury can also disrupt the capsule, secondary ligament restraints, and muscular insertions. If this occurs, joint instability in more than one direction or plane of motion results. Rotary instabilities usually denote a serious injury that is often surgically repaired. Rotary instabilities can be anteromedial, anterolateral, posterolateral, and posteromedial. Understanding the structures and mechanisms involved in these rotary instabilities will help you in your objective examination of knee ligament injuries and in interpreting your findings.

- **Anteromedial rotary instability.** Anteromedial rotary instability, the most common type of instability, occurs when the medial tibial plateau subluxes on the femur. It results when the ACL, MCL, medial capsule, and possibly the medial meniscus are torn. The posterior medial capsule and posterior oblique ligament may also be involved. The typical mechanism for this injury is lateral rotation of the tibia with valgus stress.

- **Anterolateral rotary instability.** Anterolateral rotary instability results from injury to the ACL, LCL, and lateral capsule. It is characterized by subluxation of the lateral tibial plateau with anterior translation and medial rotation of the tibia on the femur.

- **Posterolateral rotary instability.** Posterolateral rotary instability allows posterior subluxation of the lateral tibial plateau. It is caused by injury to the posterolateral compartment, PCL deficiency, or both. Posterior lateral structures usually include the LCL and popliteus tendon; they sometimes may also include the biceps femoris and lateral head of the gastrocnemius. Posterolateral rotary instability most often results from an anterior blow to the tibia with the foot laterally rotated and the knee under varus stress.

- **Posteromedial rotary instability.** Posteromedial rotary instability results from combined injury to the PCL, MCL, and medial joint capsule. The typical mechanism is an anterior blow to the tibia with the knee partially flexed and under valgus stress and the foot laterally rotated. You will note instability with valgus stress, posterior translation, and medial rotation of the tibia.

Meniscal Injuries

The menisci are two semilunar cartilages that sit on the tibial plateau, attaching only at their peripheral margins (see figure 17.2). They are thickest at their peripheral borders and thinner toward the center. They move with the tibia during flexion and extension and with the femur during rotation. They possess no nerves, and their vascular supply is primarily along the periphery. The primary functions of the menisci are to

- help stabilize the joint by deepening the tibial condyles,
- absorb the shock of weight bearing and decrease loading stress,
- lubricate the joint and reduce friction during movement, and
- make joint surfaces more congruent and improve weight distribution by increasing the contact area between the tibia and femur.

Tearing of the medial or lateral meniscus typically occurs from compression and rotation of the femur on the fixed tibia. Cutting and pivoting with the joint in full weight bearing can pinch the meniscus between the femur and tibia and tear it as the femur rotates on the joint surface. Tears to the posterior horn of the menisci can also occur with hyperflexion and compression. In addition, the menisci can be torn with ligament injuries with axial compression and excessive translation of the femur on the tibia when the ligament fails. Because the medial meniscus has a broader attachment to the tibial surface and attaches to the MCL and semimembranosus, it is less mobile and more frequently injured than the lateral meniscus. Older physically active patients are more prone to injuries of the menisci as these structures become less compliant and degenerate with age. The athlete may or may not recall the specific injury occurrence.

Signs and symptoms include pain, swelling, and joint line tenderness. Because there is virtually no sensation in the menisci themselves, the pain typically results from surrounding inflammation and synovial irritation. Delayed or persistent joint effusion may also occur with meniscal injuries. If the torn portion of the meniscus displaces or detaches, it may become impinged as the joint moves through its ROM, resulting in symptoms of clicking, catching, or locking of the joint. The athlete may complain of pain, instability, or the knee giving way during cutting or pivoting. If the tear is in the posterior horn, the athlete complains of posterior knee pain and pain with deep squatting. Special tests compressing and rotating the joint (see McMurray and Apley tests, pages 456-457) also elicit symptoms.

Strains

Muscular strains typically stem from forceful contraction of the muscle during eccentric loading or from overstretching. Inflexibility, fatigue, weakness, muscular imbalance, and inadequate warm-up increase an athlete's susceptibility to thigh muscle strains. Recurrent strains are a common problem, as the symptoms often subside and the athlete returns to activity before adequate healing has occurred.

Quadriceps Strain

The quadriceps muscle is most often overloaded during sudden acceleration or deceleration, so injuries most often occur during sprinting, kicking, and weight lifting. Injury typically involves the rectus femoris muscle. The athlete usually complains of immediate pain, spasm, and loss of function. However, with some first-degree strains the initial pain quickly subsides and so the athlete returns to activity, only to have the pain return and remain the next day. The athlete experiences pain with passive stretch into knee flexion with the hip extended. Pain and weakness with active or resistive extension are consistent with the degree of injury. The athlete is palpably tender over the injured area, and a defect may exist with second- and third-degree injuries. Second- and third-degree injuries may also result in observable swelling, ecchymosis, and a quadriceps avoidance gait.

Hamstring Strain

Hamstring strains—more common than quadriceps strains—occur most often with sprinting activities. Injury can occur in the midbelly of the muscle, at the distal myotendon junction, or at the proximal insertion on the ischial tuberosity. Proximal strains near the ischial attachment typically result from overstretching or hyperflexion of the hip with the knee extended. Unfortunately, proximal injuries heal very slowly, prolonging disability. Strains most often result when the quadriceps is forcefully contracted while the hamstrings eccentrically contract. Asynchronous muscle timing, inflexibility, and muscular imbalance (excessive quadriceps to hamstrings strength ratio) appear to be contributing factors to these injuries. At the time of injury, the athlete typically pulls up or shortens the stride on the involved leg and grabs the thigh while trying to decelerate.

The athlete experiences an immediate sharp or burning pain in the hamstrings at the time of injury. With some first-degree sprains, though, pain and stiffness may be delayed until the next day. Other signs and symptoms include palpable tenderness and spasm over and around the injured fibers. You will note pain with passive stretching and active or resistive knee flexion. There may be a palpable defect with second- and third-degree injuries. The athlete may also exhibit a shortened stride during gait on the involved side to avoid fully extending the knee and stretching the muscle. Delayed swelling and ecchymosis often occur within 24 to 48 hours following second- and third-degree strains.

Patellar Tendon Rupture

A violent, rapid quadriceps contraction can rupture the midsubstance either of the infrapatellar or suprapatellar tendon. Patellar tendon ruptures, which are infrequent, can occur in a healthy tendon as a result of an acute, single mechanism; however, more often the tear is precipitated by episodes of chronic tendinitis or inflammation that weaken the structure. At the time of injury the athlete complains of immediate, severe pain and loss of active knee extension. A pop may also be felt and heard as the tendon ruptures. The patella appears to sit more superiorly with an infrapatellar tendon rupture, and there is a palpable gap between the inferior pole of the patella and tibial tuberosity. With suprapatellar tendon ruptures, the defect is superior to the patella. Considerable swelling and ecchymosis will likely result within 24 hours following the injury. Ruptures in the midsubstance of the tendon are less common in young athletes, with failure typically occurring at the tibial apophysis where the tendon attaches (figure 17.10) (see also Osgood-Schlatter disease later in this chapter).

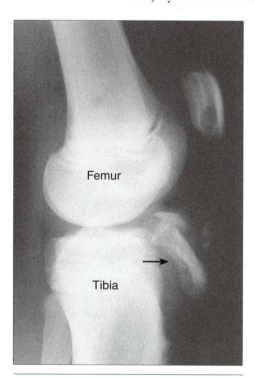

Figure 17.10 Avulsion fracture of the tibial apophysis.

Courtesy of Theodore E. Keats.

Chronic or Overuse Soft Tissue Injuries

The soft tissue structures of the knee are also prone to chronic inflammatory conditions caused by repetitive friction and overuse. The soft tissues most often overused are the numerous tendons that cross and attach at the knee joint and the bursae that reduce friction and allow free movement of the tendons. Repetitive kneeling, jumping, and flexing and extending are common mechanisms associated with inflammation of these structures. Inflammation of a tendon or bursa can cause considerable discomfort and significantly affect performance.

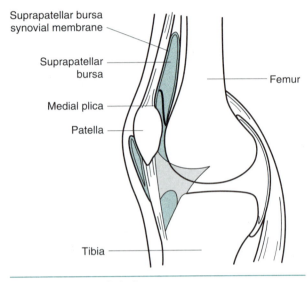

Figure 17.11   Medial plica.

Plica Syndrome

Plica syndrome is an anomaly or fold in the synovial membrane on the anterior aspect of the knee that runs from the lateral femoral condyle, superior and medial to the patella, and down toward the fat pad (figure 17.11). While a synovial fold can occur anywhere around the knee, the most typical location is along the superior medial border of the patella. Although a plica is often asymptomatic, it can cause problems if the area becomes inflamed or taut, resulting in a snapping, clicking, or jumping of the patella as the knee moves into flexion. Other signs and symptoms include pain along the medial border of the patella, swelling, and a possible locking sensation. You can often palpate the snapping or clicking of the patella by placing a finger on the patella during knee flexion and extension.

Bursitis

Roofers, carpet layers, tilers, wrestlers, distance runners, and other athletes whose activities cause repetitive trauma or friction over a bursa can experience episodes of chronic bursitis. Numerous bursae have been identified around the knee; they are typically present between tendons and other joint structures to prevent friction during knee movement. Those most prone to irritation and inflammation are the pes anserine, infrapatellar, prepatellar, and suprapatellar bursae (see figure 17.9). The suprapatellar, prepatellar, and superficial infrapatellar bursae are irritated with frequent kneeling or bending. Because the suprapatellar bursa is continuous with the synovium, irritation or inflammation affecting one affects the other. The deep infrapatellar bursa lies deep to the infrapatellar tendon and anterior to the infrapatellar fat pad and the anterior surface of the tibia. It also experiences irritation with frequent kneeling, but the subsequent swelling is more obscured and appears on either side of the patellar tendon when the leg is extended. Chronic irritation of the pes anserine bursa, which lies between the pes anserine tendons and the MCL, is typically caused by overuse and repetitive valgus loading, particularly in distance runners and cyclists.

Signs and symptoms of chronic bursitis include pain, redness, and localized swelling. The area is tender to palpation and warm to the touch. Crepitus and bogginess, or thickening of the bursal fluid, also occurs with chronic bursitis. Flexion of the knee may be painful or limited with patellar bursitis secondary to increased pressure over the bursa as the skin tightens into flexion. Extension may also be limited with suprapatellar and deep infrapatellar bursal swelling. Pes anserine bursitis is painful with knee flexion and extension and medial tibial rotation. In prolonged cases of bursitis, permanent thickening of the bursal wall may occur, and calcium deposits may also form within the bursa.

Popliteal Cyst (Baker's Cyst)

! Because popliteal cysts are commonly associated with meniscal tears and arthritic conditions, suspect intra-articular pathology when the patient presents with a posterior cyst as the primary complaint.

A popliteal cyst typically results from a herniation of the synovial cavity and fluid accumulation in the popliteal space (figure 17.12). Fluid accumulation may also result from distension of the popliteal, semimembranosus, or subtendinous bursa, all of which communicate with the

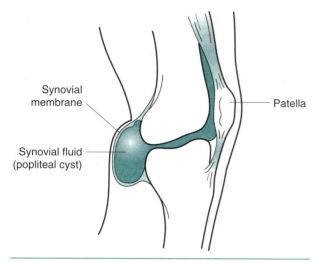

Figure 17.12 Baker's cyst.

synovial cavity. Signs and symptoms include a palpable, fluid-filled cyst in the inferomedial popliteal fossa. The cyst may or may not be tender and typically in and of itself does not restrict activity. However, significant swelling may cause discomfort and restrict knee flexion. Because popliteal cysts are commonly associated with meniscal tears and arthritic conditions, you should suspect intra-articular pathology when the patient presents with the posterior cyst as the primary complaint.

Tendinitis and Strains

Given the many tendons that cross and attach at the knee, tendinitis resulting from repetitive or overuse mechanisms is a frequent complaint in the physically active. As with most tendinitis conditions, the patient presents with an insidious onset of pain and a history of repetitive activity or significant increase in training over the past few days or weeks. Initially the patient may feel pain only after activity and cool-down; pain may also occur at the beginning of activity but improve with warm-up. As symptoms worsen, the patient complains of pain during activity as well as throughout the day.

Patellar Tendinitis (Jumper's Knee)

Patellar tendinitis frequently occurs from repetitive jumping (basketball, volleyball, long jump, triple jump), running, or weight lifting (leg extensions, squats, lunges). Overloading the extensor mechanism can cause microtearing and inflammation of either the suprapatellar or infrapatellar tendons. Patellar tendinitis is characterized by symptoms of pain, inflammation, and mild swelling either superior or inferior to the patella. Palpable tenderness and crepitus are often present over the inflamed tendon. The patient complains of pain with passive stretching of the tendon and active or resisted knee extension. In chronic cases, degeneration and scarring within the tendon can weaken its structure and increase susceptibility to patellar tendon rupture.

Iliotibial Band Friction Syndrome

Genu valgum (valgus) is excessive lateral angulation of the tibia relative to the femur. See table 17.1 and figure 17.50.

Iliotibial band friction syndrome is an overuse injury most typically seen in runners and cyclists. It is caused by excessive friction between the iliotibial (IT) band and the lateral femoral epicondyle. At approximately 30° of flexion, the IT band changes from a knee extensor to a knee flexor (figure 17.13). When the knee is flexed less than 30°, the IT band lies anteriorly to the lateral epicondyle and assists with knee extension. As the knee flexes, the IT band rides over the epicondyle at about 25° to 30° of knee flexion and then sits posteriorly past 30° of flexion, assisting with knee flexion. Irritation occurs with repetitive activity at the transitional range if there is excessive friction or snapping of the IT band as it passes over the epicondyle. Athletes with increased genu valgum, excessive quadriceps angle, excessive pronation, or leg length discrepancy are more prone than others to IT band friction syndrome.

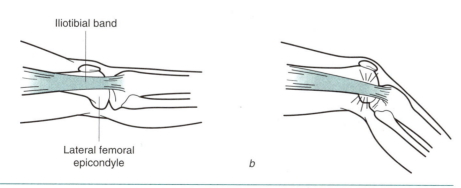

Figure 17.13 *(a)* At less than 30° the IT band is anterior to the lateral epicondyle and acts as an extensor. *(b)* As the knee flexes to more than 30°, the IT band passes posteriorly to the lateral epicondyle to act as a flexor.

Tightness in the IT band (see Ober's test, page 499 in chapter 18), training errors, downhill running, and running on a slanted surface may also be predisposing factors.

Signs and symptoms include pain and point tenderness over the lateral femoral condyle just proximal to the lateral joint line. Pain may also radiate up the lateral thigh or down the IT band to its insertion at Gerdy's tubercle. As with other inflammatory conditions, pain is often first noted only after activity and does not restrict activity initially. As inflammation and irritation increase, pain gradually appears during running and if left untreated will eventually restrict activity. Pain and snapping may also occur with walking down stairs or squatting, or with flexion and extension movements of the knee around 30° of flexion.

Hamstring Tendinitis

Hamstring tendinitis can occur in both the proximal and distal tendons. Proximal hamstring tendinitis near the insertion to the ischial tuberosity is less common, but can result either from repetitive friction and pressure over the tendon and tuberosity—as occurs in cycling with an improperly adjusted seat—or from overstretching or tensioning of the proximal attachment with straight-leg hip flexion. Because of the poor vascularization of the proximal tendon, healing is slow and symptoms often persist for a prolonged period. Signs and symptoms include an achy pain just below the gluteal fold and deep palpable tenderness just distal to the ischial tuberosity. Passive stretching in straight-knee hip flexion, resisted straight-knee hip extension, and long striding often exacerbate the pain. Distal hamstring tendinitis most often results from repetitive flexion and overuse during running and weightlifting. Signs and symptoms include insidious onset of pain, palpable tenderness, mild swelling, and crepitus in the inflamed tendon. With medial hamstring tendinitis, the athlete may complain of snapping or clicking behind the knee with flexion that occurs when the inflamed tendons ride over adjacent structures. Pain may also be noted with passive knee extension and active or resistive knee flexion.

Pes Anserine Tendinitis

The same mechanisms that result in bursitis of the pes anserine can also inflame and irritate the tendons near their attachment on the medial tibial plateau. Pes anserine tendinitis is most often seen in runners and cyclists. Anteroinferior medial knee pain, palpable tenderness over the anteromedial tibial plateau, crepitus, and local swelling are typical signs and symptoms. Pain also occurs with active knee flexion, with passive knee extension, and possibly with valgus stress.

Traumatic Fractures

Traumatic fractures occur less frequently at the knee than at other joints because the ligaments and soft tissues provide most of the stability to the knee joint and thus are more likely to fail. As is typical for other body regions, fractures of the knee and thigh are more commonly seen in young, skeletally immature athletes. When you suspect fracture, immobilize the extremity and immediately refer the athlete to a physician.

Epiphyseal Fractures

Fractures through the proximal tibial epiphysis, and less often through the distal femoral epiphysis, can result from rotational and shearing forces at the knee joint. Twisting, varus, or valgus forces directed at the knee with the foot firmly planted are the more common fracture mechanisms in the adolescent athlete. Signs and symptoms include immediate pain, tenderness along the bone, swelling, loss of function, and possible deformity. The athlete may report hearing a pop or snap at the joint. You may observe crepitus with joint motion, but the athlete will typically be unwilling to move the extremity. False joint motion, or opening of the epiphyseal joint with varus and valgus testing, may make it difficult to distinguish an epiphyseal fracture from a collateral ligament injury (figure 17.14). You should highly suspect

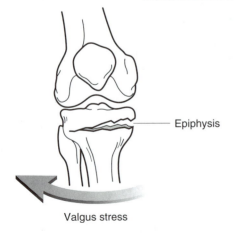

Epiphysis

Valgus stress

Figure 17.14 Epiphyseal plate injury at the proximal tibia and false joint motion with valgus testing.

fracture when examining varus and valgus injuries in the adolescent. A potential complication of epiphyseal fractures is disruption and premature closing of the growth plate, which may ultimately result in a true leg length discrepancy.

Tibial Plateau Fracture

Tibial plateau fractures can result from severe varus, valgus, or rotational forces in combination with axial compression when the foot is firmly planted. The athlete complains of severe and immediate pain and is unwilling to move the knee joint. Other signs and symptoms include swelling, tenderness over the proximal tibia, pain with percussion, crepitus, and possible deformity.

Patella Fracture

Fractures of the patella can result from direct contact, as in a fall directly on the patella with the knee flexed, or from indirect forces, such as severe tractioning produced by a forceful quadriceps contraction. The patient complains of sudden and severe pain in the kneecap and is unwilling to contract the quadriceps or extend the knee, or is unable to do so without considerable pain. You will also observe immediate tenderness, rapid swelling, and crepitus over the patella. Patellar fractures can often cause considerable and prolonged disability. Inhibition or inability to contract the quadriceps for an extended period can also result in severe atrophy and delayed rehabilitation. Fractures through the articular surface of the patella are particularly troublesome, as they create an uneven or roughened articular surface that may cause chronic pain and symptoms similar to those associated with chondromalacia patella (discussed later in this chapter).

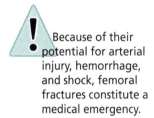

Because of their potential for arterial injury, hemorrhage, and shock, femoral fractures constitute a medical emergency.

Femur Fracture

Femoral shaft fractures resulting from athletic activity are rare because of the relative strength of the femur. When femoral fracture does occur, it usually does so in contact sports such as football as a result of a severe, direct blow to the midthigh, but such fractures may also occur secondary to severe torsional forces. Femoral shaft fractures are readily apparent. Signs and symptoms include immediate and severe pain, muscle spasm, and inability to move the extremity. Considerable hemorrhage may occur, resulting in shock. Complete fractures are usually displaced because of the strength and resultant spasm of the surrounding musculature. The characteristic deformity is typically a shortened, laterally rotated thigh.

Chondral and Osteochondral Fractures

Chondral fractures (fractures of the articular cartilage) and **osteochondral** fractures (fractures extending through the articular cartilage and into the bone) of the femoral condyle may occur by themselves or concurrently with a ligament injury. Joint compression combined with a varus, valgus, or rotational shearing force can contuse the articular surface and cause a compression or avulsion fracture (figure 17.15), resulting in loose fragments (**joint mice**) that can produce irritation, locking and clicking within the joint. Signs and symptoms of chondral or osteochondral fracture include pain, immediate or delayed swelling, locking or clicking, and pain with joint compression or weight bearing. Depending on the extent of injury, the patient may be unable to bear weight or move the knee. When the fracture extends into the underlying bone, considerable bleeding and joint effusion may result. Palpable tenderness and crepitus may also be present near the joint line and femoral condyle. Pain increases with manual joint compression combined with knee flexion, extension, or rotation.

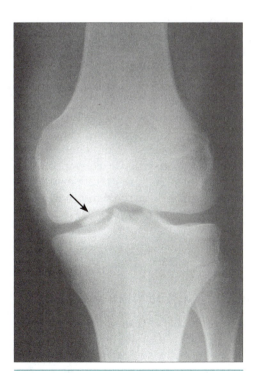

Figure 17.15 Osteochondral fracture of the femoral condyle.

Courtesy of Theodore E. Keats.

Dislocation and Subluxation

Of the three joints that make up the knee complex, the patellofemoral joint is most prone to subluxation and dislocation. Although dislocation of the tibiofemoral joint is less common, it is a much more serious and potentially limb-threatening injury.

Patellofemoral Subluxation and Dislocation

Patella alta is a patella that sits abnormally high in the femoral groove. See table 17.1.

Patellar dislocations, which can result from either direct or indirect forces, typically occur lateral to the femoral groove secondary to the more lateral angular pull of the quadriceps and the lesser height of the lateral femoral condyle compared to the medial femoral condyle. A direct blow to the medial patella and indirect forces applied by the quadriceps during cutting maneuvers with the tibia laterally rotated can force the patella to displace over the lateral femoral condyle. Patients with an abnormally shallow femoral groove, excessive Q-angle (see table 17.1), hypermobile patella, weak medial quadriceps, or patella alta are more prone to recurrent patellar dislocations. Consequently, patellar dislocations occur more frequently in females than males since females generally possess a larger Q-angle and have a greater propensity for lateral tracking problems.

When the patella subluxates or dislocates, the patient complains of a sharp pain and pop in the anterior knee and a feeling of the knee giving way at the time of injury. If the patella remains displaced, the deformity is obvious. However, often the patella spontaneously reduces, making the injury more difficult to identify. The patient is palpably tender along the medial border of the patella and soft tissue structures. The lateral femoral condyle may also be tender. You will note considerable anterior knee swelling, particularly in first-time dislocations, shortly after injury. The patient will be apprehensive when the patella is moved laterally. A physician should examine first-time dislocations or subluxations, especially those resulting from direct trauma, and obtain X rays to rule out any associated chip fractures of the patella or lateral femoral condyle.

! Knee dislocations require immediate neurovascular examination and medical referral.

Tibiofemoral Dislocation

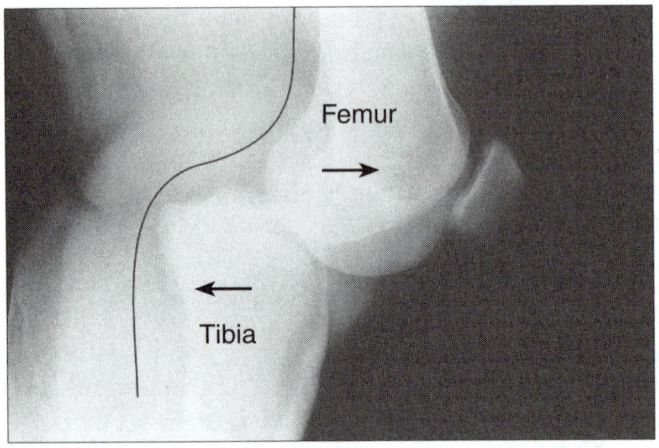

Figure 17.16 Posterior dislocation of the knee. The location of the posterior tibial artery has been drawn in to illustrate the potential for neurovascular injury.

Courtesy of Theodore E. Keats.

A total knee dislocation of the tibia and the femur is a very serious, potentially limb-threatening injury that fortunately rarely occurs in sports. Knee dislocations due to indirect forces are extremely unusual; the majority of cases are caused by large mechanical forces that force the joint well beyond its normal ROM. An example might be a running back who is running full speed and is tackled in such a way that his foot is fixed, while his opponent's weight forcefully drives his knee back into hyperextension. Given that the ligaments act as the primary stabilizers of the knee joint, multiple ligaments—including both cruciate ligaments and at least one of the collateral ligaments—must tear in order for the joint to dislocate. In addition to the significant soft tissue damage that occurs, the risk of neurovascular injury is high, particularly with posterior dislocations (figure 17.16). Knee dislocations require immediate neurovascular examination and medical referral.

Bony and Articular Defects Secondary to Repetitive Stress

Physical activity subjects the articular surfaces of the tibiofemoral and patellofemoral joints to considerable compressive forces. These forces most often affect the patellofemoral joint, particularly in patients with faulty alignment. There are additional concerns that are unique to the adolescent athlete which will be discussed as well. Since the majority of femoral stress fractures occur at the femoral neck and manifest as hip and groin pain, they are discussed in chapter 18, which covers the hip and pelvis.

Patellofemoral Pain Syndrome

Patellofemoral pain syndrome (PFPS), also known as **miserable malalignment syndrome**, or **patellofemoral stress syndrome (PFSS)**, are vague terms describing the general term *anterior knee pain*. Anterior knee pain can be caused by a variety of factors that result in patellar malalignment, increased patellofemoral compression, or poor patellofemoral tracking. These include anatomical and biomechanical abnormalities, muscular weaknesses and imbalances, and training errors. Anatomical and biomechanical abnormalities that can alter lower-extremity alignment include subtalar pronation, lateral tibial torsion, genu valgum, increased Q-angle, hip anteversion, and patella alta (see table 17.1). Weakness in the vastus medialis muscles relative to the lateral quadriceps and tightness in the lateral retinaculum and IT band can also pull the patella laterally, as shown in figure 17.17. An abrupt change in training activity, surface, intensity, or duration that substantially increases the load on the patellofemoral joint may also cause anterior knee pain. Regardless of the cause, the result is the same in each case: pain and irritation consequent to increased patellofemoral compression and pressure.

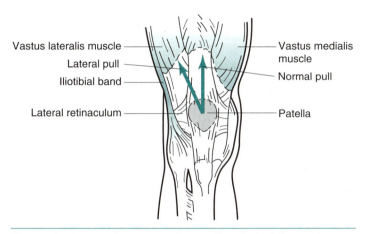

Figure 17.17 Attachments to the patella. Their tightness laterally pulls on the patella (shown by the arrow).

One of the hallmark signs and symptoms of PFPS is poorly localized anterior knee pain that is exacerbated by squatting, climbing stairs, ambulation, or other activity after prolonged sitting (**theater sign**). Most of the time there is little or no observable swelling. The patient may be palpably tender under the lateral border of the patella. There is usually no history of specific onset; instead the pain appears gradually. However, sudden changes in the training regime may initiate symptoms. PFPS is often difficult to manage; success in alleviating the patient's symptoms depends on both identifying and correcting predisposing factors. PFPS usually indicates a rehabilitation program designed to increase mobility of lateral soft tissue structures and improve lower-extremity limb alignment and muscle function.

For more information on managing patellofemoral syndromes, refer to *Therapeutic Exercise for Musculoskeletal Injuries, Second Edition,* (Houglum 2005), chapter 21.

Chondromalacia Patella

While chondromalacia patella fits within the general category of PFPS, it is a specific condition characterized by softening, roughening, and eventual degeneration of the lateral articular surface of the patella. The articular facet is most commonly affected. Chondromalacia patella can result from direct and repetitive trauma, patellar malalignment, or previous trauma such as a patella dislocation or a fracture that extends through the articular surface. Patellar malalignment, or abnormal tracking of the patella within the femoral grove, can occur due to a variety of predisposing factors, including tight lateral soft tissue structures, increased Q-angle, excessive hip anteversion, excessive pronation, or other structural and functional abnormalities of the lower extremity. These abnormalities increase compression and friction of one or more of the articular facets within the femoral groove.

Signs and symptoms include general anterior knee pain, crepitus, minor swelling, and increased pain with patellofemoral compression in activities such as deeply bending the knee, extending the knee, or walking up and down stairs. You may note palpable tenderness under the medial or lateral border of the patella.

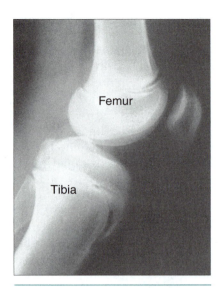

Figure 17.18 Osgood-Schlatter disease (traction tibial apophysitis).

Courtesy of Theodore E. Keats.

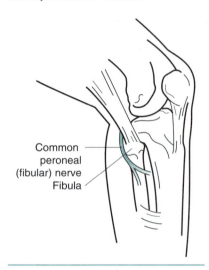

Figure 17.19 Location of the common peroneal nerve where it courses superficially around the head of the fibula.

Apophysitis (Osgood-Schlatter Disease)

In young athletes, repetitive tractioning by the patellar tendon can considerably stress the apophysis of the tibial tubercle. During adolescence, the epiphyseal line is weaker than the quadriceps muscle and tendon. Muscle tightness, repetitive jumping, and running during significant growth spurts can excessively traction the apophysis, leading to irritation, inflammation, and partial avulsion (figure 17.18). Signs and symptoms include focused anterior knee pain, swelling and tenderness over the tibial tuberosity, and increased prominence of the tibial tuberosity. The athlete complains of increased pain with knee extension exercises, squatting, kneeling, and jumping.

Osteochondritis Dissecans

Osteochondritis dissecans, or avascular necrosis of the osteochondral surface of the knee, usually involves the femoral condyle and occurs most often in adolescent athletes. The cause is often unknown but may be repetitive insult. Signs and symptoms include a gradual onset of pain and periodic swelling after activity. The athlete may complain of occasional clicking or catching in the joint if there is a loose fragment. Palpable tenderness may be present on the femoral condyle near the joint line.

Nerve and Vascular Injuries

The neurovascular structures are well protected at the knee as they pass through the popliteal space. Only severe joint disruption places these structures at risk. One exception is the common peroneal nerve as it courses superficially around the proximal fibula.

Peroneal Nerve Palsy

The common peroneal nerve is vulnerable to injury where it wraps superficially around the head of the fibula (figure 17.19). The nerve can be traumatized secondary to a direct blow (contusion), severe cold (ice bag application), or tractioning (varus injury force). Signs and symptoms of nerve palsy include pain and tenderness over the distal fibula; numbness, burning, or tingling along the lateral aspect of the leg and into the dorsum of the foot; and motor weakness of the dorsiflexors, everters, and toe extensors. A foot drop may appear immediately with severe trauma or may appear progressively over the next day secondary to delayed swelling.

Popliteal Artery or Nerve Injury

The popliteal vessels and nerves are well protected in the popliteal space. Injury to these structures, although rare, can result from a severe fracture or total knee (tibiofemoral) dislocation. Conduct distal pulse and sensory checks to examine nerve and vessel integrity with any severe knee trauma.

Structural and Functional Abnormalities

Structural abnormalities at the knee have been implicated as predisposing factors in a variety of lower-extremity ailments. You must be able to recognize these abnormalities in order to fully examine chronic conditions at the knee. The reference position for the structural abnormalities listed in table 17.1 is the patient standing with feet straight ahead and knees fully extended. Unless the abnormality is a functional deformity resulting from some pathology, you will typically note it bilaterally.

Table 17.1
Structural Abnormalities at the Knee

Abnormality	Characteristics
Genu recurvatum	Excessive knee hyperextension; normal knee extension may include a few degrees past neutral; females tend to have greater knee laxity and incidence of knee recurvatum than males; see figure 17.51
Genu valgus	Excessive valgus (lateral) angulation at the tibia relative to the femur; may be caused by hip anteversion or lateral tibial torsion; commonly referred to as knock-kneed; see figure 17.50
Genu varus	Decreased valgus or actual varus (medial) angulation at the tibia relative to the femur; may be caused by hip retroversion or medial tibial torsion; commonly referred to as bowlegged; see figure 17.48
Patella alta	The patella sits abnormally high in the femoral groove; indicated by a lengthened infrapatellar tendon relative to the height of the patella
Patella baja	The patella sits inferiorly in the femoral groove; indicated by a shortened infrapatellar tendon relative to the height of the patella
Quadriceps angle	Excessive angulation (>18-20°) of the quadriceps line (from the anterior superior iliac spine) and the infrapatellar tendon line (from the tibial tubercle) at their bisection through the midpoint of the patella; often associated with genu valgus, hip anteversion, or lateral tibial torsion; Q-angles are normally higher for females than males; see figure 17.39
Squinting patella	Medially rotated or inward-facing patellae; may be caused by hip anteversion or lateral tibial torsion
Tibial torsion	Rotation of the tibia such that when the medial and lateral condyles are in the frontal plane, the foot is angled either out or in; lateral tibial torsion will cause the feet to point outward excessively (slight outward angulation is normal); medial tibial torsion will cause the feet to angle in toward each other (pigeon-toed); see figure 17.49

OBJECTIVE TESTS

The most common thigh and knee injuries you will encounter are thigh muscle strains, internal derangement of the knee due to both contact and noncontact mechanisms, and overstress injuries due to repetitive stress and structural abnormalities at the knee. Along with the patient's history and your observations, the following objective tests will help you examine the structural integrity of the involved tissues.

Palpation

Palpation of the knee and thigh can follow any systematic routine you desire. Once again, this discussion uses a regional approach to describe palpation.

• **Anterior structures.** Anterior palpation includes examining the quadriceps muscle group, suprapatellar tendon, suprapatellar pouch, patella, infrapatellar tendon, tibial tuberosity, patellar retinaculum, and superficial bursa and includes searching for evidence of a plica. Palpate the quadriceps and oblique fibers of the vastus medialis (VMO) for muscle spasm, myofascial restriction, and tenderness. The suprapatellar pouch lies between the superior patella and the muscle belly of the quadriceps. Note any tenderness, nodules, thickening, or soft tissue restriction in this area. Palpate the patella for tenderness and irregularity, and follow its medial and lateral borders to its apex. You can palpate the medial and lateral articular surfaces of the patella by moving the patella medially and laterally and feeling under its rim. Be careful when laterally moving the patella if you suspect subluxation or dislocation, or if the patient is apprehensive (see apprehension sign, page 457). You may find tenderness and roughness if the patient has a history of patellofemoral dysfunction. From the patella, follow the patellar tendon and tibial tuberosity. Palpate bursae around the anterior knee in their locations superficial and deep to the patellar tendon and palpate the prepatella bursa that lies over the patella for tenderness, texture, and swelling. Palpate the patellar retinaculum superiorly, medially, and laterally to the patella for tenderness and restriction of normal tissue mobility. If a plica exists, you can palpate it medial to the patella as a thickened ridge that runs toward the patella either horizontally or at a slight angle.

• **Medial structures.** On the medial aspect of the knee, palpate the medial femoral condyle and epicondyle and the MCL from its origin on the femoral epicondyle to its insertion just below the joint line on the tibial flare. Palpate the adductor tubercle and pes anserine insertion, medial joint line and tibial plateau, and medial hamstring and gastrocnemius tendons for tenderness and swelling. The pes anserine is located distal to the knee joint medial to the tibial tuberosity. You can palpate the medial joint line more easily with the knee flexed; palpate it anteriorly on the medial side of the patella's apex for tenderness and irregularity. Follow the joint margin around toward the posterior knee as far as possible. As your palpation approaches the posterior joint, the joint margin will be too difficult to palpate. Medially rotating the tibia allows palpation of the rim of the medial meniscus. You can also palpate the medial tibial and femoral plateaus inferiorly and superiorly to the menisci, respectively.

• **Lateral structures.** Laterally, palpate the lateral femoral condyle, epicondyle, LCL (lateral epicondyle to fibular head), fibular head, IT band to its insertion on Gerdy's tubercle, lateral joint line, and biceps femoris and gastrocnemius tendons. You can easily palpate the LCL if the patient crosses the ankle of the palpated extremity onto the opposite knee. With your fingertips on the lateral joint margin, you should feel the ligament pop into your fingertips as the leg crosses. The IT band inserts on and just proximal to the fibular head on the tibial condyle and can be followed superiorly toward the tensor fascia lata. Normally a thick, broad band of connective tissue, the IT band should be smooth and not tender. Palpate the lateral joint line and meniscus in a similar fashion to palpating the medial meniscus; lateral rotation of the tibia permits palpation of the posterior rim of the lateral meniscus.

• **Posterior structures.** Posteriorly, palpate the hamstrings and gastrocnemius muscle bellies and tendons, as well as the soft tissue structures in the popliteal fossa. Note areas of tenderness, nodules, spasm, and swelling. You can sometimes palpate the pulse of the deep popliteal artery in the posterior center of the knee. You can palpate the biceps femoris tendon, lateral gastrocnemius tendon, popliteal muscle, and occasionally the posterior aspect of the lateral meniscus and joint margin on the posterolateral aspect of the knee. Palpating the posteromedial compartment includes identifying the flat semimembranosus tendon, the cordlike semitendinosus tendon that you can follow as it traverses medially and anteriorly into the pes anserine, the medial gastrocnemius, and occasionally the medial meniscus.

Range of Motion

ROM testing is straightforward for the knee joint, as it only involves physiological motions in two planes. The motions are flexion and extension and medial and lateral rotation. However, given the functional demands on the knee joint, even slight limitations of these motions can substantially affect knee function. Examine active ROM first; if the movement is pain free, apply overpressure to examine passive motion and gross end feel. You can add goniometric examination to more accurately quantify ROM. Goniometric examination of knee flexion along with girth measurement may be particularly helpful in monitoring the progression of swelling that accompanies acute knee injuries.

Active ROM

Active ROM testing at the knee should include flexion (about 135°) and extension (about 0°), and medial (10-20°) and lateral (20-30°) tibial rotation (figure 17.20). Because muscles acting on the ankle and hip also cross the knee joint, you may need to also examine hip (chapter 18, table 18.1) and ankle (chapter 16, table 16.1) motions.

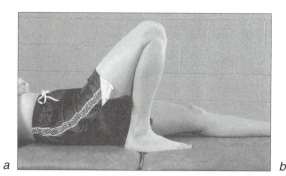

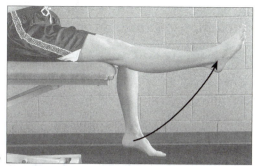

Figure 17.20 ROM of the knee, including *(a)* flexion, *(b)* extension, *(c)* medial tibial rotation, and *(d)* lateral tibial rotation.

Passive ROM

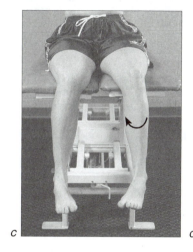

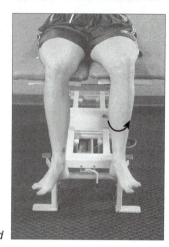

Follow active ROM with passive overpressures, or if active ROM is incomplete, examine first with full passive motion. Overpressure in flexion should be a soft tissue end feel as the calf moves against the posterior thigh. Overpressure in extension and medial and lateral tibial rotation is a firmer end feel as the soft tissue stretches at the end of the motion. ROM and end feels should be pain free for all motions. You can also examine passive patellar motion using your thumb and index fingers to glide the patella in medial, lateral, inferior, and superior directions. Medial and lateral glide excursion can occur up to half the width of the patella in each direction. Perform lateral patellar glides cautiously if you suspect patellofemoral instability or if the patient displays signs of apprehension.

Goniometric Examination of ROM

Goniometric measurement of knee motions is described in table 17.2 and illustrated in figure 17.21. Medial and lateral tibial rotation are typically not measured with a goniometer because of the difficulty in aligning the axis and arms with anatomical landmarks and the difficulty in defining neutral rotation. An indirect goniometric measurement method is described here.

Strength

Because of the knee's lack of bony stability, the muscles play a critical role in dynamic joint stabilization during physical activity. Knee extension and flexion is produced by contraction of the powerful quadriceps and hamstrings, respectively. Test knee extension while the patient is seated or supine and test flexion with the patient prone. Isolated activation of the medial (semitendinosus, semimembranosus) and lateral (biceps femoris) hamstrings produces internal and external rotation of the tibia, respectively, and together counter anterior translation of the tibia on the femur.

Manual Muscle Strength Examination

Manual muscle tests for the knee include knee flexion and extension and medial and lateral tibial rotation (table 17.3, figure 17.22). Because muscles acting on the ankle and hip also cross the knee joint, you may need to examine hip flexion, extension, abduction, and adduction (chapter 18, table 18.2) and ankle plantar flexion (chapter 16, table 16.2).

Table 17.2
Goniometric Examination of Ankle and Foot ROM

Motion	Location of goniometer	Movement	Normal range
Knee flexion	P: Supine A: Lateral femoral epicondyle S: Long axis of femur M: Long axis of fibula	Athlete flexes knee by bringing heel toward buttocks	0° to 135°
Knee extension	P: Supine A: Lateral femoral epicondyle S: Long axis of femur M: Long axis of fibula	Athlete extends knee as far as possible. Hyperextension (extension past 0°) may be present	−5°-0°
Medial and lateral tibial rotation	P: Seated, knee flexed to 90° with foot placed on markable surface A: Midcalcaneus S: Long axis of 2nd MT at start position M: Long axis of 2nd MT at end position	With the foot placed neutrally on a sheet of paper, draw an outline of the foot, marking the tip of the 2nd ray. Have the athlete maximally internally and externally rotate the tibia, keeping the thigh stable. Mark the boundaries at the end of medial and lateral ranges. Draw lines between the 2nd ray and midpoint of the heel for both start and end positions. Measure the angle between the start and end lines for both motions. (Be careful the athlete does not invert or evert the foot, or rotate the thigh during these motions).	Medial rotation = 10-20° Lateral rotation = 20-30°

P = athlete position; A = goniometer axis; M = movable arm; S = stationary arm; MT = metatarsal.

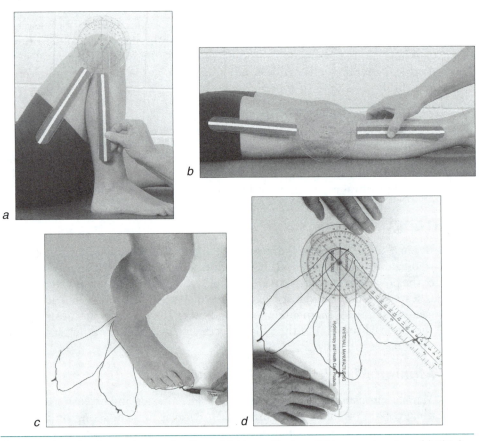

Figure 17.21 Goniometric examination of *(a)* knee flexion, *(b)* knee extension, *(c)* tibial medial rotation, and *(d)* tibial medial and lateral rotation measurement.

Table 17.3
Manual Muscle Testing for the Knee

Motion	Athlete position	Stabilizing hand placement	Resistance hand placement	Instruction to athlete	Primary muscles tested
Knee flexion	Prone, knee extended with foot off the table	Pelvis	Distal, posterior tibia	Flex knee by bringing heel toward buttock Perform also with tibia laterally and medially rotated	Neutral: Biceps femoris, semimembranosus, semitendinosus ER: Biceps femoris IR: Semimembranosus and semitendinosus
Knee extension	Seated, knee flexed to 90° and lower leg hanging off table	Upper thigh	Distal, anterior tibia	Extend knee by raising foot toward ceiling (Watch hip rotation)	Quadriceps femoris
Medial tibial rotation	Seated, knee flexed to 90° and lower leg hanging off table	Distal femur	Grasp distal medial tibia	Rotate foot toward the midline of the body	Semimembranosus, semitendinosus
Lateral tibial rotation	Seated, knee flexed to 90° and lower leg hanging off table	Distal femur	Grasp distal lateral tibia	Rotate foot away from midline of the body	Biceps femoris

ER = external rotation; IR = internal rotation.

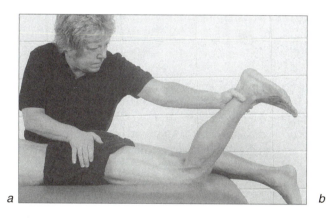

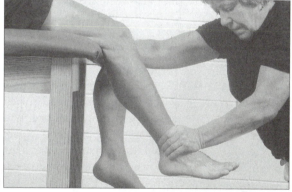

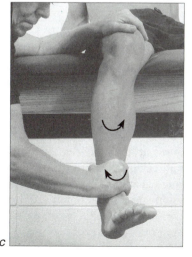

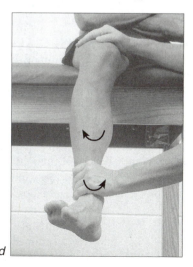

Figure 17.22 Manual muscle testing for (a) knee flexion, (b) knee extension, (c) medial tibial rotation, and (d) lateral tibial rotation.

Instrumented Strength Examination

You can quantitatively examine strength with isokinetic devices (knee flexion and extension, tibial medial and lateral rotation) and repetition maximum testing with a variety of free and machine weights (e.g., squat, leg press, leg curl, leg extension, toe raise). See chapter 7 for details on how to perform 1RM and 10RM isotonic strength tests.

Neurovascular Examination

Complete a neurovascular examination primarily with suspected femoral fractures, tibiofemoral joint dislocations, and with direct trauma to the peroneal nerve as it runs superficially around the proximal head of the fibula. Tibial nerve injury is very uncommon, as this nerve is well protected in the popliteal fossa.

Neurological Testing

If you suspect neurological involvement about or below the knee, perform sensory and motor testing for the peripheral nerves (deep peroneal, superficial peroneal, tibial, and the medial plantar). Suspected neurological involvement proximal to the knee also warrants dermatome, myotome, and reflex examination of the lumbar plexus (see chapter 8, table 8.7 and figures 8.13 and 8.15).

Sensory Testing

Peripheral sensory nerve examination should include the deep peroneal nerve in the dorsal web space, the superficial peroneal nerve on the dorsum of the foot and the lateral leg, the tibial nerve over the posteriomedial plantar heel, and the medial plantar nerve over the medial plantar surface of the foot (see chapter 8, figure 8.14). Changes in sensation over the distribution of the deep and superficial peroneal nerve may occur with direct blows to the lateral aspect of the knee. For severe trauma at the tibiofemoral joint, you should examine both tibial and peroneal nerve distributions.

Motor Testing

Motor testing includes examining each peripheral nerve (see chapter 8, figure 8.16). The posterior tibial nerve innervates the muscles in the posterior compartment and is examined with plantar flexion and toe flexion. The superficial peroneal nerve innervates the lateral compartment muscles and is tested with eversion. The deep peroneal nerve innervates the muscles in the anterior compartment and can be tested with dorsiflexion and great toe extension. If the patient receives a direct blow over the peroneal nerve causing severe neuropraxia, you may observe a foot drop and complete loss of dorsiflexion strength.

Reflex Testing

For symptoms below the knee, you can elicit a deep tendon reflex from the Achilles tendon (S1-S2). Place the ankle in slight dorsiflexion and lightly tap the Achilles tendon with a reflex hammer. If the response is absent or diminished, use Jendrassik's maneuver (see chapter 8, figure 8.2) to ensure that the patient is not inhibiting the response. If necessary, you can examine a deep tendon reflex over the posterior tibialis tendon (L4-L5) on the medial aspect of the ankle.

If you are have difficulty eliciting a reflex response, remember to use Jendrassik's maneuver to distract the patient and increase the nervous system's sensitivity (see chapter 8, figure 8.2).

Vascular Compromise

If the injury may result in vascular compromise, palpate pulses over the popliteal and tibial arteries in the popliteal fossa (for injuries proximal to the knee joint), the posterior tibial artery at the posterior medial ankle, and the dorsalis pedis artery over the dorsum of the foot. Also note changes in skin color and temperature in the lower leg. Since significant trauma to the thigh musculature can also result in a compartment syndrome similar to that described for the anterior compartment of the lower leg (see chapter 16), periodically examine neurovascular status if you suspect increased compartment swelling.

Special Tests

Special tests include those for uniplanar and multiplanar joint instability, meniscal pathology, patellofemoral dysfunction, and joint effusion, as well as other isolated tests for chronic knee conditions.

Uniplanar Ligament Stress Tests

Use the stress tests soon after the injury before muscle spasm, guarding, and swelling occur, as these can cause inaccurate test results.

When applying stress tests, always examine the uninvolved extremity first. To ensure muscular relaxation during the test, instruct the patient to relax, and monitor the muscles during the test. The stress needs to be gentle but forceful enough to produce an accurate result. Signs and symptoms of severity will be consistent with those described for first-, second-, and third-degree sprains in chapter 1. Remember that pain will likely occur during stress tests on new sprains. Practice and become proficient at these skills to avoid having to test the knee three or four times to get a good result.

Valgus Stress Test

When applying stress tests, always examine the uninvolved extremity first. This familiarizes the patient with the test and gives you the information you need in order to make a comparison.

The valgus stress test, also known as the abduction or medial instability stress test, examines the integrity of the inert and active structures providing medial joint stability. The patient is in a supine position with the injured extremity relaxed. Place one of your hands around the distal medial leg and the other hand on the lateral side of the knee. The hand on the lateral knee acts as a fulcrum while the hand on the leg applies a lateral force to the tibia to gap the medial joint (figure 17.23). Perform this test with the knee in full extension and then in 20° to 30° of flexion.

With the knee in extension, the primary structures stressed are the MCL and posteromedial capsule. Other structures, including the posterior and anterior cruciate ligaments, posterior oblique ligament, medial quadriceps muscle, and semimembranosus muscle are also stressed. When the knee is in slight flexion, the primary structure tested is the MCL, since the capsule becomes relaxed, but the medial capsule and other structures including the posterior oblique ligament and PCL can also be stressed. Laterally rotating the tibia during the stress test in knee flexion reduces stress on the PCL, and if the tibia is medially rotated, the stress increases to the cruciate ligaments and decreases to the MCL. If the maneuver causes pain or gaps the joint in extension, the injury is more severe than when the positive results occur with the knee in partial flexion. You must take care to avoid hip rotation during the stress test so that you appropriately apply the force.

Varus Stress Test

In the varus stress test, also known as the adduction or lateral instability stress test, the patient is supine with the leg relaxed. Place one hand on the patient's distal lateral lower leg and the other on the medial aspect of the knee. Using the hand on the knee as a fulcrum, apply a varus force to the knee with the other hand (figure 17.24). As with the valgus stress test, perform the test first with the knee in full extension and then in 20° to 30° of flexion. Pain or gapping on the lateral joint margin is a positive sign. A positive sign in extension indicates serious instability of the lateral knee. Although the primary structures stressed with the knee in full extension are the LCL and posterolateral capsule, other structures may also be involved, including the arcuate complex, anterior and posterior cruciate ligaments, biceps femoris tendon, IT band, and lateral gastrocnemius. With the knee in slight flexion, the capsule is more lax, so the primary structure involved when the test is positive is the LCL; but other structures such as the posterolateral capsule, arcuate complex, biceps femoris tendon, and IT band may also be involved. Laterally rotating the tibia during this test with the knee flexed applies additional stress to the LCL. Take care to avoid hip rotation during these stress tests.

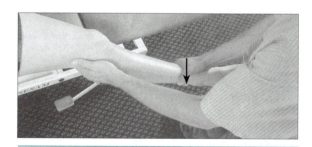

Figure 17.23   Valgus stress test.

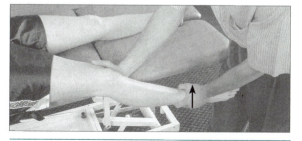

Figure 17.24   Varus stress test.

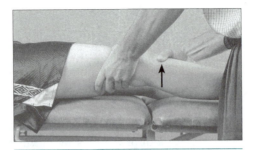

Figure 17.25   Standard Lachman test.

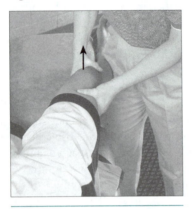

Figure 17.26   Modified Lachman test with the thigh stabilized between the examiner's leg and the side of the table.

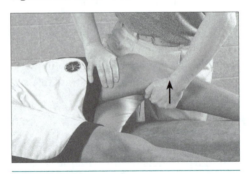

Figure 17.27   Modified Lachman test with the thigh stabilized between the examiner's knee and hand.

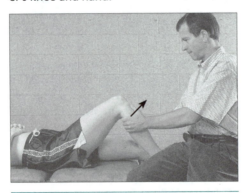

Figure 17.28   Anterior drawer test.

Lachman Test

This uniplanar instability test examines the integrity of the ACL. Also known as the **Ritchie test**, **Lachman-Trillat test**, or **Trillat test**, it has become the test of choice for examining anterior cruciate sufficiency. With the patient supine, grasp the distal thigh with one hand and grasp the medial proximal tibia just below the knee joint with the other hand. Place the knee in approximately 20° to 30° flexion, which is the resting position of the joint (loose-packed position) and which isolates the anterior cruciate as the primary restraint to anterior tibial translation. With the tibia in slight lateral rotation to clear the posterior meniscal horns from the femoral condyles, apply a posteromedial to anterolateral translational force to the tibia while stabilizing the thigh (figure 17.25). The result is positive if the tibia translates forward more than on the contralateral knee.

For examiners with small hands who are testing a patient with a large thigh, there are a number of alternative positions for the Lachman test. Two common positions are shown in figures 17.26 and 17.27. In figure 17.26, the tibia is held between the examiner's thigh and the side of the table to better stabilize the limb in 20° to 30° of flexion while the examiner pulls forward on the tibia. In figure 17.27, the examiner's knee is under the patient's distal thigh. This allows the hand on the thigh to simply stabilize the thigh against the knee while the other hand translates the tibia anteriorly.

Anterior Drawer Test

The anterior drawer test, which also determines ACL integrity, was the primary examination tool for ACL instability until the Lachman test appeared. Although many still use the anterior drawer test, it is not as reliable as the Lachman, primarily because of the knee flexion angle it uses. Whereas the Lachman test uses limited knee flexion, the anterior drawer test is performed at 90° of flexion. Increasing knee flexion pulls other capsular and ligamentous structures taut and optimally positions the hamstrings to oppose anterior tibial translation when contracted or in spasm. Because of these potential secondary restraints, an isolated ACL tear may falsely produce a negative test result. For the anterior drawer test, the patient lies supine with the hip flexed about 45° and the knee flexed at 90° so that the foot is positioned flat on a table or the ground. Place your hands around the proximal tibia with your thumbs over the joint margins anteriorly. Use your thigh to anchor the patient's foot in a neutral position. With your hands in contact with the hamstring tendons to monitor their relaxation, pull the tibia forward (figure 17.28). Normal excursion is about 4 to 6 mm (0.15 to 0.24 in.). Motion greater than that or greater than the uninvolved side indicates possible injury to the ACL, as well as possible involvement of the posterior capsule, MCL, IT band, posterior oblique ligament, and arcuate complex.

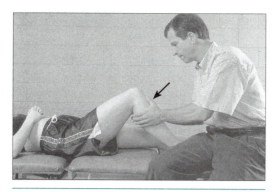

Figure 17.29   Posterior drawer test.

Posterior Drawer Test

This test identifies PCL instability. The positioning and hand placements are the same as for the anterior drawer test. Then push the tibia posteriorly on the femur (figure 17.29). Since structures other than the posterior cruciate provide posterior stability, including the posterior oblique ligament, arcuate complex, and ACL, they are also stressed in this test. If they are intact but the PCL is damaged, the test may be negative or demonstrate only moderate instability.

Posterior Sag Sign

This test is also referred to as the gravity drawer test or the drop back sign. It identifies PCL instability and related injury of the ACL, posterior capsule, and arcuate complex. A positive sign can also indicate injury to the IT band and LCL. Place the patient's lower extremity in the drawer test position with the hip flexed to 45°, the knee flexed to 90° to 110°, and the foot flat on the table. A positive sign occurs if the tibia sags posteriorly on the femur in comparison to the uninvolved side (figure 17.30). For this test the quadriceps should be completely relaxed, as contraction of the quadriceps can pull the tibia forward and make the tibial position appear normal.

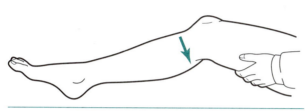

Figure 17.30   Posterior sag sign.

Multiplanar Stress Tests

These tests apply rotary forces to the ligaments to aid in examining joint stability. Generally, positive results indicate a severe injury to the cruciate ligaments and joint capsule.

Slocum Test

The Slocum test examines medial and lateral anterior rotary instabilities. The patient lies supine on the table with the involved hip flexed to 45°, the knee flexed to 90°, and the foot flat on the table (drawer test position). To test anterolateral rotary instability, rotate the tibia so that the foot is at 30° medial rotation. Anchor the foot with your thigh, and place both hands behind the proximal tibia with your thumbs on the joint margins as for the anterior drawer test. Then translate the tibia forward. If anterolateral rotary instability exists, the lateral side of the tibia moves forward more than on the uninvolved knee. Involved structures may include the ACL, posterolateral capsule, arcuate complex, LCL, PCL, and IT. When examining anteromedial rotary instability, the foot is positioned in 15° of lateral rotation (figure 17.31). The positions are otherwise the same as those just described except for the tibial rotation component. Examine anterior translation of the tibia as just described; excessive movement occurs primarily on the medial side if instability is present, indicating injury to the ACL, posteromedial capsule, MCL, posterior oblique ligament, or a combination of these.

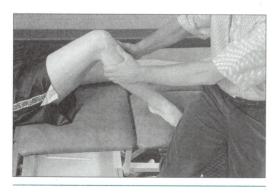

Figure 17.31   Starting position of the Slocum test for anteromedial rotary instability. Note the lateral rotation of the tibia.

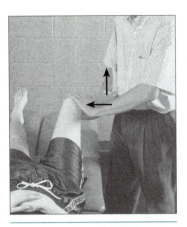

Figure 17.32 MacIntosh test.

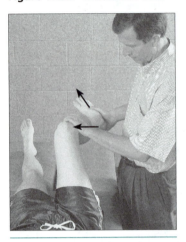

Figure 17.33 Hughston's test.

Lateral Pivot Shift Maneuver

This test, also known as the **MacIntosh test**, identifies anterolateral instability. It is used primarily to identify anterior cruciate ruptures, but positive results also indicate possible injury to the posterolateral capsule, arcuate complex, LCL, and IT. With the patient supine, position the hip of the involved extremity in 30° abduction, 30° flexion, and about 20° medial rotation. Use one hand to place the knee in about 5° to 10° of flexion by putting the heel of your hand behind the fibula, over the lateral gastrocnemius muscle. With your other hand, grasp the ankle and hold the leg in slight medial rotation. Attempt to sublux the tibia anteriorly with a shift maneuver by applying a valgus stress to the knee while maintaining the medial rotation of the tibia and moving the knee into flexion (figure 17.32). If the test is positive and the IT band is intact, between 20° and 40° the tibia slips backward as the IT band's line of pull changes from that of a knee extensor to that of a knee flexor as the knee is moved into flexion.

Hughston's Test

This test is also referred to as the jerk test of Hughston and, like the lateral pivot shift test, examines anterolateral instability of the knee. With the patient supine, the hip is flexed to 45° and the knee to 90°. While maintaining the tibia in medial rotation, apply valgus stress and simultaneous knee extension (figure 17.33). If the test is positive, at 20 to 30° of knee flexion the lateral tibia jerks forward as the lateral tibial plateau subluxes.

Meniscal Tears

As with ligament instability, several tests for meniscal injuries are available. Because the menisci are primarily aneural, these tests are not always reliable; pain is often considered the positive sign, but may not be present unless surrounding structures are also irritated or inflamed. The most commonly used tests are presented here.

McMurray Test

With the patient supine, place one hand on top of the knee with your thumb over one joint line and your index and middle fingers over the opposite joint line; with the other hand, grasp the heel to maintain tibial rotation. Beginning with the knee in full flexion, medially and laterally rotate the tibia and note any audible click. Then, with the tibia laterally rotated, extend the knee beyond 90° while maintaining lateral tibial rotation to stress the medial meniscus (figure 17.34). To stress the lateral meniscus, reposition the leg into full flexion and medially rotate the tibia before moving it into extension. While some have modified this test to include a varus or valgus stress at the knee as the knee is rotated and extended, this modification is not a feature of the original McMurray Test. While joint line pain and an audible click are both considered positive signs, the audible click is the more often associated with actual meniscal findings (Evans and Bell 1993).

Apley Test

With the patient prone, stabilize the thigh with your knee and passively flex the involved knee to 90°. Rotate the tibia into medial and lateral rotation while applying traction to the knee. Then repeat the rotational movements while compressing the knee joint (figure 17.35). If the

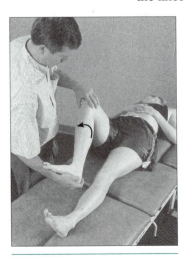

Figure 17.34 McMurray test for medial meniscus.

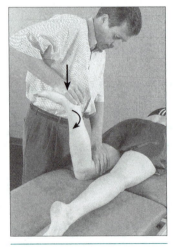

Figure 17.35 Compression and lateral rotation of the tibia with the Apley test.

patient reports pain with distraction, the injury is likely ligamentous; if she reports pain with compression, the injury probably involves the meniscus.

Patellofemoral Tests

The following tests are used to examine patellofemoral joint mobility, pain, and dysfunction.

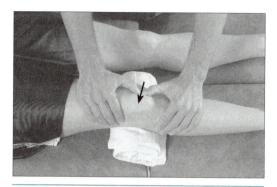

Figure 17.36 Patellar apprehension test.

Acute Patella Injury Test (Apprehension Test)

It is common for a dislocated patella to spontaneously reduce before you have the opportunity to examine the patient. Although the patient may or may not be able to describe the injury, he will recall the sensation of the dislocation. If he feels the same sensation during this test, he will reactively contract the quadriceps or stop the test to prevent the patella from dislocating again. This reaction is often referred to as an **apprehension sign**. With the patient supine and the quadriceps relaxed, position the knee in 20° to 30° flexion. Carefully and slowly glide the patella laterally (figure 17.36). A positive test occurs if the patient prevents the maneuver or stops the test in anticipation of it dislocating the patella.

Grind Test

The grind test examines the integrity of the articulating surface of the patellofemoral joint. With the thigh relaxed and the knee in full extension, place the web of one of your hands just proximal to the superior pole of the patella. Push down on the thigh and instruct the patient to contract the quadriceps (figure 17.37). A positive test occurs if the patient reports pain. This test can produce a positive sign on almost everyone if administered incorrectly. Be cautious about the amount of force you apply, as well as the location. You should apply the force in a gradual fashion, immediately superior to the patella, not directly over it. Repeat this test three to four times, each time applying greater force. Also repeat the test in different knee flexion positions to coincide with the various patellofemoral articular contacts (30°, 60°, and 90°). Because of this test's potential to cause pain in a healthy knee, you should always perform the test bilaterally and compare your findings to the opposite side.

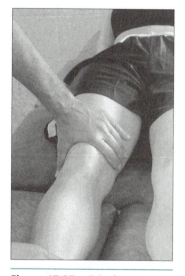

Figure 17.37 Grind test.

Lateral Glide Test

This test identifies tightness in the lateral thigh structures or muscle imbalance of the quadriceps that contributes to PFPS. The patient lies supine with the legs in extension and the thigh muscles relaxed. Instruct her to contract the quadriceps, and observe the patellar movement. Normally the patella moves to an equal extent superiorly and laterally (figure 17.38). A positive sign occurs if the patella moves laterally an excessive amount. The patient can also perform this test in a straddle squat, with the involved extremity in front and the uninvolved extremity behind, for examination of lateral glide during weight bearing.

Patellofemoral (Quadriceps) Angle

This test, also called the quadriceps angle or Q-angle, measures the angle between the quadriceps muscle and the patellar tendon. With the patient supine, the extremity in full extension, and the hip and foot in neutral positions, draw a line from the anterior superior iliac spine to the midpoint of the superior patella. Draw another line from the tibial tuberosity to the midpoint

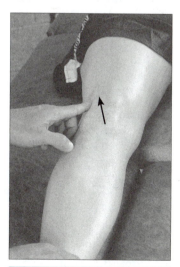

Figure 17.38 Active lateral glide test.

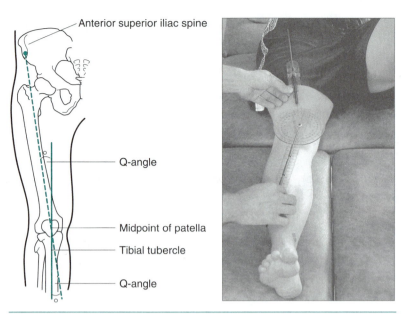

Figure 17.39   Measurement of Q-angle.

of the patella (figure 17.39). The normal patellofemoral angle for men is approximately 10° to 12° and for women is approximately 15° to 18°. Angles less than 10° or greater than 18° are abnormal and can contribute to PFPS.

Tests for Joint Effusion

Edema results from injuries around the knee. There are a few different tests you can use to identify joint effusion about the knee.

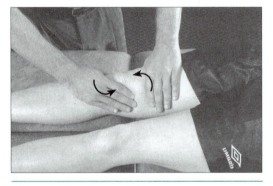

Figure 17.40   Sweep test.

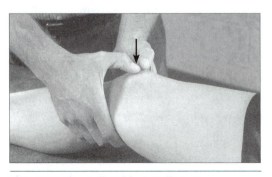

Figure 17.41   Ballotable patella test.

Sweep Test

This test, also known as the **brush test**, **stroke test**, or **wipe test**, detects minimal joint effusion. With the knee relaxed in full extension, stroke the medial aspect of the knee, beginning distal to the joint margin and moving upward into the supra-patellar pouch, in a sweeping motion toward the hip. With the other hand, stroke downward on the lateral side of the patella toward the little toe (figure 17.40). If there is any excess fluid in the knee, you will notice a small bulge or wave on the medial aspect of the knee just inferior to the patella within 1 to 2 seconds.

Ballotable Patella Test

This test, also referred to as the **patellar tap test** or the **dancing patella sign**, identifies moderate to severe effusion. With the knee in a comfortable position near full extension, apply light pressure or a tap to the top of the patella (figure 17.41). The test is positive if the patella bounces or seems to float or bob.

Other Special Tests

Since there are many structures around the knee, a number of structures can be involved in a knee injury. Specific tests used to identify unique structural injuries are discussed here.

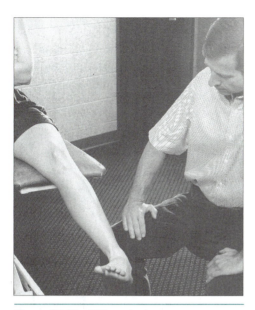

Figure 17.42   Wilson test.

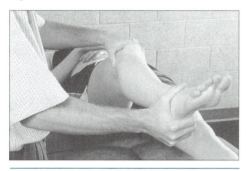

Figure 17.43   Noble compression test.

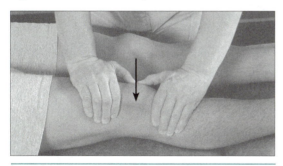

Figure 17.44   Lateral patellar glide.

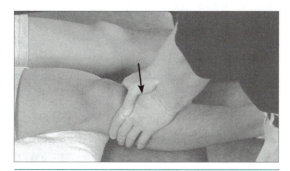

Figure 17.45   Dorsal tibial glide.

Wilson Test

The Wilson test indicates osteochondritis dissecans if the location of injury is the classic site near the intercondylar notch on the medial aspect of the medial femoral condyle. With the patient sitting with the legs over the end of the table, have her actively extend the knee with the tibia in medial rotation (figure 17.42). If the test is positive, the patient reports pain in the knee about 30° from full extension and a resolution of the pain if the tibia is laterally rotated.

Noble Compression Test

This test identifies IT band friction syndrome. The patient is supine, and the involved knee is passively flexed to 90° and the hip flexed to at least 45°. Apply and maintain pressure over the IT band just proximal to the lateral femoral condyle while the knee is passively or actively extended (figure 17.43). The test is positive if the patient reports pain over the lateral femoral condyle when the knee is approximately 30° from full extension as the IT band passes over the femoral condyle.

Joint Mobility Tests

Accessory motion at the knee is essential for full ROM. If you suspect joint restriction, use the following mobility tests for the patellofemoral, tibiofemoral, and tibiofibular joints. A positive sign for each of these tests is pain and restricted mobility in comparison to the opposite side.

Patellofemoral Joint (Patellar Glides)

This maneuver investigates patellar mobility. Restricted patellar mobility may limit knee flexion. The patient is supine with the knee extended and the muscles relaxed. Place the flat part of your thumbs against the lateral patella and glide it medially; then use the flat part of the fingers on the medial patella to move it laterally (figure 17.44). You should also examine inferior and superior glides. It is common for patellar glide restrictions to be bilateral. For this reason, comparing to the uninvolved side may tell you that the range is normal for that patient but may not indicate that mobility is sufficient. It is helpful to practice your examination techniques on multiple athletes to get a better sense of what may be considered restricted versus normal mobility.

Tibiofemoral Joint (Dorsal Tibial Glide)

This movement examines joint mobility and end feel of the knee joint. If flexion is limited, mobility is restricted compared to that for the opposite knee. The patient is supine, with a towel roll under the distal femur and the knee muscles relaxed. Place one hand over the other for leverage over the proximal tibia just distal to the knee joint (figure 17.45). Apply an anterior–posterior force parallel to the joint surface.

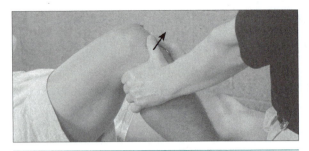

Figure 17.46 Ventral tibial glide.

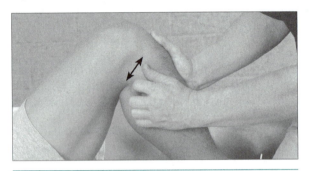

Figure 17.47 Anteroposterior fibular glide.

Tibiofemoral Joint (Ventral Tibial Glide)

This test is for tibiofemoral joint mobility, which is limited if the patient has restricted knee extension. The patient lies supine with the hip and knee flexed so that the foot rests comfortably on the table. Place both hands around the proximal tibia as close to the joint margin as possible (figure 17.46). Instruct the patient to relax the leg muscles and apply a posterior–anterior force parallel to the joint surface.

Anteroposterior Fibular Glide

This maneuver examines the mobility and end feel of the superior tibiofibular joint. Restriction of the joint, which results from knee or ankle injuries, can influence both knee and ankle mobility. With the patient supine and the hip and knee flexed so that the foot is flat on the top of the table, grasp the fibular head with your mobilizing hand and place your stabilizing hand around the superior tibia (figure 17.47). Perform a glide motion from anterior to posterior and then from posterior to anterior to examine mobility and end feel.

INJURY EXAMINATION STRATEGIES

An injury to the knee is often debilitating and can seriously jeopardize an athlete's sport career. Therefore, accurate examination, appropriate care, and applicable rehabilitation are absolutely necessary. Since many conditions can result in significant swelling within and around the joint within a few hours of injury, a thorough initial examination enables you to accurately interpret your objective tests.

On-Site Examination

You observe Molly, a point guard, running a fast break down the court. As she comes to a sudden stop to pivot and change directions around a defender, her knee appears to buckle. She goes down on the court, holding her knee.

During a soccer match, Michael collides with an opponent while lunging forward to take possession of the ball. He goes down on the field holding his left thigh. Upon your arrival, he states that he was kneed in the left thigh. He complains of severe pain and spasm.

Other than the rare occasion when a knee injury occludes the popliteal artery, the knee is not an area in which consequences typically threaten life or limb. However, because that rare occasion does exist, you must always be alert in your on-site examination to immediate signs and symptoms that indicate a medical emergency.

As you approach the athlete, note the position of the limb and the athlete's response. Often the athlete will be holding the injured muscle or joint. If the athlete is holding a flexed knee, the injury is likely a knee sprain. A position in which the knee is locked straight is more indicative of a fracture or dislocation. Upon arriving at the athlete's side, you should include in your primary survey observations for obvious deformities indicating fracture or dislocation, severe

Conduct distal pulse and sensory checks to examine nerve and vessel integrity with any severe knee trauma.

bleeding, and signs and symptoms of shock. If you note severe deformity, immediately examine neurovascular status by palpating for a posterior tibial or dorsal pedal pulse and perform a cursory sensory examination over the distribution of the tibial and peroneal nerves. If you note any of the signs and symptoms just mentioned, treat the injury as a medical emergency. If all findings are negative, proceed with your on-site examination.

Obtain a brief history from the athlete to ascertain the chief complaint, mechanism of injury (even if you witness it), type and location of symptoms, and any unusual sounds or sensations noticed at the time of injury. Since time is of the essence on the field, you need to quickly focus on the area of injury. Observe the area for immediate signs of swelling, discoloration, or deformity.

Palpate the injured area for bony tenderness or deformity, soft tissue tenderness, defects, or spasm. If you suspect a sprain, whenever possible stress test the involved ligaments immediately after injury to determine the severity or degree of ligament injury; it is important to examine sprains early on before muscle guarding and swelling settle in. When you suspect strain, perform an active ROM test. If the motion is weak and painless, you should suspect

Checklist for On-Site Examination of the Knee and Thigh

▷ Primary Survey

- ☐ Consciousness
- ☐ Airway, breathing, and circulation
- ☐ Severe bleeding
- ☐ Position of the limb and athlete's response to injury
- ☐ Obvious deformity indicating severe fracture or dislocation
- ☐ If deformity, immediately check neurovascular status
- ☐ Signs and symptoms of shock

If any of the signs listed are positive, treat as a medical emergency. If all of the signs are negative, proceed with your on-site examination.

▷ Secondary Survey

▷ History

Quickly ascertain the following:

- ☐ Chief complaint
- ☐ Mechanism of injury
- ☐ Unusual sounds or sensations
- ☐ Type and location of pain or symptoms

▷ Observation

- ☐ Immediate swelling, deformity, discoloration
- ☐ Note willingness to move the limb or position holding the limb

▷ Palpation

- ☐ Bony tenderness, abnormal contours, or subtle deformities
- ☐ Soft tissue tenderness, defects or bulges, muscle spasm or guarding

▷ Special Tests

- ☐ Perform ligament stress test if sprain suspected
- ☐ Perform active ROM if strain suspected
- ☐ Compare bilaterally

If all tests are negative, remove athlete from field with assistance as needed for a more thorough examination off-site.

a rupture; if the athlete reports pain with movement or resistance, a first- or second-degree strain is likely.

Once you have enough information to determine the nature and severity of the injury, decide on the mode of transportation from the field. If you have any doubt about the nature of the injury or the athlete's ability to ambulate off the field, use a passive or an assistive carry to avoid weight bearing on the injured extremity pending a more thorough examination.

Acute Examination

You are covering a high school football game and a player comes off the field with a slight limp. He complains of pain on the inside of his right knee. His history reveals that while his foot was planted, he was tackled from the right side, with contact made to the lateral knee and lower leg.

As Sheila sprints along the last quarter of the track during her 400m event, she appears to be running strong when you see her suddenly pull up her stride and reach toward her left thigh. She is determined to finish the race and hobbles over the finish line. As you approach, she is lying down on the inside of the track and holding her left thigh.

When an injured athlete has been removed from the field or has walked over to the sideline under his own power, you can examine the injury more thoroughly to determine its nature and severity, to decide whether the athlete can return to participation, and to select appropriate immediate treatment.

History

When obtaining a history of previous injuries, be sure to ask about both the involved and uninvolved extremities, since you will use the uninvolved knee as your reference for what is normal for that athlete.

When asking about previous injuries, determine the nature and severity of the injury, the time of onset and duration of the injury and disability, any treatment or surgical interventions, and the final outcome.

With the athlete on the sideline, complete a full injury history. If the mechanism was one of contact, note whether the pain is on the same side or on the opposite side of the limb where the contact was made. Pain on the opposite side tends to indicate a sprain, and pain on the same side more often results from a contusion. If the mechanism was one of noncontact, determine whether the athlete was weight bearing, rotating with the foot planted, or both. See if the athlete can recall whether the knee was flexed, extended, or hyperextended at the time. Was the athlete accelerating (possible meniscus injury) or decelerating (possible cruciate ligament injury)? At this time ask again about any unusual sounds or sensations, the current location and type of pain, and any radiation of pain to other areas. Note whether the pain has changed from the time of injury. Isolated meniscal injuries may cause pain when they occur, but the pain can quickly subside and then return later; in contrast, the pain of a musculotendinous injury does not subside. Ligamentous injuries are not always predictable. It is common for a third-degree ACL injury to hurt immediately, quickly ease, and then hurt considerably a few hours or a day later once swelling begins to set in. Take full advantage of this time window and obtain a thorough and accurate examination on the sideline, since examination will be much more difficult once secondary pain and swelling set in.

The history should also include questions regarding previous injuries to the lower extremity. Previous ligament or meniscal injuries are particularly important, as they may result in residual laxity or other positive signs that may confound your findings regarding the current injury. Although prior knee injury is a primary concern, you should also be interested in other lower-extremity injuries. For example, a fractured ankle that was immobilized, requiring the athlete to ambulate on crutches, may have left the knee muscles weak and atrophied and thus susceptible to injury.

Observation

By this time you have been able to observe how the athlete is responding to the injury, how the athlete moves and protects the injured part, how the athlete stands and walks, and how the athlete transfers from sitting to standing or moves onto the bench, examination table, or to the ground. Note any hesitation, evidence of guarding, unequal weight distribution, or favoring of the injured limb with standing and walking. In some cases an athlete is able to ambulate fairly well following a meniscus or ligament injury, so be careful not to underestimate the injury based on observation alone. When inspecting the knee itself, observe again for any signs of swelling, discoloration, or deformity. Check the contour and muscle tone of the thigh and lower leg for equal appearance bilaterally. Note any scars that would indicate previous injury. Observe the alignment and relationship of the femur, tibia, and patella.

Palpation

For palpation, comfortably position the leg in slight flexion. Begin with superficial structures and move to deeper tissue, palpating the injured region last. Note any temperature differences, tenderness, swelling, crepitus, incongruencies, and differences in soft tissue mobility throughout the palpation process. Perform all palpations bilaterally, comparing your positive findings to the uninvolved extremity.

Special Tests

As already mentioned, acute knee injuries often involve ligament, capsular, or meniscal structures and are best examined immediately following injury. The special tests you use in the acute examination identify and quantify the severity of acute injuries. There are a number of joint instability tests, and you will not use them all in your examination. The injury mechanism plays an important role in your selection of joint stability tests.

ROM

Active extension and flexion are best examined with the athlete supine, while medial and lateral tibial rotation are best performed with the athlete seated with the leg hanging off the edge of a table or bench. As the athlete moves the knee through its ROM, observe for equal and full movement bilaterally, noting any hesitation, pain, or audible clicks during motion. Active knee hyperextension ($-5°$--$10°$) is common but should be equal bilaterally and pain free. Passive motion should follow active motion, and flexion should slightly surpass the active motion. If pain occurs with active motion, there is no need to apply overpressure, since active motion has accomplished the goal of reproducing the athlete's symptoms. Overpressure also causes undue stress to the knee and should be avoided when pain occurs with active motion.

Strength

Unless the injury indicates otherwise, perform manual muscle tests on all knee motions. Due to the evaluative constraints of the acute examination, manual muscle testing may be limited to isometric break tests for knee flexion and extension. If you use break tests, perform them at multiple knee positions for the quadriceps and hamstrings. You can apply quadriceps resistance at $0°$, $30°$, $60°$, and $90°$. Apply hamstrings resistance with the knee flexed at $90°$ and the tibia in a neutral position and in medial and lateral rotation to differentiate between the medial and lateral hamstring muscles. Examine strength for hip flexion and ankle plantar flexion with the knee both flexed and extended, since muscles producing these motions also cross the knee joint.

Neurovascular

A blow to the lateral aspect of the knee can contuse the common fibular nerve, and the athlete may complain of pain, tingling, or numbness referred down the lateral aspect of the leg and the top of the foot. If you think the nerve may be involved, perform sensory and motor testing over the distribution of the common fibular nerve. Any abnormal result warrants a more detailed sensory examination.

Checklist for Acute Examination of the Knee and Thigh

▷ *History*

Ask questions pertaining to the following:

- ☐ Chief complaint
- ☐ Mechanism of injury (contact or noncontact)
- ☐ Position of the knee and foot at time of injury
- ☐ Unusual sounds or sensations
- ☐ Type and location of pain or symptoms
- ☐ Previous injury to involved and uninvolved extremities

▷ *Observation*

- ☐ Visible facial expressions and response to injury
- ☐ Swelling, deformity, abnormal contours, or discoloration
- ☐ Gait, willingness to bear weight
- ☐ Overall position, posture, and alignment of lower extremity
- ☐ Bilateral comparison

▷ *Palpation*

Bilaterally palpate for pain, tenderness, crepitus, defects, and deformity over the following:

- ☐ Quadriceps muscle (including VMO), suprapatellar tendon, suprapatellar pouch, patella, infrapatellar tendon, tibial tuberosity, patellar retinaculum, superficial bursae
- ☐ Evidence of plica
- ☐ Medial femoral condyle and epicondyle, MCL, adductor tubercle, pes anserine insertion, medial joint line and tibial plateau, medial hamstring and gastrocnemius tendons
- ☐ Lateral femoral condyle and epicondyle, LCL, fibular head, IT band, Gerdy's tubercle, lateral joint line and tibial plateau, biceps femoris and gastrocnemius tendons
- ☐ Hamstring and gastrocnemius muscle bellies and tendons, popliteal fossa

▷ *Special Tests*

- ☐ Patellar apprehension
- ☐ Uniplanar ligament stress tests (valgus, varus, Lachman test, anterior drawer, posterior drawer, and sag)
- ☐ Multiplanar ligament stress tests (Slocum, lateral pivot shift, Hughston's)
- ☐ Meniscal tests (McMurray's, Apley's)
- ☐ Bilateral comparison

▷ *Range of Motion*

- ☐ Active ROM for knee flexion and extension, medial and lateral tibial rotation
- ☐ Passive ROM for the same motions
- ☐ Passive ROM for medial, lateral, inferior, and superior patellar glides
- ☐ Bilateral comparison

▷ *Strength Tests*

- ☐ Perform manual resistance against knee flexion and extension, and knee internal and external rotation
- ☐ Perform manual resistance against hip flexion and extension with knee flexed and extended
- ☐ Perform manual resistance against ankle plantar flexion with knee flexed and extended
- ☐ Check bilaterally and note any pain or weakness

▷ *Neurovascular Tests (If Warranted)*

- ☐ Sensory, motor (common fibular nerve)
- ☐ Popliteal, posterior tibial, and pedal pulses
- ☐ Sensory, motor, and reflex of lumbar plexus and peripheral nerves

▷ *Functional Tests*

Functional Tests

As mentioned previously, you must consider both your subjective and objective findings when determining whether or not the athlete can return to sport participation. For example, consider a meniscal injury, which often includes immediate pain that quickly subsides and does not return until later. If you rely only on the subjective reports of no pain following injury, you may allow the athlete to return prematurely, potentially exposing the athlete to a more serious injury. In addition to considering subjective examination, you must be confident in your objective examination in order to decide the best participation status. If ever in doubt, the safer approach is to defer the functional examination, restrict participation for the remainder of the day, and see how the knee responds. If you are confident that the knee injury is minor and that the athlete may appropriately return to participation, perform functional tests before making a final decision. Since the ankle, knee, and hip encounter the same stresses during sport participation, the functional tests for the knee are similar to those discussed for ankle injuries (see chapter 16).

> Functional tests should be specific to the athlete's sport and position and should mimic the demands the activity places on the knee.

Clinical Examination

> Christina has come into the clinic on crutches with her knee wrapped in an elastic bandage. She states she and her siblings took on their cousins in a soccer game over Thanksgiving break and she injured her knee. She was going after the ball when her 200 lb cousin fell into her leg, pushing her knee backward and inward. She states she was able to bear weight on the leg, but it felt really unstable, so she borrowed her dad's old crutches to get around. You now observe gross edema in the knee joint and severe ecchymosis over the medial aspect of the knee.

> Andrew is a 14-year-old basketball player. He comes to you complaining of anterior knee pain that worsens during jumping activities. He also states that it is painful with kneeling.

Patients often do not report a knee injury until the next day, as pain and swelling are frequently delayed. The clinical examination for these injuries is similar to the acute examination, but includes a more in-depth history and differential diagnostic tests to rule out involvement of other joints. Unfortunately, these injuries are often more difficult to examine once pain, swelling, and muscle guarding have set in, so in the clinic you must rely more heavily on the history before proceeding with the examination.

You will also see many chronic and overuse injuries in the athletic training facility. These injuries warrant other investigations, including structural and postural examination of the entire lower-extremity chain, joint mobility examination, and soft tissue examination, since such factors often contribute to these types of injuries.

History

After determining the initial onset and mechanism of injury, duration of symptoms, and immediate response to the injury, investigate the patient's current complaints and symptoms. Find out how the knee pain has changed since the initial injury and what activities aggravate the symptoms. Ask the patient to describe her pain. Sharp pain may indicate a mechanical problem; an aching pain accompanied by stiffness often indicates inflammation. Generalized pain may point to partial musculotendinous tears, large joint effusions, or contusions. Knee pain with ankle movement may indicate tibiofibular joint dysfunction.

Determine whether the patient is experiencing any grating, clicking, locking, or giving out of the knee. Grating in the anterior aspect of the knee commonly occurs with degenerative patellofemoral disorders. Clicking and snapping are common complaints when inflamed tendons, such as the IT band and the hamstring tendons, ride over other structures. Locking can signal that either a loose body or a meniscal tear is interfering with normal joint motion. Giving out can be a sign of instability, meniscal injury, and patellar subluxation, or it may simply occur secondary to pain and muscle weakness. Pain that affects daily activities such as climbing stairs, squatting, standing, or prolonged sitting often relates to patellofemoral dysfunction.

Asking about the knee swelling will also yield important clues. Find out whether the swelling occurred immediately after injury or later. Swelling that occurs within 2 to 3 hours following injury most often results from blood extravasation. Swelling that occurs 8 to 24 hours after injury usually results from synovial irritation. If the swelling is chronic, determine what activities cause the knee to swell. When the swelling does occur, is it localized (i.e., bursa) or diffuse?

As with chronic injuries at other joints, always consider the patient's training history and type of footwear. Training on hills (particularly downhill) and training on slanted surfaces are commonly associated with patellofemoral pain and IT band friction syndrome. Any abrupt change in training intensity, duration, surface, or type is often a predisposing factor to chronic inflammatory conditions. By the time you complete the history, you should have a good sense of the stage, irritability, nature, and severity of the injury, as well as of how aggressive you can be in the objective portion of the examination. You should also be aware of any previous injuries to either lower extremity and any previous occurrences of the current complaint.

Observation

In addition to making the observations outlined for the acute examination, inspect for structural and biomechanical abnormalities that may contribute to or cause chronic or overuse injuries (see table 17.1). Observe posture and alignment of the lower extremities from anterior, posterior, and lateral views. Examine hip and ankle alignment for its potential effect on the knee.

Any abnormal alignment of the lower extremity or pelvis can cause compensatory changes at the knee and increase stress on its supporting structures. For example, genu varus (figure 17.48) can stem from pes cavus, medial tibial rotation (figure 17.49a), hip abduction, or excessive lateral hip rotation. Genu valgus (figure 17.50) can occur secondary to pes planus, lateral tibial rotation (figure 17.49b), hip adduction, or excessive medial hip rotation. Genu recurvatum (figure 17.51) can be related to joint laxity, excessive medial hip rotation with

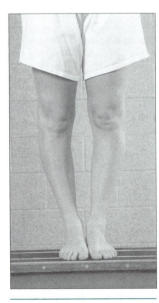

Figure 17.48 Genu varum (varus).

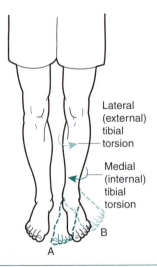

Figure 17.49 Lateral tibial rotation (a) and medial tibial rotation (b). The arrows show the direction of rotation.

Lateral (external) tibial torsion

Medial (internal) tibial torsion

A   B

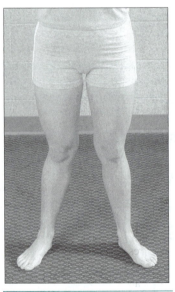

Figure 17.50 Genu valgum (valgus).

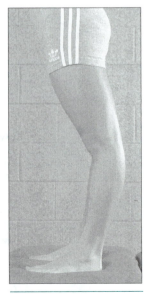

Figure 17.51 Genu recurvatum.

Genu varum (varus) *is a decrease in the normal valgus angle or a medial angulation of the tibia relative to the femur. See also table 17.1.*

Genu recurvatum *is excessive hyperextension of the tibiofemoral joint. See also table 17.1.*

pes planus, or to tightness of the ankle or gastrocnemius-restricting dorsiflexion. Therefore, focus on the overall alignment of the lower extremity and then examine its collective effect at the knee.

Examine for symmetry of the lower extremities in weight distribution, position, alignment, size, color, and definition. Observe for any swelling, atrophy, bruising, scars, or protuberances.

In young athletes with anterior knee pain, be sure to note any increased prominence of the tibial tubercle, which may indicate apophysitis or Osgood-Schlatter disease. As part of your general observation you should also note patellar alignment and location relative to the anterior knee and femur. Compare the patellar tilt and rotation left to right. Normal alignment is when the patella faces straight ahead, with no tilt or rotation and with its inferior pole at the level of the joint margin.

Observe gait with the patient in shoes and also barefoot. Determine normal gait cadence first. If there are no abnormalities and the patient can normally ambulate without pain, you can investigate the effect of increased speed with a treadmill. You should be familiar with normal gait examination for walking and running (see chapter 4). Perform this examination, as for standing posture, from anterior, lateral, and posterior views. Stride length, swing-through, and weight bearing should be equal left to right. The patient should move smoothly from heel strike to foot flat to toe-off without hesitation or imbalances from one side to the other. Shortened stride length, abbreviated weight bearing on the involved leg with reduced swing-through on the uninvolved leg, rapid foot flat, limited toe-off, and a dropping of the contralateral hip (Trendelenburg gait; see chapter 18) all indicate a reluctance to bear weight on the extremity because of pain, weakness, or limited motion.

For more explicit information on examining posture and gait and the expected normal findings, refer to chapter 4.

Differential Diagnosis and ROM

Because the back, hip, and ankle can all refer symptoms to the knee, you must eliminate each of these areas as possible causes of the patient's complaints before proceeding to a full knee examination. Use a scanning examination to rule out external causes for knee symptoms. For ruling out the back as a source of knee pain, standing ROM with overpressure is the most widely recognized technique. The patient stands and moves into full trunk flexion, extension, and side-bending, all with overpressure. Perform trunk rotation with overpressure with the patient sitting. Rule out the hip with the patient supine. Have the patient perform active hip flexion, abduction, and rotation, and apply overpressure techniques at the end of each motion. Rule out the ankle in similar fashion, using both active motion and passive overpressures. You should further examine any pain caused by these tests that refers to the knee before continuing with your knee examination.

Perform ROM examination of the knee actively and passively as discussed for the acute examination. Provide overpressure if the patient reports no pain with active motion. You should pay careful attention to the presence of an **extensor lag**. With this condition the patient is unable to fully extend the knee during active motion, but demonstrates full passive motion. An extensor lag usually results from quadriceps weakness or inhibition secondary to pain or chronic swelling. The patient should regain this active motion before returning to activity.

Strength Tests

Manual resistance is the most efficient method of strength examination off the field and is consistent with that for the acute examination. Often the patient with patellofemoral pain tolerates a series of isometric tests at varying angles better than resistance applied through a full ROM. Isometric tests at incremental angles will also help you identify the point in the ROM at which the pain or compression occurs.

Manual resistance should also include examining the ankle (chapter 16) and hip muscles (chapter 18), since prolonged disability secondary to chronic or overuse pain can result in disuse atrophy, muscle imbalance, an antalgic (abnormal) gait, or some combination of these. You must detect deficiencies in any lower-extremity muscle group so that you can correct them during the rehabilitation program.

If you desire a more objective strength examination, you can use weight machines and isokinetic equipment if they are available. Be cautious, however, in deciding to use machine and isokinetic equipment because these devices can impose additional stress on the knee. For example, the applied forces of these machines can aggravate patellofemoral dysfunction and exacerbate symptoms. Moreover, when pain is present during these tests, muscle strength results will be inaccurate because of the pain withdrawal reflex that occurs. In these instances, you may have to defer mechanical and even manual strength examination until later.

Neurological Tests

When the patient reports tingling, numbness, shooting pain, burning, or weakness, perform a neurological examination. Begin with a scan for referring lumbar pathology and then follow with a more detailed neurological examination of peripheral nerve distributions. The sensory, motor, and reflex tests are the same as those previously discussed for the lumbar plexus and peripheral nerve distributions. Refer back to chapter 8, figures 8.13 through 8.17, for details on these tests.

Special Tests

The special tests for the acute examination are also used in the clinical examination. Include tests for overuse injuries if chronic symptoms are indicated by the patient's history and previous objective tests. A list of tests is included in the Clinical Examination checklist.

Checklist for Clinical Examination of the Knee and Thigh

▷ *History*

Ask questions pertaining to the following:

- ☐ Chief complaint
- ☐ Mechanism of injury
- ☐ Unusual sounds or sensations (grating, clicking, locking, giving out, referred pain)
- ☐ Type, quality, and location of pain or symptoms
- ☐ Change in pain symptoms since initial onset to injured area
- ☐ Previous injury
- ☐ Previous injury to opposite extremity for bilateral comparison
- ☐ Previous injury to involved and uninvolved lower extremities

If chronic, ascertain:

- ☐ Onset and duration of symptoms (especially swelling)
- ☐ Aggravating and easing factors
- ☐ Training history
- ☐ Footwear

▷ *Observation*

- ☐ Visible facial expressions of pain
- ☐ Swelling, deformity, abnormal contours, scars, or discoloration
- ☐ Muscle tone and atrophy
- ☐ Bony prominences (e.g., Osgood-Schlatters)
- ☐ Gait, willingness to bear weight
- ☐ Structural or biomechanical abnormalities of the knee (genu varus, valgus, and recurvatum; Q-angle; patella alta and baja; squinting patellas)

- ☐ Observe overall position, posture, and alignment of lower extremity
- ☐ Compare bilaterally

▷ *Differential Diagnosis*

- ☐ Clear low back, hip, and ankle with active ROM and overpressure tests

▷ *Range of Motion*

- ☐ Perform active ROM for knee flexion and extension, medial and lateral tibial rotation
- ☐ Check for extensor lag
- ☐ Perform passive ROM for same motions as for active ROM
- ☐ Perform passive ROM for medial, lateral, inferior, and superior patellar glides
- ☐ Make bilateral comparison

▷ *Strength Tests*

- ☐ Perform manual resistance against knee flexion and extension, as well as hip flexion and extension and ankle plantar flexion with knee extended
- ☐ Perform isokinetic concentric and eccentric strength tests for knee flexion and extension
- ☐ Perform isometric tests at incremental angles for patellofemoral disorders
- ☐ Examine strength of hip and ankle muscles crossing the knee joint
- ☐ Compare bilaterally and note any pain or weakness

▷ *Neurovascular Tests*

- ☐ Sensory (L1-S2, peripheral)
- ☐ Motor (L1-S2, peripheral)
- ☐ Distal pulse (popliteal, posterior tibial, and dorsalis pedis)

▷ *Special Tests*

- ☐ Tests for joint effusion (ballotable patella, sweep)
- ☐ Patellofemoral tests (apprehension, grind, lateral glide, Q-angle)
- ☐ Uniplanar ligament stress tests (valgus, varus, Lachman, anterior drawer, posterior drawer, and sag)
- ☐ Multiplanar ligament stress tests (Slocum, lateral pivot shift, Hughston's)
- ☐ Meniscal tests (McMurray's, Apley's)
- ☐ Wilson test
- ☐ Noble compression test
- ☐ Compare bilaterally

▷ *Joint Mobility Examination*

- ☐ Tibiofemoral glides (dorsal, ventral)
- ☐ Patellofemoral glides (medial, lateral, superior, inferior)
- ☐ Tibiofibular glides
- ☐ Bilateral comparison

▷ *Palpation*

Bilaterally palpate for pain, tenderness, crepitus, defects, and deformity over the following:

- ☐ Quadriceps muscle (including VMO), suprapatellar tendon, suprapatellar pouch, patella, infrapatellar tendon, tibial tuberosity, patellar retinaculum, superficial bursae
- ☐ Evidence of plica
- ☐ Medial femoral condyle and epicondyle, MCL, adductor tubercle, pes anserine insertion, medial joint line and tibial plateau, medial hamstring and gastrocnemius tendons
- ☐ Lateral femoral condyle and epicondyle, LCL, fibular head, IT band, Gerdy's tubercle, lateral joint line and tibial plateau, biceps femoris and gastrocnemius tendons
- ☐ Hamstring and gastrocnemius muscle bellies and tendons, popliteal fossa

▷ **Functional Tests**

Joint Mobility

If you suspect joint restrictions, perform joint mobility tests to determine the extent and quality of accessory joint motion. The knee's capsular pattern is more limited in flexion than in extension. If this is the ROM profile of the patient with reduced ROM, you should perform joint mobility examination to determine the specific capsular restrictions. Examine joint accessory movements of the patellofemoral, tibiofemoral, and tibiofibular joints. Always compare with the contralateral joint to determine normal mobility for the patient. A positive sign for each of these tests is pain and restricted mobility in comparison to the opposite side.

Palpation

Palpation is consistent with that performed for the acute examination. For optimal palpation, palpate the knee in both extension and flexion to relax and tighten tissues as necessary. Remember that for palpating the joint line and surfaces adjacent to the joint margin, the knee is best positioned in about 90° of flexion.

Functional Tests

As mentioned for the acute examination, the functional tests for the knee are the same as those for the ankle. Specific skill tests are dictated by the patient's sport or work demands.

SUMMARY

1. Describe the etiology, signs and symptoms, and potential complications associated with acute and chronic injuries of the knee frequently encountered in the physically active.

   The knee is one of the most frequently injured joints in physically active people. It is particularly susceptible to injury because of its lack of bony stability, its reliance on soft tissue structures for stability, and the large mechanical forces it sustains during sport activity. Compressive, varus and valgus, and anterior and posterior shear and rotational forces are constantly applied to the knee joint during sport activities, particularly those that require running, jumping, cutting, and rapidly changing directions. When intrinsic or extrinsic forces exceed the structural integrity of the supporting tissues, injury results. The soft tissue structures of the knee are also prone to chronic inflammatory conditions caused by repetitive friction and overuse. Repetitive kneeling, jumping, and flexion or extension movements are common mechanisms associated with tendinitis and bursitis conditions of the knee. Lower-extremity malalignments can also contribute to overstress injuries.

2. Describe the etiology and signs and symptoms, including predisposing structural and biomechanical factors, associated with chronic patellofemoral pathologies.

   Patellofemoral pain syndrome (PFPS) is a general term that describes anterior knee pain. Patellofemoral pain can result from a variety of factors that cause patellar malalignment, increased patellofemoral joint compression, or poor patellofemoral tracking. These factors include anatomical and biomechanical abnormalities, muscle weaknesses or imbalances, and training errors. Regardless of cause, the result of PFPS is pain, irritation, and sometimes degeneration of the articular surfaces consequent to decreased patellofemoral contact area and increased patellofemoral pressure.

3. Describe and perform the stress tests for examining internal derangement of the knee joint.

   A variety of stress tests are available to examine structural integrity of the knee joint. Tests for uniplanar instability examine the primary and secondary stabilizing structures in a varus, valgus, anterior, or posterior direction. Multiplanar stress tests incorporate rotational forces to check for rotary instabilities that indicate an injury to one or more of the cruciate ligaments, the joint capsule, and possibly other ligamentous and muscular constraints. Compression tests identify meniscal involvement. You should perform all stress tests bilaterally and compare end feel. Proper positioning and stabilization of the proximal and distal segments are essential for accurate results, and mastering the technique for each test requires practice.

4. Describe and perform the special tests for examining patellofemoral dysfunction.

The patellofemoral joint is prone to chronic inflammatory and degenerative conditions, and pain in this region is a frequent complaint of the physically active. Special tests for swelling, degeneration, and mobility help determine the nature and severity of the injury. The difficulty is not so much identifying the nature of problem as understanding the potential contributing or causative factors. Careful examination of lower-extremity alignment and structural abnormalities at the knee in standing, walking, and running is an integral part of examination.

5. Describe and demonstrate the objective tests for examining the knee and thigh.

The most common injuries that you will encounter in the thigh and knee are thigh muscle strains, internal derangement of the knee due to contact and noncontact mechanisms, and overstress injuries due to repetitive stress and structural abnormalities at the knee. Along with the patient's history and your observations, objective tests help you examine the structural integrity of the involved tissues. Palpation is best performed with a regional approach. Passive, active, and resisted ROM testing at the knee should include flexion and extension and medial and lateral rotation of the tibiofemoral joint. Because muscles acting on the ankle and hip also cross the knee joint, you may need to examine hip and ankle motions. Use neurovascular examination primarily with suspected femoral fractures, tibiofemoral joint dislocations, and with direct trauma to the peroneal nerve as it runs superficially around the proximal head of the fibula. Special tests include those for uniplanar and multiplanar joint instability, meniscal pathology, patellofemoral dysfunction, and joint effusion, as well as other isolated tests for chronic knee conditions. If you suspect a joint restriction, perform mobility tests for the patellofemoral, tibiofemoral, and tibiofibular joints.

6. Perform an on-site examination of the knee, indicating criteria for immediate medical referral and mode of transportation from the field.

Most knee injuries are not life threatening, but before moving the athlete off the playing field, you must identify signs and symptoms that could indicate serious injury. Signs of shock, severe bleeding, dislocation, fracture, and compromised neurovascular supply all necessitate precise, deliberate, and efficient management and transportation. The majority of acute injuries involve the soft tissue structures of the knee. If you suspect ligament injury, perform a stress test on the field to obtain the best results, before swelling and muscle guarding set in.

7. Perform an acute examination of the knee, including functional criteria for return to activity.

Once the athlete is on the sideline, a complete examination can determine more precisely the nature and extent of the injury. Important clues to the nature of the injury come from a thorough history of the mechanism, including whether it was contact versus noncontact. You should palpate all joint line and soft tissue structures at this time and perform special tests for patellofemoral and tibiofemoral joint stability to examine ligament, meniscal, and capsular integrity. Although there may be multiple tests for a particular ligament structure, you do not need to perform all of them; you should choose those tests that best isolate the structure and, in some cases, accommodate your hand size. Degrees of injury severity for sprains and strains of the knee are consistent with those described in chapter 1.

8. Perform a clinical examination of the knee, including examination of lower-extremity alignment and considerations for differential diagnosis of referring pathologies from the back, hip, foot, and ankle.

When you see an injured patient for the first time in the athletic injury treatment facility, you often need additional examination tools to determine the nature, severity, irritability, and stage of the injury for postacute and chronic conditions. In the clinical examination, you must rule out the possibility of referring pathologies from the ankle, hip, and low back through differential diagnostic tests. Examine joint mobility if the patient has a capsular pattern of reduced ROM of the knee. Examine postural and lower-extremity alignment for possible abnormalities that may contribute to or cause chronic or overuse injuries. Always perform functional tests for dynamic lower-extremity movements required in the patient's work or sport before permitting his return to full activity.

REVIEW QUESTIONS

1. What is a potential complication of a severe quadriceps contusion? What causes this complication, and what signs and symptoms should you look for?

2. Discuss the different mechanisms associated with isolated injuries to the four major stabilizing ligaments of the knee. Which structures are involved in an "unhappy triad," and what is a common mechanism for this type of injury?

3. Describe the etiology and signs and symptoms of a meniscus injury. Why are these injuries sometimes difficult to detect, and what special tests would you use to identify injury to these structures?

4. What is the difference between the Lachman test and the anterior drawer test? Which is the preferred test for examining an isolated ACL injury? Explain your answer.

5. What tendon structures around the knee are most susceptible to chronic inflammatory conditions? Describe the repetitive mechanisms most often associated with each.

6. What are the predisposing factors for patellar dislocations? If you suspect that a patient has suffered a dislocation that has spontaneously reduced, what signs and symptoms would you look for? Include any special tests you would use to confirm your suspicions.

7. Describe the tests you would use to examine rotary instabilities of the knee. For each test, discuss what structures may be involved if the test is positive.

CRITICAL THINKING QUESTIONS

1. You are examining a 14-year-old athlete who was playing soccer. When you witnessed the injury, you noted that his foot was firmly planted and that he appeared to twist his knee while an opponent made contact against its lateral aspect. You note immediate swelling, and the athlete is complaining of severe pain and tenderness along the proximal tibia. He also reports hearing a pop at the time of injury. Given the mechanism observed and these initial findings, what injuries might you suspect, and how would you proceed with your examination?

2. What is the difference between patellofemoral pain syndrome and chondromalacia patella? In your examination, how might you differentiate chondromalacia patella from other causes of anterior knee pain?

3. A female runner comes to you complaining of anterior knee pain. She reports that she has just returned to training after taking 6 weeks off because of a tibial stress fracture. She also reports that she has had recurrent anterior knee pain for the past 5 years and does not seem to know what causes it when it occurs. Given her history of previous injury and her current complaint, describe your observational examination of this athlete and explain what you would specifically look for to obtain clues of contributing factors. Include any special tests or measurements you would use to confirm your observational findings.

CITED REFERENCES

Arendt, E., and R. Dick. 1995. Knee injury patterns among men and women in collegiate basketball and soccer. *Am J Sports Med* 23(6): 694-701.

Arendt, E.A., J. Agel, et al. 1999. Anterior cruciate ligament injury patterns among collegiate men and women. *J Athl Train* 34(2): 86-92.

Biondino, C.R. 1999. Anterior cruciate ligament injuries in female athletes. *Conn Med* 63(11): 657-660.

Boden, B.P., G.S. Dean, et al. 2000. Mechanisms of anterior cruciate ligament injury. *Orthopedics* 23(4): 573-578.

Evans, P.J., and D. Bell. 1993. Prospective evaluation of the McMurray Test. *Am J Sports Med* 21(4): 604-608.

Ferretti, A., P. Papandrea, et al. 1992. Knee ligament injuries in volleyball players. *Am J Sports Med* 20(2): 203-207.

Johnson, R.J., B.D. Beynnon, C.E. Nichols, and P.A. Renstrom. 1992. Current concepts review: The treatment of injuries of the anterior cruciate ligament. *J Bone Joint Surg* 74A: 140-151.

Malone, T.R., W.T. Hardaker, et al. 1993. Relationship of gender to anterior cruciate ligament injuries in intercollegiate basketball players. *J South Orthop Assoc* 2(1): 36-39.

Myklebust, G., S. Maehlum, et al. 1998. A prospective cohort study of anterior cruciate ligament injuries in elite Norwegian team handball. *Scand J Med Sci Sports* 8:149-153.

Oliphant, J.G., and J.P. Drawbert. 1996. Gender differences in anterior cruciate ligament injury rates in Wisconsin intercollegiate basketball. *J Ath Train* 31(3): 245-247.

ADDITIONAL RESOURCES

Harmon, K.G., and M.L. Ireland. 2000. Gender differences in noncontact anterior cruciate ligament injuries. *Clin Sports Med* 19(2): 287-302.

Hartley, A. 1990. Knee assessment. In *Practical joint assessment: A sports medicine manual*, 464-543. St. Louis: Mosby Year Book.

Hillman, S.K. 2005. *Introduction to athletic training*. 2nd ed. Champaign, IL: Human Kinetics.

Houglum, P.A. 2005. *Therapeutic exercise for musculoskeletal injuries*. 2nd ed. Champaign, IL: Human Kinetics.

Kendall, F.P., E.K. McCreary, and P.G. Provance. 1993. *Muscles: Testing and function*. 4th ed. Philadelphia: Lippincott Williams & Wilkins.

Moore, K.L. 1992. *Clinically oriented anatomy*. 3rd ed. Baltimore: Williams & Wilkins.

Hip, Pelvis, and Groin

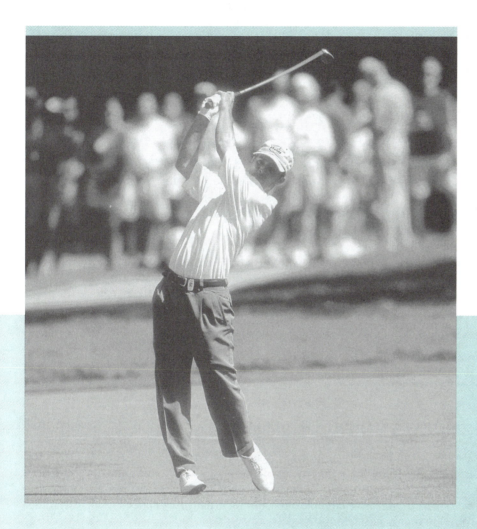

Objectives

After completing this chapter, the reader will be able to do the following:

1. Describe the etiology, signs and symptoms, and potential complications associated with acute and chronic injuries of the hip, pelvis, and groin commonly encountered in the physically active

2. Identify conditions and concerns specific to the pediatric athlete

3. Identify common structural and functional abnormalities of the hip and pelvis

4. Describe and demonstrate the objective tests for examining the hip and pelvis

5. Perform an on-site examination of the hip, pelvis, and groin, noting criteria for immediate medical referral and mode of transportation from the field

6. Perform an acute examination of the hip, pelvis, and groin

7. Perform a clinical examination of the hip, pelvis, and groin, including differential diagnosis of referring back and lower-extremity pathologies

8. Describe and differentiate potential causes and conditions of groin pain

Donna was a dually certified athletic trainer and strength and conditioning specialist working at Silver's Gym. She noticed that Nancy, one of her athletes, appeared to be limping when she came into the gym. "Hey Nancy, how are you doing today? You got a bit of a limp there?" Donna asked.

"Hi Donna! Yeah, I've had this nagging groin strain for about four weeks now and I'm getting kind of sick of it."

"How do you know it's a groin strain? How did you hurt it?" Donna asked. She was not quite so ready to dismiss the pain as Nancy was.

"I guess I must have slipped or something while running one day, but I can't really remember when. I just noticed it started hurting one day," Nancy said, trying to remember when it actually began.

"You're a pretty avid runner, right? What did you say you were running, 25 to 30 miles a week?" Donna tried to recall.

"Yes, that's about right. It's the only thing that keeps my sanity!" Nancy said.

"Is there any other activity that makes it hurt?" Donna continued.

"You know, that's what's interesting about this strain. It hurts while I'm running, but it never bothers me while I'm lifting."

"Nancy, from what you're saying, it may not be a groin strain. It could be a number of things, maybe even a stress fracture," Donna cautioned.

"A what? A stress fracture? No way!"

"I'm not saying it is for sure—I'm just saying we should take a closer look and examine what is causing your pain. You know, a number of injuries can refer to the groin area. In addition to stress fractures, bursitis and problems from your low back and sacroiliac joints can also cause groin pain. Let's examine it and see if we can find out where this pain is coming from. If we can figure that out, we can come up with the right treatment plan to get you better and back to running pain free. Deal?"

"I'd appreciate that, Donna, thanks."

Given the structural integrity of the hip and pelvis and the tremendous forces sport activity can exert on these structures, injuries in this region may range from minor strains and irritations to severe joint disruptions. It is important to appreciate the types of injuries that you may encounter in the physically active and to be able to adequately examine and differentiate these injuries for proper referral and care. The information in this chapter provides you with both the injury knowledge and the examination techniques that you will need to identify and differentiate common injuries in the hip and pelvis.

FUNCTIONAL ANATOMY

The hip and pelvis are among the strongest and most stable joints in the body. The pelvic girdle is made up of three joints, including the hip joint (acetabular femoral), the sacroiliac joint, and the pubic symphysis, which work in unison to provide both mobility for locomotion and stability to support the upper torso (figure 18.1).

Mobility is provided primarily by the hip joint, which is the only movable joint of the three. The hip is a multiaxial ball-and-socket joint in which the head of the femur fits well into the deep concavity of the acetabulum. The acetabular labrum functions to further deepen the acetabular cavity and embrace the head of the femur. The joint is strengthened by the articular capsule and the broad ligamentous support provided by the iliofemoral (Y), pubofemoral, and ischiofemoral ligaments (figure 18.2). As such, the hip is the strongest joint in the body, requiring tremendous forces to disrupt its integrity and cause injury.

Vascular supply to the head of the femur occurs through the artery that courses through the ligament of the head of the femur (figure 18.3) and upwardly from the capsular and retinacular arteries. In spite of the tremendous stability provided by the articulation of the femoral head and the acetabulum of the pelvis, unrecognized hip injuries can have devastating long-term consequences. Injury to the ligament of the head or the capsular structures about the joint can compromise blood supply to the head of the femur. Prolonged complications from avascular necrosis can result if joint injury disrupts the blood supply to the head of the femur.

An important ossification center also exists between the femoral head and neck. Injury to this epiphyseal center before complete ossification is known as slipped capital femoral epiphysis (see page 486) and tends to occur more frequently in obese adolescent boys. A persistent antalgic gait (limp) is a common sign of the injury. You have learned the importance of carefully examining gait patterns and the relevance of certain antalgic gaits to injuries of the

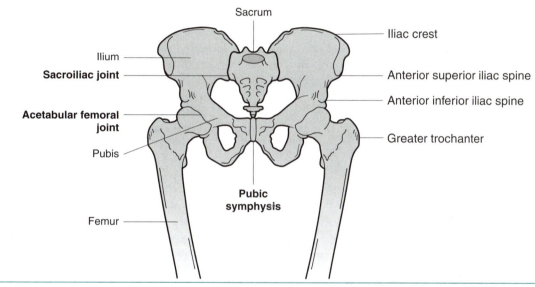

Figure 18.1   Bony anatomy and joints of the hip and pelvis.

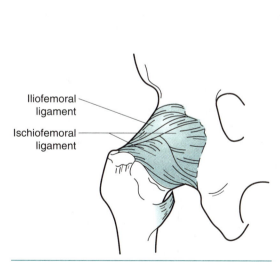

Figure 18.2   Posterior view of the ligamentous support of the hip joint. The pubofemoral ligament can only be seen in the anterior view.

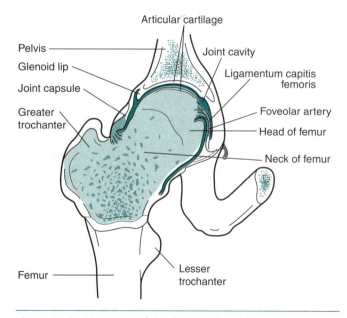

Figure 18.3   Ligament of the femoral head (ligamentum capitis femoris).

lower extremity. An unrecognized slipped capital femoral epiphysis can also result in avascular necrosis of the femoral head and can adversely affect normal growth of the femur. The hip joint is also notorious for referring pain distally along the lower extremity. For this reason, you should examine the hip when unexplained pain occurs in the thigh or knee.

The ball-and-socket configuration of the hip joint permits flexion, extension, abduction, adduction, circumduction, and rotation. The 22 muscles acting on the hip are classified by the motions they produce and include three flexors (psoas, iliacus, and rectus femoris); one flexor adductor (pectineus); three extensors (biceps femoris—long head, semimembranosus, semitendinosus); one extensor outward rotator (gluteus maximus); one abductor (gluteus medius); four adductors (gracilis; adductors longus, brevis, and magnus); two inward rotators (tensor fascia latae, gluteus minimus); six outward rotators (piriformis, obturator externus, obturator internus, gemelli superior and inferior, quadratus femoris); and one flexor-abductor outward rotator (sartorius). Review the points of origin and insertion of these muscles, as the positions of the hip and knee can affect length–tension relationships and consequently your strength examination techniques.

The pelvis or pelvic girdle forms the base of the trunk, which supports the abdominal contents and provides a link between the lumbar spine and the lower extremities. It consists of two innominate bones, each comprising three parts (the ilium, pubis, and ischium) that fuse together between 12 and 16 years of age. Anteriorly, the two innominate bones articulate with each other to form the symphysis pubis; posteriorly, they articulate with the sacrum to form the sacroiliac joints (see figure 18.1). Very little movement occurs at these joints, lending to their primary function of stability. However, these joints can become irritated or inflamed by mechanical forces or repetitive stress caused by weight-bearing activity and muscular tension.

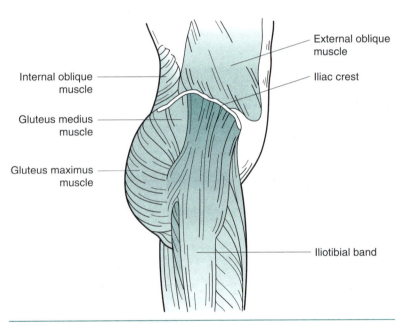

Figure 18.4 Lateral view of the muscular attachments to the hip and pelvis.

The strong muscular support provided to the hip and pelvis lends to their strength, stability, and mobility. The hip and pelvis serve as attachment sites for muscles of the trunk as well as the lower extremity, allowing forces to transfer between the lower extremity and upper torso (figure 18.4). Therefore, the muscles about the hip and pelvis play a major role in locomotion and postural stability, and muscle injury usually affects weight-bearing and locomotor functions.

The movements of the pelvic girdle result from combined movements at the lumbosacral and hip joints and are described as pelvic tilts. Forward, or anterior, pelvic tilt is a combination of hip flexion and lumbosacral hyperextension (figure 18.5a); backward, or posterior, tilt is a combination of hip extension and lumbosacral flexion (figure 18.5b); right lateral tilt is a combination of left lateral flexion of the lumbosacral joint, abduction of the right hip, and adduction of the left hip; and left lateral tilt is a combination of the opposite movements of right lateral tilt. The muscles of the abdomen, back, and thigh all move and position the pelvis. Check the strength and flexibility of these muscles when examining the pelvis, hip, and thigh. A deficiency in strength of the rectus abdominis muscles can cause excessive anterior tilt in the pelvis, while tightness of the hamstring muscles can restrict anterior tilt.

Several skeletal landmarks of the pelvic girdle are important for examining pelvic position and lower-extremity length discrepancies (see figure 18.1). In particular, the anterior supe-

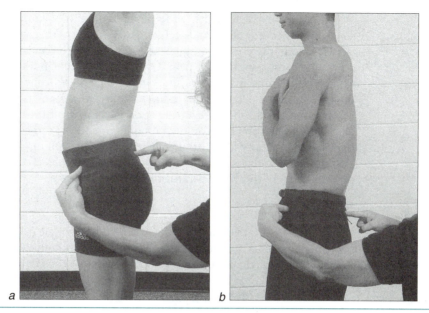

Figure 18.5   Movement of the pelvic girdle into *(a)* anterior and *(b)* posterior tilts.

rior iliac spine and the posterior superior iliac spine are palpation landmarks. Other skeletal landmarks serve as points for attachment of the major muscle groups acting on the hip and knee. In this chapter you will learn about the potential for apophysitis or avulsion injuries from these points of muscular attachment.

HIP, PELVIS, AND GROIN INJURIES

Considerable forces can be transmitted through the hip and pelvis during weight-bearing activities. Primarily because of the strength and stability of the hip and pelvis, injuries to this region are less common than those to the knee and ankle. However, when injuries do occur, even those that are minor can be painful and debilitating because of the role these structures play in weight bearing and locomotion.

Acute Soft Tissue Injuries

The most common types of acute injury are contusions, muscle strain (particularly in the groin), and sprains. Traumatic fractures and dislocations are rare; stress fractures of the femoral neck and avulsion fractures are more common. In children, acute apophysitis and epiphyseal injuries are also a concern.

Contusions

Because of their many superficial bony prominences, the hip and pelvis are prone to contusions. Most vulnerable to injury are the lateral hip, iliac crest, and coccyx. Contusions to these areas can cause considerable pain and disability, particularly when they occur near a muscular attachment. Direct contact to the lateral hip can contuse the soft tissue and bursa overlying the greater trochanter. Signs and symptoms include localized pain, swelling, and ecchymosis. The patient is point tender over the greater trochanter, and the inflamed bursa may be palpable. Because the greater trochanter serves as the attachment site for the gluteus medius and minimus and the hip rotators, pain and weakness may occur with hip abduction and medial rotation.

Even more disabling is a contusion to the iliac crest, commonly known as a **hip pointer**. A direct blow can cause considerable pain and hemorrhage along the superficial crest. The athlete complains of exquisite tenderness at the point of contact and its surrounding area. You can easily observe swelling and ecchymosis. Because of the broad attachment of the abdominal muscles along the crest (see figure 18.4), trunk flexion and rotation, as well as sneezing and coughing, cause considerable pain. Often the patient leans the trunk to the side of injury in an effort to avoid muscular tension at its insertion. Single-leg weight bearing may also be painful on the injured side. Commonly, a hip pointer severely restricts an athlete's activity until pain and inflammation subside. Proper padding can protect the area from further insult.

Landing or sitting hard on the tailbone, or coccyx, can contuse it. The athlete complains of pain and difficulty with sitting, particularly when leaning back or slouching. Point tenderness, swelling, and possible discoloration are observable. If pain persists for an extended time, refer the athlete to a physician to rule out fracture.

Sprains

Because of the relative stability of the hip and sacroiliac joints and the strength of the surrounding ligaments, sprains to this region are less common compared to other lower-extremity joints. However, when they do occur, they will most likely limit physical activity.

Sacroiliac Joint

Sacroiliac sprains most often result from jamming mechanisms—for example, when a basketball player comes down from a rebound and lands off balance on a single leg with the leg straight and the back extended. This can transmit sizable forces through the lumbosacral and sacroiliac regions, contusing the joint and possibly disrupting the ligament.

Signs and symptoms associated with sacroiliac sprains include pain, swelling, and tenderness over the affected joint and ligaments. Pain may be localized to the involved area but may also be felt as a deep ache or radiating pain into the buttock and thigh. Unilateral or bilateral hip flexion and unilateral leg stance often increase pain. You will also commonly find pain with pelvic rock or Faber's tests (see the section on special tests). You may also note an upslip of the pelvis on the affected side. An **upslip** occurs when one ilium rides higher on the sacrum than the other ilium.

Hip Joint

Direct and indirect forces that cause excessive rotation or abduction or that drive the femur posteriorly when the hip is flexed can stretch or tear the surrounding ligaments of the hip joint. Extreme rotation at the trunk and hip with the foot planted on the ground is one mechanism. A third-degree sprain that results in hip dislocation is a serious injury that can present considerable complications (see the section on dislocations and neurovascular disorders later in this chapter).

Signs and symptoms of a hip joint sprain are pain deep in the joint and difficulty with weight bearing. The athlete complains of pain with passive hip movement as the injured ligament becomes taut. Pain with passive extension and lateral rotation tensions both the iliofemoral (Y) and the ischiofemoral ligaments (see figure 18.2). Abduction stresses the pubofemoral ligament. You will also note decreased range of motion and pain with active movement. You will have to rely on the findings of your ROM assessment when examining this injury because it is impossible to palpate the ligaments due to the depth of the overlying soft tissue and muscle.

Strains

Muscular strains about the hip are relatively common, resulting from overstretching or from a rapid, forceful contraction. Explosive starts and slipping of the foot during cutting are common mechanisms for strains to the hip flexor and adductor. Abductor strains can result from quick and forceful movements such as cutting away from the side of the plant leg. Improper warm-up, muscle fatigue, and weakness are thought to increase an athlete's risk for muscle strain, as these injuries frequently occur during the beginning of practice and preseason training.

Signs and symptoms may include pain and a burning or tearing sensation at the time of injury, and the athlete may feel or hear a pop. You will note palpable tenderness and spasm in the involved muscle, and you may also palpate a defect with third-degree strains. Swelling, ecchymosis, and pain with passive stretch and active contraction are consistent with the degree of injury.

A number of other conditions can refer pain to the groin and mimic the signs and symptoms of muscular strain. Other causes of groin pain, listed in Potential Causes of Groin Pain, should be considered when examining this area.

Potential Causes of Groin Pain

Condition

- Muscle strain
- Lymph node infection and inflammation
- Inguinal and femoral hernias
- Kidney stone
- Legg-Calvé-Perthes disease
- Referred pain from lumbar region
- Sacroiliac joint dysfunction
- Stress fracture of the femoral neck
- Synovitis of the hip joint capsule
- Trochanteric and iliopsoas bursitis
- Apophysitis (young athletes)
- Epiphyseal injury (young athletes)

Chronic or Overuse Soft Tissue Injuries

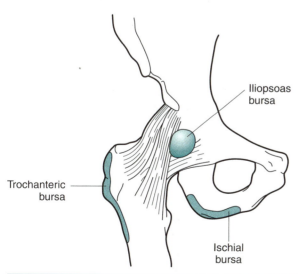

Figure 18.6 Location of the iliopsoas, trochanteric, and ischial bursae.

Because of the repetitive stresses placed on the hip and pelvis during locomotion and cutting and jumping maneuvers, chronic conditions caused by inflammation and muscle tightness are seen more often than acute injuries. Structural and functional abnormalities at the hip can significantly affect the entire lower extremity.

Bursitis and Snapping Hip Syndrome

Although numerous bursae surround the hip and pelvis, chronic bursitis usually involves the trochanteric, iliopsoas, or ischial bursae (figure 18.6).

Trochanteric Bursitis

The trochanteric bursa sits between the iliotibial (IT) band and the greater trochanter. Tightness in the IT band, repetitive insult to the lateral hip, excessive Q-angle (quadriceps angle), hip anteversion, leg length discrepancy (long leg), and running on a slanted street (downhill side) may cause abnormal friction and irritation of the bursa between these structures. The patient complains of pain or deep aching in the lateral hip, palpable tenderness, and crepitus over the greater trochanter, and is unable to lie on the involved side. Swelling and redness occur if the bursa is acutely inflamed. The patient may also complain of pain radiating down the lateral leg and a snapping sensation when the IT band travels over the greater trochanter and inflamed bursa during hip flexion and extension.

Iliopsoas Bursitis

Iliopsoas bursitis most often results from overuse activities. The patient complains of pain in the anterior groin with hip flexion. As the bursa is deep to the adductor muscles, it is difficult to examine and palpate for tenderness. Because of the difficulty in palpating the specific structures, iliopsoas bursitis is often mistaken for a muscular strain. In chronic bursitis, snapping in the groin may also occur as the iliopsoas passes over the lesser trochanter and inflamed bursa.

Ischial Bursitis

The ischial bursa, which lies over the ischial tuberosity, may become painful and inflamed with excessive friction. As the ischial tuberosities bear the weight in sitting, repeatedly flexing the hip and extending one leg and then the other (e.g., cycling with an improperly adjusted seat) can irritate the bursa. The patient complains of pain with sitting, palpable tenderness over the ischial tuberosity, and pain with passive hip flexion and active or resistive hip extension. Ischial bursitis is often difficult to differentiate from proximal hamstring tendinitis.

Piriformis Syndrome

The piriformis muscle is a lateral hip rotator that originates on the sacrum and passes through the greater sciatic notch to its attachment on the posterior superior aspect of the greater trochanter of the femur. Anatomically, the sciatic nerve usually passes underneath the piriformis as it exits the greater sciatic foramen. However, in about 12% of the population (Moore 1992), the sciatic nerve splits and the fibular portion passes through the piriformis muscle (figure 18.7). Because of the close proximity of the sciatic nerve to the piriformis muscle, it is prone to irritation in this region.

Sciatic Irritation Secondary to Piriformis Syndrome

Trigger points, tightness, or piriformis spasm resulting from overuse or repetitive activities are all characteristics of piriformis syndrome. Any of these can cause buttock pain and symptoms of sciatic nerve irritation. Muscle spasm and tightness can compress the sciatic nerve, referring pain and tingling down the posterior thigh. Other signs and symptoms include pain and limited ROM with hip medial rotation and palpable tenderness deep to the gluteals.

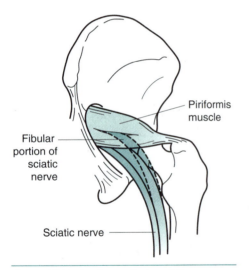

Piriformis muscle

Fibular portion of sciatic nerve

Sciatic nerve

Figure 18.7 In the majority of the population, the sciatic nerve passes underneath the piriformis, but in about 12% of the population the sciatic nerve splits, and its fibular portion passes through the piriformis with the tibial portion still passing underneath.

Traumatic Fractures and Hip Dislocation

While traumatic fractures of the hip and pelvis and hip dislocation commonly result from falls in the elderly and as a result of motor vehicle accidents, they rarely occur in the healthy athlete as a result of sport activity. While some fractures are obvious, others are not; some may mimic a muscle strain. Conversely, hip dislocations are usually easy to identify. When these injuries occur in athletes, they are seen primarily in adolescents, so you should carefully examine all hip and pelvis pain resulting from traumatic mechanisms in this population.

Hip and Pelvic Fractures

Hip fractures, which most frequently occur through the femoral neck, typically result from a direct blow to the lateral hip. Acetabular fractures may occur in conjunction with a hip dislocation or from landing hard on a single leg (e.g., hurdling) that drives the femoral head into the acetabulum. Pelvic fractures are probably the least common; but when they do occur, they typically result from high impact or crush mechanisms as seen in sports such as auto racing, skiing, or horseback riding.

Signs and symptoms include immediate pain, swelling, and loss of function. Hip fractures are usually obvious, as the involved leg appears shortened and laterally rotated. With less obvious fractures, if the athlete is able to move the hip and lower extremity at all, she will most certainly be unable or unwilling to bear weight. Pelvic fractures due to crush injuries can be life threatening, as they may cause considerable hemorrhage. Any patient with a suspected traumatic fracture should be examined and continually monitored for shock.

> ⚠ Any athlete with a suspected traumatic hip or pelvis fracture should be closely examined and continually monitored for shock.

Avulsion Fractures

Avulsion fractures, more common in sport than in other physical activities, result from a violent contraction. Kicking hard against an immovable object or performing a quick, explosive movement can produce tremendous tractioning forces at the bony attachment and pull the tendon away from the bone. Common sites for avulsion fractures are the anterior superior iliac spine (ASIS, sartorius), anterior inferior iliac spine (AIIS, rectus femoris), lesser trochanter (iliopsoas) (figure 18.8), and ischial tuberosity (hamstring). Avulsion fractures occur more commonly in younger, skeletally immature athletes who have yet to obtain closure of the apophyseal joint. The athlete complains of a sudden and sharp pain at the time of injury and may report hearing or feeling a snap or pop. Immediately after injury, the athlete will be unwilling to move the extremity. Tenderness will be noted along the bone, and a palpable defect in the myotendon unit near the attachment or a muscle bulging away from the attachment may also be evident. Swelling may be immediate or delayed.

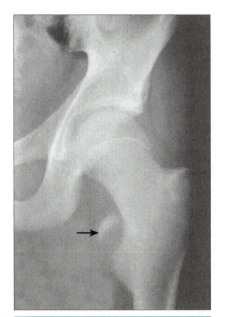

Figure 18.8 Avulsion fracture of the lesser trochanter.
Courtesty of Theodore E. Keats.

Hip Dislocation

Because of the relatively deep acetabular socket and numerous thick and strong supporting ligaments, the hip joint is one of the strongest and most stable joints in the body. It takes tremendous force to dislocate the hip.

Most dislocations occur posteriorly with the hip and knee in a flexed position. A direct blow transmitted up the shaft of the femur, or less commonly an indirect medial (internal) rotational force with the foot firmly planted, can displace the femoral head posteriorly to the acetabulum. Examples of common mechanisms include the knee hitting the dashboard during a traffic collision and landing hard on a flexed knee with the full weight directed through the long axis of the femur. In order for the hip to dislocate, significant stretching and tearing of the acetabular labrum and surrounding ligaments must occur.

Signs and symptoms include extreme pain, obvious deformity, and inability to move the extremity. The leg appears shortened and medially rotated (the opposite of fracture where the leg is laterally rotated). Immobilize the athlete and immediately transport him to emergency medical care via emergency medical services (EMS). Complications of hip dislocation include rupture of the artery to the head of the femur and avascular necrosis of the femoral head. Posterior dislocations may also injure the sciatic nerve may also result.

Defects and Abnormalities Secondary to Repetitive Stress

Given the primary weight-bearing function of the hip and pelvis, the large mechanical forces transmitted through the bone and joint structures make them vulnerable to repetitive stress injuries. Injuries of this type occur most commonly in runners. As you will see, particular concerns arise with the pediatric athlete.

General Repetitive Stress Injuries

Repetitive stress injuries include sacroiliac joint dysfunction, osteitis pubis, and stress fractures.

Sacroiliac Joint Dysfunction

The sacroiliac (SI) joint is relatively immobile, with the majority of lumbosacral and pelvic movement occurring in the lumbar spine and hip joints. However, many of the muscles acting on the lumbar spine and hip regions attach near and around the SI joint, and these can affect its function. SI joint dysfunctions can result from similar mechanisms that cause SI sprains, such as landing hard on a single leg with the knee and hip extended or falling on one buttock. However, SI joint dysfunction can also occur without significant trauma through chronic, repetitive stress resulting from biomechanical and postural faults, such as improper lifting, muscular imbalances, and chronically shifting the body weight to one side during sustained stance.

SI dysfunction typically involves a subtle rotation or upslip of the ilium on the sacrum. **Sacroiliac rotation** occurs when the ilium rotates on the sacrum unilaterally. An anterior rotation is characterized by the ilium rotating forward on the sacrum, which causes the anterior superior iliac spine (ASIS) to sit lower than the posterior superior iliac spine (PSIS) in the sagittal plane on the involved side (figure 18.9). Conversely, a posterior rotation of the sacroiliac joint presents with the ASIS sitting higher than the PSIS on the involved side. If both the ASIS and PSIS sit higher on the involved side compared to the uninvolved side, an upslip of the ilium on the sacrum has occurred (figure 18.10). Torsion can result from a combination of a rotation and upslip, and is identified by the ASIS sitting higher on one side compared to the other and the PSIS sitting lower on the same side as the elevated ASIS.

Signs and symptoms of SI joint dysfunction include a sense of joint stiffness and considerable pain with unilateral weight bearing on the involved side. The patient may feel a dull ache or heaviness in the involved lower extremity. Spasm and inhibition of the gluteus medius is common with these joint dysfunctions. Altered gait and a functional leg length discrepancy will be noted with an upslip.

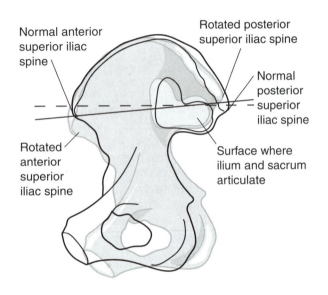

Figure 18.9 Anterior sacroiliac rotation (ASIS sits lower than the PSIS on the involved side).

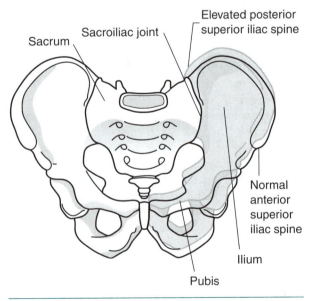

Figure 18.10 Upslip of the left sacroiliac joint (ASIS and PSIS higher on involved side).

Osteitis Pubis

Osteitis pubis is characterized by irritation and inflammation of the pubic symphysis resulting from overuse and repetitive stress of the adductor muscles at their insertion (figure 18.11). Most often seen in runners, osteitis pubis produces signs and symptoms of groin

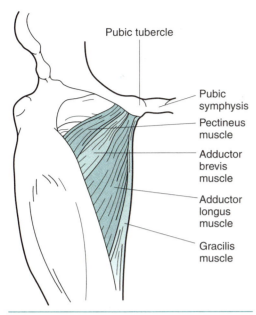

Figure 18.11 Adductor insertion near the pubic symphysis.

Labels in figure: Pubic tubercle, Pubic symphysis, Pectineus muscle, Adductor brevis muscle, Adductor longus muscle, Gracilis muscle

pain, palpable tenderness over the pubic symphysis and bone, adductor tightness, and pain with passive abduction and active adduction. Pain increases with activity and eases with rest.

Stress Fracture

Stress fractures of the femoral neck and pelvis occur most commonly in long distance runners, particularly female runners. Athletes who have been inactive for long periods of time because of injury or who have recently and abruptly changed their training routine may also be at greater risk for stress injuries.

Stress fractures of the femoral neck result primarily from chronic and repetitive overload due to weight bearing. Femoral stress fractures are more prevalent in athletes who have poor dietary habits, osteoporotic bone, leg length discrepancy, or other biomechanical abnormalities in the lower extremity that may impose abnormal stress on the bone. Signs and symptoms of femoral neck stress fracture include groin pain that may radiate out to the lateral hip or down the thigh. Initially, the athlete complains of increased pain with weight-bearing activity that diminishes or disappears completely with rest, only to return once activity is resumed. Pain becomes more constant if the offending activity and overstress continue. Palpable tenderness and pain with percussion to the greater trochanter may also occur.

The pubic ramus, which serves as the attachment site for the hip adductors, is also prone to stress fractures due to repetitive muscular stress. Endurance running activities are usually the primary cause. Signs and symptoms of a pubic stress fracture include pain in the groin radiating down the medial thigh and palpable tenderness along the bone. Initially, pain increases with activity and decreases with rest; if stress continues, the pain becomes more constant. Single-leg weight bearing, active or resistive adduction, or passive abduction may also reproduce pain.

Special Pediatric Concerns

If you are accustomed to examining adults, you may miss certain conditions in the pediatric athlete that are not typically seen in adults. These include apophysitis, epiphyseal fractures, slipped capital femoral epiphysis, and chronic synovitis. Watch carefully for these injuries when examining the young athlete, as the injuries may bear considerable consequences on later bone growth and development. Refer children or adolescents with groin pain lasting longer than a week to a physician.

Apophysitis

Before ossification, the apophyseal joints are weaker than the myotendinous unit; they can become inflamed and can separate as a result of repetitive muscular contraction and stress. In some cases, a complete avulsion of the apophysis can follow a forceful contraction of the attaching muscle. Often, apophysitis is mistaken for a muscle strain because it mimics many of the signs and symptoms of muscle strains in adults. Common sites for apophysitis are the insertions of the rectus femoris at the inferior iliac spine, the iliopsoas at the lesser trochanter, the adductors at the pubic ramus, and the proximal hamstring at the ischial tuberosity (figure 18.12).

The young athlete will complain of pain and point tenderness near the myotendinous insertion. An enlarged bony prominence and crepitus may also be observable at the point of insertion. Pain increases with passive stretch and active or resistive contraction of the attaching muscle. With complete avulsion, the athlete complains of a pop and sharp pain in the

! Refer children or adolescents with groin pain lasting longer than a week to a physician.

Anterior view   **Posterior view**

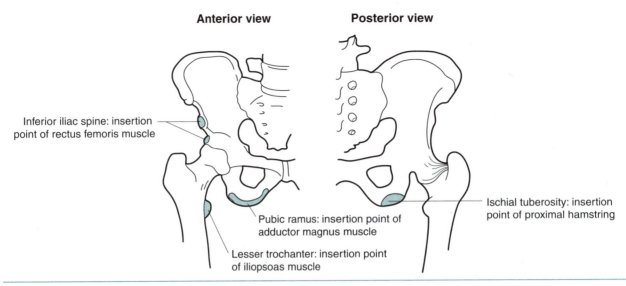

Inferior iliac spine: insertion point of rectus femoris muscle

Ischial tuberosity: insertion point of proximal hamstring

Pubic ramus: insertion point of adductor magnus muscle

Lesser trochanter: insertion point of iliopsoas muscle

Figure 18.12   Common sites for apophysitis at the hip.

hip or groin at the time of injury and may be unwilling to move the extremity. There may or may not be swelling in the area.

Epiphyseal Fractures

When sustaining traumatic forces at the hip, adolescents are more prone to fracture at the weaker epiphyseal plate than at the shaft of the bone. Epiphyseal fractures occur most commonly at the greater trochanter and capital femoral epiphysis. The fracture can be partial (separation) or complete (avulsion). With capital femoral epiphyseal fractures, the injury mechanism and signs and symptoms are similar to those of a hip dislocation. The acute fracture may have been preceded by weakening and separation of the epiphysis over time.

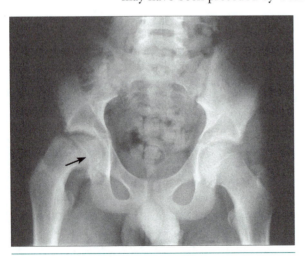

Figure 18.13   Slipped capital femoral epiphysis on right (see arrow).

Courtesy of Theodore E. Keats.

Young athletes who present with a limp and complaints of intermitted groin pain that radiates down the medial thigh to the knee and have no recall of a specific injury should be referred to a physician for examination. Separation of the epiphysis can cause a secondary chronic synovitis.

Slipped Capital Femoral Epiphysis

A similar condition to epiphyseal fracture found in children and adolescents that also manifests itself as a limp and causes pain in the groin and thigh region is a slipped capital femoral epiphysis. As the name implies, the capital femoral head slips or displaces at the epiphysis (figure 18.13). This injury results from progressive weakening of the epiphysis and not directly from athletic activity. Other signs and symptoms include decreased ROM, particularly with medial rotation, and medial knee pain. Avascular necrosis and synovitis are frequent complications.

Chronic Synovitis

Chronic synovitis is an inflammatory process at the hip joint that is characterized by chronic irritation and excess secretion of synovial fluid within the capsule. The excess synovial fluid can increase pressure within the joint capsule and occlude blood flow to the femoral head. Because of the depth of the joint capsule, this condition is very difficult to detect. Swelling is not obvious, and pain may mimic that of a groin strain. Prolonged synovitis may lead to avascular necrosis of the femoral head.

Nerve and Vascular Injuries

Although nerve injury is uncommon at the hip and pelvis, the site most vulnerable to vascular compromise is the head of the femur. Avascular necrosis can occur in both children and adults as a result of either chronic inflammatory or traumatic injury mechanisms.

Legg-Calvé-Perthes Disease

The condition known as Legg-Calvé-Perthes disease is characterized by avascular necrosis of the proximal femoral epiphysis. This is a chronic condition that develops slowly in children, more often in males than in females. For unknown reasons, vascularization to the epiphysis is diminished, causing degeneration and flattening of the femoral head articular cartilage. The child complains of pain in the hip or groin that may radiate to the knee. You will also note limping, decreased ROM, and hip flexor tightness. Remember, any time a child or adolescent complains of hip or groin pain lasting more than a week, consult a physician to rule out serious pathologies such as this.

Avascular Necrosis of the Femoral Head

Nutrition and vascular supply to the femoral head is provided primarily by the artery to the femoral head that enters through the acetabulum. Avascular necrosis (osteochondritis dissecans) of the femoral head can occur when this artery is severed or occluded for a prolonged period. This is a common complication following hip dislocations, fractures, or chronic synovitis and often necessitates a hip replacement.

Structural and Functional Abnormalities

Because of the weight-bearing function of the hip and pelvis, structural or functional abnormalities in this region can significantly alter biomechanical function in the lower extremity and may increase vulnerability to lower extremity and back stress injuries. Understanding the abnormalities common in the hip will help you examine chronic injuries in the lower extremity and trunk.

Femoral Angulation

Alterations in normal femoral angle can significantly affect biomechanics and muscle function in the lower extremity and influence Q-angle, genu varus or valgus, and patella tracking, among others. The normal alignment between the femur and hip and lower leg is determined by the degree of angulation of the femoral neck relative to the femoral shaft. The normal degree of angulation of the femoral head and neck is approximately 120° to 125° with an anterior angulation of 14° to 15° relative to the trochanters and distal femoral condyles (figure 18.14a). This angulation allows the head of the femur to be directed medially, superiorly, and slightly anteriorly to fit into the acetabulum.

Coxa valga (figure 18.14b) refers to a femoral neck to shaft angle greater than 135°, whereas in coxa vara (figure 18.14c) the degree of angulation is less than 120°. You may note a concomitant genu varus or valgus with coxa valga and vara, respectively. In hip anteversion (figure 18.14d), excessive anterior angulation results in a toe-in gait (figure 18.15). Hip anteversion will likely increase Q-angle and genu valgus at the knee. Hip retroversion occurs with a decreased anterior angle (figure 18.14e), producing a toe-out gait.

Leg Length Discrepancy and Pelvic Obliquity

Leg length discrepancies can be classified as true or apparent. A true leg length discrepancy is characterized by a bilateral difference in the measurable length of the femur or tibial shaft. In the absence of a true length discrepancy, abnormalities in the hip and pelvis may shorten

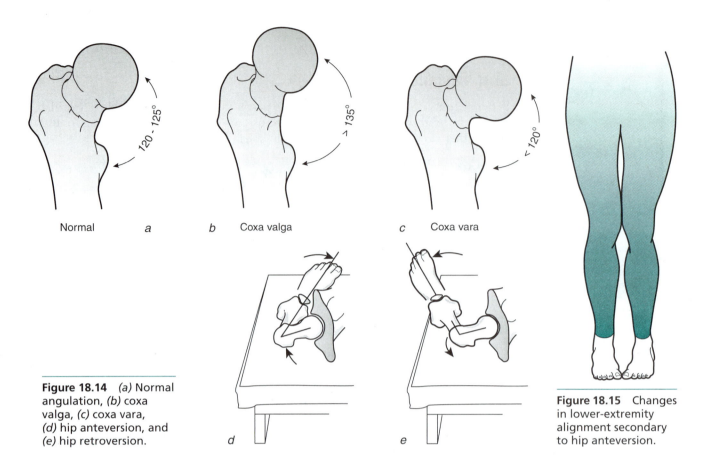

Figure 18.14 *(a)* Normal angulation, *(b)* coxa valga, *(c)* coxa vara, *(d)* hip anteversion, and *(e)* hip retroversion.

Figure 18.15 Changes in lower-extremity alignment secondary to hip anteversion.

one leg. This apparent or functional leg length discrepancy may result from pelvic obliquity or a **hemipelvis**, in which one side of the pelvis is smaller than the other. Soft tissue tightness or sacroiliac dysfunction can also draw one leg more superiorly than the other and can give the appearance of a leg length difference.

Regardless of whether the difference is true or apparent, the asymmetry can cause pain and dysfunction in the hip, pelvis, or low back with weight-bearing activities. Always investigate leg length when an athlete reports with chronic hip, pelvic, or low back pain of unknown etiology.

Gluteus Medius Weakness

Atrophy or weakness of the gluteus medius muscle results in an inability to abduct the hip and maintain a level pelvis during gait. The ability to stand on one leg and maintain the opposite hip at the same level as the weight-bearing hip relies primarily on the gluteus medius in the weight-bearing leg. The primary sign of gluteus medius weakness or dysfunction is a **gluteus medius lurch**, or **Trendelenburg gait**, a dropping of the uninvolved hip during its swing-through phase (figure 18.16). These gait alterations can also increase hip, pelvis, and low back complaints.

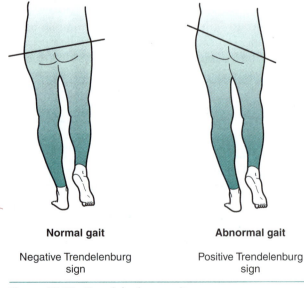

Normal gait

Negative Trendelenburg sign

Abnormal gait

Positive Trendelenburg sign

Figure 18.16 Trendelenburg gait.

OBJECTIVE TESTS

Following a thorough history, the objective segment of the examination begins with your observation. While observation is discussed specific to each examination strategy in the next section, the remaining objective tests that you will perform based on the history and observation are discussed here.

Palpation

You can palpate the anterior, lateral, and medial hip with the patient lying supine; palpate the posterior aspect with the patient lying prone. Palpate the level of the ASIS and PSIS bilaterally with the patient standing when appropriate.

- **Supine.** Starting with the iliac crests, palpate the rim of the iliac by following the crest anteriorly to the ASIS. Palpate the insertion of the abdominals and hip abductors along the iliac crest, a common site of contusions and strains. Follow the gluteus medius as it fans from the iliac crest to its insertion on the greater trochanter. A traumatic trochanteric bursitis is tender to palpation off the superior aspect of the greater trochanter. Medial to and about 1 in. (2-3 cm) superior to the ASIS, you can palpate the inguinal ligament. You can palpate an inflamed psoas bursa beneath the midsection of the inguinal ligament. Medially and inferiorly to the inguinal ligament, the femoral triangle that is formed by the sartorius laterally, inguinal ligament superiorly, and adductor longus medially frames the femoral artery, femoral vein, and femoral nerve (figure 18.17). Deep palpation of the hip joint is done indirectly, about 0.5 in. (1-2 cm) distal to the inguinal ligament on the midpoint of a line between the greater trochanter and pubic tubercle. Although direct palpation of the joint is not possible, pain from deep palpation may indicate hip joint pathology. Palpate the pelvic tubercles by following the inguinal ligament medially. Pain from pressure on the tubercles may indicate pubic symphysis or sacroiliac pathology. Palpate the lateral (gluteus medius, tensor fascia), anterior (rectus femoris, sartorius), and medial (adductor group) thigh muscles to identify areas of tenderness, defects, spasm, swelling, temperature, and other pathology.

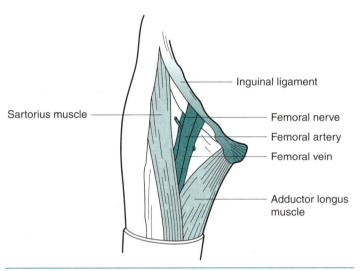

Sartorius muscle

Inguinal ligament

Femoral nerve

Femoral artery

Femoral vein

Adductor longus muscle

Figure 18.17 The femoral triangle.

- **Prone.** Identify the iliac crests and follow them posteriorly to the PSIS, which are areas usually indicated by dimples in the lower back. You can locate the ischial tuberosities in the gluteal fold region with an upward and anterior palpation. Tenderness over this area may indicate an ischial bursitis or hamstring insertion pathology. Locate the hip lateral rotators, especially the piriformis, from the greater trochanter in a superior and medial pattern toward the sacrum. The sciatic nerve lies midway between the ischial tuberosity and the greater trochanter as it exits from underneath the piriformis, and it is best palpated with the patient lying on the side and flexing the hip. You can follow the sacral joints from the PSIS inferiorly and slightly medially. Palpate the sacrotuberous ligament between the ischial tuberosity and the sacrum (figure 18.18). Unequal tension between the right and left sacrotuberous ligaments accompanied by tenderness to palpation may indicate either a ligamentous injury or sacroiliac dysfunction. You may note tenderness or spasm in these muscles. Also investigate the gluteal muscles and hamstrings for spasm, tenderness, and swelling.

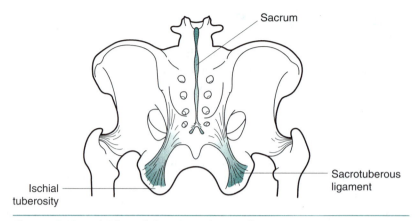

Figure 18.18   Location of the sacrotuberous ligament.

Range of Motion

Examine active and passive ROM bilaterally for all hip motions.

Active ROM

With the patient supine, perform hip flexion both with the knee extended to examine hamstring flexibility and with the knee flexed to eliminate the influence of the hamstrings on hip movement (figure 18.19). The normal ROM for hip flexion is 115° to 125° with the knee flexed and about 90° with the knee extended. Also examine hip abduction (45°-50°) and adduction (20°-30°) with the patient supine (figure 18.20), and examine hip extension while the patient is prone or side-lying. As with hip flexion, perform hip extension both with the knee flexed and extended to differentiate muscle tightness from joint restriction (figure 18.21). You can perform hip medial and lateral rotation (about 45° each) either with the patient prone (hip extended and knee flexed to 90°) or seated (hip and knee flexed to 90°) (figure 18.22).

Passive ROM

Active ROM requires repositioning for some motions, so you should immediately follow each active motion with passive ROM for efficiency. End feel for each motion should be tissue stretch. With hip flexion and adduction however, a softer end feel may occur if the segment contacts the abdomen and the opposite thigh, respectively. When examining rotation, always perform lateral rotation movements with care when the knee is flexed because of the lever (arm) length advantage you have on the hip in this position. If the hip is unstable, dislocation can occur.

Goniometric Examination of ROM

Goniometric examination of hip motion is described in table 18.1 and illustrated in figure 18.23.

Strength

You can test hip strength both manually and with free weights and weight machines. As you will see, isokinetic dynamometers are not often used for examining the healthy hip.

Manual muscle tests for the hip are described in table 18.2 and illustrated in figure 18.24. With the patient seated, test hip flexion and rotation and sartorius strength. Watch for hip rotation or abduction substitutions with hip flexion, and watch for hip flexion or abduction or adduction substitutions with rotation. Although you can perform these tests alternately with the patient supine, this position can place greater stress on the lumbar spine during resisted movement. Test abduction and adduction with the patient in the side-lying position. Make sure that the patient maintains the hip in pure abduction and does not flex it

While examining strength of hip flexion and extension, watch for hip rotation or abduction substitution.

While examining strength of hip abduction, watch for muscle substitution as indicated by flexion or lateral rotation of the hip.

Always compare strength results with the uninvolved leg to determine what is normal for the patient. Test the uninvolved hip first so the patient knows what to expect on the injured side and will be less apprehensive and more willing to produce a maximal effort.

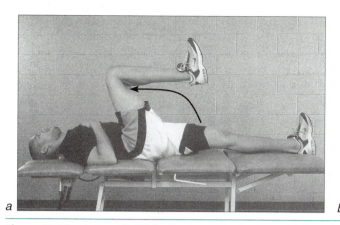
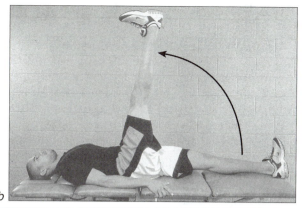

Figure 18.19 Active ROM hip flexion with the knee *(a)* flexed and *(b)* extended.

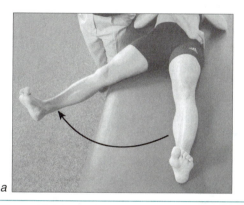
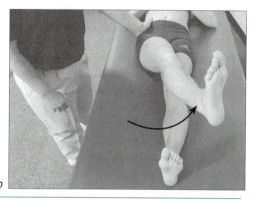

Figure 18.20 Active ROM hip *(a)* abduction and *(b)* adduction.

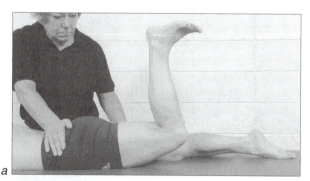
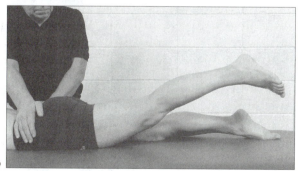

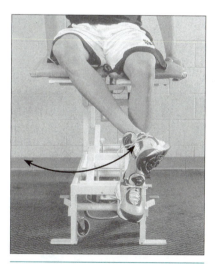

Figure 18.22 Active ROM for medial and lateral rotation of the knee while in a seated position.

Figure 18.21 Active ROM hip extension with the knee *(a)* flexed and *(b)* extended.

Table 18.1
Goniometric Examination for Hip Motions

Motion	Location of goniometer	Movement	Normal range
Flexion	P: Supine A: Greater trochanter S: Parallel to midline of trunk M: Long axis of femur	Flex hip to end of range; measure with knee flexed (KF) for joint motion and knee extended (KE) for hamstring muscle length	KF = 0° to 110-125° KE = 0° to 90°
Extension	P: Supine A: Greater trochanter S: Parallel to midline of trunk M: Long axis of femur	Stabilize pelvis and passively hyperextend hip to end range (knee in extension)	0° to 15°
Abduction	P: Supine A: ASIS S: Line connecting the left and right ASIS M: Parallel with long axis of femur	From neutral (goniometer reading 90°), abduct hip to limit of motion	0° to 45-50°
Adduction	P: Supine A: ASIS S: Line connecting the left and right ASIS M: Parallel with long axis of femur	From neutral (goniometer reading 90°), adduct hip across opposite leg to limit of motion	0° to 20-30°
Medial and lateral rotation	P: Seated A: Midpatella S: Perpendicular to floor M: Long axis of tibia	Rotate hip to limit of motion by moving the lower leg and foot laterally (internal) and medially (external)	0° to 35° (lateral) 0° to 45° (medial)

P = patient position; A = goniometer axis; S = stationary arm; M = movable arm.

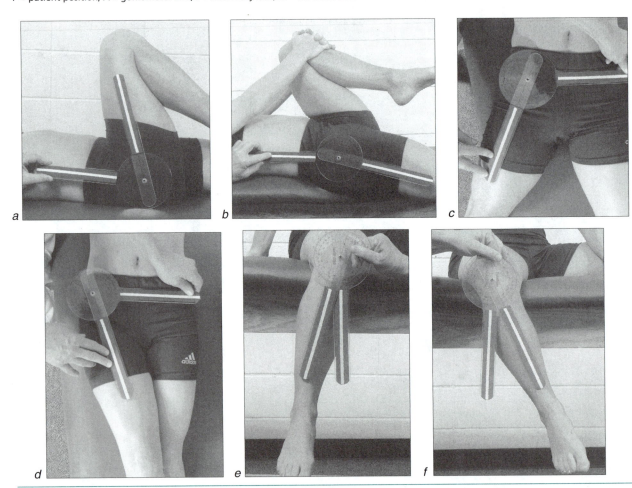

Figure 18.23 Goniometric examination for hip *(a)* flexion, *(b)* extension, *(c)* abduction, *(d)* adduction, *(e)* medial rotation, and *(f)* lateral rotation.

Table 18.2
Manual Muscle Testing for the Hip Musculature

Motion	Athlete position	Stabilizing hand placement	Resistance hand placement	Instruction to athlete	Primary muscles tested
Hip flexion	Seated or supine	Iliac crest of test leg	Distal anterior thigh above the knee	Raise knee toward chest	Iliopsoas
Hip flexion, abduction, and rotation	Seated or supine	N/A	One hand on anterolateral surface of distal thigh just above the knee and one hand grasping the posteriomedial aspect of the distal lower leg	Flex, abduct, and laterally rotate the hip by sliding the foot along the anterior medial shin of the opposite leg, bringing the foot to rest on the anterior distal thigh just above the knee	Sartorius
Medial rotation	Seated	N/A	One hand medial aspect of distal thigh, the other hand on lateral distal lower leg	Rotate hip toward midline, moving foot away from midline	Tensor fascia latae, gluteus medius and minimus
Lateral rotation	Seated	N/A	One hand lateral aspect of distal thigh, the other hand on medial distal lower leg	Rotate hip away from midline, bringing foot toward midline	Lateral hip rotators (piriformis, gemelli, obturators, quadratus femoris)
Abduction	Side-lying, test leg up	Pelvis	Distal lateral thigh above knee	Raise leg toward ceiling, leading with heel	Gluteus medius and minimus
Adduction	Side-lying on test leg, uninvolved leg in a figure-4 position with the hip and knee flexed and the foot flat on the table in front of the test leg	Pelvis and opposite leg	Distal medial thigh above knee	Raise leg toward ceiling	Adductor group (adductor longus, brevis, and magnus, pectineus, gracilis)
Hip extension	Prone with knee flexed (KF) and extended (KE)	Pelvis	Distal posterior thigh above the knee	Keep back in neutral, lift leg off table	KF = Gluteus maximus KE = Gluteus maximus, hamstrings

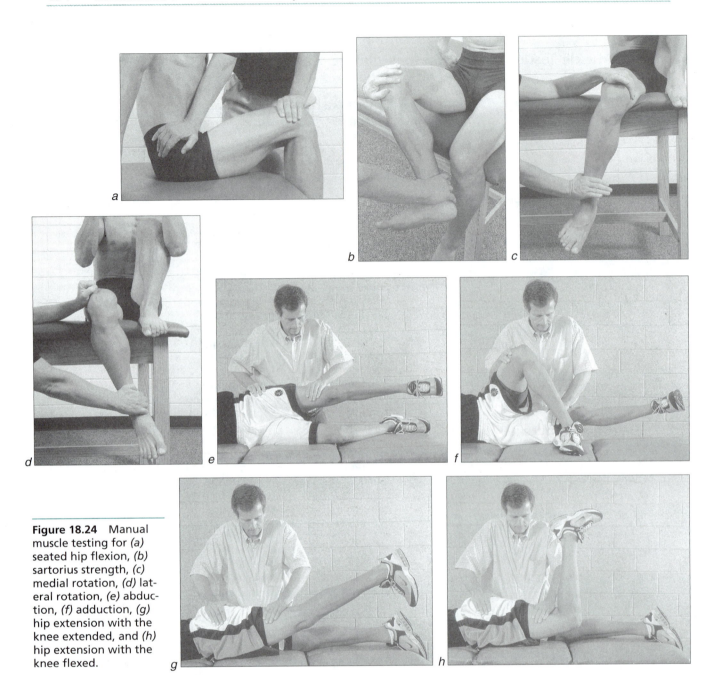

Figure 18.24 Manual muscle testing for *(a)* seated hip flexion, *(b)* sartorius strength, *(c)* medial rotation, *(d)* lateral rotation, *(e)* abduction, *(f)* adduction, *(g)* hip extension with the knee extended, and *(h)* hip extension with the knee flexed.

forward or laterally rotate it when you apply manual resistance. Test hip extension while the patient is prone.

Instrumented Strength Examination

Although some isokinetic dynamometers are designed for hip strength, many do not test a healthy hip because the high torque levels that the hip can produce may exceed the dynamometer's torque limit. As a result, the hip is not often isokinetically tested. A more functional examination of hip strength can be gained using free weights and weight machines. Squats and lunges are multiple-joint activities that require adequate hip extensor (gluteals, hamstrings) strength. Activities that isolate muscles can include weight pulleys or ankle weights to measure strength into abduction, adduction, hip extension, and hip flexion.

Neurovascular Examination

The hip and pelvis are surrounded by the nerves of the lumbosacral plexus. Sensory and motor nerves from this plexus innervate the hip and pelvis regions.

Table 8.7 and figures 8.13, 8.15, and 8.17 in chapter 8 describe and depict the sensory, motor, and reflex tests for the lumbar and sacral plexus. Since these tests are identical to those covered in chapters 8 and 15, they are not discussed here. Refer to those chapters for more detailed information.

If you suspect vascular compromise with significant trauma to the hip and pelvis, palpate the distal femoral pulse in the femoral triangle, the popliteal pulse in the popliteal space of the posterior knee, and the dorsalis pedis pulse over the dorsum of the foot in the space between the first and second metatarsals. Note pulse presence and strength bilaterally. Also look for signs of skin pallor and reduced temperatures in the lower extremity on the involved side. The potential for severe internal bleeding and shock to accompany suspected pelvic fractures is of particular importance in the hip and pelvis region.

Special Tests

Special tests for the hip and pelvis are divided into hip pathology, sacroiliac pathology, alignment, muscle weakness and dysfunction, and muscle length examination.

Hip Pathology

Joint, nerve, and bony injuries, although not common, can be seen in severe traumatic injuries. Because of the potential consequences of these injuries, you must be aware of the signs and symptoms they present.

Hip Dislocation

Although an X ray is the ultimate examination tool to determine hip dislocation, acute dislocations are not usually difficult to identify. The leg is often positioned in adduction and medial rotation. The greater trochanter is prominent, and the patient reports severe pain, especially when attempting to move the leg.

Congenital dislocations are more difficult to determine. One common test uses **Nelaton's line**, which is a line from the ischial tuberosity to the ipsilateral ASIS (figure 18.25). The test is positive when you palpate the greater trochanter above this line. This test can also determine coxa vara.

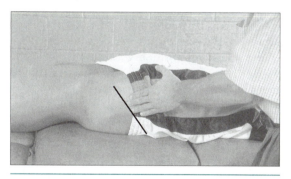

Figure 18.25 Palpation of the greater trochanter above Nelaton's line.

Femoral Nerve Traction Test

This test examines femoral nerve pathology that may emanate from the lumbosacral nerve roots (L2-L4), causing pain in the groin and hip that radiates into the anterior thigh. The patient lies on the unaffected side with the lower hip and knee flexed for stability and the top hip and knee extended (figure 18.26). While the hip is maintained in about 15° of extension, passively move the knee into flexion. The patient should maintain the head in slight flexion throughout the test. A positive sign is present if the patient complains of pain, numbness, or tingling in the anterior thigh. The thigh should remain in slight abduction during the test so that the outcome is not a positive Ober's test (see muscle dysfunction test later in chapter). The patient's history and symptoms will help you determine whether the positive sign is related to femoral nerve or IT band pathology.

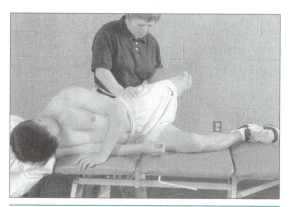

Figure 18.26 Femoral nerve traction test.

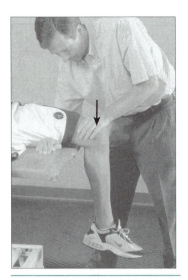

Figure 18.27 Stress fracture test.

Stress Fracture Test

The stress fracture test, or **fulcrum test**, examines for the possibility of a femoral neck stress fracture. With the patient in a relaxed sitting position on the end of a table or bench, place your forearm under the thigh (figure 18.27). With your other hand, apply a downward pressure to the proximal knee. The test is positive if the patient reports pain with the maneuver. Confirmation of a stress fracture requires a bone scan, so a positive finding warrants physician referral.

Sacroiliac Pathology

The pelvis is complex, working with multiple joints in multiple planes. Because of this, the pelvis lends itself to several examination procedures. Many tests can be used to identify sacroiliac pathology. This section presents the more common tests that identify acute sprains and chronic dysfunction.

Gaenslen's Test

Gaenslen's test is a general examination that indicates either a sacroiliac or hip pathology or an L4 nerve lesion. With the patient side-lying and the leg flexed at the hip and knee so that the knee is against the chest, stabilize the pelvis while extending the top leg (figure 18.28). Pain in the sacroiliac region is considered a positive sign. Although not as feasible for an acute examination, an alternative position for this test is the patient lying supine, with both knees drawn up to the chest and the buttock on the involved site off the edge of the table. The patient slowly extends the leg off the table. As before, pain in the sacroiliac region is a positive sign.

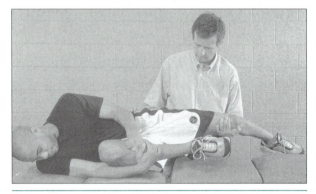

Figure 18.28 Gaenslen's test.

Sacroiliac Distraction (Iliac Crest Compression) Test

This test stresses the posterior sacroiliac ligaments. Place the patient in a side-lying position with the involved side on top. Place your hands over the proximal iliac crest and apply a downward force (figure 18.29). Pain in the sacroiliac joints is a positive sign for sacral joint irritation or sprain.

Sacral Apex Compression Test

This test places a rotational stress on the sacroiliac joints. With the patient prone, place the base of both your hands over the sacral apex (figure 18.30) and apply pressure over the apex. Pain in the sacroiliac joints is a positive sign for this test.

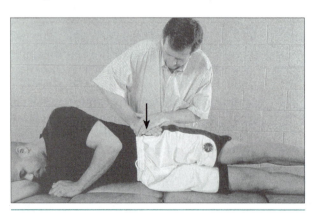

Figure 18.29 Sacroiliac distraction (iliac crest compression) test.

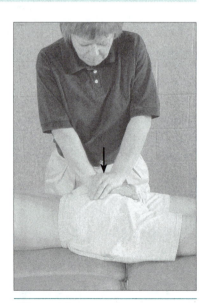

Figure 18.30 Sacral apex compression test.

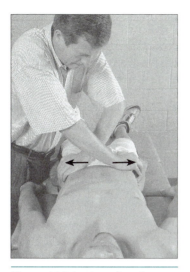

Figure 18.31 Anterior distraction test.

Sacroiliac Compression Test

This test, also known as the **anterior distraction**, or **gapping test**, stresses the anterior sacroiliac ligaments. With the patient supine, cross your arms so that your hands are on the patient's opposite ASIS (figure 18.31). Apply a downward and outward pressure to each ASIS simultaneously. A positive sign occurs if the patient reports posterior gluteal or leg pain. If the patient complains of pain over the ASIS, you may use a pad between the ASIS and your hand.

Posterior Distraction Test

The posterior distraction test, also known as **Hibbs' test**, investigates the integrity of the posterior sacroiliac ligaments. Once you have cleared any suspected hip pathology, have the patient lie prone. With the pelvis stabilized, flex the knee to 90° and medially rotate the hip to its end point while palpating the sacroiliac joint on the same side (figure 18.32). The test is positive if palpation over the sacroiliac joint reveals greater laxity or movement on the involved side than on the uninvolved side.

Patrick Test

The Patrick test is also known as the **Faber** (**F**lexion, **Ab**duction, **E**xternal **R**otation) **test** or **Jansen's test**. It identifies limited hip mobility, the possibility of iliopsoas spasm, or sacroiliac dysfunction. The patient lies supine with the involved leg flexed at the hip and knee so that the foot is crossed over the opposite knee (figure 18.33). Place one hand on the opposite ASIS to stabilize the pelvis and the other hand on the medial aspect of the knee of the involved leg. Passively move the leg into abduction, lowering the knee to the table. Mobility is normal and the response negative when you can lower the knee so that the thigh is at least parallel to the opposite leg. The response is positive when the thigh remains elevated above the opposite leg.

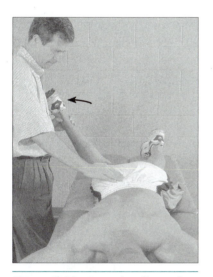

Figure 18.32 Posterior distraction test.

Alignment Tests

Malalignment of the hip can increase stress on the hip and other segments. Use the following alignment examination techniques to identify pathology.

Craig's Test

This test identifies retroversion and anteversion of the hip and is sometimes referred to as the **Ryder method** for retroversion and anteversion measurement. The patient lies prone with the knees flexed to 90°. Palpate the greater trochanter and position the hip so that the greater trochanter lies parallel to the surface of the table (figure 18.34). Measure the angle between the shaft of the lower leg (tibia) and vertical. In the adult, a measurement of greater than 15° medial rotation is considered hip anteversion. If the measurement is less than 8°, the hip is retroverted. An excessively anteverted hip also causes a toe-in stance, whereas a retroverted hip produces a toe-out stance.

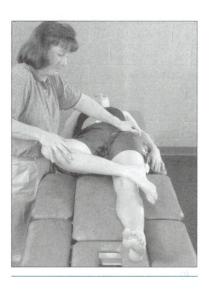

Figure 18.33 Patrick test.

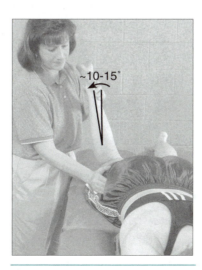

~10-15°

Figure 18.34 Craig's test noting about 10 to 15° of medial rotation.

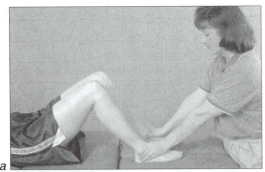

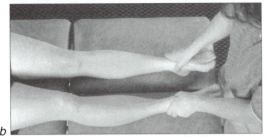

Figure 18.35   Quick check for leg length discrepancy: *(a)* hook-lying and *(b)* with legs extended.

A true leg length difference occurs when the bones of the legs are not the same length. An apparent leg length difference results from soft tissue shortening, pelvic obliquity, spinal pathology, or other lower-extremity joint dysfunction.

Leg Length Discrepancy

A difference in leg length can be a true discrepancy or an apparent limb shortening. To determine if a length discrepancy exists, have the patient lie supine in a hook-lying position (hips and knees flexed with feet flat on the table), and grasp the ankles with your thumbs on the medial malleoli (figure 18.35a). Have the patient raise the hips and lower them to the table. Passively extend the legs and compare the positions of the two medial malleoli (figure 18.35b). If the legs are unequal, you should proceed to determine whether the difference is true or apparent.

Measure a **true leg length discrepancy** with the patient supine and the legs fully extended. Place one end of a tape measure on the ASIS at its most prominent point. Place the other end on the medial or the lateral malleolus of the leg. (Using the lateral malleolus lowers the likelihood of thigh girth influencing measurements.) Draw the tape tightly from the proximal to the distal point (figure 18.36). Identify the location just distal to the malleolus and press your thumbnail onto the tape measure at that point. Repeat on the opposite leg, being careful to use the same landmark location for taking left and right measurements. Measurement differences greater than 0.6 in. (1.5 cm) are considered abnormal.

To measure **apparent leg length discrepancy**, position the patient in the same manner used for the true length measurement. Then take the measurement from the umbilicus to the left or right medial malleolus (figure 18.37). If there is a difference with the apparent test but not the true test, the leg length discrepancy results from factors (e.g., pelvic obliquity, hemipelvis) other than femoral and tibial leg length.

Muscle Dysfunction Tests

Tests for isolated muscle dysfunction identify weakness and contracture.

Trendelenburg Test

This test examines hip stability and abduction (gluteus medius) weakness. Have the patient stand on one leg while you observe the non-weight-bearing hip (figure 18.38). Normally, you should observe a slight elevation of the non-weight-bearing hip. A positive sign occurs when the non-weight-bearing hip drops because of weakness in the weight-bearing hip abductors.

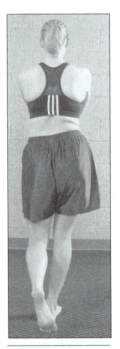

Figure 18.38   A positive Trendelenburg test. Note that the left hip has dropped, indicating right gluteus medius weakness.

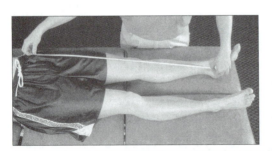

Figure 18.36   Measuring for true leg length discrepancy.

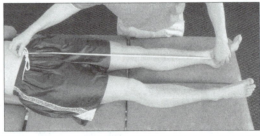

Figure 18.37   Measuring for apparent leg length discrepancy.

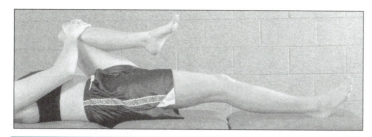

Figure 18.39   Thomas test.

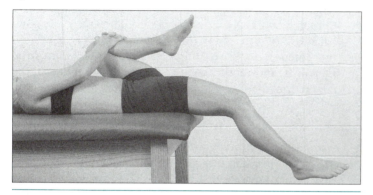

Figure 18.40   A positive rectus femoris contracture test.

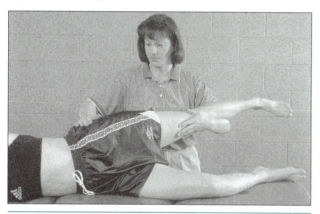

Figure 18.41   Ober's test.

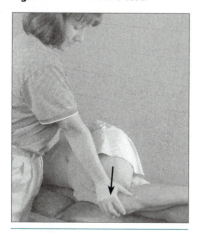

Figure 18.42   Piriformis test.

Thomas Test

The Thomas test examines the flexibility of the hip flexor muscles. The patient lies supine and brings one knee up toward the chest, then pulls the knee to the chest to flatten the back to the table. A normal response occurs when there is no change in the position of the extended leg. The test is positive if the extended leg becomes flexed so that the knee rises off the table (figure 18.39). If you push down the extended leg, the hip flexor tightness may anteriorly rotate the pelvis, and you will note an increased lumbar lordosis. Abduction or lateral rotation of the leg can indicate tightness of the IT band (**J sign**).

Rectus Femoris Contracture Test (Kendall Test)

You can perform this test, an extension of the Thomas test, to examine both hip flexor and rectus femoris tightness. The patient lies supine with the legs off hanging off the table at the midthigh (figure 18.40). The patient flexes one knee to the chest and holds it in place with both arms. The knee over the edge of the table should remain flexed at 90°. A positive sign occurs if the knee moves toward extension when the opposite knee is brought to the chest, indicating tightness in the rectus femoris.

Ober's Test

Ober's test examines tensor fascia lata and IT band tightness. With the patient in the side-lying position and the bottom hip and knee flexed for stability, position the top leg in abduction and extension. The patient should extend the knee throughout the test. Place one hand on the top pelvis, and support the top leg with your other hand (figure 18.41). Passively lower the leg into adduction. A positive sign occurs if the pelvis moves before the leg becomes adducted or if the leg remains in an abducted position. You can also perform the test with the top knee flexed, although this is not advised; a fully extended knee places a greater stretch on the IT band, whereas a flexed knee stretches the femoral nerve.

Piriformis Test

In addition to the acute tests for examining pelvis pathology, you can use the piriformis test in the clinical examination. The piriformis test checks for tightness of the piriformis muscle (see the earlier discussion of piriformis syndrome). With the patient side-lying on the uninvolved leg, position the top leg with the knee flexed and the hip in 60° of flexion. Stabilize the pelvis and apply a downward pressure to the knee (figure 18.42). A positive sign is pain in the piriformis muscle. Sciatic pain may indicate that the sciatic nerve runs through or is being compressed by the piriformis.

Joint Mobility Tests

Resting or "loose pack" position refers to the position of the joint when the ligaments are slack and under the least amount of tension.

The capsular pattern for the hip usually causes the greatest loss of motion in medial rotation; hip abduction and flexion are the second most limited motions. Lateral rotation is usually not limited.

Caudal Glide

The caudal glide (distraction) identifies gross hip joint mobility. The patient lies supine with the hip in a resting (loose pack) position of 30° flexion and abduction with slight lateral rotation. Grasp the thigh above the knee and apply a long-axis traction force by leaning backward (figure 18.43). Joint instability may be present if movement is excessive compared to that of the uninvolved joint or if you identify a telescoping of the joint during the distraction.

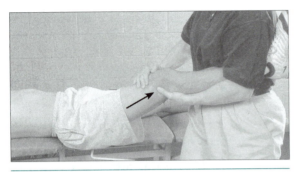

Figure 18.43   Caudal glide.

Lateral Glide (Distraction)

Lateral distraction identifies general hypomobility of the hip joint. With the patient lying supine, apply a mobilization belt around the proximal thigh and around your hips (figure 18.44). Place your hand nearest the patient's head over the greater trochanter to palpate for hip excursion while preventing thigh abduction with your far hand over the distal thigh. Use your body weight to move the patient's hip laterally. Compare with the uninvolved hip to identify abnormal mobility.

Dorsal Femoral Glide

This maneuver is used to determine anterior-posterior joint mobility. The patient lies supine with the hip flexed and adducted. Just distal to the inguinal ligament, apply a downward force through the femur to move the head of the femur posteriorly (figure 18.45). Compare bilaterally and note any restriction.

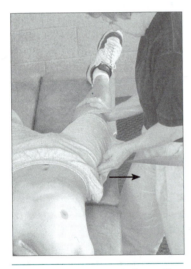

Figure 18.44   Lateral distraction of the hip joint (lateral glide).

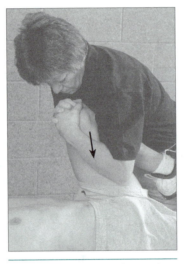

Figure 18.45   Dorsal femoral glide.

INJURY EXAMINATION STRATEGIES

The range of acute and chronic injuries of the hip and pelvis requires you to consider a number of factors when examining injuries in this area. On-site, you could be faced with only a simple disabling contusion of the hip or a painful muscle strain, or on rare occasions you may encounter a traumatic hip dislocation requiring immediate medical assistance. In all cases, you must be able to quickly determine the nature of the injury in order to properly act without delay. Off the field, injuries of the hip and pelvis are not as obvious as those on-site, as similar symptoms can indicate multiple conditions, some of them quite serious. Therefore you must acquire the examination skills to be able to differentiate the possible causes of chronic pain and dysfunction and determine which ones indicate more serious underlying injury.

On-Site Examination

Megan is a very lean forward who is going one-on-one against a defender on a fast break. When going for a layup, she is fouled by the defender and lands hard on the crest of the right hip. She is lying on the court in considerable pain.

You are covering a track meet and during the 220 hurdle heats, an athlete collapses to the track after completing the fourth hurdle. As you approach he is complaining of hip pain and a feeling of the hip giving out. He appears to be holding his leg in an awkward position and does not appear willing to move it. Other than some mild hip pain over the past few weeks, his pertinent injury history is benign.

In contrast to the knee and ankle, the hip joint is not often acutely injured in athletics, and severe acute hip injuries are rare. However, when an injury to this area does occur, it can be debilitating. As with any on-site examination, you must be able to quickly identify life- and limb-threatening conditions as well as recognize signs and symptoms of other serious injuries. As you approach the athlete, survey the surroundings and note the athlete's injury response and body position. Your primary survey is consistent with those for all other joints in that you first examine for level of consciousness, airway, breathing, circulation, and severe bleeding. If your survey reveals no life-threatening conditions, move on to examination of the hip and pelvis.

History

As always, gain a brief history from the athlete as to the mechanism of injury and the location, type, and severity of the symptoms. Remember that athletes often experience hip pain as inguinal or groin pain, whereas they more often feel lumbosacral pain in the buttocks and posterior thigh and possibly along the sciatic nerve. Because of the close communication of the sacroiliac and hip joints with the sacral plexus and sciatic nerve, respectively, be sure to ask about any unusual sounds or sensations felt at the time of injury and currently, and find out whether there is any referred pain down the leg.

Observation

Your initial observation should be for obvious and immediate signs of swelling, discoloration, and deformity. Observe bilaterally the position of the legs to see whether one leg appears shortened or medially or laterally rotated. Whereas lateral rotation is indicative of a fracture, medial rotation is characteristic of a dislocation. Observe whether the athlete is willing to move the leg or hip, as well as the opposite limb. If you suspect a serious hip or pelvis injury, call EMS and observe the athlete for signs and symptoms of shock.

Neurovascular Examination

Palpate the femoral pulse in the femoral triangle where the femoral artery is most accessible. This artery is located midway between the adductor longus and sartorius just distal to the inguinal ligament. With severe trauma and suspected occlusion, you should palpate the artery for a pulse. To examine neurological status, perform a quick sensory test of the dermatomal distributions of the lumbosacral plexus if the athlete complains of pain wrapping around the pelvis or into the lower extremity (see neurological tests in chapter 8).

Palpation

If you observe no immediate serious trauma or neurological symptoms, proceed with a brief but thorough palpation to examine for any tenderness, crepitus, or subtle deformities over

With traumatic injuries, conduct a rapid visual check of skin color and moisture, pupil size, respiration, and pulse to examine for signs and symptoms indicating shock (see chapter 9).

If you suspect a serious hip or pelvis injury or the athlete is unable to ambulate under her own power or with assistance, do not hesitate to use passive transport to remove her from the field for a more thorough examination.

Checklist for On-Site Examination of the Hip, Pelvis, and Groin

▷ **Primary Survey**

- ☐ Survey surroundings
- ☐ Information from bystanders
- ☐ Position and response of athlete as you approach
- ☐ Consciousness
- ☐ Airway, breathing, circulation
- ☐ Severe bleeding

▷ **Secondary Survey**

  ▷ **History**

  - ☐ Chief complaint
  - ☐ Mechanism, location, and severity of pain
  - ☐ Unusual sounds or sensations
  - ☐ Any referred pain

  ▷ **Observation**

  - ☐ Obvious and immediate signs of deformity, swelling, discoloration
  - ☐ Unusual positioning of the limb (shortened, rotated)
  - ☐ Signs and symptoms of shock (wet, white, weak)

  If deformity or evidence of severe trauma are present, notify EMS and monitor for signs and symptoms of shock.

  ▷ **Neurovascular Examination**

  - ☐ Pulse (femoral)
  - ☐ Sensory (L1-S2)
  - ☐ Motor (L1-S2)

  If evidence of possible fracture or significant injury, use passive transport to move athlete off-site.

  ▷ **Palpation**

  - ☐ ASIS, AIIS, iliac crest, greater trochanter, PSIS, ischial tuberosity, sacroiliac joint
  - ☐ Insertions for sartorius, rectus femoris, hamstring origin
  - ☐ Palpable defects in the adductor, abductor, and hip flexor muscle groups
  - ☐ Bilateral comparison

  ▷ **Range of Motion**

  - ☐ Perform active ROM for hip flexion, extension, abduction, adduction, medial and lateral rotation

  If all tests are negative and athlete is able to complete active ROM, move the athlete off-site and assist as pain and symptoms dictate.

the bony structures and muscular insertions as the athlete's pain and symptoms indicate. Palpate the anterior superior and inferior iliac spine, iliac crest, greater trochanter, posterior superior iliac spine (PSIS), ischial tuberosity, and sacroiliac joints. Be sure to include the insertions of the sartorius on the ASIS, the rectus femoris on the AIIS, and the hamstring origin on the ischial tuberosity. If you do not note any bony tenderness, generally examine for tenderness or palpable defects in the adductor, abductor, and hip flexor muscle groups as needed to ascertain the extent of injury.

Removal From the Field

If you do not suspect fracture or dislocation, have the athlete perform slow, active ROM of the lower extremities. If this does not significantly increase pain, allow the athlete to sit and then stand. If the athlete tolerates these movements, assist the athlete off the field. If, however, you have any doubt as to a potential fracture or dislocation, or if the athlete's pain is too severe to allow ambulation, you should have the athlete transported on a stretcher to the sideline for a more thorough examination.

Acute Examination

You are covering basketball practice and one of your athletes walks toward you with a considerable limp. He reports that during a rebounding drill, he was thrown off balance and came down on one leg with his knee and hip extended. He states he feels like he jammed his back and is experiencing pain across his right lower back and into his gluteals.

During a soccer game in the pouring rain, an 18-year-old athlete lunges for the ball. While doing so, her right foot slips on the soggy grass, and she inadvertently does the splits, causing her right hip to become hyperflexed with the knee extended. She gets up and begins to run down the field, but finds it too painful and calls for a substitution. Now on the sideline, she is complaining of pain deep in the right buttock. She states that when she began to run it was too painful to push off with the involved leg.

Before beginning the objective portion of the acute examination, obtain a more detailed injury history from the athlete.

History

From a more detailed history you gain information regarding the injury so that you can better determine its nature and severity. Ask further questions about the mechanism of the injury and the position of the limb when injury occurred. Determine whether the athlete was bearing weight at the time, and if so whether the athlete was rotating on the weight-bearing leg. If the injury was a result of impact, ask the athlete where on the body the impact occurred. Also note at this time any previous injuries or pain in the hip and pelvis, as well as any previous injuries or pain in the thigh or lower back that may be relevant.

Observation

While obtaining the history, observe for signs of pain, the position of the injured hip and the way in which the athlete moves the hip, and any difficulties or limitations with mobility and function. Observe how the athlete stands, sits, and moves from one position to another and how the hip is supported or guarded. If the athlete was able to ambulate off the field, note his ability to bear weight on the injured leg and his level of confidence in using the leg. Check the area thoroughly for discoloration and bruising, deformity, or swelling, especially over the bony prominences of the iliac crest and greater trochanter. Note any scars that would indicate previous injury or surgery.

Palpation

Palpation around the hip area involves examining temperature, skin and soft tissue mobility, tenderness, defects, muscle spasm, swelling, and bony tenderness. If there is no table on the sideline, you can perform the palpation while the athlete is standing or lying on the ground, whichever she finds more comfortable.

Checklist for Acute Examination of the Hip, Pelvis, and Groin

▷ **History**

Ask questions pertaining to the following:

- ☐ Chief complaint
- ☐ Mechanism of injury (contact or noncontact, rotational stress, weight bearing or non-weight bearing, etc.)
- ☐ Unusual sounds or sensations
- ☐ Type and location of pain or symptoms
- ☐ Previous injury
- ☐ Previous injury to opposite extremity for bilateral comparison

▷ **Observation**

- ☐ Swelling (local or general), deformity, and discoloration
- ☐ Positioning and any limitations in mobility or function
- ☐ Standing alignment: levels of greater trochanters, PSIS from behind, ASIS from front, equal weight bearing
- ☐ Gait—normal versus abnormal
- ☐ Muscular atrophy, tone, previous scars
- ☐ Bilateral comparison

▷ **Palpation**

Bilaterally palpate for pain, tenderness, and deformity over the following:

- ☐ ASIS, iliac crest including insertion of the abdominals and hip abductors, iliac tubercle, greater trochanter, trochanteric bursa
- ☐ Inguinal ligament, femoral triangle borders and contents, pelvic tubercles
- ☐ Abductor, hip flexor, and adductor muscle groups and insertions
- ☐ PSIS, ischial tuberosity, piriformis and sciatic nerve, sacroiliac joint, sacrotuberous ligament
- ☐ Gluteus maximus
- ☐ Hamstring (proximal and origin on ischial tuberosity)
- ☐ Bilateral comparison

▷ **Range of Motion**

- ☐ Perform active ROM for hip abduction, adduction, flexion (knee flexed and extended), extension (knee flexed and extended), medial and lateral rotation
- ☐ Bilaterally compare and note any pain or restricted ROM
- ☐ Perform passive ROM for the active motions listed
- ☐ Bilaterally compare and note any pain or restricted ROM

▷ **Strength Tests**

- ☐ Perform manual resistance to motions listed for ROM (may follow each active or passive test)
- ☐ Check bilaterally and note any pain or weakness

▷ **Neurovascular Tests**

- ☐ Sensory, motor, and reflex testing for lumbosacral plexus
- ☐ Femoral pulse

▷ **Special Tests**

- ☐ Test for hip pathology (femoral nerve traction test, stress fracture test)
- ☐ Test for pelvis pathology (Gaenslen's, iliac compression, sacral apex compression, posterior distraction)

▷ **Functional Tests**

Range of Motion

Perform active and passive motions bilaterally for hip flexion and extension, abduction and adduction, and medial and lateral rotation, along with motions for knee flexion and extension if you believe the hamstrings or rectus femoris to be involved. Perform hip flexion with the knee flexed and then extended to differentiate joint restriction from muscle restriction. After examining active ROM with the patient supine and then prone, perform passive ROM, including overpressure, if active motion did not produce pain.

In addition to these standard motions, you can examine functional ROM (and strength) more generally by asking the athlete to perform a full squat. The athlete should be able to squat until the knees are fully flexed with the heels on the ground and the hamstrings in contact with the calf muscles. Observe for quality and quantity of movement. The athlete should not hesitate and should move through the motion smoothly while descending and returning to standing. The hips should remain level and the buttocks should move under the athlete, not backward, which indicates a compensatory movement to avoid pain. You can perform other quick checks of functional motion with the athlete sitting by having the athlete cross the legs (hip flexion and adduction) and rest the lateral malleolus of one leg on the opposite knee (hip flexion, abduction, and lateral rotation).

> ! Always perform rotation movements with care when the knee is flexed (whether the athlete is supine or prone) because of the lever (arm) length advantage you have on the hip in this position. If the hip is unstable, dislocation can occur.

Strength

Strength examination is also performed bilaterally with the athlete lying or standing on a table or the ground. Position the athlete so that each muscle works against gravity when you test it. With the patient lying supine, resist the hip flexors manually with the knee extended (rectus femoris) and with the knee flexed (hip flexors). With the patient lying prone, resist the hip extensors with the knee extended (hamstrings) and knee flexed (gluteals).

Neurovascular

Unless the athlete reports referred pain into the lower extremity below the hip, it is not necessary to perform neurological tests during the acute examination. Should neurovascular tests be indicated, perform them as previously described on page 501.

Special Tests

As with special tests for most body segments, special tests for the hip identify or rule out injuries unique to the hip and pelvis. Test both extremities so you can compare the right and left sides. The special tests typically used to define acute injuries include those for hip pathology, nondisplaced fractures, and sacroiliac sprains.

Functional Tests

If you judge that the athlete's signs and symptoms are relatively minor, perform a functional examination to ensure that hip and pelvis pain will not return when she resumes activity. The lower-extremity functional tests described for the ankle (chapter 16) also apply here, tailored, of course, to the athlete's sport demands. A full squat also serves as a functional test. Be sure to incorporate movement (e.g., jump, landing, cutting, rotation) consistent with the demands of the sport or activity.

Clinical Examination

A 16-year-old lacrosse player comes into the athletic training facility complaining of a nagging groin pain that will not go away. His history reveals he has been having pain for about 10 days. He cannot remember a specific injury mechanism or event.

An industrial worker comes to the health care facility complaining of left lower back pain that wraps around his hip. As you obtain his history, you learn he was reaching down to pick up a hammer when he felt his back seize up. He has no complaints of numbness or tingling in his leg, but he does state the leg feels somewhat heavy. Inquiring about his job, you learn that he works on the assembly line checking for product defects and that he typically stands a great deal throughout the workday.

As with other segments, if you first see the patient in the health care facility, often the injury will be in a postacute or chronic stage, and adequate examination will require additional examination tools. Many times with sacroililac dysfunction, the pain comes on suddenly with no apparent injury episode. As with any chronic condition with insidious onset, your history and observation become increasingly important to help you select the appropriate special tests to not only identify the pathology, but also the potential underlying cause for the dysfunction. Consistent with other joints, the clinical examination procedure is presented in chronological order.

History

The history obtained from the patient in the clinic includes the same elements as the history for the acute examination. Ask additional questions to obtain a clear and accurate injury profile and to determine the stage of the injury (acute, postacute, or chronic or overuse) and, if the injury is chronic, how the pain profile has changed over time. Ask questions about the time of injury or symptom onset, any change in pain or symptoms throughout the day, aggravating and easing factors, injury response to training, and level of irritability.

Observation

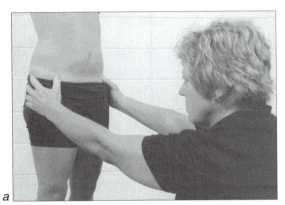

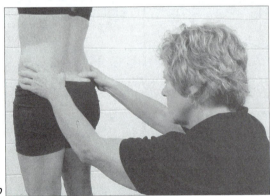

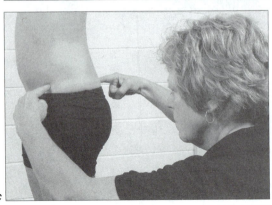

Figure 18.46 Observe the levels of the (a) ASIS, (b) PSIS, and (c) ASIS to PSIS bilaterally to identify any sacroiliac upslip or rotation.

When the patient enters the facility, observe for gait deviations (stride and cadence), stance abnormalities, unequal weight distribution side to side, and difficulties moving from standing to sitting or transferring onto and off the table. Observe for any hesitancy or guarding of the hip when the patient moves or transfers to a different position. Patients with a hip pointer may lean to the side of injury to avoid tensioning of the muscular attachments. Note how the trunk rotates and the hips move as the patient walks. Observe the stance for width, knee angulation (Q-angle, genu valgus), and feet position. Standing toe-out may indicate hip retroversion, whereas a toe-in stance and accentuated genu valgus may indicate hip anteversion. Check for obvious signs of a leg length discrepancy by comparing the levels of the greater trochanters and posterior knee creases. Check the levels of the ASIS and PSIS bilaterally by kneeling in front and then behind the patient, leveling your eyes with the pelvis; place one of your thumbs on each ASIS, then each PSIS (figure 18.46, a-b). Then, viewing from each side, palpate the ASIS and PSIS on the same side, observing whether they sit in the same plane, or if the ASIS sits higher or lower than the PSIS (figure 18.46c). If the ASIS is lower and the PSIS is higher on one side, there may be an anterior rotation of the sacrum on that side. If both the ASIS and PSIS are elevated, an upslip of the pelvis may exist on that side. In addition to studying posture, gait, and stance, observe the area of injury for swelling, discoloration, or deformities. Also

To identify postural and gait deviations, refer to chapter 4 for a complete gait and postural examination and the expected normal findings associated with these tests.

observe the erector spinae and gluteal muscle masses for equal tone and contour bilaterally, noticing any evidence of muscle atrophy or spasm.

Differential Diagnosis

Since the low back, knee, and ankle may refer to the hip, you must perform differential diagnosis tests to rule out the possibility of referred pain from other body segments. Quick tests for differential diagnosis include standing lumbar ROM in all planes with overpressure, as well as squats and active knee and ankle ROM through each movement with overpressure. You can also use the lumbar quadrant position, extension, lateral flexion, and rotation to the same side with overpressure to eliminate the low back as a referral source of hip pain (figure 18.47). None of these quick tests except the squat should reproduce the patient's pain. If any do, you should further examine the specific area as the possible source of pain before proceeding in the hip examination.

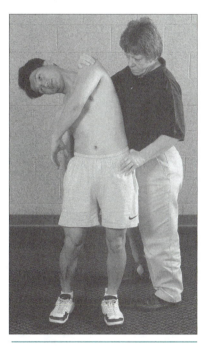

Figure 18.47 Lumbar quadrant position for clearing the low back as a source of hip pain.

Range of Motion

As with the acute examination, bilaterally examine hip ROM for hip flexion with the knee flexed and extended, extension with the knee flexed and extended, medial and lateral rotation, and abduction and adduction. Examine hip flexion, abduction, adduction, and rotation with the patient supine; examine hip extension and rotation with the patient prone. Inability to complete active hip flexion accompanied by pain in the sacroiliac region indicates sacroiliac dysfunction on the ipsilateral side.

Strength

Also examine strength in the same manner as in the acute examination. Rather than performing the complete ROM examination followed by the complete strength examination for all motions, you can perform ROM for one motion and then immediately perform the strength examination for the same motion. This sequence increases efficiency and prevents repetitive movements and unnecessary repositioning of the patient during the examination. Use gravity when testing for strength grades 3, 4, and 5 and eliminate gravity during tests for grades 1 and 2. Gradually build resistance to the maximum that the patient can tolerate, noting any strength differences bilaterally. Also carefully watch for the substitution movements previously described for each motion. Free weights and weight machines are the instruments commonly used to quantify hip strength.

Perform sensory testing using a light touch over the dermatomes of the lumbosacral nerve roots (chapter 8, figure 8.13).

Neurological Tests

Neurological tests are those previously described for the lumbar and sacral plexus. See chapter 8, table 8.7 and figures 8.13, 8.15, and 8.17. Use neurological tests to rule out lower back pathology referring to the hip and pelvis (e.g., disc and nerve root lesions) and to examine any neurological symptoms associated with nerve compression syndromes (e.g., piriformis).

Special Tests

In addition to tests for acute hip and sacroiliac joint pathology, special tests in the clinic include those for sacroiliac joint dysfunction, limb and pelvis alignment, and muscle weakness and tightness.

Joint Mobility

Restricted medial rotation, abduction, and flexion warrant investigation of the hip joint for capsular tightness. You will need to compare the right and left hips in order to determine abnormalities in joint mobility.

Palpation

If you have difficulty eliciting a reflex response, remember to use the Jendrassik maneuver to distract the patient and increase the nervous system's sensitivity (see chapter 8, figure 8.2).

Palpation of the hip and pelvis in the clinical examination is the same as that previously described on pages 501-502. It takes place after all the other tests that have been described

Checklist for Clinical Examination
of the Hip, Pelvis, and Groin

▷ *History*

Ask questions pertaining to the following:

- ☐ Chief complaint
- ☐ Mechanism of injury
- ☐ Unusual sounds or sensations
- ☐ Type and location of pain or symptoms
- ☐ Previous injury
- ☐ Previous injury to opposite extremity for bilateral comparison

If injury is chronic, ascertain:

- ☐ Duration of onset
- ☐ Changes in pain profile
- ☐ Level of irritability
- ☐ Aggravating and easing activities
- ☐ Training history

▷ *Observation*

- ☐ Visible facial expressions of pain
- ☐ Swelling, deformity, abnormal contours, or discoloration
- ☐ Gait deviations, weight distribution, difficulties with movement
- ☐ Overall stance, limb position, posture, and alignment (anterior, lateral, and posterior)
- ☐ Muscle development and tone—areas of muscular spasm or atrophy
- ☐ Bilaterally compare levels of ASIS and PSIS from front and side; greater trochanters, knee crease

▷ *Differential Diagnosis*

- ☐ Clear lumbar spine, knee, and ankle
- ☐ Examine active ROM—full squat

▷ *Range of Motion*

- ☐ Perform active ROM for hip flexion (knee flexed and extended), extension (knee flexed and extended), medial and lateral rotation, and hip abduction and adduction
- ☐ Bilaterally compare and note any pain or restricted ROM
- ☐ Perform passive ROM for the active motions listed
- ☐ Bilaterally compare and note any pain, restricted ROM, or difference in end feel

▷ *Strength Tests*

- ☐ Perform manual resistance against same motions as for active ROM (may immediately follow each active and passive motion)
- ☐ Check bilaterally and note any pain or weakness

▷ *Neurovascular Tests*

- ☐ Sensory, motor, reflex of L1-S2
- ☐ Femoral pulse

▷ *Special Tests*

- ☐ Hip pathology (femoral nerve traction test, stress fracture test)
- ☐ Pelvis pathology (Gaenslen's, iliac compression, sacral apex compression, sacroiliac compression, posterior distraction, Patrick)

☐ Alignment (Craig's, leg length discrepancy—true and apparent)

☐ Muscle restriction (Trendelenburg, Thomas, Kendall, Ober's, piriformis)

▷ *Joint Mobility Examination*

☐ Caudal glide

☐ Lateral glide

☐ Dorsal femoral glide

▷ *Palpation*

Bilaterally palpate for pain, tenderness, and deformity over the following:

☐ ASIS, iliac crest including insertion of the abdominals and hip abductors, iliac tubercle, greater trochanter, trochanteric bursa

☐ Inguinal ligament, femoral triangle borders and contents, pelvic tubercles

☐ Abductor, hip flexor, and adductor muscle groups and insertions

☐ PSIS, ischial tuberosity, piriformis and sciatic nerve, sacroiliac joint, sacrotuberous ligament

☐ Gluteus maximus

☐ Hamstrings (proximal origin on ischial tuberosity)

▷ *Functional Tests*

but precedes functional tests. By this time in the examination, you should have a reasonable suspicion of the tissue and specific segment involved and should focus your palpation on the appropriate areas.

Functional Tests

The lower-extremity functional tests outlined for the ankle (chapter 16) are appropriate here as well. Take into account the athlete's sport or work activity and consider whether deep squatting, straight plane running, rotational and cutting maneuvers, or single-leg jumping or landing maneuvers are inherent in the activity demands. Perform functional testing accordingly.

SUMMARY

1. Describe the etiology, signs and symptoms, and potential complications associated with acute and chronic injuries of the hip, pelvis, and groin commonly encountered in the physically active.

   The hip and sacroiliac joints are among the strongest and most stable in the body. As such, they are able to withstand tremendous loads and typically sustain fewer acute injuries than the ankle and knee. The most common causes of acute injury are contusions, muscle strains (particularly in the groin), and sprains. Traumatic fractures and dislocations are rare, with stress fractures of the femoral neck and avulsion fractures being more common. Because of the repetitive stresses placed on the hip and pelvis during locomotion and cutting and jumping maneuvers, chronic conditions caused by inflammation and muscle tightness are seen more often.

2. Identify conditions and concerns specific to the pediatric athlete.

   Pain surrounding the hip and pelvis in children presents a different challenge than care for physically active adults. Conditions specific to the pediatric athlete that you should consider in cases of hip and groin pain are apophysitis, epiphyseal fractures, slipped capital femoral epiphysis, and chronic synovitis. If these conditions are dismissed as a simple groin strain and proper treatment is not initiated, severe complications and permanent joint changes may result. Therefore, when a pediatric athlete complains of groin or hip pain that lasts more than a week, you should refer the athlete to a physician for follow-up and examination.

3. Identify common structural and functional abnormalities of the hip and pelvis.

Structural and functional abnormalities at the hip can significantly affect the entire lower chain as well as the lumbar spine. Abnormal hip angulation results in hip anteversion or retroversion, causing changes in knee (Q-angle, genu valgus) and foot (toe-in, toe-out) alignment that in turn may predispose the lower extremity to stress injuries. Leg length differences, also common, can result from muscle or joint dysfunction (functional, apparent length difference), or can be a true difference in femoral and tibial length (structural). It is important to recognize and examine for these abnormalities with any chronic complaints in the knee, hip, or lumbar region.

4. Describe and demonstrate the objective tests for examining the hip and pelvis.

As always, begin the examination with a thorough history and observation that will dictate the remaining objective tests. You can palpate the anterior, lateral, and medial hip with the patient supine; palpate the posterior aspect with the patient prone. Examine active and passive ROM and strength bilaterally for hip flexion and extension (both with the knee flexed and then extended), abduction and adduction, and medial and lateral rotation. Neurological examination includes sensory and motor testing of the lumbosacral plexus that innervates the hip and pelvis regions. If you suspect vascular compromise with significant trauma to hip and pelvis, check the appropriate distal pulses for presence and strength bilaterally. Special tests for the hip and pelvis are divided into those for hip pathology, sacroiliac pathology, alignment, muscle weakness and dysfunction, and muscle length examination.

5. Perform an on-site examination of the hip, pelvis, and groin, noting criteria for immediate medical referral and mode of transportation from the field.

Although the hip is not often acutely injured in sport, injuries to the hip can significantly impair an athlete's performance. On-site examination requires you to have good observation and palpation skills and to be able to accurately and efficiently examine the athlete's injury severity, condition, and transport needs. Note signs of obvious limb shortening or leg rotation, as they indicate a hip fracture or dislocation. If you observe no obvious signs of trauma, quickly palpate the bony structures, muscular insertions, and major muscle groups for signs of tenderness and defects before having the athlete perform active ROM and assisting him off the field.

6. Perform an acute examination of the hip, pelvis, and groin.

With the athlete on the sideline, you can make a more detailed examination of the injury. Take time to obtain a more accurate history and to perform a complete examination including palpation, ROM, strength, neurological, and special tests. Special tests for the hip, pelvis, and groin performed during the acute examination include those that identify femoral neck stress fractures, sacroiliac sprain, and nerve pathology.

7. Perform a clinical examination of the hip, pelvis, and groin, including differential diagnosis of referring back and lower-extremity pathologies.

When a patient presents in the athletic treatment facility, often the injury is chronic or postacute. Thus the clinical examination expands to include special tests to examine the hip and pelvis for muscle shortening or weakness, sacroiliac joint dysfunction, structural and functional abnormalities, and joint restrictions. The clinical examination also includes a differential diagnosis to rule out any referring back and lower-extremity pathologies.

8. Describe and differentiate potential causes and conditions of groin pain.

Groin pain is a common complaint in athletes who run, sprint, cut, and rapidly change direction. Although groin strains may be common, groin pain can also result from a variety of other pathologies including femoral neck stress fractures, inflamed lymph nodes, inguinal hernia, kidney stones, referred pain from the lumbar and sacroiliac regions, and chronic inflammatory conditions. Remember that groin pain in the adolescent may also indicate more serious hip joint pathologies. Therefore, when groin pain occurs without a clear injury mechanism and when it persists for a significant period of time, you should highly suspect these other conditions.

REVIEW QUESTIONS

1. Why can contusions around the hip and pelvis be so painful and debilitating?

2. What are some of the common causes and signs and symptoms of trochanteric bursitis? What are some of the other common sites of chronic bursitis?

3. What are the common sites of avulsion fractures? Discuss the mechanisms and the signs and symptoms associated with these injuries.

4. What is avascular necrosis? Discuss the cause of this condition and the types of injuries it may be associated with.

5. Describe the difference between true and apparent leg length discrepancy, and explain how you would differentiate between possible causes of a leg length difference in your examination. What potential problems are associated with a leg length difference?

6. When examining active ROM and strength for hip flexion and extension, why should you test with both a straight knee and a flexed knee?

7. What specific stress tests examine the integrity of the sacroiliac ligaments?

8. Describe the special tests used to identify muscular restrictions around the hip and pelvis. Include the specific structures that each test is designed to examine.

CRITICAL THINKING QUESTIONS

1. Think back to the scenario at the beginning of the chapter. You have learned that, among other injuries, femoral neck stress fractures, low back pathology, iliopsoas bursitis, and adductor muscle strains can all refer pain to the groin area. Discuss how you would differentiate these four conditions in your examination and the special tests you would use to identify or rule out each of these conditions.

2. You have a patient complaining of sciatic pain down the posterior thigh and lateral lower leg. You have examined the patient's lumbar spine and sacroiliac regions; there were no unusual findings, and you are unable to reproduce the patient's pain with spinal motions. What muscular condition might you suspect as the cause of this sciatic pain, and how would you proceed? Considering the special tests learned in this chapter and in chapters 8 and 15, which would you use to differentiate among possible causes of the nerve irritation?

3. A 25-year-old runner comes to you complaining of unilateral hip and back pain. As part of your examination, you wish to rule out any functional or structural abnormalities that may be causing muscular imbalance or joint dysfunction. Considering the lower extremity as a whole (chapters 16-18), describe how you would examine for alignment abnormalities that may be contributing to this runner's low back pain.

4. Consider the scenario of the soccer athlete who slips on the soggy grass while lunging for the ball. Her history reveals an injury mechanism of hyperflexion of the right hip with the knee extended. Her pain is located deep in the buttock and is most intense when she pushes off with her right leg. Palpation reveals pain directly over the ischial tuberosity, and reduced active and passive ROM pain with hip flexion when the knee is extended (but not when flexed). She also complains of pain with active hip extension with the knee straight. Given the history and symptoms, what injury might you suspect? What additional objective tests, if any, might you perform to further delineate this injury?

CITED REFERENCE

Moore, K.L. 1992. *Clinically oriented anatomy.* 3rd ed. Baltimore: Williams & Wilkins.

ADDITIONAL RESOURCES

Broadhurst, N.A., and M.J. Bond. 1998. Pain provocation tests for the examination of sacroiliac joint dysfunction. *J Spinal Disord* 12(4): 357-358.

Clarkson, H.M. 2000. *Musculoskeletal assessment: Joint range of motion and manual muscle strength.* 2nd ed. Philadelphia: Lippincott Williams & Wilkins.

Kendall, F.P., E.K. McCreary, and P.G. Provance. 1993. *Muscles: Testing and function.* 4th ed. Philadelphia: Lippincott Williams & Wilkins.

Mosby's medical, nursing, and allied health dictionary. 2002. 6th ed. St. Louis: Mosby.

CHAPTER 19

Head and Face

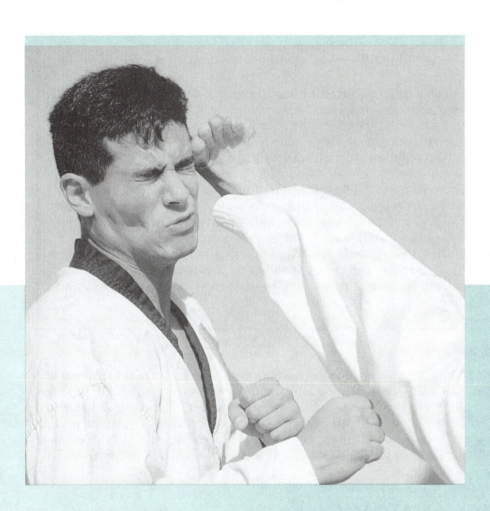

Objectives

After completing this chapter, the reader will be able to do the following:

1. Describe the mechanisms, signs and symptoms, and potential complications associated with head and facial injuries commonly encountered in the physically active

2. Differentiate among signs and symptoms of concussion, skull fracture, and intracranial hemorrhage

3. Discuss the potential complications and delayed symptoms that may result from head trauma

4. Describe and demonstrate the objective tests for examining the head and face

5. Perform an on-site examination of a potential head injury, considering the criteria for medical

referral and mode of transportation from the field

6. Perform an acute examination of a potential head injury, including special tests for cognition, balance, and coordination, considering the criteria for referral and follow-up examination

7. Perform a general examination for facial injuries, identifying differential signs and symptoms indicating associated head injury

8. Perform a complete neurological examination of the cranial nerves

Amanda was as pumped up as the rest of the team for the game that would decide whether they would make it to a bowl game this year. Late in the second quarter, Kevin, the second-string quarterback, came over to Amanda with concern about John, the first-string quarterback.

"I think something's wrong with John. He seems confused out there and isn't running the plays I'm signaling in to him—I think that hit he took in the first quarter rang his bell."

"Thanks, Kevin, I'll take a look at him," Amanda said as she headed over toward John. "Hi, John, you doing okay?" Amanda could see by his eyes that John was a bit dazed.

"Huh? Uh, yeah . . . when is the first quarter going to be over, anyway?" John said, showing frustration.

Continuing her examination, Amanda found that John had a headache and was unable to recall what plays he had just run. The team physician agreed—it was clear that John had suffered a mild concussion. Amanda promptly went over to the coach and informed him that John would have to sit out for the rest of the half, and that they would reexamine him during halftime. The coach was not happy, but he understood; he cared about the safety of his players.

Amanda continued to check John every 15 minutes. About 30 minutes after the initial examination, she noticed that he was becoming more lethargic and less oriented to his surroundings and teammates. She also noted that he was more unsteady than before and that his grip strength was weaker on one side. She called the team physician over immediately and related her findings. They called an ambulance and John was immediately taken to the emergency room, where it was found that he had a small subdural hematoma. Amanda was glad she had continued to examine John even though his initial symptoms had appeared minor. She used the incident as a lesson for the athletic training students working the sideline, emphasizing the importance of repeatedly examining athletes who suffer a head injury.

This chapter addresses the recognition and examination of injuries to the head and face and equips you to thoroughly examine these injuries and to differentiate signs and symptoms that indicate a life-threatening condition. It is important to realize, though, that head and facial pain can be caused by medical conditions unrelated to sport activity. General medical conditions of the head, eyes, ears, nose, and mouth are covered in chapter 21; keep those conditions in mind when a patient complains of head or face pain and symptoms with no known injury mechanism.

FUNCTIONAL ANATOMY

The head is a complex anatomical structure that houses the brain and the sensory organs for sight, hearing, taste, and smell. Although patients frequently complain of head and facial pain, the causes can vary widely and may sometimes indicate serious intracranial pathology. For this reason you need to understand the anatomical complexity and function of the structures in the head region in order to adequately examine injury and illness there. A complete anatomical discussion is beyond the scope of this chapter, which focuses on the most important structures of the nervous system as they relate clinically to specific injuries.

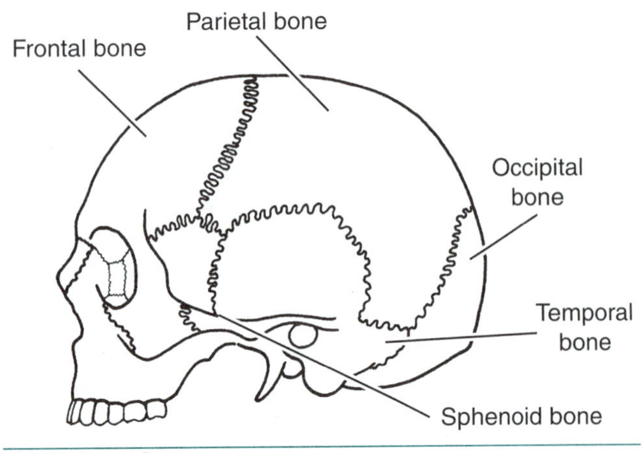

The bony structure of the head, or the skull, protects the brain and sensory organs and is divided into the cranium and facial bones. The cranium includes the frontal, occipital, ethmoid, sphenoid, and paired temporal and parietal bones (figure 19.1). The facial

Figure 19.1 Bones of the skull.

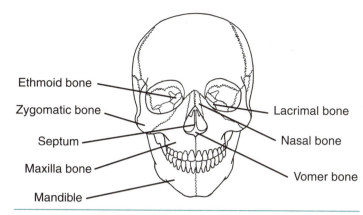

Ethmoid bone

Zygomatic bone

Lacrimal bone

Septum

Nasal bone

Maxilla bone

Vomer bone

Mandible

Figure 19.2 Facial bones. (The palantine bone which forms the palate that separates the mouth from the nasal cavity is not visible from this view.)

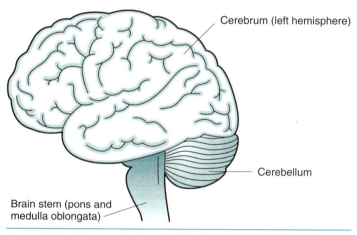

Cerebrum (left hemisphere)

Cerebellum

Brain stem (pons and medulla oblongata)

Figure 19.3 Primary divisions of the brain.

skeleton includes the mandible, palantine, and paired maxillae, nasal, zygomatic, and lacrimal bones (figure 19.2). The only movable joint in this region allowing appreciable range of motion is the temporomandibular joint, which is prone to both acute injury and chronic dysfunction.

The bony skeleton is covered by the highly vascularized scalp, which consists of layers of skin and connective tissue. Because of this rich vascular supply, lacerations of the scalp and face typically bleed profusely. Although the brain is well protected by the bony skeleton, it is not immune to severe head trauma. The brain is covered by three layers, or **meninges**, that become clinically important when vascular disruption and bleeding occurs between them. The **dura mater** is the outermost layer, consisting of a tough fibrous tissue that lines the inner skull and protects the brain. The middle meningeal artery, which is the largest of the meningeal arteries, passes through the **epidural space** between the temporal skull and the dura mater. This artery is often torn with skull fractures, causing significant bleeding and a rapid increase in intracranial pressure in the epidural space. Shearing forces can also disrupt the other vessels that cross the dura mater, causing bleeding beneath the dura mater into the **subdural space**. The **arachnoid mater** is a delicate, transparent membrane that forms the intermediate covering of the brain. It is separated from the inner meningeal membrane, the **pia mater**, by the **subarachnoid space**, which contains the cerebral spinal fluid.

Functional impairment with brain trauma depends on the brain structures involved. The primary divisions of the brain itself include the cerebral hemispheres, brain stem, and cerebellum (figure 19.3). The two cerebral hemispheres, which are divided into four lobes (frontal, parietal, temporal, and occipital), control body movement, sensation, and higher cerebral functions such as speech, learning, memory, and emotion. The two cerebral hemispheres are connected by the **brain stem**, which consists of the medulla oblongata and pons. The brain stem extends to the base of the skull and passes through the foramen magnum to become the spinal cord. The brain stem transmits information between the cerebral hemispheres and the spinal cord and controls the vital functions of respiration, heart rate, and blood pressure. On the posterior aspect of the pons and medulla is the **cerebellum**, which occupies most of the posterior cranial fossa. Consisting of a midline and two lateral lobes, the cerebellum primarily controls motor functions that regulate posture, muscle tone, and coordination. Also emanating from the brain are 12 paired cranial nerves that are numbered from anterior to posterior according to the order in which they attach to the brain (figure 19.4). The cranial nerves provide sensory and motor innervation for the head, neck, thorax, and abdomen (table 19.1). Their functions can determine the location and extent of intracranial pressure or pathology in the neurological examination of head injuries.

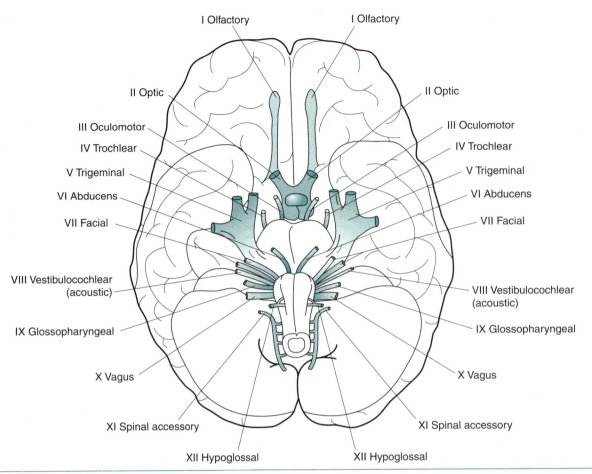

Figure 19.4 Inferior surface of the brain and the location of the 12 paired cranial nerves.

Table 19.1
Function and Examination of Cranial Nerves

Nerve	Name	Examination
I	Olfactory	Sense of smell
II	Optic	Peripheral vision, pupillary reflex to light
III	Oculomotor	Pupil size, pupillary reflex to light (consensual and direct reflex) Eyelid movement (ability to raise eyelids) Eye movement (ability to look up and in)
IV	Trochlear	Eye movement (ability to look down and in toward nose)
V	Trigeminal	Teeth clenching Side-to-side jaw movement
VI	Abducens	Lateral eye movement
VII	Facial	Expression (ability to wrinkle forehead, smile, frown)
VIII	Vestibulocochlear (acoustic)	Tinnitus, hearing, equilibrium (Romberg test)
IX	Glossopharyngeal	Sense of taste, gag reflex
X	Vagus	Voice quality
XI	Spinal accessory	Shoulder shrug
XII	Hypoglossal	Tongue movement (ability to stick tongue out; note any deviation to one side)

HEAD AND FACE INJURIES

Even with the use of protective equipment during sport activity, head and facial injuries occur frequently and can range from minor insults to serious, life-threatening conditions. You must be well versed in the etiology and signs and symptoms of each of these conditions and be able to quickly identify symptoms that indicate a medical emergency and immediate medical referral.

Head Injuries

Head injuries are common in athletics, representing the leading cause of death due to sport activity. Unfortunately, external signs resulting from head trauma have no bearing on the seriousness of the brain injury. Even apparently mild head injuries have the potential to become life threatening, and you must be able to differentiate between the signs and symptoms of mild head injury or concussion and those indicating intracranial swelling or hemorrhage. Additionally, blows to the head can result in cervical injury. Therefore it is imperative to suspect a cervical injury in the unconscious athlete until you have proof to the contrary.

Head injury can result from either direct or indirect mechanisms. There are essentially two mechanisms of direct trauma, coup and contrecoup (figure 19.5). When the head is stationary and struck by a moving object such as another player's helmet, a ball, or other sport implement, the brain is traumatized at the location of impact. This is termed a **coup-type injury**. When the head is moving and makes contact with an immovable or more slowly moving object, the result is a deceleration or **contrecoup-type injury**. Using the head to tackle, falling and striking the head on the ground, and running into a goal post are examples of decelerating injuries that cause the brain to lag in relation to the rapid deceleration of the head, affecting the brain on the side of the skull opposite the point of contact. Indirect mechanisms such as forces transmitted through the spine and jaw or blows to the thorax that whip the head while the

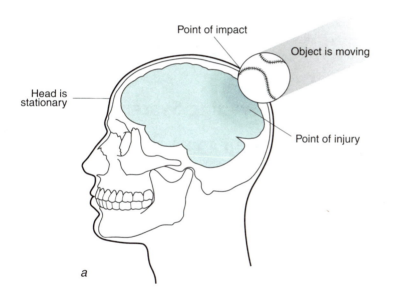

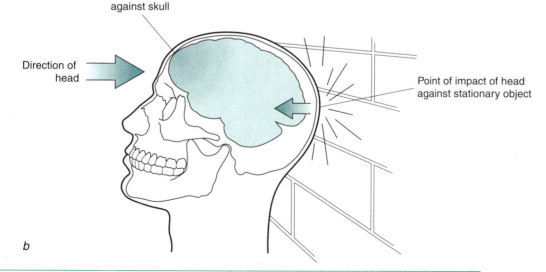

Figure 19.5 *(a)* Coup injury and *(b)* contrecoup mechanisms.

*A **compression force** places direct pressure on a surface or soft tissue.*

*A **shear force** is directed parallel to a joint or soft tissue surface.*

*A **tensile force** tractions or pulls away from the surface.*

neck muscles are relaxed can also cause head trauma. These mechanisms can place three types of stresses on the brain tissues: compressive, shear, and tensile. Because of the protection provided by the skull and the cushioning of the cerebral spinal fluid, compressive forces are usually well tolerated as force is dissipated by these structures. However, shearing forces that move the brain within the skull are poorly tolerated (Cantu 1992).

Head injuries are typically classified into three categories:

- Mild head injury or concussion
- Intracranial hemorrhage
- Skull fractures

Concussion

Amnesia means loss of memory.

A **concussion**, caused by an agitation or shaking of the brain, is defined as a transient alteration in brain function without structural damage. Clinically, it is defined by the severity of the injury. Multiple grading scales have been developed to classify the degree of mild head injury based on the duration of either unconsciousness or posttraumatic amnesia. Commonly used grading systems include the **Cantu Grading System for Concussion** (Cantu 1992), the **Colorado Medical Society Grading System for Concussion** (Colorado Medical Society 1991), and the **AAN Practice Parameter Grading System for Concussion** (Kelly and Rosenberg 1997). The Cantu grading system uses loss of consciousness, or LOC, and posttraumatic amnesia, while the Colorado Medical Society grades concussion based on confusion, amnesia, and loss of consciousness. The AAN grading system is similar to the Colorado Medical Society's.

Comparison of Three Common Grading Systems

Cantu Grading System for Concussion (Cantu 1992)

Loss of consciousness (LOC)

- Grade 1 = none
- Grade 2 = loss for <5 minutes
- Grade 3 = loss for >5 minutes

Posttraumatic amnesia

- Grade 1 = duration of <30 minutes
- Grade 2 = duration of 30 minutes up to 24 hours
- Grade 3 = duration >24 hours

Colorado Medical Society Grading System (CMS 1991)

Confusion, amnesia, and LOC

- Grade 1 = confusion, no amnesia or LOC
- Grade 2 = confusion with amnesia, no LOC
- Grade 3 = LOC

AAN Grading System (Kelly and Rosenberg 1997)

- Grade 1 = transient confusion, no LOC, with concussive symptoms or mental status abnormalities lasting <15 minutes
- Grade 2 = transient confusion, no LOC, concussive symptoms or mental status abnormalities lasting >15 min
- Grade 3 = any LOC

More recently, however, using a review of prospective studies conducted between 1990 and 2000, Cantu presented a revised **Evidence-Based Cantu Grading System for Concussion** (Cantu 2001). This system bases concussion grading on loss of consciousness, posttraumatic amnesia, and postconcussion signs and symptoms (table 19.2).

While experts do not yet universally agree on the grading and criteria for return to activity following a concussion, they do agree that any athlete suffering postconcussion symptoms during rest or exertion should not participate in contact or collision sports until symptoms clear (Cantu 2001). These signs and symptoms include headache, dizziness, nausea, ringing in the ears (**tinnitus**), loss of consciousness, confusion, and amnesia. Signs and symptoms may vary considerably from one athlete to another and according to injury severity. While it is often fairly easy to recognize second- and third-degree concussions, first-degree concussions may go unnoticed if the athlete does not report her symptoms. Often, mental confusion—of which the athlete will be unaware—is the only symptom, but it may be picked up on by an astute teammate or coach who notices that the athlete is not with the game plan.

Intracranial Hemorrhage

Although the skull provides good protection, it also acts as an unyielding casing and pressure vise around the brain when intracranial swelling or hemorrhage occurs. When head trauma results in tissue edema or hemorrhage, pressure builds in the intracranial space, forcing the contents to shift down toward the only opening, the tentorial notch (figure 19.6).

Table 19.2
Evidence-Based Cantu Grading System for Concussion

Grade	Symptoms
Grade 1 (mild)	No loss of consciousness; posttraumatic amnesia* or postconcussion signs or symptoms lasting less than 30 minutes
Grade 2 (moderate)	Loss of consciousness lasting less than 1 minute; posttraumatic amnesia* or postconcussion signs or symptoms lasting longer than 30 minutes but less than 24 hours
Grade 3 (severe)	Loss of consciousness lasting more than 1 minute or posttraumatic amnesia* lasting longer than 24 hours; postconcussion signs or symptoms lasting longer than 7 days

*Retrograde and anterograde.

Reprinted, by permission, from R.C. Cantu, 2001, Posttraumatic retrograde and anterograde amnesia: Pathophysiology and implications in grading and safe return to play. *Journal of Athletic Training* 36(3): 246.

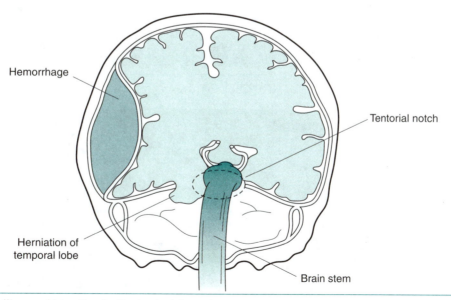

Figure 19.6   Swelling and bleeding in the tentorial notch.

This ultimately compresses the brain stem, the center for breathing, heart rate, and other life-sustaining functions. Unless pressure is relieved in a timely fashion, death will result. A space-occupying hematoma alters consciousness, vital signs, motor function, and pupillary function. Athletes with this injury vary in their level of consciousness from fully awake to drowsy or lethargic, to stuporous, to comatose. You will find it increasingly difficult to arouse and awaken the person.

Vital signs demonstrate high blood pressure, decreased pulse rate, and changes in respiration. The most common observation is **Cheyne-Stokes respiration**, characterized by a rhythmic fluctuation between **hyperpnea** (rapid, deep breathing) and **apnea** (no breathing). These altered vital signs are the opposite of those of shock, which include rapid shallow breathing, hypotension, and rapid pulse. Pupillary changes indicating increasing intracranial pressure include pupil inequality (figure 19.7) and unresponsiveness to light. Motor deficits range from weakness to paralysis. Unusual movements, such as a Babinski sign or decorticate or decerebrate posturing, also indicate severe brain damage. **Decorticate posturing** occurs with injury above the brain stem and is characterized by rigid extension of the legs and flexion of the arms, wrists, and hands in toward the chest (figure 19.8). **Decerebrate posturing**, a sign of upper brain stem injury, is a rigid extension of all four extremities, with the arms medially rotated and pronated (figure 19.9). A positive **Babinski sign**, or dorsiflexion of the great toe and splaying of the lesser toes with stroking of the plantar surface, indicates a lower brain stem injury.

You may not observe these symptoms immediately following injury; they may be delayed for minutes, hours, or even days. However, once they appear, the patient's condition can deteriorate quickly, resulting in death within minutes. Typically, the longer the period of consciousness or symptom delay following injury, the slower the hemorrhage and progression of symptoms. Therefore, it is important to observe and monitor the patient regularly for signs and symptoms of intracranial hemorrhage and to refer immediately when they occur.

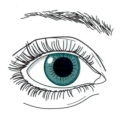
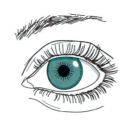

Figure 19.7 Unequal pupils indicating intracranial pressure.

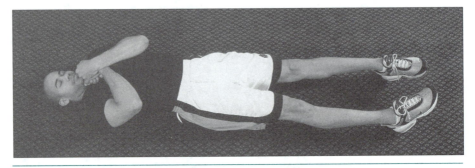

Figure 19.8 Decorticate posturing.

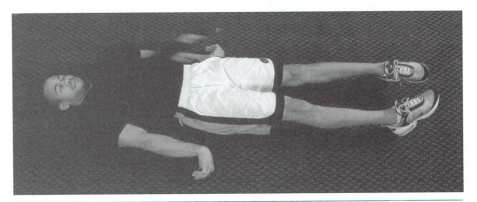

Figure 19.9 Decerebrate posturing.

In athletics, the two primary types of intracranial hemorrhage are subdural and epidural hematomas:

- A **subdural hematoma**, or bleeding in the subdural space, is a medical emergency that has a high mortality rate and is usually associated with severe closed head trauma. At the time of injury, the athlete is usually rendered unconscious and either remains unconscious or regains consciousness for a brief time before collapsing (Cantu 1991). Any athlete who loses consciousness, even for a brief time, should be closely examined and monitored following injury and throughout the next 24 hours for signs and symptoms of intracranial hemorrhage.

- **Epidural hematomas** most often result from a skull fracture in the temporal region that tears the middle meningeal artery, resulting in a rapidly expanding hematoma. The direct trauma may or may not have been sufficient to cause brain trauma or loss of consciousness at the time of injury. These injuries can be deceiving in that initially the symptoms may not be severe. However, after a brief period of consciousness, the athlete's condition deteriorates rapidly, with death occurring within minutes if pressure is not relieved.

> ⚠️ Symptoms of intracranial hemorrhage may not appear immediately following injury but may occur at some delay. However, once symptoms do appear, the patient's condition can deteriorate quickly and result in death if not immediately recognized.

> ⚠️ Any patient who loses consciousness, even for a brief period of time, should be closely examined and monitored following injury and throughout the next 24 hours for signs and symptoms of intracranial hemorrhage.

Skull Fracture

Skull fractures result from direct impact and are more common in sports utilizing a bat and ball or played on hard surfaces with the athlete not wearing a helmet. The fracture may be linear or hairline, resulting from a blunt force, or depressed, resulting from a more focused point of contact. The location of the fracture may be significant, as fractures that transverse a major artery may tear the vessel and cause an epidural hemorrhage. Other times, the fracture may aid in dissipating the force and lead to lesser brain trauma. Signs and symptoms of skull fracture include pain, palpable tenderness, swelling, discoloration, and possible depression. The overlying skin may or may not be lacerated. Additional signs include discoloration around the eyes (**raccoon eyes**) and behind the ears (**Battle's sign**), and fluid draining from the nose (**rhinorrhea**) or ears (**otorrhea**). Loss of consciousness and other signs and symptoms of concussion may also be apparent.

Second-Impact Syndrome

An athlete who returns to competition and sustains a second minor head trauma soon after an initial head injury may be at risk for second-impact syndrome. **Second-impact syndrome** is characterized by an autoregulatory dysfunction that causes rapid and fatal brain swelling. The athlete with a recent history of mild head injury who receives a blow to the head initially exhibits signs and symptoms of a mild concussion. The second impact does not usually result in loss of consciousness, and the athlete typically remains upright but may appear dazed (Cantu and Voy 1995). However, within minutes the athlete collapses into a coma and show signs of cranial nerve and brain stem pressure. The mortality rate of second-impact syndrome is high, so prevention is crucial.

Thoroughly examine athletes who sustain even a mild head injury and ensure they are symptom free before returning to activity. Unfortunately, criteria for deciding when an athlete can safely return to competition are not well defined. In 1994 the National Athletic Trainers' Association Research and Education Foundation sponsored a summit on mild head injury in sports that brought together experts from neurosurgery, neuropsychology, rehabilitation, family practice, pediatrics, and athletic training to address this important issue. Research is ongoing to establish objective criteria for determining full recovery and safe return to activity following brain trauma.

Postconcussion Syndrome

Postconcussion syndrome can follow mild head injury; the signs and symptoms are listed on page 522. These symptoms may not always be easy to recognize and can persist for days, weeks, and even months after neurocognitive functions have returned to normal. Therefore, listen to and closely observe the athlete in the days following injury for subjective complaints that may relate to the head trauma.

Signs and Symptoms of Postconcussion Syndrome

- Headache with exertion
- Dizziness
- Tinnitus
- Fatigue
- Irritability
- Frustration
- Difficulty in coping with daily stress
- Impaired memory or concentration
- Eating or sleeping disorders
- Behavioral changes
- Alcohol intolerance
- Decreased academic performance

Source: National Athletic Trainers' Association Research and Education Foundation. *Mild Brain Injury in Sports Summit Proceedings.* Washington DC, April 16-18, 1994.

Eye Injuries

Injuries to the eye, which most often result from direct contact, may involve either the corneal surface or internal eye structures. Eye injuries can be quite serious and may result in permanent damage if not recognized immediately or treated appropriately. Immediately refer serious eye injuries to an ophthalmologist for further examination and care.

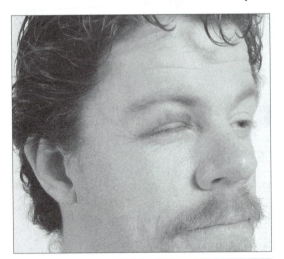

Figure 19.10   Periorbital hematoma.

Eye conditions not related to sport but resulting from infection or irritation are covered in chapter 21.

Periorbital Hematoma

A periorbital hematoma, or black eye, is caused by a direct blow and is characterized by discoloration and swelling of the orbital rim and cavity (figure 19.10). Other signs and symptoms, including pain and vision impairment, may occur secondary to severe swelling of the eyelids. Although a periorbital hematoma is rarely serious and does not require medical referral, thoroughly examine the eye itself for any associated trauma.

Corneal Abrasion

A finger poke to the eye or a foreign body under the eyelid can scratch the outer surface of the cornea, resulting in a corneal abrasion. Abrasions can also occur when an athlete attempts to remove a foreign body from the eye or removes a contact lens that has been in place too long. To prevent these types of abrasions, it is always better to flush the eye with saline, which should gently lift the foreign body off the corneal surface and out of the eye, than to try to remove the object manually. Corneal abrasions are extremely painful. The athlete is often unable to keep the eye open secondary to pain. The eye appears red (**hyperemia**) and watery, and the athlete complains of a gritty feeling, as if the object were still in the eye even after the foreign body has been removed. Visual acuity may be temporarily impaired. Fortunately, the eye heals quickly, and symptoms diminish significantly over the first 24 hours. Often the pain alone causes the athlete to seek medical attention.

Corneal Laceration

Lacerations through the full thickness of the cornea are much less common than corneal abrasions but can occur when a sharp object, such as a fingernail, cuts the eye. The patient complains of acute pain and visual impairment. Distortion or disruption of the corneal surface is observable, and the pupil may appear tear shaped (figure 19.11). Immediately refer patients with a corneal laceration to an ophthalmologist for further examination.

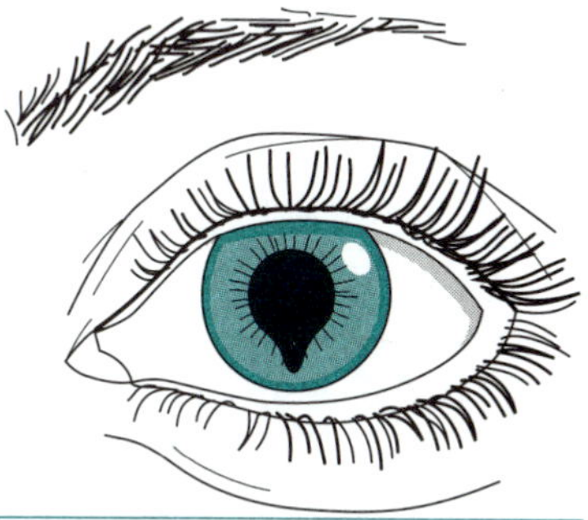

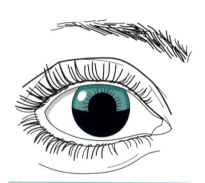

Figure 19.11 Corneal laceration and tear-shaped pupil.

Detached Retina

A sudden blow to the head or eye can cause the pigment layer of the retina to tear away or detach from its neural layer on the inner, posterior surface of the eye. A detached retina is not readily observable, but symptoms indicating a possible detached retina include blurred vision, flashes, floating spots, and blind areas in the patient's field of vision. These symptoms may occur immediately after injury but may also delay for a period ranging from a few days to a few months. Suspected detached retinas warrant immediate referral.

Hyphema

Direct trauma to the eye can also result in **hyphema**, or an accumulation of blood in the anterior chamber of the eye (figure 19.12). The chamber sits anterior to the iris and is normally filled with a clear, watery fluid (aqueous humor). Blood in the anterior chamber is readily apparent, as it obscures the iris and pupil. The patient complains of impaired vision, pain, and a feeling of pressure in the eye. Hyphemas indicate a serious eye injury that can cause excessive pressure within the eye or can be associated with further underlying pathology. Keep the patient upright and immediately refer her to an ophthalmologist or emergency room.

Figure 19.12 Blood in the anterior chamber (hyphema). Patients with a suspected hyphema should be kept upright and immediately referred to an ophthalmologist or emergency room.

Orbital Blow-Out Fracture

A fracture of the orbital floor, also known as a **blow-out fracture**, occurs from a sudden increase in orbital pressure due to a direct blow to the eye. Blunt trauma such as being struck in the eye with a baseball or racquetball is a common mechanism. The pressure from the blow fractures the thin, inferior wall of the orbit and displaces the wall inferiorly. Signs and symptoms include swelling, discoloration, and point tenderness along the inferior aspect of the eye. The injured eye may appear to sit lower than the uninjured one, and the athlete is unable to look up because the inferior eye muscles are trapped at the fracture site (figure 19.13). The athlete also complains of double vision (**diplopia**).

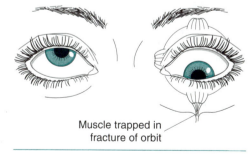

Muscle trapped in fracture of orbit

Figure 19.13 Orbital blow-out fracture with the inability to look upward.

Ear Injuries

Injuries to the ear include lacerations and hematoma caused by blunt trauma to the side of the head. Chapter 21 covers ear conditions associated with illness and infection that patients may experience but that are not a direct result of sport participation.

Auricular Contusions and Cauliflower Ear (Auricular Hematoma)

The auricle, or external ear, is made up of a single, elastic cartilage covered by a thin layer of skin that provides nutrition to the underlying cartilage. Contusions, friction, or repetitive trauma to the external ear can result in bleeding between the skin and cartilage. An observable hematoma forms, and the athlete complains of considerable pain and tenderness. If the hematoma is left untreated, separation of the cartilage from its nutritional supply results in necrosis and degeneration of the cartilage. Permanent scarring and deformity resembling cauliflower also results (figure 19.14).

Lacerations

Lacerations of the ear, though uncommon, can result from a severe direct impact or tension force. Athletes who wear earrings during sport participation are particularly at risk for lacerations of the earlobe, as the earring can get caught on a jersey and be violently torn from the ear. Signs and symptoms include pain and bleeding. Transient hearing loss may also occur with a laceration that is secondary to direct impact, but hearing should return within minutes following injury.

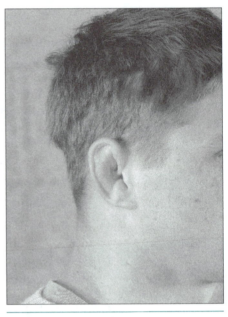

Figure 19.14   Cauliflower ear.

Nasal Injuries

Nasal injuries are the most common facial injury in sport. Nasal fractures are the most common facial fracture, and nosebleeds (epistaxis) frequently occur because of the rich blood supply in the nasal mucosa.

> You should consider general medical conditions of the nose and sinuses, covered in chapter 21, in your differential diagnosis when a patient cannot recall a mechanism of injury.

Epistaxis

Although the majority of nosebleeds (**epistaxis**) result from direct trauma to the nose or face, some patients can experience recurrent nosebleeds as a result of mucosal irritation, infection, exertion, or hypertension. The primary sign is mild to profuse bleeding from the nose. The patient may also complain of pain and difficulty breathing secondary to swelling. Refer patients with recurrent nosebleeds to a physician for further examination.

Nasal Fracture

The prominence of the nose on the face and its thin bony structure increase its susceptibility to fracture. Common scenarios include contact with an opponent's elbow during a rebound and a softball bouncing up into the face from a bad hop. The fracture may involve the bony bridge or the more distal movable cartilage. Bony displacement, usually lateral, is common. Signs and symptoms include pain, palpable tenderness, epistaxis (often profuse), probable deformity and crepitus, and immediate swelling. The nasal septum may also be damaged or severely deviated; this may restrict airflow through one of the nasal passages. Initially, breathing through the nose following a fracture is often difficult because of swelling. However, if an athlete continues to complain of restricted breathing once swelling subsides, you should rule out deviations in the nasal septum. Also examine athletes with suspected nasal fractures for associated maxillary fractures and possible concussion and refer to a physician as appropriate.

Deviated Septum

The nasal septum is a bony and cartilaginous structure that separates the nasal passageway into two narrow cavities. Minor deviations in the septum to one side or the other are common. However, severe deviations can occur as a consequence of congenital malformation or of direct trauma as already described. Severe deviations can restrict airflow, and the patient will complain of difficulty exchanging air through one side of the nose. In this case, surgery may be necessary to repair the deviation.

Face and Jaw Injuries

Direct contact and glancing blows to the face and chin can result in traumatic injury of other facial bones or the temporomandibular joint (TMJ). Chronic TMJ dysfunction may also occur in patients and may be the source of other head and facial pain.

Mandibular Fracture

Fractures to the mandible or jaw result from a direct blow, for example being struck by a ball or another player or contacting the ground when falling. Often, two fractures occur, one on either side of the jaw. The most common fracture site is the mandibular angle, near the socket of the third molar (Moore 1992) (figure 19.15). Fractures more proximal at the neck and coronoid process are usually associated with a dislocation. The athlete complains of pain with jaw movement and is palpably tender along the jaw line. Gentle tapping of the chin may also increase pain. You will also note swelling, discoloration, malocclusion, bleeding around the teeth, and possible bony crepitus and deformity.

Malocclusion is an inability to approximate the upper and lower jaw and teeth in a normal bite.

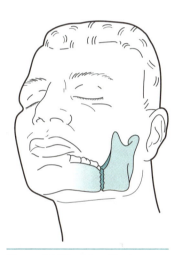

Figure 19.15 Mandibular fracture at the mandibular angle near the socket of the third molar.

Maxilla Fracture

The maxilla is a paired bone that comprises the bony surface between the mouth and the eyes. Blunt or direct trauma to the anterior face can fracture the upper jaw and mouth. Signs and symptoms include pain, swelling, bleeding around the upper teeth, and discoloration below the eyes. The face will be tender to palpation and the athlete will complain of increased pain when biting down. You may also observe malocclusion, loose teeth, and crepitus. Fractures to the maxillae may also occur concurrently with a nasal fracture, and epistaxis may result.

Zygomatic Arch Fractures

The inferolateral orbital rim is formed by the zygomatic or cheek bones. Zygomatic fractures are among the more common facial fractures and usually result from a direct blow to the cheek (figure 19.16). Signs and symptoms include pain, swelling, discoloration, and tenderness over the bony prominence. If the fracture is

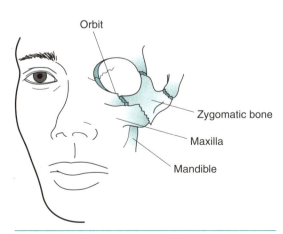

Orbit

Zygomatic bone

Maxilla

Mandible

Figure 19.16 Zygomatic arch fracture.

displaced, the cheek appears flattened. Because the zygomatic bone forms part of the orbit, fracture here may also affect visual acuity and ocular alignment.

Temporomandibular Joint Dislocation

Dislocations of the TMJ usually occur anteriorly. As the mouth opens, the proximal head of the mandible and the articular disc glide forward (Moore 1992). A blow to the chin or too much downward pressure on the lower jaw when the mouth is open may dislocate the proximal heads of the mandible. Simply opening the mouth too wide can also cause dislocation. Dislocation is usually bilateral, and the patient is unable to close the mouth. There is considerable pain and obvious deformity at the TMJ. A lateral or angular blow to the chin may also result in a unilateral dislocation or subluxation. In this case, you will observe restricted range of motion and a malocclusion of the teeth (figure 19.17).

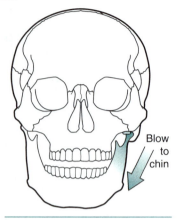

Figure 19.17 Malocclusion and lateral shift of the jaw.

Temporomandibular Joint Dysfunction

Temporomandibular joint dysfunction is characterized by chronic joint pain and crepitus that may also produce headaches and neck pain. Causes of TMJ dysfunction are direct trauma, arthritic conditions, poor approximation of the teeth when biting down, muscular tension, and grinding of the teeth at night. If the articular disc is displaced, clicking may also occur with opening or closing the mouth or with chewing. If the patient complains of chronic headaches or neck pain with no history of injury, you should always examine the TMJ and include it in the differential diagnosis examination.

Dental Injuries

> Dental injuries related to athletic participation are discussed here; dental disease is discussed in chapter 21 within the context of general medical conditions.

Patients may present a variety of dental complaints that may or may not be related to sport participation or work activity. They can experience dental pain and injury secondary either to direct trauma to the mouth or to tooth and gum disease resulting from poor hygiene.

Injuries to the teeth caused by direct trauma to the mouth are classified as fractures, intrusions, luxations, or extrusions.

Tooth Fracture

Tooth fractures may involve a simple chipping of the enamel or may extend into the dentin, pulp, or root (figure 19.18a). Involvement of only the enamel usually does not produce pain and is merely a cosmetic disruption, but fractures through the enamel into the structure of the tooth cause considerable pain. In addition, the fracture may be visible and there may be bleeding around the gum secondary to trauma. Root fractures are not readily apparent, as the root is below the gum line and cannot be seen. However, the tooth will appear loose and crepitus may occur when the patient attempts to mobilize the tooth.

Tooth Intrusion, Luxation, and Extrusion

> Instruct athletes who sustain a tooth fracture or displacement to report any increases in pain, sensitivity, or fever in the days following the injury that would indicate a secondary infection.

Traumatic forces to the mouth can also loosen a tooth in its **alveolar process** (socket). An axial force applied to the tooth may cause an **intrusion**, in which the tooth is driven into the socket (figure 19.18b). Bleeding and tenderness of the tooth and gum results, and the tooth appears shorter than the adjacent teeth. You should not attempt to move an intruded tooth.

If force is applied to the side of the tooth, the tooth may be displaced (luxation) or dislocated (figure 19.18c). The tooth appears out of alignment or crooked, and the gums may bleed. Dislocated teeth may also be partially extruded, or pulled from the socket. In this case, the tooth may appear longer than the adjacent teeth.

Complete **extrusions** result in avulsion of the entire tooth from the socket (figure 19.18d). In cases of tooth extrusion or dislocation, the tooth can be gently returned to its normal position. In all cases, refer the athlete to a dentist for further examination. An abscess may form

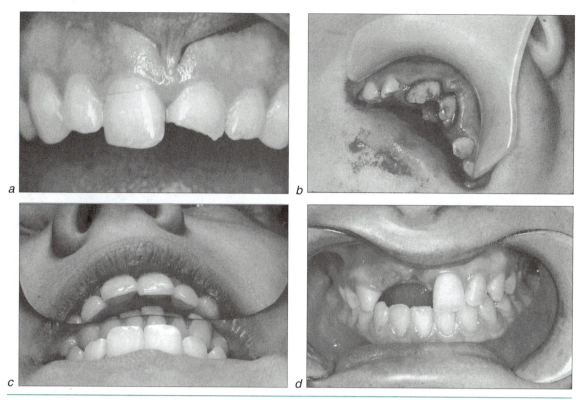

Figure 19.18   *(a)* Fracture, *(b)* intrusion, *(c)* luxation, and *(d)* extrusion (avulsion) of a tooth.

secondary to dental injuries. For this reason, instruct athletes who sustain a tooth fracture or displacement to report any increases in pain, sensitivity, or fever in the days following injury.

OBJECTIVE TESTS

Objective tests for the head and face are somewhat different from those for other areas of the body. ROM examination is primarily limited to active motion, which examines neuromuscular function in lieu of strength tests. Neurological examination deviates from the standard sensory, motor, and reflex tests that are specific to each nerve, as cranial nerves are typically tested with a single functional examination that may test either sensory or motor skills. Reflex testing focuses more on superficial and pathological reflexes when brain injury is suspected. Special tests identify the neurological and cognitive effects of head injury, identify facial fractures, and identify dysfunction of the primary senses (eyes, ears, and nose). The objective tests you include in your examination will depend on the type of trauma and the direction in which your history and observation examinations lead you.

Observation and Palpation

Observe the skull and facial bones for contour, swelling, and symmetry. Palpate for tenderness, swelling, deformity, and abnormal contour (e.g., depressions). Palpate the forehead, orbital rims, zygomatic arches, maxillae, nasal bones, and mandible bilaterally for tenderness, contour, and crepitus (refer to figure 19.2 for facial bone anatomy). Observe the TMJ for symmetry, smoothness of jaw motion, and excursion during jaw opening (see the section on AROM on page 528). Palpate the TMJ in the external ear canal while the patient opens and closes the mouth, noting any clicking, locking, or tenderness with movement (figure 19.19). Observe the teeth for alignment and symmetry, and then palpate for looseness and fracture. Perform all palpations bilaterally.

Range of Motion

Active ROM examines the functional integrity of the facial muscles and tests the degree of eye and jaw motion the patient can achieve.

Active ROM of the Temporomandibular Joint

Active ROM examination for the temporomandibular joint (TMJ) should include opening and closing the mouth, moving the jaw side to side, and protruding the mandible (figure 19.20). Normal ROM for opening the mouth is approximately two to three finger widths. Note any pain, decreased range, catching, or difficulty with movement. Side-to-side movement should be equal bilaterally.

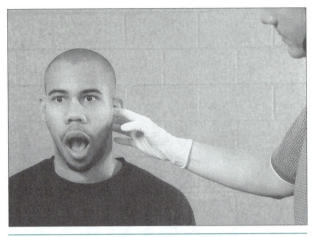

Figure 19.19   Palpation of the temporomandibular joint.

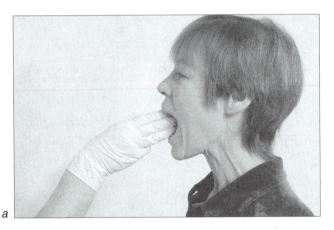

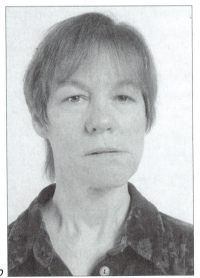

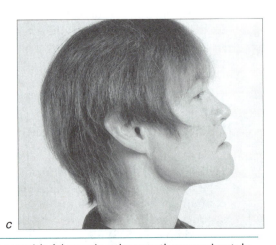

Figure 19.20   Active ROM of jaw movement with *(a)* opening the mouth approximately 2 to 3 finger widths, *(b)* moving the jaw side to side, and *(c)* protruding the mandible.

Active ROM of Eye Movements

Examine eye movement bilaterally, noting any motion restrictions, difficulty in tracking, or bilateral differences. Ask the patient to track your finger superiorly, inferiorly, and side to side. To test the various ocular muscles, have the patient look side to side, up and outward, down and outward, up and inward, and down and inward (figure 19.21, a-c). The eyes should move together, smoothly tracking your finger with ease and without head movement.

Active Movement of Facial Muscles

Perform active motion testing of the facial muscles to determine muscle function. Have the patient open and close the eyelids, smile, frown, wrinkle the forehead, protrude the tongue and move it side to side, and purse the lips. Some of these motions serve as the primary test for specific cranial nerves (see table 19.1).

Neurovascular Examination

Use neurovascular examination for the head and face primarily when you suspect brain trauma. These tests examine cranial nerve function, the presence of a brain lesion, and the development of intracranial hemorrhage. Concern for an associated cervical injury also warrants a neurological examination of the cervical and brachial plexuses.

Cranial Nerve Function

A cranial nerve check examines the integrity of each of the 12 cranial nerves. The name, function, and appropriate test for each cranial nerve are presented in table 19.1. If any one cranial nerve test produces a positive sign, you should suspect serious brain trauma and refer the patient for emergency care immediately.

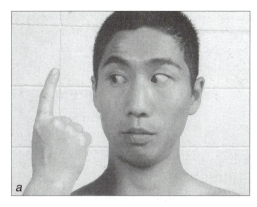

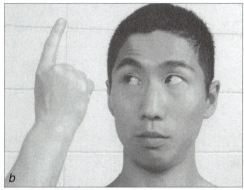

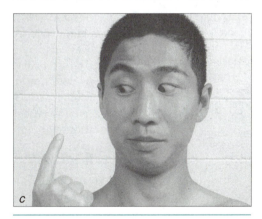

Figure 19.21   Active ROM of eye movement (a) side to side, (b) up and to the side (right eye) and up and inward (left eye), and (c) down and to the side (right eye) and down and inward (left eye).

Upper Motor Neuron Lesion

The tests described in chapter 8 (table 8.4) for upper motor neuron lesions are used to confirm a brain lesion. As previously discussed, signs and symptoms associated with an upper motor neuron lesion include hemiplegia, paraplegia, or quadriplegia, depending on the injury's extent and location, and may also include loss of voluntary control, spasticity, sensory loss, and abnormal superficial and pathological reflexes. When the brain is the source of the lesion, you will usually note these symptoms bilaterally.

Superficial reflexes are cutaneous reflexes that are elicited by stimulating the skin over areas where the central nervous system mediates movement. Examine superficial reflexes for upper motor neuron lesions by lightly stroking the skin with a pointed object (e.g., the sharp end of a reflex hammer). An absent superficial reflex indicates an upper motor neuron lesion. **Pathological reflexes** such as those examined in the Babinski, Chaddock, Gordon, and Oppenhiem tests (chapter 8, table 8.4) are also mediated by the central nervous system; for these tests, however, the presence of the reflex is considered a positive test for an upper motor neuron lesion.

Associated Cervical Spine Pathology

Perform sensory and motor testing of the cervical and brachial plexuses if you suspect an associated cervical spine injury with any head trauma. These tests are consistent with those previously discussed for injuries to the cervical spine (chapter 11, table 11.3) and are described in detail in chapter 8, tables 8.5 and 8.6 and figures 8.3, 8.4, 8.5, 8.7, and 8.9.

Vascular Compromise

Vascular examination includes tests that detect intracranial bleeding. Test pulse, blood pressure, and respirations as soon as possible following a head injury and then retest periodically to monitor the progression of any cardiorespiratory symptoms. Chapter 9 covers the examination of vital signs in detail.

Special Tests

Special tests for the head and face include those that examine neurological and cognitive deficits following head injury, that monitor postconcussion symptoms, that identify facial fractures, and that examine the eyes, ears, and nose for trauma.

Neurocognitive Tests

⚠ Failure to note deficits during cognitive tests does not rule out neurological dysfunction. Consider the results in conjunction with the overall findings of your objective and subjective examinations.

Neurocognitive testing determines cognitive function for immediate memory, delayed memory, and concentration. According to some researchers, athletes with mild head injury do not always display significantly poorer performance on neuropsychological tests than the uninjured controls display (Guskiewicz et al. 1997). Failure to note deficits during these cognitive tests does not in itself rule out neurological dysfunction, and you should consider the results in conjunction with the overall findings of your objective and subjective examinations. However, if you observe profound confusion or memory loss, or if the athlete shows signs of deterioration, immediately refer him to a physician for further examination.

Retrograde Amnesia Examination

Retrograde amnesia is determined through questions testing the patient's ability to remember or recall events that occurred just prior to the injury. Retrograde amnesia may range from not remembering the injury event to a total loss of orientation to person, self, place, and time (orientation × 4). Although any list of questions works, it is helpful to develop a standard list of questions that focus on recalling recent events; using the same questions allows you to compare the patient's responses over time. Order the questions so that they deal first with the injury event and progress back in time to activities immediately before injury, then to earlier in the day, and then to the previous day. Repeat the questions every 5 to 15 minutes following injury and then daily during the recovery process to check whether memory is improving or worsening. A positive sign for retrograde amnesia is any loss of memory, and severity is based on how far back the loss of memory extends.

Anterograde Amnesia Examination (Five-Object Recall)

Examination of **anterograde amnesia** concerns the patient's immediate memory and ability to recall events that have occurred since the injury. Anterograde amnesia may lead to decreased attention and inaccurate perception (Cantu 2001). A **five-object recall** test examines for anterograde amnesia through the verbal presentation of five unrelated objects (e.g., baby, dog, perfume, sunset, hammer). To examine immediate memory, instruct the patient that you are going to test her memory and read a list of five words. When finished, ask the patient to repeat back to you as many words as she can remember. Then have her perform the same task two more times, each time repeating as many words as she can recall. Note any incorrect response or missed word. To examine delayed recall, wait 2 to 5 minutes and then ask the patient to recall the list of words that you read a few minutes earlier. Record any missed or incorrect word. For either test, an incorrect response or an inability to remember the words is a positive sign.

Digit Span Test

A digit span test can consist of a one- or two-part protocol that determines concentration and immediate memory recall. Tell the patient that you are going to read him a series of numbers. When finished, ask him to repeat the series of digits in the same order (part one) and in reverse order (part two). Start with a string of 3 numbers and progress on successive trials to strings of 4, 5, and 6 numbers. If the patient responds correctly on one string, proceed to the next string, which will include one more number. If he responds incorrectly, repeat the test using the same string length but a different set of numbers. Record the number of successful trials. The Weschler Digit Span Test (Psychological Corporation, San Antonio, TX) is a digit span test that is commonly used in neuropsychological testing following mild head injury (Guskiewicz, Ross, and Marshall 2001).

Serial 7 Test

The serial 7 test examines concentration and analytical skills. Ask the patient to count backward from 100 to 0 in increments of seven (i.e., 100, 93, 86, 79, and so on). Inability to perform this or similar math skills is a positive sign.

Standardized Assessment of Concussion (SAC)

The **Standardized Assessment of Concussion (SAC)** is a valuable tool for examining the immediate and prolonged effects of mild head injury on mental status, and it tracks symptom resolution over time to assist with informed decisions on return to play (McCrea 2001). The SAC may help you pick up subtle deficits that may not otherwise be readily detected when injury occurs without loss of consciousness, posttraumatic amnesia, or gross neurological abnormalities. It requires no equipment, so it can be used on the sideline immediately following injury. When postinjury measurements were compared to preinjury baseline tests, the SAC had a reported 95% sensitivity and 76% specificity in accurately classifying injured and uninjured athletes examined on the sidelines (McCrea 2001). The SAC is not intended as a stand-alone concussion examination or a measurement of readiness to return to play. Rather, it provides a standardized, quantifiable measurement of neurocognitive abnormalities that complements other aspects of the concussion examination, including postconcussive symptom reports, neuropsychological examination, and postural stability testing.

The SAC test examines orientation, immediate memory, concentration, and delayed recall and can be used for both acute and follow-up examination of mild head injury. The athlete answers a series of questions, a check is placed by each correct answer, and the checks are then totaled for each section and for the complete assessment (refer to the SAC checklist on page 532). Exertional maneuvers, also included in the assessment, are used only during follow-up examination when the athlete is ready to simulate sport participation. Never use exertional maneuvers when the athlete is clearly dazed or is already exhibiting signs and symptoms of head injury.

Dr. Jeffrey Barth of the University of Virginia adds his own neurological questions to the SAC checklist (see Neurological Questions) on page 533.

STANDARDIZED ASSESSMENT OF CONCUSSION (SAC)

1. ORIENTATION

Month: _____ 0 1

Date: _____ 0 1

Day of week: _____ 0 1

Year: _____ 0 1

Time (within 1 hour): _____ 0 1

Orientation total score: _____ / 5

2. IMMEDIATE MEMORY

(All 3 trials are completed regardless of score on trial 1 and 2; total score equals sum across all 3 trials.)

List	Trial 1	Trial 2	Trial 3
Word 1	0 1	0 1	0 1
Word 2	0 1	0 1	0 1
Word 3	0 1	0 1	0 1
Word 4	0 1	0 1	0 1
Word 5	0 1	0 1	0 1
Total	0 1	0 1	0 1

Immediate memory total score: ____ / 15

(Note: Subject is not informed of delayed recall testing of memory.)

NEUROLOGICAL SCREENING:

Loss of consciousness: (occurrence, duration)
Pre- and posttraumatic amnesia: (recollection of events pre- and postinjury)

Strength:

Sensation:

Coordination:

3. CONCENTRATION

Digits backward. (If correct, go to next string length. If incorrect, read trial 2. Stop after incorrect on both trials.)

4-9-3	6-2-9 _____	0	1
3-8-1-4	3-2-7-9 _____	0	1
6-2-9-7-1	1-5-2-8-6_____	0	1
7-1-8-4-6-2	5-3-9-1-4-8_____	0	1

Months in reverse order: (entire sequence correct for 1 point)

Dec-Nov-Oct-Sept-Aug-July
June-May-Apr-Mar-Feb-Jan _____ 0 1

Concentration total score: _____ / 5

EXERTIONAL MANEUVERS:

(when appropriate)

5 jumping jacks   5 push-ups
5 sit-ups   5 knee-bends

4. DELAYED RECALL

Word 1   0   1

Word 2   0   1

Word 3   0   1

Word 4   0   1

Word 5   0   1

Delayed recall total score: _____ / 5

SUMMARY OF TOTAL SCORES:

Orientation _____ / 5

Immediate memory_____ / 15

Concentration _____ / 5

Delayed recall _____ / 5

Overall total score _____ / 30

Neurological Questions

Neurological Part A

Vomiting present	Yes ____
Dizziness present	Yes ____
Normal pupil reaction to light	No ____
Normal eye tracking	No ____
Equal pupil size	No ____
Finger to nose 5 ×	No ____
Heel to toe 10 steps	No ____

Neurological Part B

Nausea (since head injury)	Yes ____
Headache (since head injury)	Yes ____

Neuropsychological Test Battery

While not conducive to acute testing, more sophisticated neuropsychological tests can be performed in the athletic training facility, comparing preinjury baseline examination results to postinjury recovery scores. While a number of these tests are available, a few of the more common tests for mild head injuries are described briefly in this chapter.

Trail-Making Tests A and B

Trail-Making Tests A and B (Halstead-Reitan Neuropsychological Test Battery, Reitan Neuropsychological Laboratory; Tucson, AZ) examine visual and auditory attention as well as information-processing speed. For Trail-Making Test A, the patient must trace 25 numbers sequentially on a piece of paper, and the time to completion is recorded. A modification of this scoring system adds 1 additional second for each sequential error committed (Guskiewicz, Ross, and Marshall 2001). Trail-Making Test B further challenges working memory and processing speed by having the patient connect numbers (1-13) and alphabet (A-L), in alternating, sequential order.

Stroop Color Word Test

The Stroop Color Word Test (Stoelting Company; Wood Dale, IL) takes approximately 5 minutes to complete and tests cognitive flexibility and attention. The test consists of three components: a word page with the names of colors printed in black ink; a color page with meaningless symbols (X) printed in colored ink; and a word and color page with the names of colors printed in colors that match the color names. The patient moves down the columns of each sheet, reading words or naming the ink colors as quickly as possible within a given time limit (e.g., 45 seconds). The test yields three scores based on the number of items completed on each component. In addition, you can calculate an interference score, which is useful in determining the athlete's cognitive flexibility, creativity, and reaction to cognitive stress.

Hopkins Verbal Learning Test—Revised (HVLT-R)

The Hopkins Verbal Learning Test (John Hopkins University; Baltimore, MD) examines verbal memory and learning. The test consists of a list of 12 nouns that fit into three categories. The list is read to the patient one word every 2 seconds and the patient is asked to immediately recall as many of the words as possible, in any order. This task is repeated two more times and the total number of correct words recalled over the three trials is recorded. Delayed recall is examined by asking the patient to recall the word list after a 20-minute delay.

Balance and Coordination Tests

Balance and coordination tests examine brain function through the patient's ability to maintain postural equilibrium. Although there are sophisticated computer devices for examining postural control and coordination, the more common field tests available for the sideline examination include the Romberg, modified Romberg, Balance Error Scoring System, heel-to-toe walking, heel-to-knee, and finger-to-nose tests.

Romberg Test

The traditional Romberg test identifies cerebellum dysfunction by examining balance and equilibrium. The patient performs the test with the feet together, eyes closed, and arms at the sides (figure 19.22). In this position, the patient should be able to stand stationary with minimal postural sway. A positive sign occurs if the patient substantially sways or loses his balance.

Modified Romberg Test

Many variations of the Romberg test have been employed to examine postural equilibrium. A common modification has the patient standing with the legs shoulder-width apart, eyes closed, arms stretched out, and head tilted back (figure 19.23). You can make the test more challenging by having the patient (1) stand in tandem (heel to toe), (2) lift one leg off the ground, or (3) touch his finger to his nose. A positive sign is excessive sway or loss of balance.

Balance Error Scoring System (BESS) Test

The challenge with the Romberg and the Modified Romberg tests is to objectively score excessive sway or loss of balance. The Balance Error Scoring System, or BESS, is a more objective, clinical postural stability examination that you can perform on the sidelines without sophisticated equipment. The test was first validated and proved reliable on healthy subjects (Reimann, Guskiewicz, and Shields 1999), then later was found to be sensitive to postural deficits following mild head injury when compared to preseason baseline measures and matched controls (Guskiewicz, Ross, and Marshall 2001).

The test consists of three stance variations of the standard Romberg test: narrow double-leg stance, single-leg stance with the opposite limb in about 20° of hip flexion and 45° of knee flexion, and a tandem (heel-to-toe) stance. The patient performs each of these stances in order of increasing difficulty on two surfaces (a firm surface and a 46 cm² (7 in.²) piece of foam of medium density) for a total of six testing conditions (figure 19.24). For each condition, the patient stands as still as possible while keeping the eyes closed and resting the hands on the iliac crests for 20 seconds. If she loses her balance during the course of the 20-second trials, she is instructed to regain her balance and return to the original test position as soon as possible. Time begins when the patient closes the eyes, and the test is scored by counting the number of balance errors that occur through the course of each 20-second trial (see Scoring for BESS). Before testing, patients are informed how to perform each stance and how errors are scored.

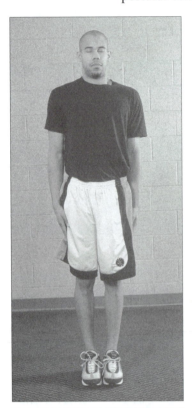

Figure 19.22 Romberg test.

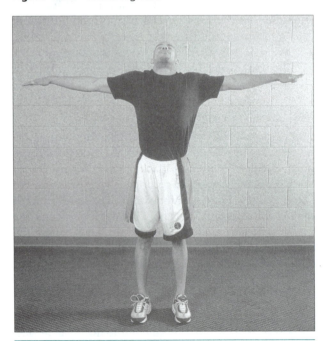

Figure 19.23 Modified Romberg test.

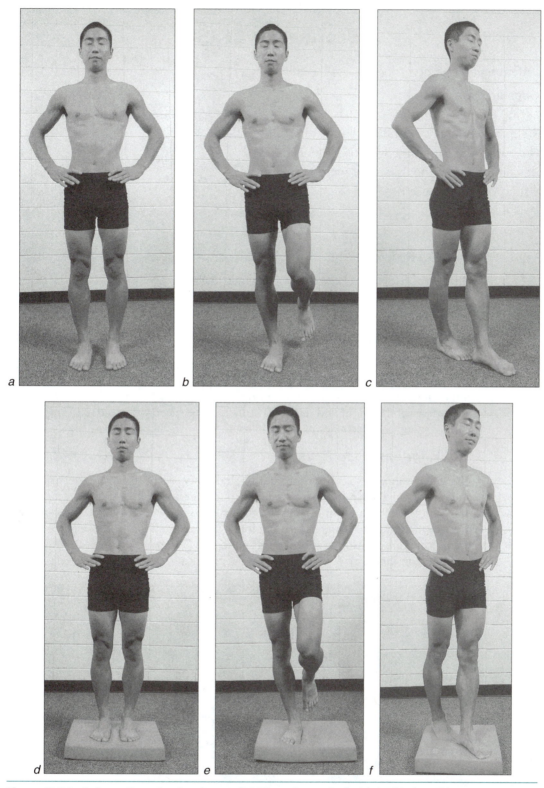

Figure 19.24 Balance Error Scoring System (BESS) testing order is *(a)* double-leg, *(b)* single-leg, and *(c)* tandem stance on a firm surface and then *(d)* double-leg, *(e)* single-leg, and *(f)* tandem stance on a foam surface.

535

Scoring for BESS

The patient scores one point for each of the following errors:

- Opening the eyes
- Lifting the hands off the iliac crests
- Stepping, stumbling, or falling out of the stance
- Flexing or abducting the hip more than 30°
- Remaining out of the stance for more than 5 seconds
- Lifting the forefoot or heel

Heel-to-Toe (Tandem) Walking

Having the patient walk a straight line with a heel-to-toe gait is another way to examine balance and equilibrium (figure 19.25). Inability to walk a straight line, unsteadiness, or loss of balance is considered a positive test.

Heel-to-Knee Test

If the patient is supine, you can determine coordination by having him touch the heel of one foot to the opposite knee (figure 19.26). The patient performs the test with his eyes open and then with his eyes closed. You can repeat the test by having the patient alternate movement between the right and left sides at increasing speeds. A positive sign is any difference in movement between sides or an inability to perform the task smoothly and efficiently.

Finger-to-Nose Tests

To examine upper-extremity coordination, have the patient stand with the arms outstretched and eyes open. Then ask her to alternately touch her nose with her left and right index finger, first with the eyes open and then with the eyes closed (figure 19.27). You can make the test more challenging by having the patient touch her nose and then your finger as you move your finger from one position to another in front of her. Compare the results of the test bilaterally; coordination difficulty or a difference between sides is a positive sign.

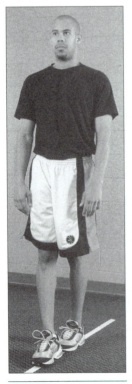

Figure 19.25 Heel-to-toe (tandem) walking.

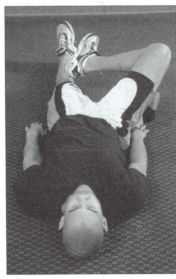

Figure 19.26 Supine heel-to-knee test.

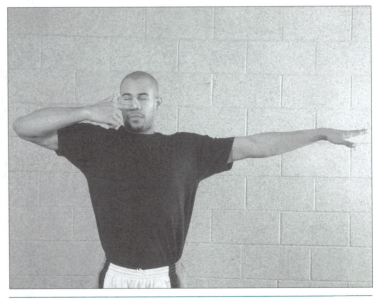

Figure 19.27 Finger-to-nose test.

Postconcussion Symptom Checklist

Postconcussion symptom checklists are used to document and compare over time the subjective reports of the athlete (Cantu 2001; Oliaro, Anderson, and Hooker 2001). You can administer the test in the preseason to gain baseline data, administer it again at the time of injury, and then again in the hours and days following injury. The athlete rates each checklist symptom on a scale of 0 (none) to 6 (severe). Table 19.3 provides a sample checklist.

Tests for Facial Fractures

Blunt trauma to the face can result in a variety of fractures. The following tests will assist you in identifying facial fractures.

Table 19.3
Postconcussion Symptom Checklist
Check all that apply.

Symptom	Preseason	Time of injury	2-3 hour follow-up	1 day follow-up
Headache				
Dizziness				
Drowsiness				
Fatigue				
Difficulty sleeping				
Excessive sleep				
Depression				
Nausea				
Vomiting				
Tinnitus (ringing in ears)				
Difficulty with balance				
Sensitivity to noise				
Sensitivity to light				
Blurred vision				
Difficulty concentrating				
Impaired memory				
Sadness				
Irritability				
Nervousness				
Change in eating habits				

*Rate symptoms on a 0 (= none) to 6 (= severe) scale.

Bite Test

To examine for malocclusion or pain caused by fracture or dislocation, have the patient bite down on a tongue blade (figure 19.28). Positive signs include pain, weakness, and malocclusion of the jaw and teeth with biting.

Maxillary Fracture Test

Gently moving the upper jaw while stabilizing the forehead can help you identify a possible maxillary fracture (figure 19.29). Positive signs include pain, mobility, and crepitus.

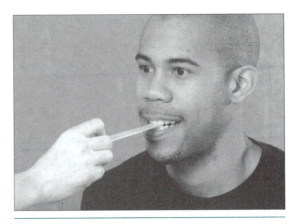

Figure 19.28 Bite test.

Percussion or Vibration Tests

Applying percussion or vibration to any bone can help you determine a fracture. Percussion and vibration tests include applying a tuning fork or gently tapping the orbit, cheekbone, or mandible away from the area of tenderness. A positive sign occurs when the patient feels pain at the site of injury.

Examination of the Eyes, Ears, and Nose

On occasion, your examination may require that you test the integrity of senses for sight, hearing, and smell. Other information can be gained by visually inspecting the interior structures of the eyes, ears, and nose.

Vision

A Snellen eye chart, named after Dutch ophthalmologist Herman Snellen, is relatively inexpensive and simple to use. It lists 11 lines of letters in decreasing size from top to bottom (figure 19.30). Modified charts may use numbers or a tumbling E chart for which patients must identify the direction

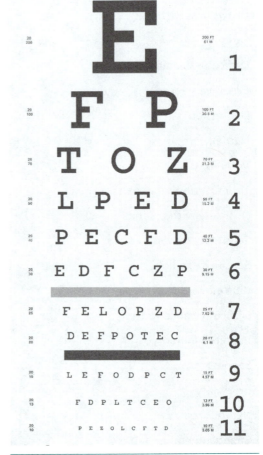

Figure 19.30 Snellen eye chart.

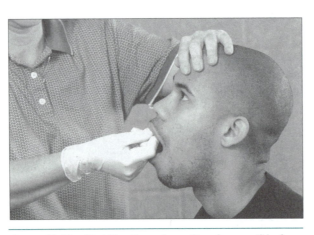

Figure 19.29 Mobilization of maxillae for possible fracture. Wear gloves when palpating mouth structures.

that the "E" faces (up, down, right, or left). To test visual acuity, position the patient 20 feet (6 m) in front of the Snellen eye chart. Test each eye individually by covering the other, and also test both eyes together. Each line represents an acuity fraction typically ranging from 20/20 to 20/200, and the patient is scored based on the lowest line he can clearly read from 20 feet away. Normal vision is considered 20/20. A visual acuity of 20/50 indicates the patient can read from 20 feet what a person with normal acuity (20/20 vision) can read from 50 feet. Immediately refer any patient showing a loss of visual acuity or blurred or double vision to an ophthalmologist for further examination.

If a Snellen chart is not readily available, you can grossly examine visual acuity by having the patient read the scoreboard for distance vision. You can test near vision acuity by having the patient identify the number of fingers you hold in front of her.

Interior Eye Examination Using an Ophthalmoscope

An **ophthalmoscope** (figure 19.31) is an instrument used in a routine eye exam to detect injury or disease in the interior structures of the eye. It consists of a light source combined with a set of lenses of graded focal lengths designed to inspect the structures of the eyeball. The lenses are calibrated so that shorter (black scale, positive values from 0 to +16) and longer focal lengths (red scale, negative values) can be used to isolate the various structures by moving them in and out of focus. With experience, you will become familiar with the various scale settings and which focal length best visualizes each structure. In general, shorter focal lengths focus on structures in the anterior globe (e.g., lens and cornea) while longer focal settings exam-

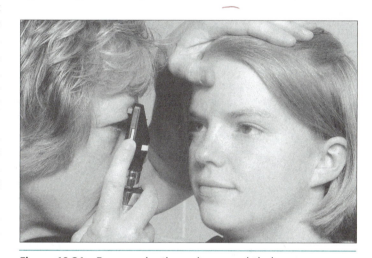

Figure 19.31   Eye examination using an ophthalmoscope.

ine the internal structures (e.g., retina and optic nerve). There are two types of ophthalmoscopes, direct and indirect. In the clinical setting, you will more commonly use the direct ophthalmoscope, a handheld instrument with a light source that is battery powered.

To examine the internal structures of the eye, hold the instrument in one hand, keeping the index finger free to manipulate the focal length, beginning with the lens setting at zero. To examine the right eye, sit on the right side of the patient and use one hand to stabilize the forehead and the other to hold the instrument. The room should be dimly lit during examination, and the ophthalmoscope should be approximately 3 in. (7.6 cm) from the eye surface. Resting your hand on the patient's cheek may help you maintain a steady hand and the correct distance from the eye surface. With the patient holding her gaze at a stationary point on the far wall, view the retina through the pupil using your right eye. A minor adjustment in the focal length should bring the retina into focus. A nearsighted patient requires a more negative setting to focus deeper into the elongated globe; the opposite is true for a farsighted patient (Munger and Baird 1980). The optic disc, retina, and blood vessels should all appear normal. Understanding the appearance of normal is best accomplished through practice with a trained professional.

To examine structures in the anterior globe, increase the setting to approximately +6 to bring the lens into focus, and progressively increase magnification to +15 to view structures through the anterior chamber, including the cornea (Munger and Baird 1980). Note any inconsistencies or evidence of debris. As with the internal structures, practice with a trained professional will develop your examination skills.

Smell and Breathing

Loss of smell or difficulty breathing can occur with epistaxis and nasal fractures, but smell and breathing should return to normal once bleeding and swelling subside. Loss of smell can also result from injury to the first cranial nerve (olfactory) and may be evidence of brain trauma. To determine the presence of smell, have the patient close both eyes and describe or identify a particular scent that you wave under the nose. The scent should be one that the patient is familiar with and able to identify under normal circumstances.

Hearing

Transient hearing loss is common with blows to the head or ear, but hearing should return to normal shortly following injury. Sustained hearing loss may indicate rupture of the tympanic membrane, infection, swelling, or impacted cerumen. You can examine diminished or loss of hearing bilaterally by rubbing two fingers together or by snapping your fingers beside the patient's ear. Patients with lost or diminished hearing in one ear may turn their head while you speak to align the good ear with the direction of the sound. Whenever loss of hearing persists or is profound, you should refer the patient to a physician for further examination.

Inner Ear Examination Using an Otoscope

An **otoscope** (figure 19.32) is a light source combined with a magnifying lens and specula used to examine the inner ear. The specula are usually disposable for hygienic purposes and adjustable in size to accommodate adults and children. The examiner holds the otoscope with the hand corresponding with the ear to be examined.

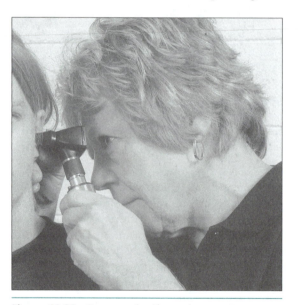

First inspect the outer ear for swelling and other abnormalities. Use your free hand to grasp the outer aspect of the ear, gently pulling it upward, backward, and outward to allow you to view the canal and eardrum. Be careful to introduce the speculum gently into the canal to avoid friction or pressure, as the canal is very sensitive and rough insertion may cause pain or a gag or cough reflex. Note the condition of the skin, evidence of foreign bodies, redness, or swelling in the canal. If the canal is clear, you can observe the tympanic membrane (eardrum) as a pale or grayish structure deep in the canal that is pulled inward at its center by the malleus. Inspect the membrane for evidence of scarring, which appears as a white, thickened area, or signs of erythema, a pattern of small blood vessels that indicates inflammation (Munger and Baird 1980).

As with use of the ophthalmoscope, considerable practice is required to distinguish normal from abnormal findings. Refer patients if you note swelling, redness or disruption of the external canal and ear drum, excessive wax occluding the canal, and excessive swelling trapped in the external ear (pinna).

Figure 19.32   Ear examination using an otoscope.

INJURY EXAMINATION STRATEGIES

A major blow to an athlete's head or chin should immediately arouse suspicion of potential head injury. When examining potential head injuries, your concern is not only whether the athlete exhibits any characteristic signs and symptoms, but also whether the signs and symptoms change or worsen over time. Your observation skills must be particularly keen in this examination, as the behavior and response of the athlete provide important clues to injury severity.

The examination portion of this chapter is divided into on-site and acute examination of head injury and acute examination of facial injuries. The on-site examination of facial injuries is similar to that for head injury, as your primary concern on-site is identifying life threatening conditions and the need to rule out brain trauma. Clinical examination for head and facial injuries is essentially the same as the acute examination; thus instead of clinical examination guidelines, the discussion presents information on the follow-up examination for head injuries. In fact, in any clinical or follow-up examination, you should deliberately use the same examination techniques used in your on-site and acute examination so that you can compare your findings over time and determine whether the athlete's symptoms have improved or worsened.

On-Site Examination of Head Injury

The men's ice hockey match against the cross-town rival was rougher than usual, and the referees did not seem to be doing much to curtail the rough bodychecking. Late in the second period, Patrick was checked hard by an opponent, sending him crashing into the boards headfirst. He slumped to the ice and appeared to be unconscious.

Elyse was a hard-charging guard for Western High School. While running a two-on-one fast break, she went up for a lay-up and was knocked off balance by her defender. As she landed hard on the court, you could audibly hear her head bounce off the floor. She attempted to stand, but then laid back down on the court, holding her head.

You should begin on-site examination of a suspected head injury with a primary survey to immediately determine the athlete's level of consciousness and the presence of life-threatening conditions. Throughout the acute examination, you should closely monitor vital signs, level of consciousness, and signs and symptoms of intracranial hemorrhage.

Primary Survey

As you approach the athlete, note the environment and surroundings and check for any potential hazards that may place the athlete at risk for further injury. Also note the position and any response of the athlete.

Establish Level of Consciousness

Treat any unconscious athlete with a suspected head injury as if he has a cervical spine injury until there is proof of the contrary. Stabilize the head and neck throughout the examination process.

An athlete with a head injury may range from conscious, coherent, and ambulatory to completely unconscious and unresponsive; your initial goal is to establish the level of consciousness. Determine the baseline level of consciousness by observing the athlete's eye opening and motor and verbal response to a verbal command or pain stimulus. Many use the Glasgow Coma Scale to objectively communicate an athlete's level of consciousness (table 19.4). If the athlete does not respond spontaneously or to verbal commands, use a pain stimulus to evoke a response or arouse the athlete by applying supraorbital pressure just below the eyebrow, by rubbing your knuckle on the sternum, or by pinching the upper trapezius or inner aspect of the arm. The point system of the Glasgow Coma Scale, based on the athlete's response, provides both an initial determination of level of consciousness and a means of monitoring changes in level of consciousness over time.

Examine Vital Signs

If the athlete is moving and immediately speaks to you, you are assured that airway, breathing, and circulation are present. However, if the athlete is unconscious, you should immediately examine vital signs. As with any unconscious athlete, suspect a cervical spine injury and immobilize the head and neck throughout your examination. If it is necessary to move the athlete to appropriately examine or care for him, you must follow cervical spine precautions. When establishing an airway, you should use a modified jaw thrust.

Table 19.4
Glasgow Coma Scale
Rate best response in each category

Eye opening		
Spontaneous	4	
In response to voice	3	
In response to pain	2	
Does not open eyes	1	
		Score _____
Verbal response		
Oriented and easily converses	5	
Confused, but converses	4	
Inappropriate words	3	
Incomprehensible words	2	
No verbal response	1	
		Score _____
Motor response		
Obeys verbal commands	6	
Localized pain	5	
Withdraws from pain	4	
Abnormal flexion response (decorticate rigidity)	3	
Abnormal extension response (decerebrate rigidity)	2	
No pain response	1	
		Score _____
Total score	15	_____

- **Respirations** are examined for presence, rate, depth, and rhythm. Respiration is influenced by many parts of the brain and is a key vital sign that should be checked before anything else. Shock produces rapid and shallow respirations; in contrast, intracranial hemorrhage causes slow and irregular respirations. You may also observe Cheyne-Stokes respiration, characterized by a rhythmic fluctuation between rapid, deep breathing (hypernea) and slow or absent breathing (apnea).

- Examine **pulse** for presence, strength, rate, and rhythm. A rapid pulse may be the result of the level of exercise just prior to injury, or it may indicate shock or increased pressure at the base of the brain. A decreased (less than 60 beats per minute), bounding pulse indicates intracranial hemorrhage.

- You should also take **blood pressure**. A rise in blood pressure (hypertension) occurs with intracranial hemorrhage due to a compensatory response by the body to maintain blood flow through the brain as intracranial pressure increases. The blood pressure response to shock is hypotension—opposite that for intracranial hemorrhage.

Other Immediate Observations

As with any primary examination, you should immediately observe and care for any severe bleeding and shock. As just mentioned, signs and symptoms of shock are essentially the opposite of those for an intracranial hemorrhage. Shock rarely develops from head injury alone and usually indicates that other trauma also exists. Although you will examine pupillary reflexes and for any evidence of lateralizing signs or unusual posturing (decorticate, decerebrate) in the secondary survey, your primary observation should also include these. If the athlete remains unconscious or exhibits any positive signs, summon emergency medical services (EMS) immediately. While waiting for EMS to respond, continually monitor vital signs and reexamine the patient every 5 minutes.

Secondary Survey

If there is no immediate evidence of life-threatening injury, proceed with the secondary survey. In the on-site examination of a suspected head injury, the secondary survey includes history, observation, palpation, and neurological examination.

History

If the athlete is unconscious, ask bystanders what happened to get a sense of the mechanism of injury as well as the direction and point of contact. If the athlete is conscious, ask about the mechanism of injury and find out whether she recalls losing consciousness; also include questions about the location, type, and severity of symptoms and any unusual sensations or feelings. Unusual sensations may include ringing in the ears (tinnitus), headache, or dizziness. Before moving the athlete, be sure to ask whether there is any cervical pain or radiating symptoms into the extremities. If any of these symptoms are present, you should immobilize the head and neck and perform a cervical spine examination. Taking a history not only helps you determine the nature and severity of the symptoms, it also examines the athlete's orientation × 4 (place, person, self, and time). Although you will examine this more thoroughly on the sideline, the athlete's ability to articulate symptoms and recall what happened or whether loss of consciousness occurred will give you an initial impression of brain function.

Observation

Your on-site observation of the athlete should include a check for any immediate signs of skull fracture and brain trauma. Observe for unusual body movements (posturing) or unusual behavior. Check for unusual facial expressions such as drooling, drooping of one eyelid, or drooping of the corner of the mouth (lateralizing signs). Observe the athlete's level of consciousness and overall behavior. Is the athlete alert and responsive, or is the athlete restless, lethargic, or combative? Is the athlete aware of the surroundings, or is he dazed and confused? Your observation should also include an examination of eye movement and responsiveness. Check the pupils for size, equality left to right, and reaction to light. Specifically, the pupils should be equal in size and should constrict when a beam of light is shone in the eye. Examine both direct (same eye) and consensual (contralateral eye) reflex. Also observe for unusual eye movements that indicate cranial nerve pressure such as nystagmus (involuntary eye movement), lateral drift of one eye, or a downward and inward positioning of the eyes (cross-eye). If any of these signs are positive, you should assume serious brain injury and immediately summon EMS.

Also observe for swelling, deformity, discoloration, and bleeding or drainage from the nose or ears that would indicate a skull fracture. To determine whether drainage from the ears or nose contains cerebral spinal fluid, use gauze to absorb some of the drainage. If cerebral spinal fluid is present, a yellowish halo forms around the blood stain. Rhinorrhea (drainage from the nose) and raccoon eyes (discoloration around the eyes) may indicate a nasal fracture or a frontal skull fracture, while Battle's sign (discoloration behind the ears) and otorrhea (drainage from the ears) may indicate a basilar skull fracture. During your observation, continuously monitor the athlete's respiration and level of consciousness, carefully noting any changes from your earlier examination. If the symptoms change for the worse rather than improve, call EMS immediately.

Palpation

Carefully palpate the entire face and skull for tenderness, swelling, deformity, or depressions. If you find a depression or deformity on the skull, be very careful not to apply additional pressure to the area. With any deformities or depression, you should suspect a fracture. If the athlete is unconscious or incoherent, or is conscious and complains of cervical pain, you should also palpate the cervical spine for tenderness, swelling, and deformity.

Neurological Tests

The need to perform neurological tests on the field depends on your examination thus far. If you are still unsure of the athlete's condition and ability to ambulate off the field, perform a series of neurological tests. As described earlier in this chapter, neurological tests include those for checking cranial nerve integrity, detecting an upper motor neuron (brain) lesion, and screening the upper quarter if you need to rule out cervical spine injury. If you have not yet ruled out cervical spine injury, perform a cervical spine check for sensory and motor function. The procedures for the on-site examination of cervical spine injuries are appropriate here (see chapter 11). Also use general **motor tests** to determine unilateral weakness and the athlete's ability to respond to commands. Ask the athlete to move all four extremities. Note any pain, unwillingness to move, unusual movements, or inappropriate responses. You can examine upper- and lower-extremity strength quickly with bilateral grip strength and resisted dorsiflexion and plantar flexion strength tests. Any positive tests indicate neurological pathology and mean that the athlete should be immobilized and passively transported for emergency medical care.

Continuous Monitoring and Decision for Emergency Medical Referral

The condition of an athlete with a serious brain injury can quickly deteriorate, and death can occur within minutes. It is imperative that you monitor vital signs and level of consciousness every 5 minutes until you have ruled out serious head trauma or are sure the athlete is stabilized or improving. Even then, you should reexamine the athlete every 15 to 30 minutes. Because the athlete's condition can deteriorate so quickly, if you have any doubt as to the severity of the head trauma, you must not hesitate to seek emergency medical assistance. In addition to the positive signs already mentioned, any one of the following changes is reason for immediate referral:

- Decreasing level of consciousness (decreasing score on Glasgow Coma Scale)
- Increasing blood pressure
- Decreasing or irregular respirations
- Decreasing or irregular pulse
- Unequal, dilated, or unreactive pupil(s)

Acute Examination of Head Injury

Refer to the opening chapter scenario where it was initially determined that John had suffered a mild head injury. As Amanda continued to check John every 15 minutes on the sideline, she noticed that he was becoming increasingly lethargic, was less oriented to his surroundings and teammates, and was showing signs of unilateral weakness.

Acute examination of a potential head injury serves as a follow-up to the on-site examination, providing a more complete picture of neurological function. In some cases, your initial examination may take place on the sideline; for example, an athlete may suffer a mild head injury that goes unnoticed until she comes to you complaining of a headache—or until you, the coach, or teammates notice a change in the athlete's behavior or concentration. This scenario demonstrates the importance of constant alertness on the sidelines, particularly in contact sports, to signs and symptoms of unusual behavior in the athletes.

Checklist for On-Site Examination of Head Injury

▷ Primary Survey

☐ Check surroundings and environment and gain history of event as necessary from bystanders if you did not witness

When you reach the injured person, establish level of consciousness by checking:

☐ Eye opening

☐ Verbal response

☐ Motor response

If athlete is unconscious, immediately:

☐ Examine in the position found

☐ Check airway, breathing, and pulse (rate, rhythm, strength), and take blood pressure

☐ Observe and control severe bleeding

☐ Observe for lateralizing signs and evidence of decorticate or decerebrate posturing

☐ Examine pupillary reflexes

☐ Observe for shock (signs and symptoms opposite those of intracranial hemorrhage)

It is of utmost importance that you:

☐ Assume cervical spine injury until proven otherwise

☐ Summon EMS if you note any positive signs

☐ Reexamine vital signs every 5 minutes

▷ Secondary Survey

▷ History

If athlete is conscious, ask questions pertaining to the following:

☐ Mechanism of injury

☐ Loss of consciousness

☐ Location, type, and severity of symptoms

☐ Unusual sensations (tinnitus, dizziness, headache)

☐ Complaints of cervical pain or any radiating symptoms into extremities

☐ Orientation to time, person, place, and self

▷ Observation

☐ Unusual body movements or behavior

☐ Unusual facial expressions (drooling, drooping of one eyelid or corner of mouth)

☐ Level of consciousness (alert, restless, lethargic)

☐ Pupils for size, equality, and reaction to light

☐ Unusual eye movements (nystagmus, cross-eye, or lateral drift)

☐ Otorrhea, rhinorrhea

☐ Swelling, deformity, bleeding, or discoloration (Battle's sign, raccoon eyes)

☐ Continued monitoring vital signs (pulse, respirations, blood pressure, level of consciousness)

▷ Palpation

☐ Face and skull for tenderness, swelling, deformity, or depressions

☐ Cervical spine for tenderness, swelling, and deformity (as indicated)

▷ Neurological Tests

☐ Upper motor neuron lesions tests (table 8.4)

☐ Cranial nerve check (table 19.1)

☐ Cervical spine check

(continued)

(continued)

☐ Active ROM of all four extremities

☐ Grip strength and dorsiflexion strength

Continue to monitor vital signs every 5 minutes, and refer immediately if changes in the following:

☐ a. Level of consciousness (decrease)

☐ b. Blood pressure (increase)

☐ c. Pulse (decrease, irregular)

☐ d. Respiration (decrease, irregular)

☐ e. Pupils (unequal, dilated, unreactive)

If the athlete is stable and there are no signs of serious head injury, the athlete can be transported off-field with assistance as needed for a more thorough examination.

History

The history obtained on the sideline is essentially the same as that on the field but is more detailed. You should repeat the questions you asked the athlete on the field to examine memory before and after the injury event. Throughout the history portion of the examination, remember that you are also examining the athlete's cognitive function through her responses. You should question the athlete about previous head injuries and concussions, including the date of the most recent episode.

In investigating the mechanism of injury, ask the athlete about the point of contact and the activity he was engaged in when the injury occurred. Ask the athlete to recall recent events (e.g., describe the play the team was running); the answers will help you determine his memory function and the possible presence of **retrograde amnesia**. Also ask the athlete if he recalls losing consciousness, and if so, for how long. You can compare the athlete's recollection with your own observations or with those of other witnesses. If the athlete complains of unusual sensations such as tinnitus, dizziness, blurred vision, or headache, ask if these symptoms have improved or worsened since the injury occurred. A headache will almost always occur, and you should ask the athlete to describe the location and quality of the pain. Is the pain on the same side (coup mechanism) where the contact was made or on the opposite side (contrecoup mechanism)? Is the headache diffuse (concussion) or localized (skull contusion or fracture), or is it a pressure headache? If the athlete complains of an increasing headache, suspect intracranial edema and hemorrhage and closely observe the athlete for associated signs and symptoms.

The history portion of the acute examination should also include questions relating to the athlete's orientation to place, person, self, and time. To determine orientation to place, ask the athlete to tell you where the two of you are and what was going on at the time of injury. If the injury occurred during the game, have the athlete tell you the name of the opposing team and what the score is. To determine orientation to person, ask the athlete to identify you, a teammate, or a coach. Orientation to self is reflected in the athlete's response to her own name and her ability to tell you her age and birth date. Examine orientation to time by asking what period of play the game is in.

Once you have completed the history, you should have a better sense of the nature and severity of the injury, as well as an impression of the athlete's mental status in relation to memory and appropriateness of verbal response (confusion).

Observation

If the athlete left the field without assistance, observe for any unsteadiness or imbalance. Once on the sideline, visually inspect again for signs of otorrhea, rhinorrhea, Battle's sign, or raccoon eyes that indicate a skull fracture. Note any swelling, discoloration, deformity, or bleeding from the scalp that you may have previously overlooked. Look for obvious fracture by observing for bilateral symmetry of all facial structures and contours. Continue to observe for unusual body posturing, movement, or behavior that would indicate brain trauma. Note any signs such as nausea, vomiting, yawning, or unilateral weakness. If you are familiar with the athlete's normal behavior, note any changes in his attitude. Examples of unusual behavior include confusion, lethargy, restlessness, and aggressiveness, or the athlete may appear argumentative or repeat the same questions again and again. Observe facial expressions for drooping of the eyelid or of the corner of the mouth that would indicate cranial nerve dysfunction. Check appearance of the pupils bilaterally for size (dilation), equality, and shape. If any of these symptoms were present on the field, are they worse now, the same, or improved?

As in the on-site examination, you should closely observe the athlete's eyes for unusual movements and reaction to light. To further observe eye movement, ask the athlete to track your finger. Observe the movements of the eyes as they follow your finger superiorly, inferiorly, and left to right. Note any sluggishness, deviation from midline, difficulty in tracking, or nystagmus.

Your observational examination should continue throughout the entire examination process, including continuous monitoring of respirations for depth, rate, and rhythm.

Palpation

Palpation, which is the same as for the on-site examination, involves carefully palpating the skull and facial bones for evidence of trauma.

Neurovascular Tests

Neurological tests at the sideline are the same as on the field. Depending on the athlete's condition, you may perform them here for the first time or as follow-up to your on-site examination to note any change in the athlete's condition. You will use other special tests during the acute examination to examine postconcussion symptoms and neurological function in relation to cognition, balance, and coordination. You should also monitor pulse rate, strength, and rhythm periodically throughout the examination.

Special Tests

Special tests used to examine brain function are classified as

- cognitive tests for memory and concentration and
- tests of balance and coordination.

A postconcussion checklist will help you determine more objectively the severity of the athlete's reported symptoms and whether these symptoms improve or worsen over time. These tests are detailed on pages 537 through 540. Remain consistent in the administration of these tests to allow accurate examination with repeated testing over time. In an effort to improve the sensitivity of these tests to deficits following mild head injury, baseline measurements are often performed before the season begins in athletes engaging in sports at risk for head injury, so that a more reliable, within subject comparison can be made in the event of injury.

Repeated Testing

Reexamine vital signs, pupillary response, and level of consciousness every 15 to 30 minutes if the athlete is stable, or once every 5 minutes if the athlete is unstable, until serious head injury is ruled out. It is essential that you are able to differentiate the signs and symptoms of a concussion from those of an expanding intracranial lesion, as the latter indicates a life-threatening medical emergency and makes immediate referral imperative.

Referral Decision

When your examination shows only signs and symptoms of a concussion, your decision regarding referral will depend on the degree of injury. Any athlete who exhibits signs and symptoms of a first-degree concussion for longer than 5 minutes should be removed from activity for the remainder of the day and closely watched for increasing signs and symptoms. Any athlete exhibiting signs and symptoms of a second- or third-degree concussion should be removed from activity and referred to a physician for a medical examination regardless of duration or improvement of symptoms.

Checklist for Acute Examination of Head Injury

▷ History

- ☐ Previous head injuries
- ☐ Mechanism of injury and activity at time of injury
- ☐ Chief complaint
- ☐ Unusual sensations (tinnitus, dizziness, blurred vision, headache, unsteadiness)
- ☐ Location, type, and quality of pain (including headache symptoms)
- ☐ Loss of consciousness
- ☐ Orientation to place, person, self, and time

Throughout history, examine memory, appropriateness, and quality of verbal response.

▷ Observation

- ☐ Gait (unsteadiness, imbalance) if ambulated off-field
- ☐ Otorrhea, rhinorrhea, Battle's sign, raccoon eyes (skull fracture)
    - ☐ Halo effect for cerebral spinal fluid
- ☐ Swelling, deformity, discoloration, or bleeding of skull, scalp, or face
- ☐ Bilateral symmetry of facial structures
- ☐ Unusual body posturing (decerebrate, decorticate)
- ☐ Unusual movement (vomiting, seizures, yawning, unilateral weakness)
- ☐ Unusual behavior (violent, combative, argumentative, repeating questions, confused)
- ☐ Unusual facial expressions (drooping of eyelid or corner of mouth)
- ☐ Level of consciousness (alertness, restlessness, lethargy)
- ☐ Pupil appearance (size, shape, equality)
- ☐ Pupil reaction to light (consensual and direct light reflex)
- ☐ Unusual eye movement (nystagmus, tracking difficulty, deviation from midline)
- ☐ Continued observation of vital signs (respiration depth, rate, and rhythm)

▷ Palpation

Bilaterally palpate for pain, tenderness, and deformity over the following:

- ☐ Skull and face
- ☐ Continued monitoring of pulse rate

▷ Neurological Tests

- ☐ Cranial nerve check
- ☐ Bilateral grip strength

▷ Special Tests

- ☐ Standardized Assessment of Concussion (SAC)
- ☐ Other cognitive tests
    - ☐ Memory
    - ☐ Retrograde examination (memory of events prior to injury)
    - ☐ Anterograde examination (five-object immediate and delayed recall)
    - ☐ Concentration (Serial 7)
- ☐ Balance and coordination
    - ☐ BESS
    - ☐ Romberg test
    - ☐ Finger-to-nose test
    - ☐ Heel-to-toe walking
- ☐ Postconcussion checklist

Repeat testing of the following every 15-30 minutes if stable, every 5 minutes if unstable, until serious head injury is ruled out:
- ☐ Vital signs
- ☐ Pupils
- ☐ Level of consciousness

▷ *Functional Tests*

Performed only in cases in which athlete is otherwise symptom free under resting conditions.

Follow-Up (Clinical) Examination of Head Injury

Follow-up examination of mild head trauma during the first 24 to 48 hours after injury should include home instructions for the athlete and a roommate or family member to watch for signs and symptoms that indicate a worsening condition. It is useful to have a prepared instruction sheet that you can give to the person who will be staying with the athlete over the 24 to 48 hours following injury (see box below). Even in mild cases that appear to warrant little concern about serious brain injury, you should provide this information as a precaution, as signs of intracranial hemorrhage may be delayed or may progress slowly.

As already mentioned, clinical examination of head injuries should be the same as acute examination. Repeated testing is fundamental to the examination of head injury in order to determine whether symptoms are worsening, staying the same, or improving. It is helpful to have a standardized examination protocol that allows clear documentation of your examination and subsequent findings; this enables you or another health professional to make objective comparisons over time. Examples of standardized tests include the Standardized Assessment of Concussion (SAC) for determination of mental status (see page 532), daily examination of postconcussion symptoms (see page 537), and objective postural stability tests such as the BESS (see pages 534-536) or more sophisticated instrumented tests. You can perform each of these examinations before the season to gain a baseline measurement for each athlete by which to compare later injury. As previously noted, none of these tests are intended as a stand-alone concussion examination or return-to-play measurement; you should consider their results along with physical examination findings.

Take-Home Instructions for Head Injury

There are times when signs and symptoms of serious head injury may be delayed following injury; therefore it is important that you observe the athlete frequently over the next 24 to 48 hours for any changes in condition or behavior. Call your athletic trainer or team physician if you have any questions, and seek medical attention immediately if you note any of the following signs and symptoms:

- A severe headache that increases in intensity and pressure
- Vomiting more than 2 to 3 times
- Any evidence of seizures or unusual body movements
- Unilateral weakness or inability to move one or both arms and legs
- Changes in facial expressions
- Changes in behavior such as increased irritability, agitation, or restlessness
- Increased mental confusion or loss of memory
- Increased lethargy, decreased level of consciousness, or difficulty awakening
- Unusual eye movements or changes in size or position of one or both pupils
- Breathing rate that decreases below 12 breaths per minute or becomes irregular
- Pulse that decreases below 60 beats per minute or becomes irregular

! Never use exertional maneuvers to examine head injuries when the athlete is clearly dazed or is already exhibiting signs and symptoms.

Functional Tests

Functional tests enable you to determine whether the signs and symptoms of head injury have cleared and to establish the athlete's readiness to return to activity. Often, the athlete's symptoms (e.g., headache) dissipate under resting conditions but reappear with exercise. The SAC test initially provides for this functional examination by using exertional maneuvers of jumping jacks, push-ups, and crunches before cognitive and neurological testing. If symptoms are clear with these simple exercises, the athlete can perform activities more specific to his sport in progressively increased intensity and duration.

Criteria for Return to Play

The decision for return to play should be based on the subjective and objective findings of your follow-up examination and should always be made in concert with the team physician. While advancing research continues to identify more objective criteria for testing injury recovery through cognitive and balance testing, comparable evidence-based criteria do not exist. However, it is universally agreed that the athlete should be completely free of all signs and symptoms during both rest and exercise before returning to play. The length of rest mandated before the athlete returns to activity free of symptoms depends on the nature and severity of the injury, the duration of lingering symptoms, and the number of previous head injuries. Tables 19.5 and 19.6 provide sample lists of return-to-play guidelines established by Cantu (2001) and the University of North Carolina at Chapel Hill (Oliaro, Anderson, and Hooker 2001).

Until evidence-based criteria are established, exercise caution and err on the conservative side if you have any doubt about an athlete's readiness to return to participation. Athletes who exhibit signs and symptoms of a concussion greater than the first degree should always be examined and cleared by a physician before being allowed to return to play. This is particularly true of athletes who have suffered a previous head injury. It is recommended that the medical team (team physician, athletic trainer, and so on) meet periodically to review the current research on head injury and to develop and periodically update a written protocol for determining return to play based on current knowledge.

Table 19.5
Cantu Guidelines for Return to Play After Concussion

	First concussion	Second concussion	Third concussion
Grade 1 (mild)	May return to play if asymptomatic* for 1 week	Return to play in 2 weeks if asymptomatic for 1 week	Terminate season; may return to play next season if asymptomatic
Grade 2 (moderate)	Return to play after asymptomatic for 1 week	Minimum of 1 month; may then return to play if asymptomatic for 1 week; consider terminating season	Terminate season; may return to play next season if asymptomatic
Grade 3 (severe)	Minimum of 1 month; may then return to play if asymptomatic for 1 week	Terminate season; may return to play next season if asymptomatic	

*Asymptomatic in all cases means no postconcussion symptoms, including retrograde amnesia experienced at rest or with exertion.

Reprinted, by permission, from R.C. Cantu, 2001, Posttraumatic retrograde and anterograde amnesia: Pathophysiology and implications in grading and safe return to play. *Journal of Athletic Training* 36(3): 246.

Table 19.6
University of North Carolina Return to Play Guidelines After Concussion

Grade	Suggested action
0	Remove the athlete from contest. Examine immediately for abnormal cranial nerve function, cognition, or coordination or for other postconcussive symptoms at rest and with exertion. Athlete may return to contest if examination is normal and asymptomatic for 20 minutes. If any symptoms develop within 20 minutes, return that day is not permitted.
1	If athlete is removed from contest after developing symptoms, daily follow-up evaluations are necessary. Athlete may begin restricted participation when asymptomatic at rest and after exertional tests for 2 days. Unrestricted participation allowed if asymptomatic for 1 additional day and neuropsychological and balance testing normal.
2	Remove the athlete from contest and prohibit return that day. Examine immediately and at 5-minute intervals for evolving intracranial pathology. Reexamine daily. Athlete may return to restricted participation when athletic trainer and physician are assured the athlete has been asymptomatic at rest and with exertional testing for 4 days. Unrestricted participation if asymptomatic for an additional 2 days and performing restricted activities normally and comfortably.
3	Treat the athlete on field or court as if cervical spine injury has occurred. Immediate examination and reevaluation at 5-minute intervals for signs of intracranial pathology. Reexamine daily. Return is based on resolution of symptoms: 1. If symptoms totally resolve within first week, return to restricted participation when the athlete has been asymptomatic at rest and with exertion for 10 days. If asymptomatic for an additional 3 days of restricted activity, the athlete may return to full participation. 2. If symptoms do not resolve within the first week, the athlete may return to restricted participation when asymptomatic at rest and with exertion for 17 days. Return to unrestricted participation if asymptomatic an additional 3 days.

Note: If the athlete suffers a second concussion within 3 months of the first concussion, the athlete must be removed for twice the maximum time for the respective grade of concussion.

Reprinted, by permission, from S. Oliaro, S. Anderson, and D. Hooker, 2001, Management of cerebral concussion in sports: The athletic trainer's perspective. *Journal of Athletic Training* 36(3): 260.

NATA's Position Statement on Management of Sport-Related Concussion

Research in the area of sport-related concussion continues to evolve. In an effort to assist athletic training and medical professionals in the care and management of sport-related concussion, the National Athletic Trainers' Association recently published a position statement titled "Management of Sport-Related Concussion" (Guskiewicz et al. 2004). This document reflects the current knowledge and consensus in

- "Defining and Recognizing Concussion,"
- "Evaluating and Making the Return-to-Play Decision,"
- "Concussion Assessment Tools,"
- "When to Refer an Athlete to a Physician After Concussion,"
- "When to Disqualify an Athlete,"
- "Special Considerations for the Young Athlete,"
- "Home Care," and
- "Equipment Issues.

Examination of Facial Injuries

Tammy was pitching in her first NCAA regional softball championships. When she threw a fastball to the first batter in the third inning, the batter connected with a hard line drive that came straight back at Tammy. Unfortunately, Tammy was not able to get her glove up quickly enough, and the softball glanced off the tip of her glove and right into her nose.

Fran, the university women's basketball coach, was an avid recreational racquetball player. When meeting a colleague for a match after work, she realized she had forgotten her protective eyewear. She decided to play anyway and just be careful. Unfortunately, being careful did not prevent the ball from hitting her directly in the left eye following a hard return by her friend. She walked into the athletic training room in severe pain.

The goal of examining facial injuries is to determine the structures involved and the nature and severity of the injury. Whereas facial examination is presented here as a single, generic examination, your actual examination will be tailored to the athlete's complaint and your observations. Whenever an athlete sustains significant trauma to the face (i.e., nasal, maxillary, or mandible fracture), you should also maintain a high suspicion of associated head injury and should rule it out during your injury examination.

History

History should include typical questions addressing the mechanism of injury; the location, type, and quality of pain; unusual sounds or sensations; and previous injury. Since bleeding from the ears or nose and discoloration around the eyes and behind the ears can also result from skull fractures, determine the mechanism and the point of contact to the head or face. When you suspect eye or head trauma, you should also question the athlete about visual disturbances such as visual impairment, blurred vision, blind spots or decreased peripheral vision, flashes or floating spots (retinal detachment), and double vision (blow-out fracture). Also ask whether the athlete has any hearing loss, headache, dizziness, or tinnitus.

Observation

Visually inspect bilaterally for signs of swelling, discoloration, flattening, or deformity of the facial structures. Observe the facial structures in three planes: from in front of the athlete (frontal), from the side (lateral), and from a position above the head (superior) that allows you to see nose alignment. Facial structures including the forehead, cheeks, orbits, and jaw angles should be symmetrical, and the chin and nasal bones should be midline. Observe for any bleeding from the nose (nasal or maxillary fracture) or around the teeth (tooth, maxilla, or mandibular fracture). Note the position of the eyes bilaterally for symmetry and midline position. An eye that exhibits a downward gaze or sits lower than the other may indicate an orbital blow-out fracture. You should also closely inspect the eyes for any change in size or shape of the pupil and evidence of hyperemia or hyphema. When observing the mouth and jaw, note the position and alignment of the teeth, the position of the jaw, and any malocclusion during approximation of the upper and lower teeth. Inspect the ear and auditory canal for signs of infection, swelling, discoloration, and hematoma formation. Throughout the observation, you should also look for any signs and symptoms of head injury, including those relating to level of consciousness, body movements or posturing, and respirations.

Throughout the observation, you should check for any signs and symptoms of head injury, including those relating to level of consciousness, body movements or posturing, and respirations.

Palpation

Carefully palpate the soft tissue and bony structures of the skull, face, temporomandibular joint, and teeth for signs of swelling, deformity, crepitus, depression, and tenderness.

Checklist for Examination of Facial Injuries

▷ *History*

- ☐ Mechanism of injury
- ☐ Unusual sounds or sensations
- ☐ Location, type, and quality of pain
- ☐ Previous injury
- ☐ Complaints of impaired, blurred, or double vision
- ☐ Complaints of headache, dizziness, tinnitus (evidence of associated concussion)
- ☐ Complaints of loss of hearing

▷ *Observation*

- ☐ Swelling, deformity, flattening, or discoloration of facial structures
- ☐ Symmetry of facial structures
- ☐ Bleeding from nose or around teeth
- ☐ Position of eyes bilaterally
- ☐ Eyes for pupil size and shape, corneal surface, hyphema, hyperemia
- ☐ Jaw position, malocclusion
- ☐ Position and alignment of teeth
- ☐ External ear and auditory canal
- ☐ Signs and symptoms of head injury (particularly with blows to the jaw)
- ☐ Bilateral check

▷ *Palpation*

Bilaterally palpate for swelling, depressions, deformity, crepitus, and point tenderness:

- ☐ Forehead, orbital rim, zygomatic arch, maxilla, nasal bones, mandible
- ☐ Temporomandibular joint (clicking, locking, tenderness with movement)
- ☐ Soft tissue cartilage of the external ear
- ☐ Teeth for looseness, fracture

▷ *Special Tests*

- ☐ Examination of smell
- ☐ Examination of breathing (nasal passageway)
- ☐ Examination of hearing
- ☐ Examination of vision
- ☐ Opthalmascope and Otoscope examination
- ☐ Fracture tests (bite, maxillary fracture, percussion)

▷ *Range of Motion*

- ☐ ROM of temporomandibular joint
    - ☐ Opening and closing of mouth (2-3 finger widths)
    - ☐ Side-to-side movement of jaw
    - ☐ Mandible protrusion
- ☐ Eye movement (compare bilaterally and note restriction of movement)
- ☐ Facial movements

▷ *Neurological*

- ☐ Sensory for smell, taste, or hearing (may indicate symptoms of head injury)
- ☐ Cranial nerve check if you suspect associated head injury

Special Tests

Special tests of the head and face are limited; they include examination for fractures and general inspection of the eyes (vision, opthalmascope), ears (hearing, otoscope), and nose (breathing, nasal speculum). These tests were described on pages 538 through 540.

Range of Motion

Test active movement of the jaw, eyes, and facial muscles to rule out joint, muscle, or nerve injury as appropriate. You should examine active ROM of the temporomandibular joint with trauma to the mouth or jaw. Examine eye movement whenever there is direct trauma to the eye or orbit, or when you suspect an orbital blow-out or maxillary fracture. Perform active facial movements when trauma to facial nerves (e.g., contusions, lacerations) is of concern.

Neurological Tests

Perform neurological examination of the cranial nerves when you suspect head injury or when you note loss of hearing, taste, or smell. The examination is the same as that for head injury (see also table 19.1).

Functional Tests

You may want to perform functional tests to further examine the extent of the athlete's injury and to determine whether the athlete is safe to return to participation. Pain with biting and chewing may indicate temporomandibular dysfunction or maxilla, mandible, or tooth pathology. Examining visual and auditory acuity during sport activity will help you determine whether the athlete's senses are sufficient to allow safe resumption of activity. Examples of functional tests for vision and hearing are having the athlete catch a ball, shoot a basket, or respond to a command from across the field or when distracted. You can also examine vestibular function through functional balance tests.

SUMMARY

1. Describe the mechanisms, signs and symptoms, and potential complications associated with head and facial injuries commonly encountered in the physically active.

   Even with the use of protective equipment during sport activity, head and facial injuries are common and range widely from minor insults to life-threatening conditions. Head injuries, which can result from both direct and indirect mechanisms, are the leading cause of death due to sport participation. Facial injuries typically result from direct insult and most commonly take the form of contusions, fractures, and lacerations. Although the majority of the injuries you will encounter may not be life threatening, it is necessary to treat any injury resulting in neurological or sensory organ deficits as a medical emergency and to refer the athlete immediately to a physician for further examination.

2. Differentiate among signs and symptoms of concussion, skull fracture, and intracranial hemorrhage.

   Head injuries are classified into three categories: concussion, intracranial hemorrhage, and skull fractures. It is imperative that you be able to differentiate between the signs and symptoms of these different types of head injuries. A concussion will typically result in signs and symptoms of diffuse headache, dizziness, nausea, and tinnitus and may produce confusion, amnesia, and loss of consciousness. Intracranial hemorrhage leading to swelling and pressure on the brain will cause characteristic changes in vital signs, motor function, and pupillary function. Skull fractures may or may not result in intracranial hemorrhage; these are identified by palpable tenderness and possible bony deformity as well as by the presence of discharge or discoloration of the eyes, ears, and nose.

3. Discuss the potential complications and delayed symptoms that may result from head trauma.

Prompt recognition of neurological complications or evidence of increasing intracranial pressure is paramount to any examination following head trauma. Symptoms of intracranial hemorrhage may not be observable immediately after injury but may be delayed for minutes, hours, or even days. However, once symptoms of serious brain injury appear, the athlete's condition can quickly deteriorate. Any time an athlete's symptoms worsen over time or neurological deficits are present, the athlete should be immediately referred for emergency medical care. Because the athlete's condition can deteriorate so quickly, you must not hesitate to seek emergency medical assistance if you have any doubt as to the severity of the head trauma.

4. Describe and demonstrate the objective tests for examining the head and face.

Objective tests for the head and face are performed somewhat differently than those for the joints. Range of motion examination is primarily limited to active range of motion, which also functions to examine neuromuscular function in lieu of strength tests. Neurological examination departs somewhat from the standard sensory, motor, and reflex tests for specific nerves, as the examination of cranial nerves are typically tested with a single functional examination that may be either sensory or motor. Reflex testing focuses more on superficial and pathological reflexes when the potential for brain injury is suspected. Special tests are categorized as those that identify the neurological and cognitive effects of head injury, those that identify facial fractures, and those that identify dysfunction of the eyes, ears, and nose. Inclusion of these objective tests in your examination will depend on the type of trauma and the direction that the history and observation lead you.

5. Perform an on-site examination of a potential head injury, considering the criteria for medical referral and mode of transportation from the field.

The athlete with a head injury may range from conscious, coherent, and ambulatory to completely unconscious and unresponsive. The on-site examination of a suspected head injury begins with a primary survey to immediately determine level of consciousness and the presence of life-threatening conditions. In athletes who are unconscious, a cervical spine injury should also be suspected until there is proof to the contrary. Obtain a history from the athlete or from bystanders who witnessed the injury to determine the mechanism and nature of the injury. The observation includes examination for unusual body movements, facial reactions, and pupillary responses, as well as a visual check for signs of swelling, deformity, discoloration, or drainage from the nose or ears. The skull and facial bones are then palpated for evidence of fracture and pulse is monitored for changes in rate or strength. Neurological tests are performed to examine cranial nerve and motor function. Throughout the examination you should closely monitor vital signs, level of consciousness, and be alert for signs and symptoms of intracranial hemorrhage.

6. Perform an acute examination of a potential head injury, including special tests for cognition, balance, and coordination, considering the criteria for referral and follow-up examination.

The acute examination is similar to the on-site examination but includes a more complete history and neurological examination. The history is helpful for determining not only the mechanism and nature of injury, but also the athlete's level of consciousness and orientation. Special tests examine postconcussion symptoms and any loss of cognitive function such as memory, concentration, or analytical skills or any loss of equilibrium or balance. Examination of head injury at the sideline is unique in that it is imperative to repeatedly monitor vital signs and level of consciousness until serious head trauma has been ruled out or until it is clear that the athlete is stabilized or improving. This examination uses the same history questions and the same protocol as on the field to aid in determining whether symptoms are improving or worsening over time and to allow more effective follow-up.

7. Perform a general examination for facial injuries, identifying differential signs and symptoms indicating associated head injury.

The goal in acute examination of facial injuries is to determine the structure involved, the nature of the injury, and the injury's severity. If the structures of the ears or eyes are involved, the history should include questions regarding any difficulty with vision and hearing. Observe for any change, asymmetry, deformity, swelling, or discoloration of the facial structures and palpate all structures for tenderness, crepitus, and deformity. There are very few special tests for this region, with most used primarily as a functional examination of the sensory organs. Movement of the jaw and eyes should also be examined, if these structures are involved, for any restriction or difficulty with movement. Whenever an athlete sustains significant trauma to the face (i.e., nasal, maxillary, or mandible fracture), it is important to maintain a high suspicion of associated head injury and to rule this out during the injury examination.

8. Perform a complete neurological examination of the cranial nerves.

A cranial nerve check examines the integrity of each of the 12 cranial nerves. It is important to memorize the functional test for each cranial nerve and include these tests in the neurological examination of the head and face. Any time a positive sign is present with any one cranial nerve, serious brain trauma should be suspected and the athlete referred immediately. Neurological examination of the trigeminal and facial nerves should also be included in examination of facial trauma, as these nerves are sometimes traumatized or injured.

REVIEW QUESTIONS

1. What are the two primary mechanisms of head injury? What types of stresses do these mechanisms place on the brain tissues, and which are least and best tolerated?

2. What are the two primary types of intracranial hemorrhage, and what structures are commonly involved in each? What changes in vital signs indicate an expanding lesion?

3. What are the general classifications and signs and symptoms of concussion? How are these signs and symptoms different from those of an intracranial hemorrhage, and which ones indicate a medical emergency?

4. What are the signs and symptoms of a corneal abrasion, and how would you differentiate this condition from a corneal laceration?

5. Describe the difference between hyperemia and hyphema. Which of these conditions represents a medical emergency?

6. How are level of consciousness and orientation determined in an examination? Describe the examination procedure and list the questions you would ask to determine an athlete's orientation to her surroundings.

7. Pupillary position, size, and response are important in the examination of head and eye injuries. What would be considered abnormal in your observations of size, shape, and responsiveness, and what conditions might these abnormalities indicate?

8. Describe the common fractures of the facial bones and their general signs and symptoms. What special tests can be performed to help identify the presence of a fracture?

CRITICAL THINKING QUESTIONS

1. Consider the scenario where Fran sustains a blunt trauma to the eye with a racquetball and is in considerable pain. Discuss the various structures and conditions that may be associated with this mechanism. Which conditions and symptoms would warrant immediate medical referral, and how you would differentiate between minor and eye-threatening conditions in your examination?

2. While providing a history on the sideline, an athlete reports that this is the second concussion he has had in the past month. How might this information affect your injury examination and your follow-up examination and return-to-play criteria?

3. An athlete receives a hard blow to the chin and complains of jaw pain and an inability to completely close her mouth. She also complains of a severe headache and dizziness. How would your examination proceed?

4. One of the football players on your college team is an incredibly tough athlete with a high tolerance for pain. Your experience from working with this athlete in the past tells you that he often minimizes the reporting of his symptoms to avoid the risk of you or the coach pulling him out. On one occasion, you are concerned that he has sustained a mild head injury after a hard hit, but he tells you in front of the coach that he has no headache or other complaints. Of course, the coach believes him and wants him in the next play. You, however, are still not convinced. Describe how would you handle this situation. What would you tell the coach, and how would you go about determining whether it is safe for this athlete to return to play?

CITED REFERENCES

Cantu, R.C. 1991. Minor head injuries in sports. In *Sports and the adolescent*, ed. P.G. Dyment, 141-154. Philadelphia: Hanley and Belfus.

Cantu, R.C. 1992. Cerebral concussion in sport: Management and prevention. *Sports Med* 14: 64-74.

Cantu, R.C. 2001. Posttraumatic retrograde and anterograde amnesia: Pathophysiology and implications in grading and safe return to play. *J Athl Train* 36(3): 244-248.

Cantu, R.C., and R. Voy. 1995. Second-impact syndrome. *Phys Sports Med* 23: 27-34.

Colorado Medical Society's Report of the Sports Medicine Committee. 1990 (revised May 1991). *Guidelines for the management of concussion in sports*. Denver, CO: Colorado Medical Society.

Guskiewicz, K.M., S.L. Bruce, R.C. Cantu, M.S. Ferrara, J.P. Kelly, M. McCrea, M. Putukian, and T.C. Valovich McLeod. 2004. National Athletic Trainers' Association position statement: Management of sport-related concussion. *J Athl Train* 39(3): 280-297. Available at http://www.nata.org/publicinformation/files/concussion.pdf. Accessed November 2, 2004.

Guskiewicz, K.M., B.L. Riemann, D.H. Perrin, and L.M. Nashner. 1997. Alternative approaches to the assessment of mild head injury in athletes. *Med Sci Sports Exerc* 29: S213-221.

Guskiewicz, K.M., S.E. Ross, and S.W. Marshall. 2001. Postural stability and neuropsychological deficits after concussion in collegiate athletes. *J Athl Train* 36(3): 263-273.

Kelly, J.P., and J.H. Rosenberg. 1997. The diagnosis and management of concussion in sports. *Neurol* 48: 575-580.

McCrea, M. 2001. Standardized mental status testing on the sideline after sport-related concussion. *J Athl Train* 36(3): 274-279.

Moore, K.L. 1992. *Clinically oriented anatomy*. Baltimore: Williams & Wilkins.

Munger, B.L., and I.L. Baird, I.L. 1980. *Anatomy-Px: A practical introduction to anatomical correlates of the physical examination*. Baltimore: Williams & Wilkins.

National Athletic Trainers' Association Research and Education Foundation. 1994. *Mild brain injury in sports summit proceedings*, April 16-18. Washington, DC: National Athletic Trainers' Association.

Oliaro, S., S. Anderson, and D. Hooker. 2001. Management of cerebral concussion in sports: The athletic trainer's perspective. *J Athl Train* 36(3): 257-262.

Reimann, B.L., K.M. Guskiewicz, and E.W. Shields. 1999. Relationship between clinical and forceplate measures of postural stability. *J Sport Rehabil* 8(2): 71-82.

ADDITIONAL RESOURCES

Hillman, S.K. 2004. *Introduction to athletic training*. 2nd ed. Champaign, IL: Human Kinetics.

McCrea, M., J.P. Kelly, J. Kluge, B. Ackley, and C. Randoph. 1997. Standardized assessment of concussion in football players. *Neurol* 48(3): 586-588.

CHAPTER 20

Thorax and Abdomen

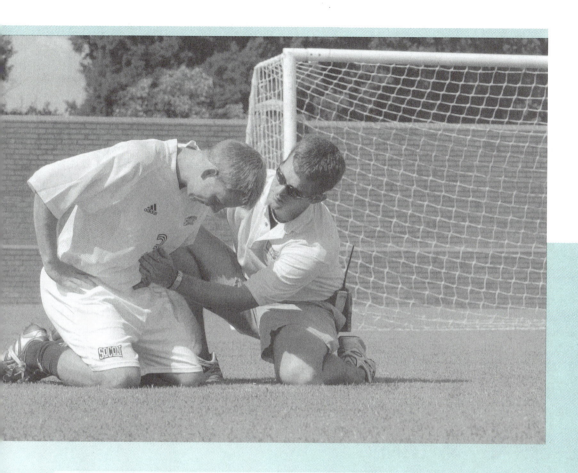

Objectives

After completing this chapter, the reader will be able to do the following:

1. Describe the common mechanisms, signs and symptoms, and potential complications associated with injuries to the thorax commonly encountered in the physically active

2. Describe the common mechanisms, signs and symptoms, and potential complications associated with injuries to the abdomen commonly encountered in the physically active

3. Differentiate among pathologies and signs and symptoms of cardiac contusion, tamponade, and concussion

4. Appreciate the potential for life-threatening injury resulting from direct and indirect trauma to the thorax and abdomen

5. Describe and demonstrate the objective tests for examining the thorax and abdomen

6. Perform an on-site examination of the thorax and abdomen, indicating criteria for immediate medical referral or continued observation

7. Perform a clinical examination of the thorax and abdomen, indicating considerations for differential diagnosis

Jeremy was in his third year of lacrosse at Tucker University. As he was going for the ball during practice, a collision with a teammate sent him sprawling, and he landed hard on his back. Sharon, the athletic trainer who was covering practice, saw the collision and started to go over to him, but then Jeremy got up and appeared to be okay.

"I'm okay," Jeremy yelled over to Sharon with a grimace on his face as he slowly trotted over to the rest of the team to continue practice. Even so, Sharon kept an eye on him. No more than five minutes later Jeremy came over to see her. "Sharon, I don't feel so good."

Sharon noticed that Jeremy appeared a bit pale and clammy. "Tell me exactly what happened and where your pain is."

"I collided with John going for the ball and he hit me hard, right in the stomach, and knocked me flat. Now I feel kind of weak and nauseated. My stomach hurts, too."

Sharon continued to question Jeremy as she inspected his abdominal region for signs of swelling or discoloration. "Are you having pain anywhere else?"

"Yeah, my left shoulder kind of hurts too." Sharon became concerned; she checked Jeremy's vital signs and found that his respirations were rapid and shallow and his pulse was fast. His blood pressure was about 90/50. It appeared that Jeremy was going into shock, and his symptoms indicated a potential spleen injury. Sharon immediately called 911 for emergency transport to the local hospital. As she waited for EMS to arrive, his symptoms continued to worsen, and his abdomen became rigid. She hoped EMS would arrive soon.

You will often be presented with patients complaining of chest and abdominal pain. Although most of these complaints will be associated with minor injuries and illnesses, others may indicate serious underlying pathologies. This chapter introduces you to the complexities of chest and abdominal trauma and helps you recognize the signs and symptoms of both common and life-threatening injuries, as well as provides you with the tools for both on-site (emergent) and clinical (nonemergent) injury examination. Chapters 21 and 22 address the general medical conditions associated with this region, which you should also consider and rule out when a patient complains of pain in the absence of trauma.

FUNCTIONAL ANATOMY

To understand and properly examine chest and abdominal injuries, you must first be familiar with the anatomical orientation and physiological function of the organs and structures of the thorax and abdomen. Although this chapter presents anatomical orientation where appropriate within the context of various pathologies, you are encouraged to review the general anatomy and physiology of this region before proceeding.

Thoracic Cavity

The thoracic cavity is divided into three sections or spaces: two separate pleural cavities housing the left and right lungs, and the **mediastinum**, which houses the heart, the thoracic parts of the great vessels, the trachea, the left and right bronchi, and other important structures (figure 20.1). Some injuries to the musculoskeletal system can injure the internal structures of the thoracic cavity. For example, a posterior dislocation of the sternoclavicular joint can compress or perforate the great vessels of the heart. For this reason, you should take great care when moving a patient with this injury. Rib fracture also carries the potential for injury to the lungs and deserves careful examination and management.

The heart is slightly larger than the athlete's clenched fist. Its position within the thorax varies depending on the person's body type (narrow and slender versus broad and stocky), body position (recumbent versus upright), and lung status (inspiration versus expiration). In general, one-third of the heart lies to the right and two-thirds lie to the left of the median plane of the sternum. The inferior border of the heart is approximately level with the xiphisternal junction.

The heart produces two quick sounds that correspond with valve closure. The first sound corresponds to closure of the atrioventricular valves and the second to semilunar valve closure. Abnormal heart sounds, known as murmurs, occur occasionally in athletes who otherwise appear to be completely healthy. These sounds may represent relatively benign conditions or may represent heart abnormalities that place a physically active person at great risk. **Auscultation**, or listening to the heart sounds with a stethoscope, is a complex process that requires the skills of a cardiologist to differentiate between benign and pathologically abnormal heart sounds.

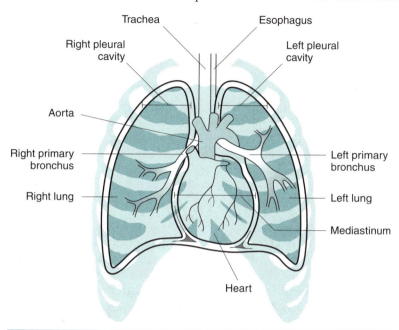

Figure 20.1 Thoracic cavity and skeletal rib cage. Note the two pleural cavities and the structures of the mediastinum.

Abdominal Cavity

The abdominal cavity contains both hollow and solid organs that can be injured during sport activity. The hollow organs, which allow solid and fluid materials to pass through the body, include the stomach, large and small intestines, ureters, and bladder (figure 20.2a). The solid organs include

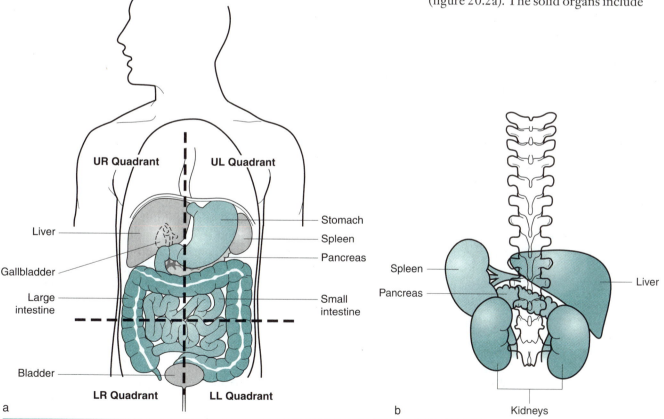

Figure 20.2 Organs of the abdominal cavity from an (a) anterior (note the four quadrants of the abdominal cavity) and (b) posterior view.

the liver, spleen, pancreas, and kidneys (figure 20.2, a-b); because of their rich blood supply, injury to these organs can cause considerable hemorrhage. Injuries to the hollow organs are less common than injuries to the solid visceral organs because the hollow organs are able to give when trauma is directed at the abdomen.

The abdominal cavity is divided into quadrants (see figure 20.2a), and within each quadrant lies important internal organs with which you should become familiar. Contusions to the quadrants combined with characteristic signs and symptoms can help you diagnose injury to the internal organs. You should review the location of the internal organs in the abdominal cavity. Later in this chapter you will learn the signs and symptoms associated with injury to these organs that are so essential to normal living.

One controversy you may encounter as a health care professional is whether or not you should permit a competitive athlete to participate in his chosen sport despite the loss of a paired organ. In the case of the abdominal cavity, this controversy normally involves the absence of a kidney or testicle. This is a complex decision that should include the athlete, his parents if he is a minor, his personal physician, and the team physician.

INJURIES OF THE THORAX AND ABDOMEN

Injuries to the thorax and abdomen can result from a variety of mechanisms. Injury can occur as a consequence of violent muscle contractions and can even occur spontaneously without evidence of direct trauma. Blunt trauma or direct insult is the most common mechanism and the one that presents the greatest concern for serious injury. Although the internal organs of the thorax and abdomen are well protected, they are vulnerable to injury during sport. Internal injuries often result from a hard fall; a helmet to the chest, lower back, or abdomen; or impact from a baseball, softball, or other sport implement. Because of the potential for life-threatening complications arising from these injuries, you should suspect underlying pathology throughout your examination any time a patient sustains a significant blow to the chest or abdomen.

Thorax

Injuries to the chest wall and organs of the thoracic cavity can result from direct insult or violent muscle contractions; they also may occur spontaneously as a consequence of intense exercise. The most common injuries resulting from these mechanisms are contusions, strains, sprains, and fractures of the chest wall. However, the same mechanisms can also traumatize the heart and lungs or cause internal bleeding—all of which can have life-threatening consequences.

Contusions

Because of the superficial nature of the anterior and lateral chest wall, rib and sternal contusions are common in contact sports with no or inadequate chest protection. Signs and symptoms include localized pain, swelling, discoloration, periosteal irritation, and point tenderness. Deep inspiration may cause pain if the adjacent intercostal muscles or costochondral joints are irritated or injured. Although severe contusions may be difficult to distinguish from fracture, contusions typically do not display signs of bony crepitus or pain with indirect compression of the chest wall.

Sprains

Sprains or separation of the costochondral joint can result secondary to anteriorly directed trauma to the sternum or lateral compression of the chest wall. Bouncing the barbell off the chest during bench press can also cause costochondral injury. Severity can range from a mild sprain or irritation to separation and complete dislocation (figure 20.3). The patient complains of pain and point tenderness at the costochondral junction. With separation or dislocation, he will also complain of increased pain with deep inspiration, of crepitus or clicking, and of increased prominence of the joint. You may also observe swelling and discoloration.

Costochondritis

Chronic irritation and inflammation of the costochondral junction (**costochondritis**) can occur following acute, traumatic injury or as a result of chronic stress or repetitive activities such as coughing, rowing, or lifting. The patient may have no history of trauma but complains of a gradual onset of pain in the anterior chest wall and tenderness over the affected joint. Crepitus and mild inflammation may also be present. Rest, ice, and anti-inflammatory medication typically resolve symptoms within a few weeks.

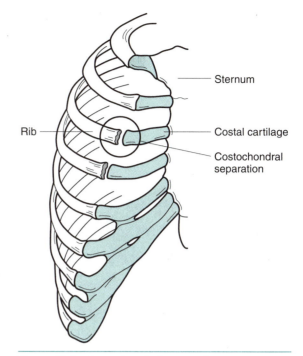

Figure 20.3   Costochondral separation.

Traumatic Fractures and Dislocations

Traumatic fractures can result from a direct blow, indirect compression of the chest wall, or muscular tension. Rib fractures are much more common than sternal fractures. Depending on the mechanism of trauma associated with fractures of the thorax, you must be keenly aware of underlying pathology and potential complications, particularly if the direction of force compresses the chest wall or displaces the fracture inwardly.

Ribs

While the first through fourth ribs are well protected by the shoulder girdle and the 10th through 12th ribs are more mobile, the rigidly fixed fifth through ninth ribs are prone to fracture. Fractures most commonly occur at the weaker, posterior angle (figure 20.4). Signs and symptoms include localized pain, point tenderness, swelling, discoloration, crepitus, and muscle guarding. Pain increases with indirect chest wall compression, deep inspiration, and coughing, sneezing, laughing, or jarring. Because deep inspiration increases pain, the patient often presents with rapid, shallow breathing to avoid pain. The patient may also rotate the trunk and lean toward the injured side to prevent muscle tensioning and pain.

Severe trauma can cause a **flail chest injury**, characterized by multiple fractures of three or more adjacent ribs. Direct trauma fractures are often more serious, as the fragment is more likely to be driven into the thoracic or abdominal cavity, leading to secondary visceral injury. For instance, when you suspect a lower posterior rib fracture, you should also suspect potential kidney trauma (figure 20.5). Signs and symptoms associated with secondary lung injury include chest pain, difficulty breathing, cyanosis, and shock (see the sections on pneumothorax and

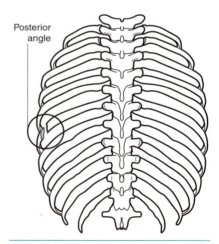

Figure 20.4   Rib fracture at the posterior angle.

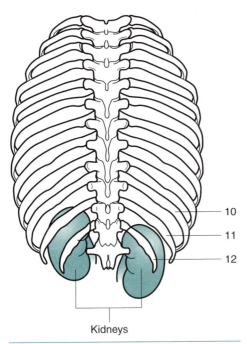

Figure 20.5 Anatomical orientation of the left kidney to the posterior margin of the rib cage.

Kidneys

10
11
12

Cyanosis *is a bluish or purplish discoloration of the skin due to deficient oxygenation of the blood.*

! Lower rib fractures may subsequently lacerate the upper abdominal viscera and result in internal hemorrhage.

! Because of the severity of the blow needed to cause a sternal fracture, always check for underlying pleural (hemothorax, pneumothorax) and cardiac (contusion, tamponade) injury, particularly if the sternum displaces posteriorly.

hemothorax). It is imperative that you look beyond the suspected rib fracture and monitor the patient carefully for signs and symptoms of internal injury.

Nontraumatic or stress fractures of the rib also occur commonly in athletes, secondary to a violent twisting or muscle contraction frequently associated with violent coughing, overhead throwing, swinging a golf club, or rowing activities. As with traumatic fractures, the athlete complains of localized pain and tenderness that increases with deep inspiration and trunk movement. Displacement is uncommon with a stress injury, and underlying pathology is rarely a concern. Although the first rib is well protected, nontraumatic fractures of this rib have been documented in sport, occurring secondary to falling on an outstretched or hyperabducted arm or to a sudden, violent contraction of the scalenus anterior muscle (Fruh 1993). Signs and symptoms include sharp pain in the anterior triangle of the neck and palpable tenderness of the surrounding musculature (trapezius and scalenes). The athlete may also complain of radiating pain into the shoulder or scapular region, as well as possible neurological symptoms due to secondary irritation or injury to the brachial plexus.

Sternum

Fractures of the sternum are rare in contact sports and more often occur secondary to high-velocity impact of the chest with the steering wheel in motor vehicle accidents. However, sternal fractures can result from a severe, direct blow to the anterior chest (e.g., when another player's helmet or a sport implement, such as a baseball, hits the chest at a high velocity). The patient will likely complain of losing his breath immediately following injury as well as feeling pain with deep inspiration. Examination will reveal localized pain, tenderness, ecchymosis, swelling, and possible deformity.

Because of the severity of the blow that is necessary to cause a fracture, there is always a concern for underlying pleural (hemothorax, pneumothorax) or cardiac (contusion, tamponade) injury, or both, particularly if the sternum displaces posteriorly. If underlying pathology exists, the patient may exhibit signs and symptoms of respiratory or circulatory distress. However, these signs and symptoms may not be present initially and can be delayed. Any time a patient receives a significant blow to the chest, thoroughly examine him and monitor carefully for signs and symptoms of shock and respiratory and cardiac dysfunction following injury.

Internal Injuries

Internal injuries in the thoracic region are serious and often life threatening. Although the thoracic cavity is well protected circumferentially by the sternum, ribs, and vertebral column, both blunt and penetrating trauma can injure these vital structures and compromise pulmonary or circulatory function, or both. It is imperative that you recognize the signs and symptoms of the following conditions and ensure immediate medical referral as appropriate.

Pneumothorax

Surrounding each lung is a pleural sac. Its outer wall, the **parietal pleura**, adheres to the external wall of the pleural cavity. The inner layer, the **visceral pleura**, adheres to the surface of the lung. Between these two layers is a **serous fluid** that reduces friction and allows the two layers to move freely on one another as the lungs inflate and collapse with normal breathing. A **pneumothorax** occurs when air enters this cavity, separating the lung from its chest wall and reducing its volume (i.e., **lung collapse**) (figure 20.6).

A pneumothorax can result from traumatic injury or can occur spontaneously in the absence of trauma. A penetrating injury such as a rib fracture can rupture or lacerate lung

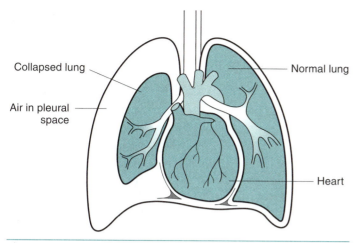

Figure 20.6 Pneumothorax.

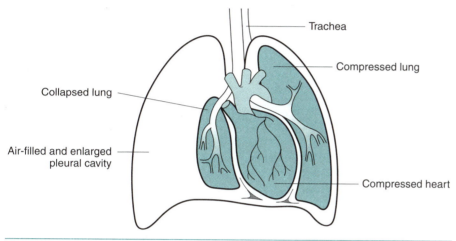

Figure 20.7 Tension pneumothorax and shift of the mediastinum with compression of the heart and healthy lung.

tissue and allow inspired air to escape into the pleural space. A hard blow to the chest with the glottis closed can result in rupture of the alveoli, or a blow-out injury. More common in sport, however, is a spontaneous pneumothorax; this most often occurs in young, healthy athletes with no history of trauma and may follow an intense bout of activity that causes small ruptures in the outer surface of the lung tissue. Signs and symptoms associated with a simple pneumothorax include upper chest pain, **dyspnea** (difficulty breathing) or shortness of breath, light-headedness, and decreased breath sounds with auscultation. If compromise is severe, the athlete may also be cyanotic. Immediately refer athletes with a suspected pneumothorax for emergency medical care.

Severe, life-threatening complications can arise if the air in the pleural cavity continues to increase, progressing to a tension pneumothorax. With a **tension pneumothorax**, the increasing pressure caused by the trapped air shifts the mediastinum away from the injured side, compressing the heart and healthy lung and compromising their function (figure 20.7). Fatal hypoxia and acidosis will occur due to compression of the vena cava, decreased cardiac filling and output, and severely compromised lung volume. Signs and symptoms of a tension pneumothorax include acute respiratory distress, distended neck veins, circulatory compromise, tracheal deviation, decreased breath sounds, and severe restlessness and agitation. You must immediately refer the patient for emergency medical care.

Hypoxia is a lack of oxygen.

Acidosis is an excess accumulation of acid in the body caused by cardiorespiratory compromise.

Hypovolemic shock is caused by internal hemorrhage resulting in decreased blood volume.

Hemothorax

Traumatic chest injuries, such as laceration of lung tissue or an intercostal artery secondary to a penetrating rib fracture, can result in a hemothorax in which blood, rather than air, fills the pleural space. Signs and symptoms of a hemothorax include lung collapse and reduced or absent breath sounds on the involved side, severe chest pain, dyspnea, cyanosis, hypotension, and the coughing up of frothy blood. If bleeding is severe, **hypovolemic shock**, shift of the mediastinum, and collapse of the uninvolved lung may also result.

Cardiac Contusion

Blunt trauma to the chest that compresses the heart between the sternum and the spine can result in a contusion to the heart muscle. High-velocity chest impact with a baseball, hockey puck, lacrosse ball, or softball is a common mechanism in sport. Signs and symptoms of cardiac contusion include chest pain, neck vein distension, possible rhythm disturbance (**arrhythmia**), muffled heart tones, and electrocardiogram changes indicating muscle injury. Signs and symptoms associated with shock and respiratory and cardiac distress may also occur, but these can vary considerably according to severity. Severe and life-threatening complications can result if the impact is sufficient to cause ventricular, coronary artery, or intraventricular septum rupture. Again, any blunt trauma to the chest should raise your suspicion of underlying internal injury, and you should refer the athlete for immediate medical care.

Cardiac Tamponade

Blunt trauma to the chest can also cause **cardiac tamponade**, or hemorrhage within the enclosed, inelastic pericardial cavity, if trauma is sufficient to rupture the myocardium or coronary artery. Fortunately, this occurs rarely in sport, but since the cause is often a penetrating injury such as a stab wound, this injury could potentially occur in sports such as fencing or javelin throwing. Cardiac tamponade is characterized by compression of the heart and pulmonary veins, which prevents venous return to the heart. Signs and symptoms include neck vein distension (due to the backup of venous flow), shock, hypotension, cyanosis, severe chest pain, and difficulty breathing. Cardiac tamponade is clearly life threatening and warrants immediate emergency medical care.

Cardiac Concussion (Commotio Cordis)

A condition that has aroused considerable interest in recent years is cardiac concussion. Cardiac concussion, or commotio cordis, is characterized by immediate cardiac arrest and sudden death following a localized blunt, but seemingly inconsequential, blow to the chest (near the region of the heart) during sport activity (Maron et al. 1995). Many cases have been documented in which a blow to the chest from a sport implement—insufficient to cause structural injury to the sternum, ribs, or underlying heart—results in immediate collapse (or collapse within seconds) and sudden death in young athletes with no previous history or evidence of heart abnormality or disease (Curfman 1998; Haq 1998; Maron et al. 1995). The most common offending projectiles are baseballs, softballs, and hockey pucks (Curfman 1998); but cardiac concussion has also resulted following impact from a lacrosse ball, cricket ball, helmet, hockey stick, body check in ice hockey, and karate kick (Haq 1998; Maron et al. 1995).

Although the precise mechanism for cardiac arrest resulting from cardiac concussion is still uncertain, the primary cause is thought to be a premature heart beat precipitated by the impact, which in turn elicits ventricular fibrillation (Maron et al. 1995). Unfortunately, in most cases, resuscitation attempts have failed and death usually results. When an athlete collapses following blunt trauma to the chest, you should immediately examine for airway, breathing, and circulation and should summon emergency medical services (EMS).

> ⚠ Any blunt trauma to the chest should raise your suspicion for underlying internal injury, and you should refer any athlete displaying symptoms of cardiorespiratory distress for immediate medical care.

> ⚠ When an athlete collapses following blunt trauma to the chest, you should immediately examine airway, breathing, and circulation and should summon EMS.

Abdomen

Traumatic injuries to the abdominal region include soft tissue injuries of the abdominal muscles, genitalia, and internal organs. While the thoracic cavity is protected by the skeletal rib cage, the abdomen is protected primarily by soft tissue structures; thus contusions and muscular strains are more common injuries in this region. Although these injuries are usually minor, they can cause considerable pain and disability if they are acute. Internal injuries, particularly to the solid organs, are also a concern with mechanisms of blunt trauma and most often involve the spleen and kidney. If internal hemorrhage results, the injury becomes life threatening if you do not immediately recognize it and manage it appropriately.

Contusion

As with any other structure left unprotected during sport activity, the abdomen is prone to contusions secondary to direct contact. External abdominal structures most vulnerable to contusions include the abdominal muscles, solar plexus, and external genitalia.

Abdominal Muscles

The abdominal muscles, which provide the chief protection to the abdominal cavity, are often exposed to direct trauma during sport activity. Severe muscular contusions are rare, since the underlying abdominal contents are soft and can "give" to dissipate blunt forces. Even so, injury to the muscle can result from direct trauma and gives rise to the typical signs of localized pain, swelling, tenderness, and ecchymosis. Blunt trauma of sufficient magnitude can also contuse the underlying abdominal viscera. Any time a patient presents with a history of direct or blunt abdominal trauma, you should complete a thorough examination to rule out any signs and symptoms of visceral trauma before return to activity.

Solar Plexus

A direct blow to the abdomen over the solar (celiac) plexus can momentarily paralyze the diaphragm and impair breathing. This syndrome, often referred to as getting the wind knocked out of you, commonly results from the impact of a knee or helmet to the abdomen or from falling on a ball. This relatively minor condition typically requires no treatment or referral, but it can produce considerable anxiety in the athlete, as he will find it difficult or impossible to breathe for a brief period of time. Signs and symptoms include abdominal pain, fear, anxiety, and difficulty breathing. The symptoms should dissipate quickly and normal breathing should resume without the need for medical intervention or treatment. By immediately recognizing the signs and symptoms of a blow to the solar plexus, you can calm and reassure the athlete until normal breathing resumes.

Testicular Trauma

Testicular trauma or scrotal contusion is relatively common among physically active males, resulting from a direct blow to the external genitalia such as getting kicked or kneed in the groin. This injury can cause considerable pain, spasm, ecchymosis, and swelling. The patient may also complain of nausea and may vomit or faint if pain is severe. Except with severe contusions, the symptoms are usually short-lived and are often relieved when you place the patient in supine and bring his knees toward his chest. The patient is typically able to return to activity after a few minutes. However, swelling and mild pain may linger for a few days. A **hydrocele** (swelling due to the accumulation of fluid within the tunica vaginalis, the membrane surrounding the testicle) or **hematocele** (rapid accumulation of blood) may also form following trauma (figure 20.8). Refer the patient for medical examination whenever severe swelling

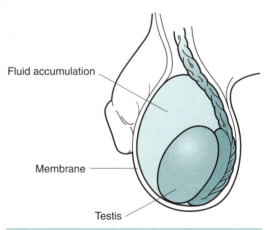

Figure 20.8 Testicular hydrocele. A hematocele may appear the same from the outside, but the fluid involved is blood rather than serous fluid.

occurs or when pain persists or symptoms worsen rather than improve. It is always wise to have the patient examine the testicle following injury to check for changes in its appearance or position.

A potential complication of testicular trauma is torsion of the spermatic cord, in which the trauma rotates the testicle in the scrotum. Torsion can also occur spontaneously in young males in the absence of trauma (see chapter 22, page 620). Signs and symptoms of testicular torsion include immediate or gradual onset of groin pain, heaviness in the scrotum, and change in the normal position or appearance of the testicle. This condition constitutes a medical emergency and requires immediate referral, as blood flow to the testicle is compromised.

Strains

The abdominal muscles stabilize, flex, and rotate the trunk during sport activity as well as restrain the abdominal contents. Sudden muscle contractions or overstretch can strain these muscles and cause considerable disability because of their postural function. Strains and weakness in the lower abdominal region can also result in a herniation of the small intestines through the abdominal wall.

Abdominal Muscles

Strain of the abdominal muscles (rectus abdominis, internal and external obliques) can result from a violent muscle contraction or trunk twisting. Chronic or repetitive overuse can also cause muscular strain. Signs and symptoms include pain, muscle spasm, and palpable tenderness. Swelling and discoloration may or may not be present. As with all muscle strains, the patient complains of increased pain with muscle contraction or with passive stretching of the involved muscle. Because the abdominal muscles are postural muscles and are involved in virtually every trunk movement, abdominal strains can be particularly bothersome and slow to heal. Often, complete rest is necessary.

Side Stitch

A side stitch or side ache is characterized by a sharp pain or spasm along the lateral abdominal wall, typically on the right side. This transient pain occurs most often with intense running activities and occurs more commonly early in the season. Although the exact cause is unknown, the side stitch is typically associated with muscle ischemia and poor conditioning but has also been attributed to intestinal gas or to consumption of a large meal just before activity. The pain often quickly subsides with reducing activity or with deep, steady breathing. Stretching away from the side of pain or raising the arm overhead also relieves symptoms. Once the pain dissipates, the patient is usually able to return to activity without further problems.

Hernia

A hernia is characterized by the protrusion of the small intestine through a weakened area in the anterior abdominal wall. The two most common sites of herniation are the femoral ring and the inguinal region. Hernias can be congenital or acquired. Acquired hernias occur in sport when lifting or other strenuous activities strain the already weak area of the abdominal wall. Herniation can also result from intense lifting, pushing, or coughing, or from straining during defecation.

- **Femoral hernia.** The femoral ring is an opening at the superior end of the femoral canal through which the femoral artery, vein, and lymphatic vessels pass into the lower extremity. The canal is widest at the femoral ring. With a femoral hernia, the abdominal viscera (usually small intestine) protrudes through the femoral ring and into the femoral canal (figure 20.9) (Moore 1992). It becomes visible or palpable just inferior to the inguinal ligament. It presents as a bulge or mass in the femoral triangle inferolateral to the pubic tubercle and medial to the femoral vein. The mass may or may not be painful, but the patient typically complains of discomfort. Because of the rigid and defined boundaries of the femoral ring, strangulation of a femoral hernia is a concern. Strangulation occurs when the herniated contents become compressed, compromising blood flow. If a strangulating hernia is left untreated, tissue necrosis occurs. Femoral hernias are more commonly seen in females because females typically have a wider femoral ring than males.

- **Inguinal hernia.** Inguinal hernias, in which protrusion occurs through the inguinal canal, are commonly seen in males. The spermatic cord passes through the

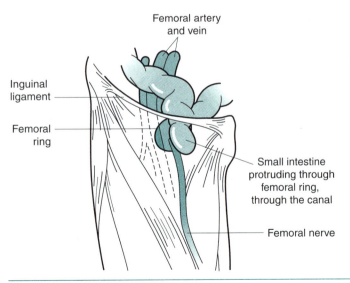

Femoral artery and vein

Inguinal ligament

Femoral ring

Small intestine protruding through femoral ring, through the canal

Femoral nerve

Figure 20.9   Femoral hernia.

inguinal canal, which runs obliquely along the anterior inferior abdominal wall. The abdominal musculature provides much of the protection to the inguinal canal. There are two types of inguinal hernia: direct and indirect; the indirect type is the more common (75% of cases) (Moore 1992). A direct hernia usually results from weakening of the anterior abdominal wall and protrudes anteriorly through the inferior portion of the inguinal (Hesselbach's) triangle. An indirect hernia enters through the deep inguinal ring, inguinal canal, and superficial inguinal ring (figure 20.10). An indirect

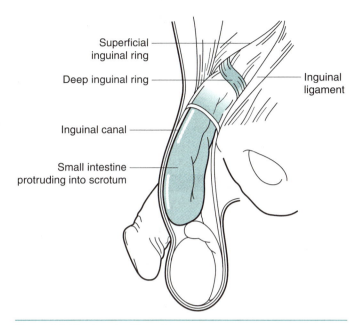

Superficial inguinal ring

Deep inguinal ring

Inguinal ligament

Inguinal canal

Small intestine protruding into scrotum

Figure 20.10   Inguinal hernia.

inguinal hernia presents as a mass in the inguinal region and may extend into the scrotum. The patient may or may not complain of pain or tenderness in the region, depending on the extent of herniation. Having the patient cough or bear down further protrudes the herniation momentarily by increasing the intra-abdominal pressure. If the herniation does not retract and remains distended, strangulation of the herniated contents can occur secondary to restriction by the inguinal ring or twisting of the intestine. A strangulated hernia causes severe pain and represents a medical emergency.

Internal Injuries

When a patient presents with a history of severe blunt trauma to the abdomen, you should highly suspect internal injury or hemorrhage. It is imperative for you to recognize the signs and symptoms associated with internal injury and hemorrhage and immediately refer the patient for a thorough medical examination.

Keep in mind the location and orientation of the gastrointestinal organs in the abdominal cavity when considering what structures may be involved in various mechanisms of injury, particularly with regard to the location and direction of impact. To aid in identifying and reporting symptoms and problems in the abdominal region, the abdominal cavity is divided by imaginary transverse and horizontal lines that bisect the umbilicus vertically and horizontally into the right and left upper and lower quadrants (see figure 20.2a on page 561). However, injuries to structures in one quadrant may cause pain or symptoms in another quadrant or may even refer symptoms to other body regions. For this reason you need to know not only the locations of these structures, but also their referral patterns (see figure 20.15 later in this chapter).

Bladder Rupture

The most common cause of a ruptured bladder is a direct blow to the abdomen with the bladder fully distended. This is rare in athletics simply because participating with a full bladder is too uncomfortable for most athletes. Athletes can easily prevent bladder ruptures by emptying the bladder prior to any athletic activity. The bladder can also be injured secondary to fracture of the pelvis. Signs and symptoms of a bladder rupture include a history of a direct blow or severe trauma to the abdomen, complaints of lower abdominal pain, and palpable tenderness and abdominal rigidity. Hematuria occurs, and the athlete has difficulty with urination.

Hematuria is blood in the urine.

Kidney Contusion

In contact sports, kidney contusions can occur secondary to a severe blow to the lower back. The kidneys sit on either side of the vertebral column between the levels of T12 through L3 (see figure 20.2b on page 561). The primary signs and symptoms of kidney trauma include deep aching in the lower back and flank region and possible muscle guarding. The pain may also wrap around anteriorly to the lower abdomen. Severe contusions can result in nausea, vomiting, and possible shock. Hematuria is a hallmark of kidney trauma but may not be visible to the naked eye and may require urinalysis for identification. Ask the athlete to check the urine for a change in color. Remove athletes with a suspected kidney contusion from activity and refer them immediately to determine the extent of injury.

Splenic Rupture

Rupture of the spleen can be a rapidly progressive injury that, if not recognized early, can lead to internal hemorrhage and possible death. In fact, splenic rupture is the most common cause of death due to abdominal trauma in sport. The spleen sits in the upper left quadrant and is protected by the 9th through 11th ribs (see figure 20.2a on page 561). It functions as a reservoir of red blood cells and produces antibodies and lymphocytes to fight illness and infection. The spleen is most vulnerable to injury after a systemic illness, such as mononucleosis, that enlarges the organ. Injury to the spleen can result from a direct blow to the left upper abdominal quadrant or a hard fall. Patient complaints typically include left upper quadrant and flank pain, and nausea and vomiting. The athlete may exhibit signs and symptoms of shock including a wet (cold, clammy skin), white (pale), and weak (weak, rapid pulse) appearance. Other signs and symptoms of hemorrhage include abdominal rigidity and rebound tenderness. If bleeding causes pressure or irritates the diaphragm, a **Kehr's sign** also occurs, characterized by pain radiating into the left shoulder and partially down the arm. Immediately refer patients exhibiting any of these signs. Removal of the spleen may be necessary. Although spleen removal was routinely performed in the past, the current trend is to save the organ whenever possible.

While some splenic ruptures are rapidly progressing, others can be deceiving and not readily apparent. The spleen can splint itself for a period of time, delaying hemorrhage for hours, days, or even weeks after injury, until a subsequent lesser or inconsequential blow activates the hemorrhage. It is imperative that you thoroughly examine a patient who sustains blunt trauma to the abdomen and instruct the patient to watch for signs and symptoms of delayed hemorrhage and to seek medical attention immediately if they appear. Because the risk of splenic rupture increases when the organ is enlarged, patients with mononucleosis who are involved in contact, jarring, or running types of sports are restricted from these activities until the spleen has returned to its normal size. This may be difficult for patients to understand, as their symptoms of illness often disappear before the spleen recovers.

OBJECTIVE TESTS

Objective tests for the abdomen and thorax are primarily aimed at distinguishing musculoskeletal injury of the chest and abdominal walls from injury to the internal organs. Led by your history and observation, you will rely heavily on your palpation skills and examination of vital signs for identifying these injuries, as there are very few special tests for this region.

Palpation

Palpation of the thorax and abdominal regions is divided into the superficial palpation of the chest wall, and the superficial and deep palpation of the abdomen.

- **Chest wall.** Palpate the chest wall for tenderness, swelling, deformity, crepitus, and asymmetry. Bony landmarks include the clavicle, sternum, xiphoid process, costochondral cartilage, thoracic vertebrae, scapula, and each rib (anterior, lateral, and posterior aspects of the chest wall). Soft tissues include the pectoralis major and minor; the intercostals on the anterior chest wall; the serratus anterior and intercostals on the lateral chest wall; and the latissimus dorsi, erector spinae, and scapular muscles on the posterior chest wall. Palpate for tenderness or defects. The inability to reproduce the patient's chest pain when palpating the superficial structures of the chest wall indicates internal pathologies.

• **Superficial abdominal wall.** Palpate the superficial abdomen for tenderness, distension, guarding, and rebound tenderness. It is best to palpate the abdomen with the patient in a supine hook-lying position, which relaxes the abdominal muscles. Begin gently, with your fingers flat and together, starting at the umbilicus and then moving into each quadrant toward the costal, lateral, and iliac margins. Note any pain, tenderness, or defects of the abdominal musculature or their origins. If the abdomen in general is tender and distended, you should suspect internal bleeding and refer the patient immediately. Also note any muscle guarding or rigidity. **Guarding** is characterized by voluntary muscle spasm to protect injury of the abdominal wall and its contents. **Rigidity**, or a boardlike feeling that does not decrease when the muscles are relaxed, indicates internal bleeding. **Rebound tenderness** indicates irritation or inflammation of the peritoneum. You can observe rebound tenderness by depressing and then releasing the abdominal wall. The depression stretches the peritoneum and causes pain when the pressure is released.

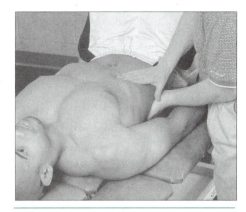

Figure 20.11 Palpation technique for the liver.

• **Abdominal viscera.** Deeper palpation of the abdomen takes practice and requires a sound knowledge of the anatomical orientation of the abdominal viscera. Although direct palpation of these structures is difficult, it can be done (Munger and Baird 1980). To palpate near the liver, firmly place the digits of one hand under the right costal margin and have the patient take a deep breath (figure 20.11). This causes the diaphragm to descend and the lower right tip of the liver to move into the palpating hand. Lifting the patient's right flank with your free hand also improves the chance of liver palpation. To palpate the spleen, lift the left flank with your nondominant hand; keeping your other hand flat, depress the palpating digits just below and anterior to the 11th and 12th ribs and ask the patient to take a deep breath (figure 20.12). A normal, healthy spleen will not be palpable. You can palpate the right kidney by raising the flank with your free hand in order to move the kidney anteriorly toward your palpating hand on the anterior abdominal wall (figure 20.13).

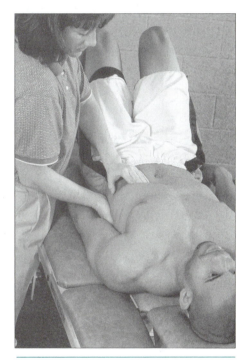

Figure 20.12 Palpation technique for the spleen.

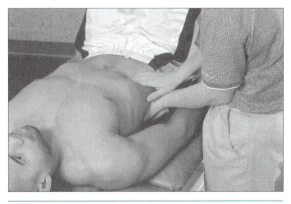

Figure 20.13 Palpation technique for the right kidney.

Range of Motion and Strength

Test active ROM when you suspect that muscles attaching to the upper and lower trunk may be injured. If you suspect muscular involvement or strain of the anterior or posterior chest wall muscles, perform active shoulder extension (latissimus dorsi and teres major), adduction (pectoralis major, latissimus dorsi, teres major) and horizontal adduction (pectoralis major), as well as scapular motions as appropriate (see chapter 12, figures 12.16 and 12.17). Injuries to the lower trunk and abdomen may warrant active ROM testing for trunk flexion (rectus abdominis), extension (erector spinae), lateral flexion (abdominal obliques and erector spinae on injured side), and rotation (internal and external abdominal obliques) (see chapter 15, figures 15.17-15.21).

Examine strength for the same muscles and motions tested during active ROM. Resisted ROM testing will help you determine the extent to which the contractile tissue is involved. To review the manual muscle tests that pertain to the thorax and abdomen, refer to chapter 12 for shoulder motions (tables 12.2 and 12.3 and figures 12.20 and 12.21) and chapter 15 for trunk motions (table 15.2 and figure 15.23).

Neurovascular Examination

Examine neurological status whenever you suspect thoracic nerve root involvement. Check cardiorespiratory status primarily to monitor signs of shock and internal hemorrhage.

- **Cardiorespiratory status.** Record and monitor vital signs if you suspect internal hemorrhage or trauma. Refer to chapter 9 to review the proper testing technique and normal expected values for pulse, respirations, blood pressure, and skin color, moisture, and temperature. The specific examination strategies discussed later in this chapter review what deviations from normal ranges should cause alarm.

- **Neurological status.** Neurological examination in the abdominal and thoracic region is primarily sensory, with considerable overlap in the dermatomal distributions (figure 20.14). While there is no clear myotome for the thoracic nerve roots, table 20.1 indicates

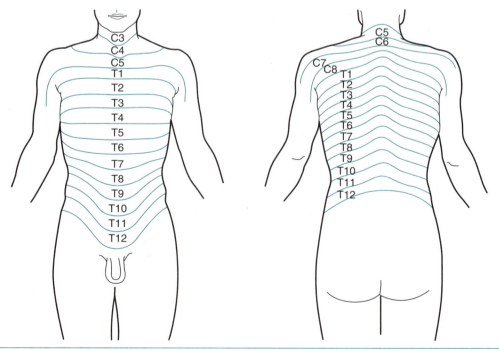

Figure 20.14   Cutaneous dermatome patterns for thoracic nerve roots over the abdominal and thorax region.

the innervation for critical muscles of the thoracic and abdominal walls (Kendall, McCreary, and Provance 1993; Moore 1992).

- **Referred pain from viscera.** Neurological examination of the thorax and abdomen also includes identifying referred pain patterns emanating from the internal organs. Common referral patterns for these structures are shown in figure 20.15.

Table 20.1
Thoracic Spinal Segment Innervations for the Trunk Musculature

Muscle	Spinal segment
Serratus posterior superior (elevation of superior ribs to aid inspiration)	T1-T4
Serratus posterior inferior (depression of lower ribs to aid inspiration)	T9-T12
Intercostals (elevation of ribs to aid inspiration)	T1-T12
Rectus abdominus (trunk flexion)	T5-T12
External oblique (trunk rotation and flexion)	T7-T12
Transverse abdominus (compression of abdominal viscera and trunk stabilization)	T7-L1
Internal oblique (trunk rotation and flexion)	T7-L1
Upper erector spinae (back extension)	T1-T12

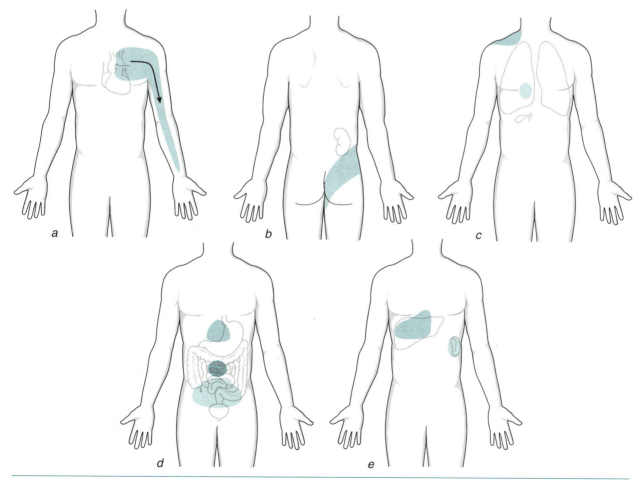

Figure 20.15 Referral patterns for abdominal and thoracic viscera.

Special Tests

Very few special tests are available for identifying pathologies in the thorax or abdominal region. The primary tests are compression tests for rib fractures; auscultation for abnormal heart, bowel, and lung sounds; and a urine dipstick test to examine the urine for abnormal elements, such as blood or bacteria.

Rib Compression (Spring) Tests

To examine for fractures of the lateral ribs, compress the chest wall by placing your hands on the anterior and posterior chest wall and squeezing them together (figure 20.16). This compression causes tensioning of the lateral ribs. Pain or crepitus is a positive sign for fracture. You can use the same compression test for anterior or posterior rib fractures or for costochondral separation by applying a lateral compression stress with your hands placed on the lateral sides of the chest wall (figure 20.17). As before, pain or crepitus is a positive sign.

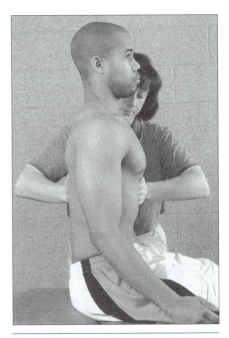

Figure 20.16 Anterior-to-posterior rib compression test.

Auscultation

Listening to heart, lung, and bowel sounds through auscultation may be appropriate and provides further information about cardiopulmonary function or abdominal injury (figure 20.18). You will need training and practice in auscultation techniques to be able to discern abnormal sounds such as decreased bowel sounds, decreased breath sounds, muffled heart tones, and arrhythmias. An Internet search reveals a number of excellent Web sites that allow you to listen to and compare normal and abnormal sounds heard via auscultation (see additional resources at the end of this chapter). You should be able to identify normal heart, lung, and bowel sounds. Any time an abnormal sound is apparent, refer the patient to a qualified physician for a medical diagnosis.

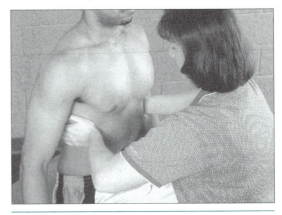

Figure 20.17 Lateral rib compression test.

Abdominal sounds result from peristalsis or the movement of food as it passes through the intestines. To listen to the abdomen, place the stethoscope over each quadrant. Gurgling and bubbling sounds are normal and vary in intensity according to the time of day and the time the patient last ate. In the case of diarrhea, the sounds are louder and more frequent.

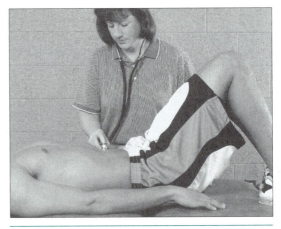

Figure 20.18 Auscultation of the abdomen with a stethoscope.

Rales are crackling, popping, or bubbling sounds heard with auscultation of the lungs.

Rhonchi are loud whooshing sounds heard with auscultation of the lungs, indicating air rushing over mucus in the bronchi.

Wheezing is a high-pitched whistling sound heard with auscultation, commonly noted with bronchial restriction in association with asthma.

Decreased or absent bowel sounds indicate slowing or complete inactivity in the intestines. Reduced intenstinal activity can be caused by a variety of conditions, including obstruction, internal injury, and other serious underlying pathology and warrants immediate referral for further medical examination.

Examine **breath sounds** over the entire thoracic surface while the patient inhales and exhales. Lung sounds are categorized as normal, decreased, absent, and abnormal. Normal breath sounds are quiet and occur at a rate of 8 to 20 breaths per minute. Check for decreased (i.e., quieter than normal) breath sounds that may indicate a pneumothorax. Abnormal sounds include rales (clicking, bubbling, or rattling), rhonchi (snoring), and wheezing (high pitch) that may indicate other nontraumatic restrictive airway or pulmonary conditions.

Auscultation of **heart sounds** should reveal a lub-dub. Rhythm should be regular, ranging from 60 to 80 beats per minute (bpm). Irregular rhythm that occurs consistently with inspiration and expiration is probably normal. Muffled or soft, faint heart tones indicate cardiac tamponade. Murmurs (blowing, whooshing, or rasping) or other sounds that occur between beats suggest vessel or heart valve dysfunction. You may note irregular heart rhythm (arrhythmia) following cardiac contusion. Figure 20.19 shows the best locations for listening to aortic, pulmonic, tricuspid, and mitral valve areas (Munger and Baird 1980).

Urine Dipstick Test

Urine dipsticks are a quick and inexpensive means for identifying hematuria and other abnormal substances in the urine that are invisible to the naked eye. A urine dipstick is a strip of plastic that is saturated with various reagents that identify elements in the urine such as glucose, protein, bacteria, ketones, white blood cells, and blood (figure 20.20). These and other substances are indicated when the appropriate portion of the strip reacts when exposed to the urine. The urine dipstick is very sensitive to blood and assists in identifying blood in the urine when invisible to the naked eye. Because of the potential for false positives, patients with a positive urine dipstick test should be referred to a physician for follow-up examination and further laboratory analysis.

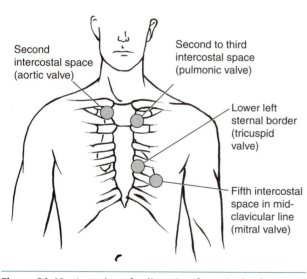

Figure 20.19 Locations for listening for valvular function.

Reprinted, by permission, from G.L. Landry and D.T. Bernhardt, 2003, *Essentials of primary care sports medicine* (Champaign, IL: Human Kinetics), 10.

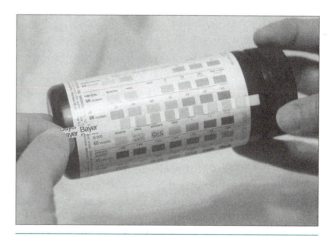

Figure 20.20 Urine dipstick.

INJURY EXAMINATION STRATEGIES

Examination of the thorax and abdomen is rather complex in that symptoms of underlying pathology may not appear immediately, masking the seriousness of the situation. The ability to recognize the signs and symptoms of internal injury and cardiorespiratory compromise can mean the difference between life and death, and often you will need to repeat examinations over time. Since the vast majority of injuries in this region will be acute or traumatic, and since the acute and clinical examinations for this region are essentially the same, the discussion of thorax and abdomen examination is divided into on-site and clinical examinations. The major difference between these examinations is their primary focus on emergent (on-site) versus nonemergent (clinical) conditions.

On-Site Examination

You are covering a soccer game when you see an athlete get kicked accidentally in the groin and go down on the field. As you approach the athlete, he is clearly in a great deal of pain.

A young pitcher collapses after sustaining a blow to the anterior chest from a line drive. As you arrive on the scene, he is conscious but appears to be having difficulty breathing. His respirations are rapid and shallow, at a rate of 30 breaths per minute.

Your goal in the on-site examination is to examine for vital signs and life-threatening conditions and then to gain an initial impression of the nature and severity of the injury. From this thorough but efficient examination, you can appropriately determine medical referral and mode of transportation from the field.

Primary Survey

As you approach the athlete, observe the surroundings as well as the position and response of the athlete, which may provide important clues to the nature and extent of the injury. Is the athlete lying still or clutching the chest or abdomen? Your first goal is to establish whether the athlete is conscious. Obviously, if the athlete is doubled over in pain or is thrashing about, you will establish this before you arrive at the athlete's side.

If the athlete is not moving, immediately examine for airway, breathing, and circulation. If the athlete is breathing and has a pulse, check next for evidence of severe bleeding or trauma. When an athlete sustains blunt trauma to the thorax and abdomen, there is always a chance of internal injury. Therefore, early in your examination you should check vital signs for cardiorespiratory distress, internal bleeding, and shock. Although symptoms of these conditions may not appear immediately, this examination provides a baseline for later comparison. How thoroughly you examine vital signs on the field will depend on the athlete's condition.

Pulse

If the athlete has been exercising, her pulse will be higher than normal and you must consider this in your interpretation. A normal pulse rate under resting conditions is 60 to 80 bpm; perhaps lower in a highly trained runner (see chapter 9). A rapid, weak pulse indicates internal injury, shock, or both. The carotid artery at the neck is the best location for pulse examination. Also note rhythm for evidence of arrhythmias, which may indicate a cardiac contusion or other cardiac trauma.

Respirations

Respiratory distress is obvious upon observation. As discussed in chapter 9, normal respirations should fall between 12 and 20 breaths per minute. Again, this value is likely to be higher after exercise. Dyspnea, or difficulty breathing, may be due to airway obstruction, chest wall injury, lung collapse, or chest compression. Deep quick (labored) respirations also indicate respiratory compromise (e.g., asthma), and rapid and shallow respirations are characteristic of rib fractures, shock, and internal injury. In cases of abdominal trauma, the athlete will purposely limit respirations within the upper chest to avoid moving the abdominal region; this limited movement is one reason for rapid and shallow respirations. Respiration rates below 10 per minute or above 24 per minute are considered abnormal. Any signs of dyspnea demand prompt medical referral.

Blood Pressure

Blood pressure can also indicate shock and internal injury. A normal blood pressure should fall between 100 and 120 mmHg systolic and 70 and 80 mmHg diastolic. A blood pressure that falls below 100/60 may indicate shock or internal hemorrhage. Remember not to wait for significant changes in blood pressure to summon EMS, as abnormal findings may not appear until later stages of hemorrhagic shock.

Skin Appearance

Expect the skin of an exercising athlete to be warm, moist, and somewhat red. Changes in skin toward a pale, cool, and wet appearance indicate shock and internal hemorrhage. When these signs are present along with changes in respiration and pulse, refer the athlete immediately.

Secondary Survey

Once you are assured that the athlete's vital signs are stable, proceed with your secondary survey. Again, because the severity of the condition may not be immediately evident, you will need to periodically reexamine vital signs following significant trauma.

History and Observation

If you did not do so as you approached, ask the athlete or bystanders, or both, about the mechanism of injury. If the mechanism was blunt trauma, try to determine the location, direction, and severity of the impact. Identify the athlete's chief complaint and the location, type, and quality of pain or symptoms. Is there any chest or abdominal pain? Nausea? Difficulty breathing? Does the pain increase on inspiration? All these are relevant questions. Keep in mind the orientation of the underlying structures, and remember that pain from the abdominal viscera may refer to other areas. For example, if the athlete complains of upper left quadrant and left shoulder pain, you should suspect a ruptured spleen. Chest pain and difficulty breathing are complaints consistent with a pneumothorax or hemothorax. Flank or groin pain characterizes kidney trauma, and pain in the upper right quadrant may indicate liver injury. Any time you suspect organ trauma, you should refer the athlete immediately to emergency care.

Continue to observe the athlete's overall response for signs of pain, respiratory or cardiac distress, and shock. Note the athlete's position and willingness to move. Is there any movement, or is the athlete doubled over or restless and agitated? Pain or avoidance of movement may indicate internal abdominal injury or peritoneal irritation. Abdominal pain and cramping causes the athlete to double over; an athlete in respiratory distress is often restless and agitated.

Note the athlete's skin color. Immediately following exercise, the face should be flushed. A pale, moist appearance (wet and white) indicates shock and internal injury. Note the color of the skin around the lips and fingernails; a bluish tint (cyanosis) characterizes respiratory compromise and inadequate oxygenation. Screen the chest and abdomen for signs of swelling, discoloration, laceration, deformity, and asymmetry. Note the position of the trachea and check whether it is in midline or shifted to one side (tension pneumothorax). Observe the neck veins for distension (cardiac contusion, tension pneumothorax).

Note any areas of discoloration at the site of trauma that may give you a sense of the severity or area of the impact. Consider whether the pain is near the site of impact or away from it; this may provide additional clues to the nature of the injury or the structure involved. Watch the chest during respirations for complete expansion and for equal rise and fall on the two sides. If the athlete has multiple rib fractures and a flail chest, the movement of the fractured ribs will be the opposite of what you would expect during inspiration and expiration. Observe the abdomen for signs of guarding (pain, spasm) or distension (blood, fluid accumulation). If the athlete sustained significant trauma to the groin region, check the testicles for normal size and shape. You may also observe nausea and vomiting; these signs are common with abdominal and groin trauma. If the athlete is coughing up blood (hemoptysis), there may be damage to the lung or bronchial passageway. Throughout your observation you should continue to monitor respirations and vital signs as necessary, particularly if the athlete appears unstable.

Palpation, Vital Signs, and Special Tests

Once you have determined the mechanism of injury and the athlete's chief complaint and have completed your observation, you should have a better sense of the location and nature of the injury. You will then proceed with palpation to quickly examine the potentially involved structures.

Periodically monitor vital signs, as signs and symptoms of shock and internal hemorrhage may not appear immediately. Note any changes and continue to monitor for arrhythmia, decreased blood pressure, increased respirations, or a rapid and weak pulse.

There are no special on-site tests for this region; your impression will be based primarily on the mechanism of the injury, the athlete's vital signs, and the signs and symptoms identified in your history, observation, and palpation. If all signs are negative, you can remove the athlete from the field for further examination on the sideline.

When to Refer

Severe abdominal or chest trauma is uncommon in athletics, but you always should be prepared to examine and rule out such conditions, particularly when the athlete sustains blunt trauma to the flank, chest, or abdomen. To review, the cardinal signs of internal injury and shock include the following:

- Decreased blood pressure
- Rapid, weak pulse
- Wet, white, and weak appearance
- Rapid and shallow respirations

When you note any of these signs, refer the athlete immediately for emergency medical attention.

Other signs and symptoms that warrant immediate medical referral include any signs of respiratory distress (dyspnea); abnormal vital signs; cardiac arrhythmia; abdominal tenderness, rigidity, or distension; or any other signs that may indicate severe trauma. Many of these signs and symptoms may not be observable immediately and may occur at some delay; therefore it is necessary to reexamine the athlete periodically for any change in vital signs or symptoms. If all of the signs just listed are negative, the athlete can leave the field for continued monitoring on the sidelines.

Checklist for On-Site Examination of the Abdomen and Thorax

▷ **Primary Survey**

☐ Consciousness

☐ Airway, breathing, circulation

☐ Signs of severe bleeding, evidence of severe trauma

☐ Vital signs

    ☐ Pulse (rate, rhythm, strength)

    ☐ Respirations (dyspnea, rate, depth)

    ☐ Blood pressure

    ☐ Skin appearance

▷ **Secondary Survey**

  ▷ *History*

    ☐ Mechanism of injury

    ☐ Location, direction, and severity of impact if blunt trauma

    ☐ Chief complaint

    ☐ Location, type, and quality of pain

    ☐ Presence and location of referred pain

    ☐ Difficulty breathing or pain with inspiration

    ☐ Feelings of nausea

  ▷ *Observation*

    ☐ Response and position of athlete, willingness to move

    ☐ Signs of respiratory or cardiac distress (dyspnea, cyanosis, neck vein distension, tracheal shift)

    ☐ Signs of shock (wet, white, weak)

    ☐ Skin coloration

    ☐ Signs of swelling, discoloration, lacerations, deformity, or asymmetry (superficial screen)

    ☐ Expansion and equal rise of the chest wall

    ☐ Abdomen for signs of guarding, rigidity, or distension

    ☐ Genitalia for swelling and abnormal appearance

    ☐ Continued monitoring of vital signs

  ▷ *Palpation*

    ☐ Chest wall for tenderness, swelling, deformity, crepitus, asymmetry

    ☐ Bony landmarks: clavicle, sternum, xiphoid process, costochondral cartilage, thoracic vertebrae, scapula, and ribs (anterior, lateral, and posterior)

    ☐ Soft tissue: pectoralis major and minor, intercostals, serratus anterior, erector spinae, scapular muscles

    ☐ Absence of palpable signs may indicate internal injury.

    ☐ Palpate abdomen in all four quadrants for the following:

       ☐ Soft tissue tenderness or muscle guarding

       ☐ Rigidity and distension

       ☐ Rebound tenderness

    ☐ Continued monitoring of vital signs (pulse, respirations, blood pressure, and skin appearance)

  ▷ *Special Tests (None)*

(continued)

(continued)

When to refer:
- ☐ Decreased blood pressure
- ☐ Rapid and weak pulse
- ☐ Wet, white, weak appearance
- ☐ Rapid and shallow respirations
- ☐ Dyspnea or cyanosis
- ☐ Cardiac arrhythmia
- ☐ Abdominal tenderness, rigidity, or distension
- ☐ Any abnormal vital signs

Acute and Clinical Examination

A football player receives a blow to the left side of his lower back from an opponent's helmet. Although he has some initial pain, it is not enough to hold him out. Later, he comes to you complaining of not feeling well and he appears quite pale.

A women's basketball player has just completed an intense conditioning session on the track. She comes to you complaining of shortness of breath and pain in her upper right chest. She denies any injury.

A young baseball player comes to you complaining of anterior chest wall pain that increases with inspiration. He can't recall a specific injury other than feeling a "pop" in his chest during a heavy bench press session with his teammates yesterday. While it did not hurt initially, it is quite painful today.

The goal of your clinical examination is to determine the SINS of the injury: *S*everity, *I*rritability, *N*ature, and *S*tage.

Not all injuries of the thorax and abdomen are immediately emergent, and some may be reported postacutely. Your goal in the clinical examination is to establish the SINS of the injury, to differentiate other possible causes of the athlete's pain, and to rule out any latent underlying pathology that may manifest at some delay following the injury.

History

All aspects of the history portion of the on-site examination apply here. Since you may have not witnessed the injury or the athlete may report it at some delay, other questions will also be relevant. Explore the mechanism of the injury and determine whether it was one of contact or noncontact. If it was noncontact mechanism, did the injury result from a sudden twist or muscle contraction that would indicate a soft tissue or muscle injury? For a contact injury, try to determine as closely as possible the location and area of impact as well as the direction and intensity of the force. As the athlete describes the location, type, and quality of pain, is the location of pain consistent with the site of injury, or is it at some remote site, indicating secondary indirect trauma or referred symptoms?

Also explore other complaints at this time. If the injury is postacute, ask about the onset and duration of symptoms and any change in symptoms since the initial injury. Find out what activities increase or decrease symptoms, and establish the pain pattern. Has the athlete suffered any episodes of nausea, vomiting, or difficulty breathing? A sharp, sticking chest pain with inspiration is often associated with pleural irritation. If the injury was to the flank or abdominal region, ask the athlete whether there has been any blood in the urine; if the athlete has not paid attention to this, provide instructions for the athlete to check the next time he voids. Rather than looking only for blood, ask also about any changes in urine color. Bleeding is not always frank, and the athlete may be unable to detect blood that is in the urine.

Finally, does the athlete with chest wall or rib pain complain of increased pain with deep inspiration, coughing, or sneezing? If so, there may be an intercostal muscle strain, abdominal strain, or rib fracture, depending on the location of injury. Gaining a history of previous injury and overall general health is also important. Other general medical conditions unrelated to sport activity may cause pain or symptoms in the thorax or abdominal region. You should rule out factors such as asthma, upper respiratory illness, or gastrointestinal conditions that may be the source of the athlete's complaints (see chapters 21 and 22).

Observation

Your inspection of the athlete will be consistent with that described for the on-site examination and should include observation for abnormal respirations, skin color, abdominal guarding, athlete response, and signs of external trauma. With postacute injuries, swelling and discoloration will likely be more pronounced than they would normally be immediately following injury. Whether the athlete walks over to you on the sidelines or seeks your assistance in the athletic training room, note her position and posture. An athlete who is having difficulty breathing may be bent forward, with her hands resting on her knees. To relieve muscle strain and stretch, an athlete often leans to the side of injury. This, as well as guarding or splinting of the arm or chest to protect the rib cage, may indicate a rib fracture. If the athlete is able to urinate and you suspect kidney trauma, inspect the urine yourself for hematuria.

Palpation

Off the field, you will palpate the chest wall and abdomen as described for the on-site examination. Place the athlete in a comfortable position (usually supine with knees and hips flexed) for maximal athlete relaxation and optimal palpation. Note areas of tenderness and consider both superficial and internal structures that may be involved. In addition to superficial palpation of the abdomen, you may also proceed with deeper organ palpation for any pain or enlargement of the spleen, liver, or kidney. If the athlete sustained severe testicular trauma that has not eased following injury, palpate or have the athlete palpate bilaterally for signs of swelling, tenderness, masses, changes in consistency, or asymmetries. If there are any abnormalities, immediately refer the athlete to a physician for further examination.

Special Tests

As previously discussed, special tests are limited for the thorax and abdominal region, and are only used for specific situations. If you suspect the athlete may have a rib fracture, you perform a compression (spring) test to help confirm your suspicions. If the athlete sustained direct trauma to the lower back and you suspect a kidney contusion, use a urine dipstick test along with gross observation to check for hematuria. Auscultation will be used less frequently to examine heart, lung, or bowel sounds as warranted.

Range of Motion

If you suspect muscular involvement or strain within the trunk or chest wall, perform active ROM to examine for the presence of pain, guarding, or restricted motion with active muscle contraction. Visceral pain can refer to various superficial regions of the abdominal and thoracic wall and may be misinterpreted as muscle pain. Pain that is unaffected by active movement is probably not of muscular origin.

Strength

Examine strength of the trunk, abdominal, and chest wall muscles by resisting the same motions tested for active ROM.

Neurovascular Examination

Perform neurological and cardiovascular examination whenever you suspect thoracic nerve root irritation or injury, or any internal injury. Thoracic nerve irritation commonly refers pain to the chest and abdomen. Because of the overlapping patterns of the thoracic nerve roots, it may be difficult to identify the specific nerve root involved, but if you note any abnormal sensations or pain that wraps around the thoracic or abdominal region, refer the athlete to a physician for further examination. See table 20.1 on page 573 and figure 20.14 on page 572 for sensory and motor distributions of the thoracic spinal nerves.

You must have a thorough knowledge of the pain referral patterns of the abdominal and thoracic viscera (see figure 20.15 on page 573) to accurately interpret the athlete's complaints. Because it is common for internal injuries to present themselves at some delay following the initial trauma, when the athlete reports a history of a forceful, direct blow to the lower abdomen and trunk, carefully examine referred pain. Also examine vital signs at this time as warranted.

Functional Examinations

You should determine functional performance only when all tests are negative and you are deciding the athlete's readiness and ability to return to activity. This examination may include aerobic exercise to ensure normal heart and lung function and sport-related movements to determine normal, painless muscular function. You should reexamine signs and symptoms associated with the injury during and after the activity, noting any return of symptoms.

Follow-Up Examinations

As has been mentioned, signs and symptoms of internal injuries may not manifest themselves until hours or even days following injury. Ongoing or follow-up examination and care of an athlete who has sustained blunt trauma should thus include frequent examination and instructions to the athlete about signs and symptoms to watch for.

Checklist for Clinical Examination of the Abdomen and Thorax

▷ *History*

Ask questions pertaining to the following:
- ☐ Mechanism of injury (contact or noncontact)
- ☐ Location, direction, and severity of impact if blunt trauma
- ☐ Chief complaint
- ☐ Onset, duration, and change in symptoms if injury is postacute
- ☐ Activities that increase or decrease symptoms
- ☐ Location, type, and quality of pain
- ☐ Presence and location of referred pain
- ☐ Pain with coughing, sneezing, or deep inspiration
- ☐ Complaints of nausea, vomiting, difficulty breathing
- ☐ Presence of hematuria
- ☐ Previous injury history
- ☐ General medical health and history

▷ *Observation*

- ☐ Response, position, and posture of athlete
- ☐ Breathing pattern (dyspnea; respirations for rate, rhythm, and depth; chest wall expansion)
- ☐ Signs of cardiac distress (neck vein distension, tracheal shift)
- ☐ Skin color and moisture (cyanosis, white and wet)

- ☐ Abdomen for signs of guarding, rigidity, or distension
- ☐ Genitalia for swelling or abnormal appearance
- ☐ Blood in urine (hematuria) or sputum (hemoptysis)
- ☐ Signs of swelling, discoloration, lacerations, deformity, or asymmetry (superficial screen)
- ☐ Vital signs
    - ☐ Respirations for rate, rhythm, and depth
    - ☐ Blood pressure
    - ☐ Pulse
- ☐ Signs of internal hemorrhage or shock

▷ Palpation

Bilaterally palpate for pain, tenderness, and deformity over the following:
- ☐ Chest wall
    - ☐ Bony landmarks: clavicle, sternum, xiphoid process, costochondral cartilage, thoracic vertebrae, scapula, and ribs (anterior, lateral, and posterior)
    - ☐ Soft tissue: pectoralis major and minor, intercostals, serratus anterior, erector spinae, scapular muscles
- ☐ Abdomen and genitalia
    - ☐ Soft tissue tenderness or muscle guarding
    - ☐ Rigidity and distension
    - ☐ Rebound tenderness
    - ☐ Deep organ palpation (spleen, kidney, liver)
    - ☐ Testicles for swelling tenderness, masses, abnormalities

▷ Special Tests

- ☐ Rib compression tests
- ☐ Auscultation of heart, lungs, and bowel
- ☐ Urine dipstick test

▷ Range of Motion

- ☐ Perform active ROM for trunk motions
- ☐ Perform active ROM for shoulder and scapular motions for muscles of the chest wall
- ☐ Compare bilaterally

▷ Strength Tests

- ☐ Perform resistance on same motions performed for active ROM
- ☐ Note weakness or difference bilaterally

▷ Neurovascular Tests

- ☐ Sensory for thoracic dermatomes
- ☐ Visceral referral patterns
- ☐ Vital signs

▷ Functional Tests

- ☐ Cardiorespiratory
- ☐ Musculoskeletal

▷ Follow-Up Examination

- ☐ Instruct athlete about signs and symptoms to watch for
- ☐ Perform periodic reexamination for emerging signs and symptoms of internal injury

SUMMARY

1. Describe the common mechanisms, signs and symptoms, and potential complications associated with injuries to the thorax commonly encountered in the physically active.

   Injuries to the chest wall and structures in the thoracic cavity can result from direct insult or violent muscle contractions or may occur spontaneously as a result of intense exercise. The most common of these injuries are contusions, strains, sprains, and chest wall fractures. These same mechanisms can also traumatize the heart and lungs or result in internal bleeding, which can have life-threatening consequences. It is essential for you to be able to identify signs and symptoms of cardiorespiratory distress and differentiate those that indicate a medical emergency and immediate medical referral.

2. Describe the common mechanisms, signs and symptoms, and potential complications associated with injuries to the abdomen commonly encountered in the physically active.

   Traumatic injuries to the abdominal region include soft tissue injuries of the abdominal muscles, genitalia, and internal viscera. While the thoracic cavity is well protected by the skeletal rib cage, the abdomen is protected primarily by the surrounding muscular wall. Consequently, contusions and muscular strains are the more common injuries in this region. Although these injuries are usually minor, when acute they can cause considerable pain and disability. Internal injuries, particularly to the solid organs, are also a concern with blunt trauma; these injuries most often involve the spleen and kidney. If internal hemorrhage results, the injury becomes life threatening if not immediately recognized and managed appropriately.

3. Differentiate among pathologies and signs and symptoms of cardiac contusion, tamponade, and concussion.

   Blunt trauma to the anterior chest can injure the heart. Cardiac contusion can result when the heart is compressed between the sternum and the spine. Cardiac tamponade is characterized by hemorrhage in the pericardial cavity, compressing and compromising the heart and pulmonary veins. Cardiac concussion, more common in adolescents, most often results from a blunt but seemingly inconsequential blow over the region of the heart. Each of these conditions represents a medical emergency; cardiac concussion often results in cardiac arrest and death. Any time an athlete receives blunt trauma to the anterior chest near the heart, suspect cardiac injury and immediately examine vital signs.

4. Appreciate the potential for life-threatening injury resulting from direct and indirect trauma to the thorax and abdomen.

   The abdominal cavity contains both solid and hollow organs that can sustain injury during sport activity. When an athlete presents with a history of severe blunt trauma to the abdomen, you should highly suspect internal injury or hemorrhage. It is imperative that you are able to recognize the signs and symptoms associated with internal hemorrhage and shock. Suspicion of internal trauma warrants immediate referral of the athlete for a thorough medical examination.

5. Describe and demonstrate the objective tests for examining the thorax and abdomen.

   Objective tests for the abdomen and thorax primarily aim at distinguishing musculoskeletal injury of the chest and abdominal walls and injury to the internal organs. Led by your history and observation, you will rely heavily on your palpation skills and examination of vital signs, as there are very few special tests for this region. Palpation of the thorax and abdominal regions is divided into the superficial palpation of the chest wall and superficial and deep palpation of the abdomen. Test active ROM and strength when you suspect that muscles attaching to the upper and lower trunk may be involved. Examine neurological status whenever you suspect involvement of the thoracic nerve root or internal injury. Neurological examination of the thorax and abdomen also includes identifying referred pain patterns emanating from the internal organs. Check cardiorespiratory status primarily to monitor signs of shock and internal hemorrhage. The primary special tests include compression tests for rib fractures; auscultation for abnormal heart, bowel, and lung sounds; and a urine dipstick test to examine the urine for abnormal elements, such as blood or bacteria.

6. Perform an on-site examination of the thorax and abdomen, indicating criteria for immediate medical referral or continued observation.

   Severe abdominal or chest trauma is uncommon in athletics, but you should always be prepared to examine and rule out such conditions, particularly when the athlete sustains blunt trauma to the flank, chest, or abdomen. The goal in the on-site examination is to examine for vital signs and life-threatening conditions and then to gain an initial impression of the nature and severity of the injury. From this thorough but efficient examination you can appropriately determine medical referral and mode of transportation from the field. If all of these signs are negative, the athlete can leave the field for continued monitoring on the sidelines. Remember that many signs and symptoms may not be immediately observable and may occur at some delay; it is necessary to reexamine the athlete periodically for any change in vital signs or symptoms. The ability to recognize signs and symptoms of internal injury and cardiorespiratory compromise can literally mean the difference between life and death, and these conditions often require repeated examination over time.

7. Perform a clinical examination of the thorax and abdomen, indicating considerations for differential diagnosis.

   Most injuries of the thorax and abdomen are not immediately emergent, and some may be reported postacutely. Therefore the goal of the clinical examination is to establish the SINS of the injury, to differentiate other possible causes of the athlete's pain (including general medical conditions), and to rule out any latent underlying pathology that may manifest at some delay following the injury.

REVIEW QUESTIONS

1. Describe the common fractures of the chest wall. When would a suspected fracture concern you about the potential for underlying pathology?

2. Describe the differences among a pneumothorax, a spontaneous pneumothorax, and a tension pneumothorax. How do their signs and symptoms differ, and which condition represents an immediate life-threatening injury?

3. What is commotio cordis? Describe the etiology and signs and symptoms of this condition and identify the populations most susceptible to this injury.

4. Testicular trauma is relatively common among physically active males. How would you differentiate between a minor and a serious injury?

5. What is a hernia, and what types of hernias are commonly seen in males versus females? What signs and symptoms indicate these conditions?

6. What are the signs and symptoms of a kidney contusion?

7. As part of the primary survey, you are asked to take a patient's vital signs. What vitals do you examine, and what are the cardinal signs and symptoms of internal hemorrhage?

8. From what you have learned in this chapter, list as many signs and symptoms as you can that indicate immediate medical referral.

CRITICAL THINKING QUESTIONS

1. During football practice you see an athlete receive a blow to the anterior abdomen. He is having difficulty catching his breath and is panicked. What conditions might you suspect, and how would you proceed in your examination to rule out serious pathology?

2. Recall the scenario of a basketball player who has just completed an intense conditioning session on the track. She comes to you complaining of shortness of breath and pain in her upper right chest. She denies any injury. Describe your examination of this athlete, including your pertinent history questions and your objective examination.

3. A wrestler is taken down hard on the mat, with his opponent landing on top of him. He complains of pain in his lateral chest wall and increased pain with inspiration. You suspect a rib fracture. To confirm your suspicions, how would your examination proceed from the history through the special tests?

4. Consider the scenario of the young baseball player who comes to you complaining of anterior chest wall pain that increases with inspiration. He can't recall a specific injury other than feeling a pop in his chest during a heavy bench press session with his teammates yesterday. While his chest did not hurt initially, it is quite painful today. What potential injuries would you consider, and how would your examination proceed? After obtaining a thorough history, where would you begin your palpations?

CITED REFERENCES

Curfman, G.D. 1998. Fatal impact—concussion of the heart [Editorial]. *N Eng J Med* 338(25): 1841-1843.

Fruh, J.M. 1993. Fracture of the first rib in a collegiate soccer player. *J Sport Rehab* 2(3): 196-199.

Haq, C.L. 1998. Sudden death due to low energy chest wall impact (commotio cordis) [Correspondence]. *N Eng J Med* 339(19): 1398-1399.

Kendall, F.P., E.K. McCreary, and P.G. Provance. 1993. *Muscles: Testing and function.* 4th ed. Philadelphia: Lippincott Williams & Wilkins.

Maron, B.J., L.C. Poliac, J.A. Kaplan, and F.O. Mueller. 1995. Blunt impact to the chest leading to sudden death from cardiac arrest during sport activities. *N Eng J Med* 333(6): 337-342.

Moore, K.L. 1992. *Clinically oriented anatomy.* 3rd ed. Baltimore: Williams & Wilkins.

Munger, B.L., and I.L. Baird. 1980. *Anatomy-Px: A practical introduction to anatomical correlates of the physical examination.* Baltimore: Williams & Wilkins.

ADDITIONAL RESOURCES

Cable, C. 1997. The auscultation assistant. Available at www.med.ucla.edu/wilkes/intro.html. Accessed August 20, 2004.

Gudmundsson, G., and T. Asmundsson. 2000. Lung sounds: Chest auscultation. Virtual Hospital. Available at www.vh.org/adult/provider/internalmedicine/LungSounds/LungSounds.html. Accessed August 20, 2004.

Cardiac auscultation of heart murmurs. 2003. GeneralMedical.com. Available at http://stethoscopemerchant.com/listohearmur.html. Accessed August 20, 2004.

Recognition of General Medical Conditions

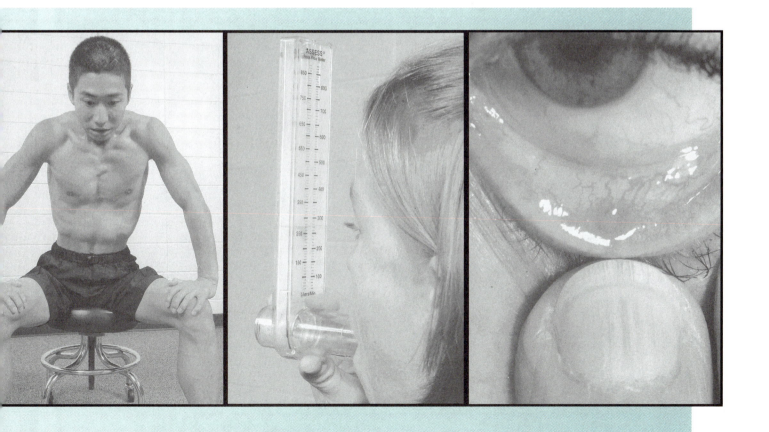

Part III consists of three chapters that cover the general medical conditions you are most likely to encounter in physically active individuals. Chapter 21 covers medical conditions of the eyes, ears, nose, and throat (EENT), respiratory and cardiovascular systems, and viral conditions that often involve signs and symptoms affecting these systems. Chapter 22 then covers conditions affecting the digestive, endocrine, reproductive, and urinary systems. Disordered eating and sexually transmitted diseases are also discussed here. Chapter 23 closes out part III with the presentation of general medical conditions affecting the musculoskeletal, nervous, and integumentary systems, and other systemic diseases of the blood and lymph. The topics in these chapters are discussed according to body systems as presented in *Athletic Training Educational Competencies* (National Athletic Trainers' Association 1999). In some cases, the order has been slightly altered to enhance comprehension and understanding of related conditions. Since the goal of this chapter is recognition, the discussion does not follow the general examination procedure framework presented in part II. Instead, such examinations are usually the responsibility of the physician and require diagnostic tests to identify the condition. It is paramount, then, that you are able to readily recognize these conditions and make the appropriate referral based on your history and observation.

CHAPTER 21

EENT and Cardiorespiratory Conditions

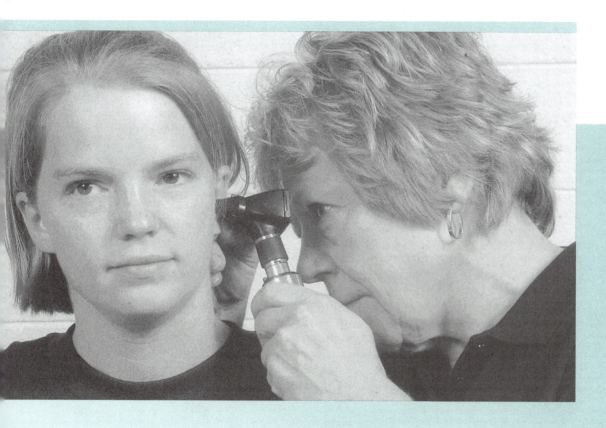

Objectives

After completing this chapter, the reader will be able to do the following:

1. Describe and recognize the signs and symptoms of medical conditions of the eyes, ears, nose, and throat that may be encountered in the physically active

2. Describe and recognize the signs and symptoms of medical conditions of the respiratory system that may be encountered in the physically active

3. Describe and recognize the signs and symptoms of medical conditions of the cardiovascular system that may be encountered in the physically active

4. Describe and recognize the signs and symptoms of viral conditions that may be encountered in the physically active

5. Appreciate the complications that may result from many of these conditions if they are not recognized and if they are left untreated

6. Determine which medical conditions require emergency medical referral and which require physician referral for diagnosis and treatment

Rhonda was completing an afternoon treatment when Brenda, one of the basketball players, walked in.

"Brenda, do you have a minute?" Rhonda asked. "I understand from one of the other players that you had a little trouble out on the track this morning after some early-morning conditioning. What exactly happened?"

"I just fainted. It's no big deal," Brenda said with some embarrassment.

"Has this happened before?" Rhonda inquired.

"Yeah, I guess a couple of other times over the past year or so. But I feel fine. There's nothing wrong with me. I think I just pushed a little too hard trying to get ready for the upcoming season," Brenda replied.

Rhonda was concerned. "Brenda, fainting after activity is not normal, and you should be checked out by a physician to make sure there is no serious underlying cause for this fainting. Let's schedule an appointment with Dr. Titan for this afternoon just to be sure you're okay."

When caring for the physically active, you may encounter a variety of general medical conditions and disabilities that are not directly related to physical activity but that can affect performance or overall health. Many of these conditions are of short duration and are accompanied by only minor signs and symptoms or disabilities. However, some can have severe, life-threatening consequences or can result in permanent disability if not recognized and treated appropriately. Other conditions represent permanent and preexisting disease states that require you to be aware of the athlete's history, as complications may arise during sport activity.

Although the majority of the conditions discussed in this and subsequent chapters are beyond the scope of your ability to care for the athlete, you must be able to recognize their signs and symptoms in order to make the appropriate medical referral and ensure proper care for the athlete. When athletes participating in physical activity exhibit such signs and symptoms, it may be necessary to provide immediate first aid or emergency care, but referral to a physician is your ultimate responsibility. In many cases, you will not see the outward manifestations of these conditions but will learn of the problem from the concerned athlete. Because of the close relationship that develops through daily interaction, it is not uncommon for athletes to confide in you rather than a physician. This is especially true in the case of more sensitive or potentially embarrassing symptoms when the athlete is unsure of what they signify or what to do about them.

This chapter addresses conditions affecting the eyes, ears, nose, and throat (EENT) and the cardiovascular and respiratory systems. Viral syndromes are also discussed here, as their signs and symptoms often involve the EENT and cardiorespiratory systems.

EYES, EARS, AND MOUTH

Irritation and infection in the eyes, ears, and mouth are common complaints in the physically active. These conditions can cause considerable pain, hampering performance until they are resolved. Most are caused by bacterial or viral infections.

Eye Conditions

Redness and irritation of either or both eyes, which can be quite painful, can result from infection, the presence of foreign bodies, or allergens. Two common eye conditions are conjunctivitis and sties.

Conjunctivitis

Conjunctivitis, or pinkeye, is irritation and inflammation of the outer surface of the eye or inner eyelid. It can be caused by allergies, infection (viral or bacterial), or direct contact (e.g., contact with an airborne substance, hand contact). While allergic conjunctivitis typically involves both eyes, viral or bacterial conjunctivitis usually begins in one eye but may spread to the other. The athlete complains of pain, itching, and burning or a scratchy sensation in the eye, and the eye appears red and swollen. Sensitivity to light (**photophobia**), blurred vision, and a yellowish discharge from the eye may also occur secondary to the irritation and infection. Viral conjunctivitis, which frequently accompanies an upper respiratory infection, is quite contagious and can easily spread to the unaffected eye or to teammates. It is imperative that the athlete avoids touching the eye when possible and immediately washes her hands after having done so in order to avoid spreading the infection. Treatment includes removal of the irritant, eye washes, and referral to a physician for an ophthalmic solution.

Sties

The glands and hair follicles of the eyelid can become irritated and swollen as a consequence of infection or obstruction. A **sty** is an infection or obstruction of a ciliary gland of the eyelid. **Chalazia**, or cysts of the sebaceous glands, may also form. Both result in focal redness and swelling that gradually appear as a small nodule or bump along the margin of the eyelid (figure 21.1). A painful pustule may develop over subsequent days. Pain and general eye discomfort are the primary complaints.

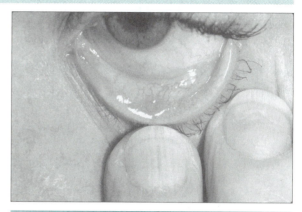

Figure 21.1 Sty.
Courtesy of Kenneth E. Greer.

Ear Conditions

Earaches can be caused by a variety of conditions. Pain can be referred from the jaw or teeth but is most often caused by inflammation in the external auditory canal. These conditions can be quite painful and can result in temporary loss of hearing due to inflammation.

Impacted Cerumen

> Neither you nor the athlete should attempt to remove excessive wax buildup with a cotton swab, as it could cause further impaction and discomfort.

Excessive wax buildup in the external auditory canal can lead to hearing loss, tinnitus, and feelings of pressure or pain within the ear. On observation, the wax accumulation is visible in the ear canal. While you may be tempted to remove the wax with a cotton swab, this is contraindicated, as it could cause further impaction and discomfort. Refer the athlete to a physician and flush the ear with warm water for gentle wax removal.

Otitis Externa (Swimmer's Ear)

Otitis externa, or bacterial infections from water accumulation in the swimmer's ear, are a common cause of inflammation in the external ear canal. Signs and symptoms of otitis externa include pain, itching or burning, and possible drainage from the ear. The external ear may be tender to palpation, and pulling on the earlobe increases pain. Inappropriate or aggressive use of a cotton swab can irritate the external canal. Refer the athlete to a physician for the appropriate medication.

Otitis Media

Otitis media is characterized by inflammation or infection of the tympanic cavity or middle ear. Within this cavity are the auditory ossicles (malleus, incus, and stapes) as well as tympanic muscles and nerves. Infections of the middle ear and tympanic membrane (eardrum) can be extremely painful. Signs and symptoms include severe earache, swollen and red eardrum, fever, dizziness (vertigo), tinnitus, and possible hearing loss. Middle ear infections are often associated with viral upper respiratory infections. The pain alone typically drives the athlete to a physician for examination and treatment. Athletes with suspected otitis media should always consult a physician before flying.

Dental and Gum Disease

Frequently athletes neglect dental hygiene and may suffer from tooth and gum conditions or disease. When signs and symptoms of tooth or gum disease appear, refer the athlete to a dentist for examination and care.

Gingivitis

Gingivitis is an inflammation of the gum that results from bacteria in and around the gums caused by food deposits and inadequate brushing or flossing. Brushing the teeth too aggressively or in a lateral versus up-and-down motion can also irritate the gums. The gums appear red and swollen, and the athlete complains of pain and bleeding when brushing the teeth. If hygiene does not improve, gingivitis can progress to periodontitis (**pyorrhea**).

Periodontitis

Periodontitis, a more serious condition caused by bacteria, results in loss of alveolar bone and recession of the gum line. Signs and symptoms include pain and bleeding with brushing, tooth sensitivity to cold and hot drinks or foods, red and swollen gums, breath odor, and possible loosening of the teeth.

Dental Caries

Tooth pain may result from **dental caries** (cavities) or **abscess**. Dental caries are caused by decay and degeneration of the tooth enamel, allowing exposure, irritation, and infection of the tooth's pulp. The athlete may complain of a toothache and sensitivity with chewing or with drinking hot and cold fluids. If the infection passes through the root of the tooth into the periodontal tissues, an abscess may form in the adjacent gum. Signs and symptoms include a severe, unrelenting toothache that may radiate into the sinus, jaw, or ear depending on the location of the infected tooth. Pain worsens when the athlete drinks hot or cold fluids. The gum will likely be swollen and red, and the tooth may be tender and loose when mobilized. A fever may also be present.

RESPIRATORY SYSTEM

Irritation and infection (viral and bacterial) can occur throughout the respiratory system and passageways. Upper respiratory conditions are common and may affect the nose, throat, tonsils, and sinuses. A less frequent but more serious condition is infection of the lower respiratory system (bronchi and lungs). Other respiratory conditions not associated with infection include allergic rhinitis, asthma, hay fever, and hyperventilation. You should be able to recognize and differentiate those conditions that can result in serious respiratory compromise, as they can be life threatening if the athlete does not receive timely and appropriate treatment.

Upper Respiratory Conditions

An upper respiratory infection (URI) is any infection that affects any portion of the upper respiratory system (conducting pathway) including the tonsils, nose, throat, sinuses, and neck lymph nodes. As previously noted, middle ear infections can also be associated with URIs. Upper respiratory infections can be viral or bacterial. The common cold, flu, sinusitis, laryngitis, pharyngitis, and tonsillitis are examples of these conditions. Specific signs and symptoms and treatments vary according to the area involved and the cause of the infection. If a URI affects one area, you must be aware that other aspects of the upper respiratory system

! Athletes with a high fever (>100° F, 38° C) who engage in activities that further increase core temperature are at risk for febrile seizures.

Antipyretics are fever-reducing agents.

Analgesics are pain-reducing agents.

can become involved and you must watch closely for changes in signs and symptoms. Refer the athlete to a physician if any URI does not appear to follow a normal course or duration. Additionally, referral to a physician may be indicated for medication to relieve symptoms.

Often the athlete continues to work or engage in physical activity despite symptoms. Although the signs and symptoms associated with these conditions are relatively minor and may have a limited effect on performance, adequate rest is essential for quick resolution. Moreover, whenever a high fever accompanies these conditions, remove the athlete from participation until the fever reduces. Any athlete with a fever over 100° F (38° C) should not be allowed to participate until the fever has gone down or a physician has given clearance. Athletes with a high fever who engage in activities that further increase core temperature may be at risk for **febrile seizures**.

Systemic Infections

General URI conditions are multisymptomatic, as they typically affect both the nose and throat and may also involve the eyes and ears.

Common Cold

Common colds are viral infections that affect the upper respiratory system and are sometimes referred to as **rhinoviruses**. The incubation time is short, 18 to 48 hours, with the onset typically heralded by a scratchy throat, sneezing, nasal discharge, and general malaise. Fever can sometimes accompany a cold, especially in children. Congestion headache, reduced smell and taste sensations, nasal congestion, cough, and general achiness are frequent complaints. Symptoms usually run their course in 4 to10 days, but additional factors such as sinusitis, bronchitis, or tonsillitis can extend their duration.

Treatment is symptomatic relief with the use of antipyretics, antihistamines, decongestants, and analgesics. Since a cold is caused by a virus, antibiotics are not recommended unless it is apparent that a bacterial infection accompanies the cold. Increased fluid intake and rest are an important part of treatment.

Influenza

Influenza, or flu, is a viral infection that affects the body in general and the upper respiratory system in particular. It is highly contagious and spread by infected persons through coughing and sneezing. According to the Centers for Disease Control (CDC), as many as 20% of United States residents contract the flu each year, with an average of 114,000 people hospitalized and 36,000 people dying each year from complications of the flu (2004). Symptoms include high fever, chills, general weakness, fatigue, body aches and pains, and inflammation of the upper respiratory system with moderate signs and symptoms of runny nose, sore throat, and dry cough. Children may also experience symptoms of nausea, vomiting, and diarrhea. Mild cases last 2 to 3 days, whereas more severe cases last for 4 to 5 days with residual symptoms of weakness and fatigue persisting for up to a few weeks. Because the signs and symptoms of influenza are similar to other respiratory infections, the flu may require a laboratory test to diagnose it. Treatment consists of rest, symptom relief with over-the-counter medications, and antiviral medications to reduce symptom duration. Bed rest is recommended until after body temperature has returned to normal; increase in fluid intake is strongly recommended, and medications for relief of pain and temperature can increase the patient's comfort. Additional complications such as sinusitis, ear infection, and staphylococcus infections can occur; these require antibacterial therapy. You should therefore carefully monitor symptoms and refer to the physician. The best prevention against influenza is receiving a flu vaccine at the beginning of each fall. This is especially important for young children, adults over the age of 65, and those with chronic medical conditions (e.g., diabetes, pulmonary or cardiac disease) who are at greater risk for complications, hospitalizations, and death from influenza (CDC 2004).

Nose and Throat

Signs and symptoms of URIs may also appear more localized, involving primarily the nose or throat.

Rhinitis

Acute inflammation or infection of the nasal passageways, usually virus or allergy based, results in annoying nasal mucosa discharge. Obstructed breathing (congestion) can occur with excessive mucosal discharge and swelling of the nasal passages. A runny nose and sneezing are often the first signs of a URI. Medications are used to control mucosal discharge and decrease congestion.

Sinusitis

Inflammation of the nasal and facial sinuses can result from either viral or bacterial exposure but is also commonly associated with predisposing conditions such as chronic rhinitis, obstructive drainage, allergy exposure, general debilitation, dental abscess, or exposure to extreme temperature and humidity. Those with a previous history of sinus infections seem to be more susceptible to repeat URI episodes. Periorbital pain and edema, frontal headaches, nasal congestion, tenderness to pressure over the sinuses, fever, and general malaise are frequent complaints. Refer the patient to a physician for symptomatic relief with the use of antipyretics, decongestants, or analgesics. Sinus irrigation may be necessary in lingering cases. Antibiotics are used for cases that are bacterial based or that develop secondary to bacterial infections. It is important, particularly with sinus infections, that an athlete who is on antibiotics follow the physician's directions and take the medication until it runs out. Because of the closed sinus spaces, sinus infections are slow to clear, and if it is not completely resolved, the infection returns.

Pharyngitis

Dysphagia is pain with swallowing.

Inflammation of the pharynx can result from either a viral or a bacterial infection and is often an extension of sinusitis, tonsillitis, or adenoid infection. Chills, fever, hoarseness, and dysphagia commonly accompany a burning or dry throat. Treatment includes rest, fluid intake, and medication for symptomatic relief. Antibiotics are used for bacterial infections.

Laryngitis

Acute inflammation of the larynx usually results secondary to a common cold, sinusitis, pharyngitis, or tonsillitis. A tickling sensation or rawness in the throat with a frequent need to clear the throat is often accompanied by hoarseness or a change or loss of voice. If edema of the larynx occurs, the athlete may have difficulty breathing (dyspnea). Treatment includes bed rest, fluid ingestion, and resting the voice; bacterial conditions indicate antibiotic medication. Steam inhalation and cough or anesthetic lozenges can also encourage symptomatic relief.

Tonsillitis

Adenoiditis is an inflammation of the glandular lymph tissue at the back of the pharynx.

Although acute inflammation of the tonsils often results from a bacterial infection, chronic tonsillitis is frequently related to predisposing factors such as a common cold or adenoiditis. Acute tonsillitis presents with signs and symptoms of chills, fever, malaise, headaches, body aches, and severe pain in the throat with difficulty swallowing. Symptoms of chronic tonsillitis, on the other hand, include a sore throat, mild fever, and nasal discharge. In either case, the tonsils will be red and edematous, and a whitish pus may be observable at the back of the throat. Acute tonsillitis is treated with antibiotics and symptomatic relief. Chronic tonsillitis may be best treated with a tonsillectomy.

Bronchial and Lung Infections

Infections of the bronchials and lungs are more serious than URIs. Although bronchitis can be caused by both infections and irritants, pneumonia is a serious lung infection that requires immediate medical referral and treatment.

Bronchitis

Inflammation of the bronchial tree, either acute or chronic, can result from an infection or a reaction to an irritating agent. Acute bronchitis is associated with a URI such as a common cold or other viral infection of the nasopharynx, throat, or upper bronchial tree. It may also be associated with a secondary bacterial infection. While acute bronchitis can affect children or adults, chronic bronchitis occurs commonly in adults and results from chronic diffuse obstructive pulmonary diseases such as emphysema or pulmonary fibrosis. Cigarette smokers frequently have chronic bronchitis.

Symptoms of acute bronchitis are the same as those of most URIs, including nasal mucous discharge, malaise, slight fever, general achiness, and sore throat. A cough is usually dry and nonproductive in the first few days but becomes productive with a mucoid secretion in later stages. A hissing or crackling (rales) may be heard with auscultation (see chapter 20). A lingering cough may continue for weeks after other symptoms subside.

An expectorant is a drug used to increase flow and decrease the viscosity of mucus in the respiratory passageway.

Refer the athlete to a physician to ensure proper treatment of possible complications and proper administration of appropriate medications. An athlete with systemic symptoms should be placed on bed rest until the fever ends. Fluid ingestion is encouraged. Administering a variety of drugs including antipyretic, analgesic, expectorant, and bronchodilator medications can offer symptomatic relief.

Pneumonia

Pneumonia is an infection of the alveolar spaces that is usually bacterial but can be viral. Bacterial infections are grouped as pneumococcal and include group A hemolytic streptococcus and types 1 and 2 staphylococci. A URI frequently precedes pneumonia in an athlete. Other factors that influence pneumonia onset in adults include alcoholism, malnutrition, debilitation (being bedridden), aspiration, coma, or bronchial tumor.

Pneumococcal pneumonia is the most common form of pneumonia. Pneumococci enter the lungs through the respiratory passages and lodge in the alveoli, initiating an inflammatory process. The edema formation serves as a rich culture medium within which the pneumococci proliferate; they spread to other alveoli and lobes. Signs and symptoms include fever, chest pain, tachycardia, difficulty breathing (dyspnea), respiratory distress (tachypnea), and a nonproductive hacking cough that advances to a cough with sputum (mucus) that is pinkish in the early stages and rusty colored in later stages. The rusty color is a hallmark of

Tachypnea refers to rapid respirations.

Tachycardia means rapid pulse.

pneumococcal pneumonia, as is an expiratory grunt. Rales in the affected lobe can be heard with a stethoscope. As the infection progresses, the alveoli fill with fluid, which severely limits gas exchange; therefore, it is imperative that the athlete receive treatment as soon as any of these symptoms appear.

Treatment includes bed rest, fluids, oxygen administration, and medications including antibiotics, analgesics, and antipyretics. Many cases require hospitalization.

Other Respiratory Conditions

Not all respiratory conditions are infectious. Chronic and acute respiratory conditions can be caused or exacerbated by allergens in the environment or can be induced by exercise or stress. These include hay fever, asthma, and hyperventilation.

Hay Fever

Hay fever is an allergic rhinitis that occurs seasonally because of the athlete's reaction to airborne pollens. Depending on the allergy, the athlete may be most susceptible in the spring, summer, or fall. A profuse watery nasal discharge accompanies itching of the eyes, nose, and mouth. Sneezing is common, along with conjunctivitis, frontal headaches with increased sinus pressure, and irritated nasal mucous membranes.

Remove the allergen if the reaction is allergy based. Medications may be prescribed to minimize irritating symptoms; these may include antihistamines in nose drop, inhalant, or

Sympathomimetic refers to medications that mimic the actions of the sympathetic nervous system to cause vasoconstriction and to open respiratory passageways.

oral form; decongestants; and sympathomimetic oral medications. Sometimes severe allergies require surgical or chemical treatments to alter discharge ability or nasal sensitivity.

Asthma

Asthma is a reactive airway disease characterized by paroxysms of dyspnea, coughing, and wheezing that has been seen in increasing frequency over the past few years. Millions of Americans experience asthma; many deaths occur each year due to complications of untreated conditions. True asthma is usually triggered by an environmental irritant, allergen, medication, or exercise that causes a reactive narrowing of the trachea, bronchi, and bronchioles and is accompanied by an inflammatory component. The result is a widespread, reversible narrowing of the airways (bronchospasm). Oxygen and metabolic wastes (mucus) improperly exchange as the airway narrows, and breathing becomes more labor intensive with increasing airflow resistance. Resulting signs and symptoms of an acute, severe asthma attack include spasmodic coughing, chest pain and tightness, wheezing, high pulse rate, rapid and shallow respirations, retraction of the neck muscles on inhalation, restlessness and agitation, and possible fainting. The athlete usually stands upright and leans forward with his hands on the knees (tripod position) (figure 21.2), using the accessory muscles in the shoulder and neck to aid labored breathing. You may also note chest hyperinflation, which represents air trapped in the lungs secondary to the bronchospasm. If the attack is severe and little or no air is moving, wheezing may be absent and the athlete appears cyanotic.

When the symptoms of reactive airway disease occur only with exercise, the condition is typically referred to as **exercise-induced asthma** or EIA. EIA usually does not include lung inflammation unless the athlete also suffers from chronic asthma. Although EIA is being seen in increasing frequency, its cause is essentially unknown. It can occur in young adult athletes who have no other history of asthma. The signs and symptoms, often more subtle than regular asthma, may consist of only a repetitive cough or slight wheezing either during intense exercise or after activity. Even more subtle symptoms may cause athletes to feel they lack endurance or to experience undue fatigue or a perception of being out of shape.

EIA diagnosis includes measuring the speed and volume of air flow out of the lungs. Peak expiratory flow rate (PEFR) or forced expiratory volume (FEV) (Weiler 1996) can confirm EIA. These measurements are taken before and after exercise and compared to see if air outflow significantly decreases. A peak flow meter (figure 21.3) is a common, easy to use, inexpensive device that measures PEFR. The athlete blows into the device as forcefully and quickly as possible, and you read the resulting peak flow. Comparing changes in peak flow between rest and postexercise or during acute symptoms can aid in determining the severity of the asthma condition or attack and the response to treatment, and it can help detect worsening lung function, among other things (National Asthma Education and Prevention Program 1997). When using the peak flow meter, the level on the device should begin at zero. Have the athlete stand and take as deep a breath as possible, seal their lips around the mouthpiece, and then blow out as hard and as fast as possible to achieve their highest possible reading. Repeat the test if the athlete spits, coughs, or blocks the mouthpiece with the tongue. Repeat the test three times and record the best of

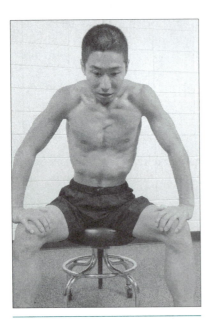

Figure 21.2 Tripod position and use of accessory muscles to aid breathing.

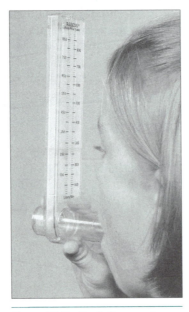

Figure 21.3 Peak flow meter for measuring expiratory flow rate.

the three trials. If the athlete gives a maximal effort, the measurements across the three trials should be reasonably close.

Screening for asthma and EIA in the preparticipation physical examination (PPE) helps identify those at risk and may include asking the athlete about common asthma indicators and performing lung function tests (e.g., peak expiratory flow rate) before and after exercise. When immediately caring for an athlete with asthma, maintain a calm, reassuring attitude to relax him, as he undoubtedly will be anxious and panicky. If asthma is part of an allergic response, the athlete should avoid the allergen whenever possible.

A variety of medications effectively treat asthma, whether exercise induced or pathogenically related. Usually, the athletes you encounter will have a previous history of asthma and will be well versed in the use of their medications. Bronchial dilators and bronchial smooth muscle relaxers (anticholinergics) along with anti-inflammatories and corticosteroids are commonly prescribed asthma medications. Although medication can be dispensed in inhaled, oral, or intravenous form, the inhaler is the most common mode of delivery, with the inhalant self-administered. Take athletes who do not respond to their inhaler medication to a physician without delay. Table 21.1 lists the common drug therapies for bronchial asthma. Become familiar with these medications, actions, and side effects, as you will encounter this condition often and may need to help athletes obtain their medication when an attack occurs.

Anticholinergic refers to medication used to block the action of the neurotransmitter acetylcholine in order to relax smooth muscle.

Hyperventilation

Hyperventilation is characterized by a breathing rate or depth exceeding that required to eliminate carbon dioxide (CO_2). Usually transient, it typically results from factors such as metabolic disturbances, panic, or fear and may occur in unconditioned athletes during exercise. An athlete who is hyperventilating breathes off too much CO_2, which results in respiratory alkalosis. This causes numbness or tingling around the mouth and in the hands and feet, as well as light-headedness. A sharp, stabbing chest pain is also a frequent complaint, causing athletes to panic further because they think they may be having a heart attack. Breathing into a paper bag to take CO_2 back in has been effectively used to rapidly reverse the condition. However, this technique is no longer recommended, as overcompensation (hypoxia) may ensue if the athlete continues to breathe excess CO_2 for too long (Caroline 1995). The best course of action is to simply calm and reassure the athlete in an effort to restore normal respiration rate and depth. When examining an athlete who appears to be hyperventilating, you should monitor the rate and depth of respirations and rule out other pathological conditions that may also produce rapid respirations (see chapter 20).

Respiratory alkalosis is a deficiency of carbonic acid in the blood caused by excessive CO_2 elimination. It is also referred to as metabolic alkalosis.

Table 21.1
Common Drug Therapies for Bronchial Asthma

Drug type	Examples	Action
Anticholinergic	Ipratropium bromide (e.g., Atrovent)	Dilates bronchial tubes by relaxing smooth muscle
Beta agonist	Albuterol (e.g., Proventil, Ventolin), isoetharine metaproterenol (e.g., Alupent, Metaprel), terbutaline (e.g., Brethine)	Dilates bronchial tubes
Corticosteroid	Beclomethasone (e.g., Anti-Beclomethasone), prednisone	Fights inflammation and prevents narrowing of airways
Mast cell inhibitor	Sodium cromoglycate	Inhibits release of chemical mediators of inflammation
Methylxanthine	Theophylline, triamcinolone (e.g., Azmacort)	Dilates bronchial tubes, increases diaphragmatic contractility, and stimulates respiratory center

CARDIOVASCULAR SYSTEM

Cardiovascular conditions are often serious; they may involve either the heart itself or the peripheral vascular system. A balance of sympathetic and parasympathetic nervous system control closely monitors and maintains blood pressure and volume throughout the body. However, illness, injury, and chronic disease states may alter or compromise cardiovascular function. You will need to understand the following cardiovascular conditions and the populations they more often affect so that you can recognize athletes at risk and provide appropriate medical referral and care.

Coronary Artery Disease

Coronary artery disease (CAD), also known as coronary heart disease, is a chronic cardiovascular condition characterized by hardening and narrowing (**atherosclerosis**) of the coronary arteries, the vessels supplying blood to the heart. It is the most common form of cardiovascular disease in the United States. CAD can reduce blood flow to the heart (cardiac ischemia), during which time the athlete may not experience any symptoms (silent ischemia). When symptoms are noted, they include varying degrees of pain (angina), pressure, or discomfort in the chest; shortness of breath; and arrhythmias. In cases of severe or prolonged ischemia, cardiac arrest or heart failure may occur. In fact, CAD is the leading cause of heart attacks and death in those aged 65 or older.

Unfortunately, the majority of those who die suddenly from CAD exhibit no previous symptoms. CAD begins to develop during childhood and progresses into adulthood, more aggressively in some than in others. The American Heart Association (2003) identifies the following controllable risk factors for atherosclerosis:

- High blood cholesterol (especially when LDL levels exceed 100 mg/dL)
- Cigarette smoking and tobacco smoke exposure
- High blood pressure
- Diabetes mellitus
- Obesity
- Physical inactivity

Males and those with a family history of CAD are also at greater risk.

Heart Murmurs

Heart murmurs most often occur due to a defective heart valve (American Heart Association 2003). Valves may be stenotic, having an atypically small opening that prevents them from opening completely, while other valves may be unable to close completely. The later condition leads to regurgitation, or the leaking of blood back through the valve when it should be closed. Murmurs can also be associated with pregnancy, fever, an overactive thyroid gland, and anemia (American Heart Association 2003). Benign (functional or innocent) murmurs are common in children and usually disappear (but may persist) into adulthood. They are completely harmless, usually unapparent to the athlete, and typically identified during a routine physical examination.

Murmurs present as an abnormal heart sound upon auscultation (see chapter 20), such as a gentle blowing, fluttering, or humming sound. A murmur heard during heart contraction is termed a systolic murmur; diastolic murmurs occur between contractions. Continuous murmurs are heard throughout the cardiac cycle. When murmurs result from cardiovascular pathology, they may be accompanied by signs and symptoms such as fatigue, syncope, shortness of breath, and arrhythmias. When you note a murmur, refer the athlete to a physician for a medical diagnosis to determine the source of the murmur and any underlying cardiovascular condition. Diagnosis is made through auscultation, chest X rays and echocardiograms to image the heart, blood tests, and cardiac catheterization.

Hypertension

High blood pressure is the common term for **hypertension**, which involves an elevated systolic or diastolic blood pressure and is associated with generalized arteriolar vasoconstriction. Pressure consistently measuring over 140/90 mmHg at rest is considered to be high. Heredity can play a predisposing role in its onset. Other determining factors include renal, adrenal, and neurogenic pathologies. Hypertension generally begins to affect adults in their early 30s. In the early stages, cardiac output, pulse rate, and blood volume do not change because of a concomitant increase in arterial blood pressure. In fact, the only symptom for many years may be an elevated blood pressure. Lesser symptoms can occur, including periodic fatigue, dizziness, headaches, weakness, and insomnia. Over time, cardiac hypertrophy and changes in electrocardiogram readings are common. Hypertension is a major contributor to renal dysfunction, angina pectoris (chest pain), myocardial infarction (heart attack), cardiovascular accidents, congestive heart failure, stroke, and retinal changes.

Neurogenic means originating in or controlled by the nervous system.

Prevention includes a variety of lifestyle changes such as a diet low in fat and high in complex carbohydrates, regular exercise, weight control, and control of stress influences. The athlete needs to avoid excessive use of substances that produce hypertension, such as coffee, tea, tobacco, salt, and alcohol. Treatment goals with prescribed medication include reducing blood pressure to within normal limits.

Many factors such as exercise, anxiety and tension, illness, or pain can temporarily increase blood pressure. Therefore, a single reading is not usually sufficient to determine high blood pressure, particularly when it is taken when the athlete is less than resting and relaxed. It is often helpful to take an athlete's blood pressure over consecutive days and to have the athlete quiet and relaxed for at least the previous 5 minutes. You should document these recordings and provide them to the physician when you refer the athlete; this valuable information will aid in the diagnosis. Athletes with mild hypertension should be examined by a physician prior to athletic participation.

Hypertrophic Cardiomyopathy

Hypertrophic cardiomyopathy is a serious disease of the myocardium (heart muscle), resulting in enlarged muscle cells in the ventricular septum and left ventricular walls. It is also referred to as **asymmetrical hypertrophy**, idiopathic hypertrophic subaortic stenosis, and muscular subaortic stenosis. Although the specific etiology is unknown, many believe that it occurs because a genetic mutation in the code for the heart muscle's cross-bridges causes changes in the important chemomechanical transduction of impulses through the heart. The enlarged left ventricular wall has more stiffness than normal, causing blood to backflow into the atrium and lungs and reducing blood flow to the body. Although many patients have no symptoms, others experience shortness of breath, chest pain, and dizziness. Shortness of breath (dyspnea) occurs because of the backflow of circulation from the left ventricle to the pulmonary circulation. Chest pain (angina) occurs because of the inadequate flow of oxygenated blood to the heart muscle. Dizziness and fainting (**syncope**) occur because of reduced blood flow to the brain.

The disease, often undetected, has a wide range of effects. Some athletes have no symptoms and lead a normal life, never realizing they have hypertrophic cardiomyopathy. Others develop progressive symptoms that limit their activity level. In extreme cases, the condition can result in sudden death during physical activity in otherwise healthy athletes who do not suspect that they have it. While this condition points to the importance of a cardiovascular screen in the preparticipation physical exam, it may not always be identified. Any time you observe or are aware of signs and symptoms associated with cardiovascular compromise or distress, immediately refer the athlete to a physician before allowing further participation.

If you are working with a physically active patient who is not a competitive athlete and has hypertrophic cardiomyopathy, first consult with her physician to find out what level of activity she may safely maintain. Treatment includes proper diet and personal health habits. The athlete with this condition should avoid isometrics as well as all forms of strenuous exercise, keeping to moderate exercise such as walking or biking. The athlete should avoid dehydration and also avoid hot tubs and saunas, which increase heart rate and blood pressure and encourage dehydration. Beta blockers and calcium channel blockers are common drugs of choice to relax the heart muscle and maintain good heart rhythm in those diagnosed with hypertrophic cardiomyopathy.

Hypotension

Hypotension is a subnormal (low) blood pressure. The most common type is orthostatic hypotension, in which the blood pressure drops when the athlete suddenly stands. Orthostatic hypotension is defined as a decrease of at least 20 mmHg in systolic blood pressure upon movement from a supine to standing position. It can be caused by cardiac pump failure, diminished blood volume available within the vascular system, venous pooling, medication, and neurogenic pathologies. The condition is transient but produces a brief period of light-headedness, dizziness, weakness, or nausea. A physician should examine persistent episodes or episodes that result in syncope for underlying causes before the athlete returns to participation.

Treatment includes relieving causative factors by changing position slowly, avoiding alcohol, avoiding hot showers or baths, increasing salt intake to increase intravascular blood volume, and taking medications. Medications usually include over-the-counter sympathomimetics or prescription doses of sympathetic agonists to increase blood pressure; fludrocortisone to promote renal sodium reabsorption and arteriole sensitivity to norepinephrine; or erythropoietin to restore normal hematocrit.

Migraine Headache

Migraines are recurring vascular headaches of sudden onset with associated gastrointestinal and visual disturbances. The exact cause is unknown, but it is believed that migraines may be related to allergies, stress, hormonal imbalance, toxins, or vasomotor disturbances. There is often a family history of migraines. It is believed that the migraine process starts with head pain that results from extracranial vasoconstriction in the scalp and dura. Vasoconstriction in intracranial circulation also takes place, reducing oxygen to the brain to cause neurogenic symptoms such as vision changes and speech difficulty. A reactive vasodilatation to meet the brain's oxygen needs affects the neck and scalp arteries, triggering a release of prostaglandins and other chemicals that produce inflammation, swelling, and increased pain sensitivity. Stimulation of nociceptors resulting from scalp artery dilation causes the throbbing pain.

Migraines are divided into the classic and common types:

- **Classic migraine attacks** are preceded 10 to 30 minutes beforehand by an aura that produces neurological symptoms. The person may experience visual disturbances such as flashing lights, sometimes with a temporary loss of vision. Photophobia is common. Common symptoms of classic migraines are speech difficulty; tingling of the face or hands; weakness on one side of the body; and intense, throbbing pain that starts on one side of the head around the temple, forehead, eye, ear, and jaw and advances to the other side. Classic migraines last for 1 to 2 days, whereas common migraine symptoms last for 3 to 4 days.

- **Common migraines**, which are more prevalent, do not have an aura preceding onset. The standard symptom, photophobia, is often accompanied by other symptoms including throbbing around the eye, nausea, vomiting, mood changes, and severe headache.

You may need to refer the athlete to a physician for analgesic medications administered orally, rectally, or intravenously. If analgesic medication can be administered early enough, full migraine symptoms can sometimes be avoided. Fluid ingestion, rest in a darkened room, and stress relief can help minimize symptoms.

Mitral Valve Prolapse

The mitral valve is a bicuspid (two-flap) valve that separates the left atrium from the left ventricle and allows blood to flow from the atrium to the ventricle during diastole and prevents backflow into the atrium with ventricular contraction. With mitral valve prolapse, one or both cusps are enlarged, and the supporting chordae tendineae (the strands that anchor the cusps to the papillary muscles of the ventricle walls) may be too long (American Heart Association 2003). Hence, when the heart contracts, the mitral valve cusps collapse backward into the left atrium, allowing blood to leak backward through the valve. A heart murmur upon auscultation indicates mitral valve prolapse; it is heard best with the stethoscope positioned over the fifth left intercostal space, about 8 cm (3 in.) from the midsternal line (the line descending from the midclavicle). More atypical signs and symptoms include chest pain (angina pectoris) and abnormal heart rhythms (arrhythmias).

Mitral valve prolapse is also known as click-murmur syndrome, Barlow's syndrome, balloon mitral valve, and floppy valve syndrome (American Heart Association 2003). An important consideration for those with mitral valve prolapse is the potential for infection, which is typically prevented by a course of antibiotics before any surgical or dental procedures likely to cause bleeding.

Syncope

Syncope, or fainting, is a sudden, temporary loss of consciousness most commonly resulting from either a physiological or an emotional stress that causes a vasovagal reaction. Syncope most often occurs when standing or with sudden changes in position (sudden sitting or standing). Syncope can also result from reduced blood volume produced by heavy sweating, violent coughing spells that rapidly change blood pressure, heart or lung disorders, side effects of medications, seizures, or any condition that results in inadequate glucose or oxygen supply to the brain.

Vasovagal refers to a reflex dilation of blood vessels and a pooling of blood in the extremities.

Syncope is a transient incident that results from a sudden increase in vasodilation of peripheral blood vessels without a concomitant increase in cardiac output. These events cause reduced blood flow to the brain and consequently fainting. Preceding symptoms include a sudden change in position, weakness, cold sweat, nausea, abdominal discomfort, dimming vision, and a roaring sound in the ears (Caroline 1995). Once the person is supine, blood flow to the brain is restored, and consciousness quickly returns. Although there are few residual effects, take care to examine for possible injury that is the consequence of any fall during fainting.

Syncope can result from a variety of factors, some cardiac in origin. Fainting should never be dismissed or considered a normal response. Refer the athlete to a physician to determine the underlying cause of the episode.

VIRAL SYNDROMES

Viral syndromes are systemic conditions caused by viral infections. They are often highly contagious and may have prolonged symptoms. Infection usually occurs well before signs and symptoms appear, with incubation periods lasting 2 weeks or more. Complications such as enlarged visceral organs and sterility may result from one or more of these conditions. Viral syndromes include mononucleosis, mumps, and measles. Chicken pox (herpes zoster), described in relation to skin conditions in chapter 23, is also classified as a viral syndrome (page 637).

Epstein-Barr Virus

The **Epstein-Barr virus (EBV)** was first discovered in 1964, and it is a member of the herpes virus family (Taber 1997). It is common worldwide and the Center for Infectious Diseases estimates that as many as 95% of adults between 35 to 40 years of age have been infected. The virus is spread via saliva and is the cause of infectious mononucleosis. But while the symptoms of mononucleosis typically resolve in 1 or 2 months, EBV remains latent in cells of the throat and blood for the rest of the person's life. The virus can periodically reactivate in infected persons, usually without symptoms of illness. Although the Epstein-Barr virus has been blamed for chronic mononucleosis symptoms lasting more than 6 months, laboratory tests have seldom found continued active EBV infection in these patients; it is recommended that these patients be examined for other causes of chronic illness or chronic fatigue syndrome (National Center for Infectious Diseases 2003).

Infectious Mononucleosis

Most cases of infectious mononucleosis, or mono, are caused by the EBV. This condition can affect any age group, but most cases are seen in patients aged 15 to 30. The disease is transmitted through direct contact with the saliva of an infected patient. A common means of transmission is sharing beverage containers or food utensils.

Incubation is 2 to 7 weeks after contact, and symptoms can last a few days or several months. Most commonly, they disappear in 1 to 3 weeks. Symptoms are vague and include general malaise, headache, fatigue, chilliness, appetite loss, and puffy eyelids. As the disease progresses, additional symptoms—swollen and tender lymph glands, sore throat, and fever—emerge. Tenderness and enlargement of the spleen, difficulty swallowing, and bleeding gums can also occur. Adults over the age of 30 who contract the disease can have a more severe episode and longer lasting symptoms. Additional symptoms for this age group can include ruptured spleen, pericarditis, and liver involvement. If an athlete of any age competes while the spleen is enlarged, there is a chance of rupture; thus an enlarged spleen contraindicates physical activities requiring contact or jostling.

Refer suspected cases to the physician for a diagnosis. A heterophil antibody blood test (monospot) confirms the diagnosis and eliminates other differential diagnoses. Treatment includes restricting vigorous activity until all symptoms have disappeared. Since an enlarged spleen is susceptible to injury, athletes should be restricted from weight lifting and competitive sport until completely recovered. There is no specific medication for mononucleosis, but the athlete should maintain a balanced diet, prevent dehydration with adequate fluid intake, and take over-the-counter analgesics for symptomatic relief of head and muscle aches. Antibiotics are not prescribed since the disease is caused by a virus and does not respond to such medication.

Measles

Measles is a highly contagious viral infection (**rubeola**) transmitted through the air; an athlete can contract measles by breathing the same air as an infected person. Because of its ease of transmission, epidemics—usually occurring in the spring in a cycle of 2 to 3 years—are common. The incubation period is about 9 to 11 days, with about 2 weeks passing between exposure and the appearance of the measles rash. The time of infectivity begins 2 to 4 days before the rash appears and ends 2 to 5 days after its appearance.

Symptoms include a fever as high as 105° F (40.6° C), rash, runny nose, photophobia, watery eyes, and hacking cough. Small, irregular spots with a red periphery and blue-white centers (Koplik spots) appear in the mouth 1 to 2 days before the rash and are a hallmark of measles. The rash, which begins about 3 or 4 days after the other symptoms, takes the form of irregular papules around the hairline of the face and neck and rapidly spreads to the trunk and extremities. The rash fades in the same way, first in the face and neck and then through the rest of the body, usually completing its course in about 6 days. The disease takes 10 to 14 days to run its course.

Complications such as croup, bronchitis, pneumonia, conjunctivitis, hepatitis, and encephalitis can occur with measles. Symptoms and complications are more severe in adults. A vaccine should be routinely administered to infants after 13 months of age. Public schools in most states require immunization prior to admission. A vaccine either before or within 3 days after exposure to the disease effectively prevents illness. Vaccines made before 1979 may not be effective, so people who were vaccinated before 1980 should receive another measles vaccine if an outbreak occurs.

Vaccinations are not given to pregnant mothers or to patients who have depressed immune systems. Athletes who are allergic to eggs or neomycin are also in danger of severe reactions from the vaccine.

Patients with measles can take over-the-counter medications to reduce the fever, but children should not take aspirin because of the risk of developing Reye's syndrome. Clear

Reye's syndrome is a rare, often fatal childhood disease that can damage the brain and other vital organs. Reye's syndrome has been linked to using aspirin in children.

fluids maintain hydration and reduce the chance of lung infections. A cool mist vaporizer may relieve cough symptoms. Rest in a darkened room and abstention from reading and watching television are advisable because of photophobia.

Mumps

Mumps is a highly contagious viral infection that affects the salivary glands, especially the parotid glands. It is spread through droplet infection or direct contact with saliva. Most cases are seen in children ages 5 to 15 and occur with greatest frequency in the late winter and early spring. The incubation period is 14 to 28 days, after which symptoms appear. These include chills, headache, malaise, swelling of salivary glands, and exquisite tenderness over the angle of the jaw where the salivary glands are located. Fever and sore throat with difficulty swallowing or chewing also occur and last for 24 to 72 hours.

Complications associated with mumps most often affect patients past puberty and can affect the testes or ovaries, resulting in sterility. Males may suffer from painful inflammation of the testicles, with up to 25% of these cases resulting in sterility. Other rare complications include facial nerve palsy and effects on the central nervous system, pancreas, kidneys, or breasts.

The mumps vaccine is usually provided in a single injection as part of the MMR (mumps, measles, rubella) immunization. When people do contract mumps, treatment is for relief of symptoms and includes bed rest until the fever subsides, analgesics for pain, clear fluid intake to prevent dehydration, and a soft diet to minimize pain caused by chewing.

SUMMARY

1. Describe and recognize the signs and symptoms of medical conditions of the eyes, ears, nose, and throat that may be encountered in the physically active.

   Irritation and infection in the eyes, ears, nose, and throat (EENT) are common complaints in the physically active. While these conditions can cause considerable pain, hampering performance until they are resolved, they are rarely life threatening. Most are caused by bacterial or viral infections.

2. Describe and recognize the signs and symptoms of medical conditions of the respiratory system that may be encountered in the physically active.

   Irritation and infection (viral and bacterial) can occur throughout the respiratory system and passageways. An upper respiratory infection (URI) is any infection (bacterial or viral) that affects any portion of the upper respiratory system (conducting pathway) including the tonsils, nose, throat, sinuses, and neck lymph nodes. Middle ear infections can also be associated with URIs. Examples of URIs include the common cold, flu, sinusitis, laryngitis, pharyngitis, and tonsillitis. Specific signs and symptoms and treatment vary according to the area involved and the cause of the infection. Infections of the bronchials and lungs are more serious than URIs. Although bronchitis can be caused by both infections and irritants, pneumonia is a serious lung infection that requires immediate medical referral and treatment. Other respiratory conditions not associated with infection include allergic rhinitis, asthma, hay fever, and hyperventilation.

3. Describe and recognize the signs and symptoms of medical conditions of the cardiovascular system that may be encountered in the physically active.

   Cardiovascular conditions involve either the heart itself or the peripheral vascular system and include coronary artery disease, murmurs, hypertension, hypertrophic cardiomyopathy, hypotension, mitro valve prolapse, syncope, and even migraine headaches. A balance of sympathetic and parasympathetic nervous system control closely monitors and maintains blood pressure and volume throughout the body. However, illness, injury, and chronic disease states may alter or compromise cardiovascular function. You should have a good understanding of these cardiovascular conditions and the populations they often affect so that you can recognize those at risk and provide appropriate medical referral and care.

4. Describe and recognize the signs and symptoms of viral conditions that may be encountered in the physically active.

Viral syndromes are systemic conditions caused by viral infections. They are often highly contagious and may have prolonged symptoms. Infection usually occurs well before signs and symptoms appear, with incubation periods of 2 weeks or more. Complications such as enlarged visceral organs and sterility may result from one or more of these conditions. Viral syndromes include chicken pox (covered in chapter 23), Epstein-Barr, mononucleosis, mumps, and measles.

5. Appreciate the complications that may result from many of these conditions if they are not recognized and if they are left untreated.

Many of the conditions affecting the EENT or the cardiorespiratory system are of short duration and are accompanied by only minor signs and symptoms or disabilities. However, some can have severe, life-threatening consequences or can result in permanent disability if not recognized and treated appropriately. Other conditions represent permanent and preexisting disease states that require you to be aware of the athlete's history, as complications may arise during sport activity. You should understand the complicating factors that can result in these conditions and know the populations that may be at greater risk for developing serious complications.

6. Determine which medical conditions require emergency medical referral and which require physician referral for diagnosis and treatment.

Although the majority of the conditions discussed in this and subsequent chapters are beyond the scope of your ability to care for the athlete, you must be able to recognize their signs and symptoms in order to make the appropriate medical referral and ensure proper care for the athlete. When athletes participating in physical activity exhibit such signs and symptoms, you may need to provide immediate first aid or emergency care, but referral to a physician is your ultimate responsibility. Hence, it is important that you recognize and differentiate those conditions that can result in serious cardiorespiratory compromise, as they can be life threatening if the athlete does not receive timely and appropriate treatment.

REVIEW QUESTIONS

1. Describe the differential signs and symptoms of influenza and the common cold. Under what circumstances should you prohibit an athlete experiencing these conditions from practice?

2. What causes bronchitis? How would you differentiate this condition from pneumonia?

3. What are the signs and symptoms of an acute asthma attack? How would you manage this condition initially, and when would you refer the athlete for medical care?

4. What causes a syncopal episode? When should you refer an athlete who has fainted for a medical examination?

5. How does mononucleosis differ from other viral conditions? What are the potential complications of mono, and what signs or symptoms contraindicate physical activity?

CRITICAL THINKING QUESTIONS

1. A thorough medical history obtained during the preparticipation physical examination at the beginning of the year can provide valuable information regarding previous medical conditions that may resurface or affect physical activity. If you were asked to design a health history questionnaire, what questions would you include?

2. You are employed in an industrial clinic and during a late summer meeting with the allied health staff the discussion turns to how the company can prevent a serious outbreak of influenza in the coming year. During the last two flu epidemics, clinic records indicate that as many as 30% of the workers missed multiple work days due to this highly contagious disease. What are some strategies that you might suggest the health staff consider for reducing influenza in the workplace?

3. You notice an athlete standing on the sidelines who is leaning forward and having difficulty breathing. As you approach her, you can see a panicked look on her face and can hear wheezing. What conditions might you suspect, and how would your examination proceed? What questions might be particularly important to ask her that may aid your immediate care?

4. You have a soccer athlete that has been diagnosed with mononucleosis 4 weeks before the start of the season. Is this sufficient time for the condition to resolve and allow the athlete to return to activity? Why or why not? What information do you need to make this determination?

5. You have an athlete who suffers from common migraine headaches. Although you many not be able to prevent these attacks, what strategies might you use in an effort to reduce the effects of the symptoms once they begin to appear?

CITED REFERENCES

American Heart Association. 2003. Atherosclerosis. Available at www.americanheart.org/presenter.jhtml?id entifier=4440. Accessed November 2, 2004.

Caroline, N.L. 1995. *Emergency care in the streets.* 5th ed. Boston: Little, Brown.

Centers for Disease Control (CDC). 2004. Influenza. Available at www.cdc.gov/flu/professionals/diagnosis/. Accessed August 20, 2004.

National Asthma Education and Prevention Program. 1997. *Clinical Practice Guidelines, Expert Panel Report 2: Guidelines for the diagnosis and management of asthma.* National Institutes of Health; National Heart, Lung and Blood Institute. NIH Publication No. 97-4051, July 1997. Available at www.nhlbi.nih.gov/guidelines/asthma/asthgdln.pdf. Accessed November 3, 2004.

National Athletic Trainers' Association. 1999. *Athletic training educational competencies.* 3rd ed. Dallas: National Athletic Trainers' Association.

National Center for Infectious Diseases. 2003. Epstein-Barr virus and infectious mononucleosis. Available at www.cdc.gov/ncidod/diseases/ebv.htm. Accessed August 20, 2004.

Weiler, J.M. 1996. Exercise-induced asthma: A practical guide to definitions, diagnosis, prevalence, and treatment. *Allergy Asthma Proc* 17:315-325.

ADDITIONAL RESOURCES

Hillman, S.K. 2005. *Introduction to athletic training.* 2nd ed. Champaign, IL: Human Kinetics.

Mosby's Medical, Nursing, and Allied Health Dictionary. 2002. 6th ed. St Louis: Mosby.

Taber, C.W. 1997. *Taber's cyclopedic medical dictionary.* 18th ed. Philadelphia: F.A. Davis.

Digestive, Endocrine, Reproductive, and Urinary Conditions

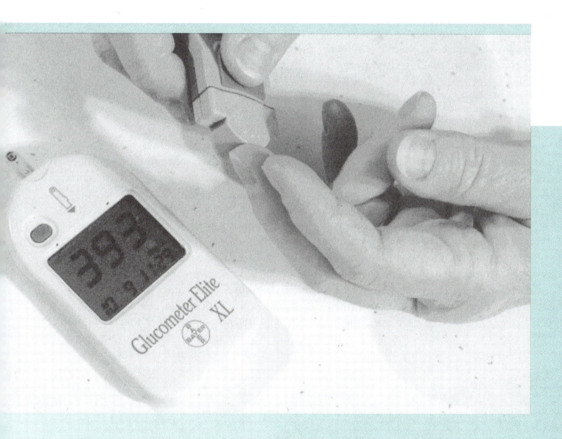

Objectives

After completing this chapter, the reader will be able to do the following:

1. Describe and recognize the signs and symptoms of medical conditions of the endocrine system that may be encountered in the physically active

2. Describe and recognize the signs and symptoms of medical conditions of the digestive system that may be encountered in the physically active

3. Describe and recognize the signs and symptoms of disordered eating behaviors that may be encountered in the physically active

4. Describe and recognize the signs and symptoms of sexually transmitted diseases that may be encountered in the physically active

5. Describe and recognize the signs and symptoms of genitourinary and gynecological conditions that may be encountered in the physically active

6. Determine which medical conditions require emergency medical referral and which require physician referral for diagnosis and treatment

Chelsea was an outgoing varsity lacrosse player. She always gave 100% and worked hard in practice. That is why it didn't take long for the coach to notice that something was wrong and to summon Patty, the athletic trainer, from the nearby athletic training room. As Patty approached, she noticed that Chelsea seemed disoriented and wasn't focused on any one thing.

"Chelsea, are you feeling all right?" Patty asked, even though it was apparent she was not. Chelsea did not respond; she seemed agitated and confused, and was pacing. Patty remembered that Chelsea had revealed in her preparticipation examination that she had insulin-dependent diabetes. Patty smelled Chelsea's breath but didn't notice any odor. When taking Chelsea's pulse, she noted that it was rapid and weak and that her skin was pale and clammy. From her symptoms, it was likely that Chelsea was hypoglycemic and was going into insulin shock. Knowing Chelsea's condition, Patty had put a glucose packet in the field athletic training kit. Chelsea was not very cooperative, but she allowed Patty to place the glucose under her tongue. Within minutes, Chelsea was acting more like herself.

"Do you know what happened?" Patty asked Chelsea.

"No, I don't really remember anything. I was practicing fine and then all of the sudden I got weak and light-headed. I thought maybe I needed some sugar, but I thought I could wait until after practice. I'm glad you knew what to do. Thanks, Patty!"

This chapter addresses conditions affecting the digestive, endocrine, reproductive, and genitourinary systems. Some of these conditions are preexisting and do not preclude the athlete from participation but may result in complications arising during activity. While athletes with preexisting conditions typically understand their disease quite well and take precautionary measures to minimize the risk of complications, it is equally important for you to be aware of these conditions and recognize signs and symptoms of complicating factors. Other conditions, such as those of the gastrointestinal tract, can be more acute or intermittent in nature and can cause considerable pain and discomfort when they occur. Your ability to differentiate conditions associated with common gastrointestinal irritation versus more serious conditions will ensure the athlete receives proper care in a timely fashion. Other topics included in this chapter are disordered eating, sexually transmitted diseases, and gynecological and genitourinary conditions. These conditions are often sensitive in nature and potentially embarrassing to the athlete. Your ability to communicate with an athlete in a professional, understanding, and confidential manner will greatly ease the athlete when discussing sensitive issues with you.

ENDOCRINE SYSTEM

Sometimes an athlete under your care has an endocrine disorder that necessitates daily medication and continual monitoring. Pancreatic (diabetes) and thyroid dysfunction are the most common conditions you will encounter. Although they do not prevent an athlete from participation, they may give rise to complications during or apart from exercise. You should understand these conditions and be able to recognize signs of complications in order to provide emergency assistance to the athlete when needed. Endocrine complications can occur in athletes with both good and poor disease management. A complication in and of itself does not indicate poor disease management; it may convey a temporary problem or an unplanned event like a developing cold virus, infection, or stress, or it may indicate that the treatment or medication regimen needs to be adjusted. Knowing the history of the athletes under your care and the medications that they take will help you provide optimal care.

Diabetes Mellitus

Diabetes mellitus is an autoimmune disorder that causes a deficiency in glucose metabolism. Insulin, a peptide hormone responsible for glucose utilization, is either not secreted by the islets of Langerhans in the pancreas or is prevented from being utilized in the body. Diabetes mellitus occurs as one of two types: insulin-dependent diabetes mellitus (IDDM), or type 1 diabetes, and non-insulin-dependent diabetes mellitus (NIDDM), or type 2 diabetes. IDDM usually occurs in nonobese children and adults, whereas NIDDM most often occurs in obese adults and children. IDDM results from insufficient insulin production in the pancreas. Patients with NIDDM have an insulin-producing pancreas, but their body's sensitivity to the insulin hormone is significantly diminished. In both types of diabetes, glucose, rather than being metabolized by target tissue, remains in the bloodstream where it is partially filtered through the kidneys. Prolonged blood glucose elevation eventually damages organs and tissues and can lead to blindness, kidney failure, recurring infections, and cardiovascular insufficiency that can in turn cause cardiac complications, neuropathy, and extremity amputation.

Signs, Symptoms, and Control

Several early signs and symptoms of diabetes are prevalent in IDDM; signs and symptoms in NIDDM are slower to progress and can remain subtle and unnoticed for extended periods of time, even months. Frequent urination, a hallmark, occurs because glucose draws large amounts of water when excreted. Rather than using glucose, the body utilizes other sources of energy, primarily fats. Fat metabolism generates acetone and other ketone waste products that change the blood's pH (**ketoacidosis**). In an attempt to restore normal pH, the body increases its elimination of carbon dioxide through deep expirations. Acetones are expired, producing a characteristic odor on the breath usually described as sweet, fruity, or like fingernail-polish remover. Rapid weight loss occurs as the body excretes glucose and uses fat stores for metabolism. Excessive thirst and dry skin result from the dehydration caused by frequent urination. Fatigue and weakness occur; and in the absence of treatment, shock and diabetic coma ensue.

Early diagnosis and control with diet, exercise, and medication are key to proper diabetes management. Normal blood glucose levels range between 70 and 120 mg/dL. The patient with diabetes should attempt to maintain as nearly normal levels as possible to minimize diabetes side effects. Medication for IDDM requires from one to several daily subcutaneous insulin injections. Insulin pumps are also available that allow insulin to be administered continuously as well as provide multiple boluses of insulin as needed through a soft catheter implanted beneath the skin in the subcutaneous layer. Patients with NIDDM typically control blood glucose levels through diet, oral medication, or both. Diet and exercise are important components of diabetes control for both type 1 and type 2 groups.

A bolus is the rapid administration of an injectable medication.

Glycemic Reactions

If a patient with diabetes has too much insulin in the body, the blood glucose levels drop below normal and a **hypoglycemic** reaction occurs. If there is too little insulin, glucose levels are elevated above normal levels and the body becomes **hyperglycemic**. You must be aware of the differences in the signs and symptoms between these two conditions, since the treatments are opposite (see table 22.1).

Hypoglycemia (Insulin Shock)

Hypoglycemia, or **insulin shock**, can be life threatening. The symptoms, which are nonspecific, include sweating, trembling, fatigue and weakness, light-headedness, irritability, headache, intoxicated behavior, apprehension, mental confusion, and—in advanced stages—convulsions and coma. Memory loss, lack of coordination, and slurred speech may also be noted. Since activity lowers blood glucose levels, you should closely monitor athletes with diabetes during times of unexpected increased activity and during early-season workouts when diet, insulin, and activity balances may not yet be established.

Many athletes who have had diabetes for some time understand the disease and take precautionary measures to minimize the risk of hypoglycemic reactions. There are times, however, when unanticipated schedule changes or altered activity levels may precipitate a hypoglycemic reaction. You should keep a supply of glucose tablets or glucose packets, designed for hypoglycemic episodes, in the athletic training kit, or have quick and easy access to sweetened drinks or foods. If candy is the only sweet substance available, hard candy with a high sugar

! If the athlete in insulin shock is unable to swallow, do not attempt to force liquids or foods; instead, arrange for immediate transportation to an emergency care facility for intravenous glucose administration to avoid possible brain damage or death.

Table 22.1

Comparison of Hypoglycemia and Hyperglycemia

Signs and Symptoms	Hypoglycemia	Hyperglycemia
Onset	Rapid onset, occurring within minutes	Slow onset, occurring over hours and even days
Neurological changes	Irritability, mental confusion, dizziness, bizarre behavior, slurred speech, memory loss, headache, dilated pupils; in severe cases, seizures and coma	Lethargy, mental confusion, listlessness
Skin	Cold, clammy; profuse sweating	Warm and dry
Muscular changes	Weakness, fatigue, muscle tremors, incoordination, ataxic gait	Weakness and fatigue
Cardiorespiratory changes	Weak, rapid pulse; no breath odor	Rapid pulse (tachycardia); deep, rapid breathing (Kussmaul respirations); characteristic odor of acetones on breath
Genitourinary and gastrointestinal changes	None	Nausea and vomiting; excessive urination, thirst, or eating

content should be ingested, not chocolate candy, which has a high fat content. Immediately administer candy, fruit juice, sugar-sweetened soft drinks, sugar, or other glucose-containing substances when you observe changes in the athlete's behavior. If the athlete is unable to swallow, do not attempt to force liquids or foods; instead, call EMS for immediate medical care and transportation to an emergency care facility for intravenous glucose administration to avoid possible brain damage or death.

Good diabetes control minimizes hypoglycemic reactions. Eating a snack about 30 minutes before exercise helps reduce insulin reactions. If activity is prolonged, the athlete should ingest about 10 g of carbohydrate every 30 minutes. Routine exercise programs allow the athlete to anticipate the necessary balance between exercise, food, and insulin, providing an optimal condition for controlling blood glucose levels.

Again, if you have an athlete with diabetes on one of your teams, maintain a supply of glucose tablets (available from drug stores) or other sugar substance in the athletic training kit, or have quick and easy access to fruit juice, sweetened soft drinks, or food during practice and games and while on the road.

Hyperglycemia (Diabetic Coma)

In its advanced stages, hyperglycemia is referred to as **hyperglycemic shock**, or **diabetic coma**. This condition develops over a period of days as the patient's blood glucose levels rise. Failure to take insulin, severe illness or infection, physical or emotional stress, or poor dietary control can disrupt glucose levels and lead to this condition. The symptoms include those mentioned earlier as onset symptoms. You will smell the characteristic odor of acetones (a fruity or sweet smell) on the patient's breath, and the patient will be lethargic. When you suspect hyperglycemia, you should refer the athlete to a physician. Most athletes who have good control over their condition do not suffer hyperglycemic shock. However, illness significantly increases the body's physical stress level and presents special concerns for athletes with diabetes in terms of glucose regulation, especially if the ill athlete is unable to eat food or drink fluids. Even a relatively mild illness such as a cold or the flu can cause a person with diabetes in normally good control to have excessively high glucose levels. When athletes with diabetes become ill, you should routinely refer them to a physician for proper management and care.

Differential Diagnosis and Immediate Care

It is sometimes difficult to distinguish between the symptoms of hyperglycemia and hypoglycemia. Lethargy, listlessness, and confusion can occur with either condition. If you are unsure which condition the athlete has, you should assume the athlete is hypoglycemic and administer glucose tablets or sugar. If the athlete is hypoglycemic, administering sugar immediately is necessary; if the athlete is hyperglycemic, ingesting glucose tablets or sugar will not significantly advance the condition. If the condition is a hypoglycemic reaction, the athlete should respond to the treatment within a few minutes, but if it is hyperglycemic, the condition will not change. If the athlete does not start to respond within 2 or 3 minutes following administration of sugar, candy, or sweetened beverages, you should suspect hyperglycemia and transport the athlete to an emergency care facility for immediate treatment.

Hyperthyroidism

Hyperthyroidism can develop during times of emotional or physical stress. It is an autoimmune condition in which an excessive amount of thyroid hormone exists in the body. This increases the body's metabolic activity and causes weight loss regardless of increased food intake. With an increase in metabolic activity comes a concomitant increase in body temperature, so the athlete does not tolerate hot environments, suffers from excessive sweating, and must significantly increase fluid intake. Increased sympathetic activity results in an increased heart rate, tremors, and protruding eyeballs. Impaired muscle function and weight loss contribute to muscle weakness. You will often find increased appetite and hyperkinesis. Other frequent manifestations of hyperthyroidism are goiters, bursitis, and systolic hypertension. If a goiter is present, the athlete may have difficulty breathing or swallowing.

Treatment is ablation of the thyroid tissue with surgery or radiation, or control of thyroid levels with medication. Antithyroid drugs bring the hyperthyroidism under control within 8 weeks, but continued intake of medication is often necessary for a year or longer. Radiation with iodine is a common treatment but increases the risk for hypothyroidism; repeated treatments may be necessary. Surgical removal of the thyroid has a 90% cure rate, but surgical risks include nerve damage and hypothyroidism.

Hypothyroidism

Hypothyroidism may result from an iodine deficiency but can also occur following radiation exposure or from hypothalamic or pituitary damage. Many of the symptoms are the opposite of those seen with hyperthyroidism. Since thyroid hormones regulate the rate at which the body utilizes calories for energy expenditure, hypothyroidism reduces body metabolism and causes weight gain even without any change in caloric intake. Additional effects are loss of appetite, intolerance to cold, decreased sweating, reduced heart rate, constipation, coarse and dry hair, premature graying in young adults, thick and dry skin, swollen eyelids, numbness and tingling in the hands, lethargy, slowness of movement, and sleepiness. In the very young, the condition is known as **cretinism**; it stunts growth, reduces hair growth, and causes improperly developed reproductive organs and mental retardation. If hypothyroidism is left untreated, more profound symptoms can occur including heart enlargement, psychiatric disorders, dyspnea, slowed mental processing, inability to maintain normal body temperature, and loss of consciousness. Several years of untreated hypothyroidism leads to **myxedema**, a condition marked by drowsiness, cold body temperature, and possible coma.

Hypothyroidism is treated with regular administration of synthetic thyroid hormone medication to deliver normal thyroxin levels throughout the body. Although most symptoms of hypothyroidism disappear after a week of medication, the patient must continue daily medication throughout life. Correct dosage administration is critical, since too much thyroxin can promote coronary artery disease and osteoporosis.

Pancreatitis

Pancreatitis, an inflammation of the pancreas, can be either acute or chronic. The most common cause is a partial obstruction of the pancreatic duct because of a penetrating duodenal

A duodenal ulcer is a disruption in the mucosal membrane of the duodenum (first part of the small intestine).

ulcer, edema following surgery or abdominal trauma, peritonitis (chapter 20), or systemic disease. An acute attack often follows a precipitating factor such as alcohol or opiate ingestion or a large meal. The escaped pancreatic enzymes cause a severe reaction of the surrounding tissues. Symptoms include nausea, vomiting, and severe pain that can be cramping and dull or poorly defined. The pain can radiate to the back, substernum, or flanks. It usually worsens when the patient attempts to lie down. Constipation or diarrhea can be present, as can diminished bowel sounds and abdominal distension. Vascular collapse and death can ultimately occur. Most cases are mild, but severe cases have a high mortality rate. Physician referral is indicated any time there are reduced bowel sounds (see chapter 20). Refer suspected pancreatitis to the physician for diagnosis and treatment with antibiotics, analgesics, or surgery.

DIGESTIVE SYSTEM

Gastrointestinal complaints are among the most common medical conditions that you will encounter in physically active people. They can be caused by inflammation, viruses, bacteria, and diet. They are particularly troublesome and often restrict participation secondary to the pain and discomfort created by the accompanying symptoms.

Appendicitis

Inflammation of the appendix can occur in an athlete of any age. You must be aware of signs and symptoms, since immediate referral to a physician is necessary to avoid dangerous and life-threatening situations. Appendicitis can be acute or chronic but is triggered by a bacterial infection lodged within the appendix. A low-grade fever accompanies lower abdominal cramps or sharp pains that centralize over the right lower quadrant. Nausea and vomiting are also common. There will be muscle guarding and rigidity of the abdominal wall, pain, and rebound tenderness in the right lower quadrant and around the umbilicus. Immediate physician referral is necessary for either administration of antibiotic medication or surgical intervention.

Colitis

Glucocorticoid is an adrenal cortical hormone primarily used to protect against stress and to affect protein and carbohydrate metabolism (Taber 1997).

Inflammation of the colon typically occurs during the second through fourth decades of life as a result of certain food hypersensitivities, bacterial or viral infections, psychogenic disorders, or autoimmune processes. Onset can be sudden but most often is slow and insidious, beginning with bowel urgency, abdominal cramps, or bloody mucus in the stools, before progressing to looser stools, frequent bowel movements, and severe cramps. Fever, nausea, vomiting, and moderate malaise are common systemic symptoms. Lower abdominal tenderness also occurs. Physician referral is recommended, and treatment often includes bed rest; fluid intake; change in diet; intravenous medication and supplements; medications such as anticholinergics (to reduce intestinal motility), antibacterial agents, and glucocorticoids; and stress management techniques.

Constipation

Constipation can result from a variety of factors, including poor hydration, stress, poor diet, medications, and neurogenic disorders. Constipation is frequently asymptomatic but can cause cramps and general abdominal discomfort. Prevention of constipation includes adequate hydration, achieved by drinking several glasses of water daily. It also includes a dietary reduction in simple carbohydrates and an increase in complex carbohydrates and fresh fruits and vegetables, as well as balance in the diet. Use of bulk laxatives can increase bulk within the colon and encourage regular bowel movements. Laxatives, suppositories, and enemas can relieve constipation, but it is generally not wise to take them on an ongoing basis.

Diarrhea

Diarrhea is characterized by loose, liquid, or frequent bowel movements. Diarrhea is usually short-term, but if it lasts for more than 2 weeks it is considered persistent or chronic. It is a symptom of many conditions, including ulcerative colitis, parasitic infections, bacterial infections, diverticulitis, irritable bowel syndrome, malabsorption syndrome, gastroenteritis, medication reactions, food additives such as sorbitol or fructose, food allergies, travel with exposure to contaminated water or food, excessive use of laxatives, or stress and anxiety.

The key to managing diarrhea is identifying its cause to remove or reduce it rather than merely treating the symptoms. Proper medication to manage diarrhea can be prescribed once the underlying cause has been determined. Many over-the-counter antidiarrheal drugs such as Lomotil (diphenoxylate with atropine) or Pepto-Bismol are effective in managing acute diarrhea related to irregular or indiscriminate eating as often occurs on team road trips. Additional steps in the care of athletes with diarrhea include preventing dehydration, having the athletes avoid beverages containing caffeine or alcohol (since caffeine promotes diarrhea and alcohol dehydrates the body), and having the athletes maintain good nutrition. Chronic diarrhea can be prevented with sensible steps such as drinking only clean or purified water, properly handling food, and maintaining good hand-washing habits.

Refer athletes who have prolonged diarrhea (more than 2-3 days) to a physician for further examination and treatment. Not only can diarrhea be a sign of more serious conditions, when prolonged, it can cause dehydration and electrolyte imbalances that can lead to metabolic shock.

Esophageal Reflux

Esophageal reflux occurs when the esophageal sphincter between the esophagus and stomach does not close completely. Acid from the stomach can enter the esophagus and cause what is commonly termed heartburn. The condition is aggravated when the patient lies recumbent. The patient is encouraged to sleep in a semirecumbent position and to seek medical attention for medication to help reduce acid in the esophagus. The greatest danger with esophageal reflux is the possibility that gastric acid will be aspirated into the trachea and cause pulmonary complications.

Gastritis

Gastritis is an acute or chronic condition in which the mucous membrane of the stomach becomes irritated or inflamed. Acute gastritis can result from ingestion of abrasive substances such as alcohol, salicylates (e.g., aspirin), antibiotics, sulfur products, excessively acidic or spicy food, or allergenic foods. Acute gastritis is usually of short duration, subsiding within 24 to 48 hours, and presents with symptoms of nausea, vomiting, headache, vertigo, sensation of fullness, malaise, and possible fever. Treatment includes abstaining from solid foods and ingesting only clear liquids. Soft foods are gradually introduced and then a bland diet is consumed for at least 2 weeks. Antiemetics and analgesics provide symptomatic relief as needed.

Antiemetics are drugs that control nausea and vomiting.

Chronic gastritis is the consequence of a bacterial infection that stimulates a cellular and humoral response, irritating the mucosa and possibly leading to ulcer disease. The bacteria are unique in that they thrive in an acidic environment. Treatment includes antibiotic therapy along with medication that reduces hydrochloric acid secretion to sensitize the bacteria to the antibiotic.

Humoral refers to a bodily fluid or semifluid such as a hormone.

Gastroenteritis

Gastroenteritis is an inflammation of the stomach and intestine mucous membrane—an acute condition that people commonly refer to as food poisoning. The cause is ingestion of virus or bacteria or excessive intake of irritating substances such as alcohol, salicylates, cathartics, or heavy metals. The severity of the symptoms directly relates to the nature and dose of the irritant ingested. There is a sudden onset of nausea, as well as vomiting, malaise, abdominal cramps, and diarrhea. A fever usually occurs if the condition is infection based. Gurgling bowel sounds can be heard with a stethoscope. Dehydration and electrolyte imbalances can occur with vomiting and diarrhea. Treatment includes intravenous therapy for restoring electrolyte balances and hydration until vomiting has stopped. Medications for symptomatic relief are usually prescribed. Once the patient has started drinking fluids, gradual introduction of soft foods and a bland diet is the usual protocol.

Indigestion

Indigestion is a nonspecific term that refers to either improper digestion or deficient absorption of food in the digestive tract. Also known as digestive upset, or **dyspepsia**, it can result from irregular eating, ingestion of foods to which the athlete is unaccustomed or allergic, and anxiety or stress. Symptoms include upset stomach, nausea, or flatulence. Treatment commonly includes one of a large selection of over-the-counter medications for relief of symptoms, including Pepto-Bismol, Tums, Rolaids, and Gaviscon. Avoiding irritating foods and controlling anxiety and stress are prevention steps advisable for patients who experience regular episodes of indigestion.

Ulcers

Ulcers involve a more severe form of gastritis and include an erosion of the mucous membrane of the stomach, duodenum, or lower esophagus. Ulcers can take the form of duodenal or gastric ulcers and are also referred to as peptic ulcer disease. They are thought to be caused primarily by the helicobacter pylori (*H. pylori*) bacterium. Prior to their discovery in 1982, ulcers were thought to result from ingestion of spicy foods, hyperacidity, or increased stress. The hallmark symptom is a gnawing or burning pain in the epigastrium, the upper middle abdominal region. Pain occurs most often when the stomach is empty, can last from minutes to hours, and is relieved by eating or taking antacids. Bleeding can result from erosion of the stomach wall and presents as a coffee-colored emesis (vomitus) if the bleeding is slow or as a more distinct red if the bleeding is more rapid. Additional but less common symptoms include nausea, heartburn, vomiting, weight loss, and diarrhea. Physician referral for antibiotic medication accompanied by medication to reduce stomach acid is the usual treatment protocol.

Irritable Bowel Syndrome

Irritable bowel syndrome is a noninflammatory, nonserious disorder that affects the large bowel. The accompanying symptoms reflect the failure of the large bowel to function smoothly. The cause is unknown, but the syndrome occurs more often in women than in men; symptoms are seen more often during menstruation and times of stress and are aggravated with ingestion of fats, chocolate, milk products, alcohol, and caffeine. A significant number of people with irritable bowel syndrome demonstrate depression, anxiety, or other psychological problems. Symptoms include abdominal cramps with painful constipation or diarrhea. Although most often the condition involves constipation, influences such as bacteria, virus, toxins, or prolonged antibiotic use can cause diarrhea. Typically, bowel movements produce hard stools covered with mucus and may be interspersed with episodes of diarrhea. Bloating and gas may also occur. Palpation reveals lower quadrant tenderness.

Physician referral for differential diagnosis to rule out more serious conditions is advisable. Treatment includes resolving possible stress and anxiety issues. The treatment protocol should also include encouragement and education for regular diet and eating habits with adequate fluid and fiber intake. Reduced laxative use should be encouraged. Antispasmodic drugs, fiber supplements, or stool softeners are commonly prescribed.

EATING DISORDERS

The eating disorders known as anorexia and bulimia can be serious and life threatening. You must be aware of their signs and symptoms and report any suspected cases to a physician for care and treatment.

Anorexia Nervosa

Anorexia is a severe psychological disorder characterized by a self-induced food aversion and extreme weight loss. Although the condition can affect males, females are 10 times more often affected and usually experience amenorrhea as a side effect. Anorexia typically begins either in the preteen years or early in the teen years but may not manifest until the 30s or

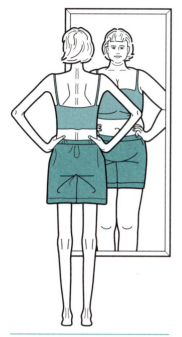

Figure 22.1 People with anorexia see themselves as overweight when they actually are severely underweight.

40s; females from professional or managerial families are most often affected. Athletes involved in activities in which body image is important and small size is advantageous, such as gymnasts, dancers, divers, jockeys, wrestlers, and crew coxswains, are particularly vulnerable.

Anorexia may appear initially as normal dieting and concern about weight loss but becomes an obsession to be thin. Patients with anorexia do not see themselves as thin, even when their appearance is emaciated and they are grossly underweight (figure 22.1). Food and caloric intake and expenditure become their central focus; they often limit food intake to 300 to 600 calories daily. They show a need and compulsion to exercise often and excessively. Signs and symptoms include weight loss greater than 25% of body weight, behavior directed toward weight loss, peculiar patterns of handling food, intense fear of gaining weight, disturbances in body image, and amenorrhea in women. Secondary symptoms include constipation, pale and dry skin, dry and brittle hair, low blood pressure, electrolyte imbalances, dehydration, subnormal temperature, broken sleep, reduced pulse rate, brittle bones, and slight edema around the ankles. The athlete may become withdrawn and may have difficulty concentrating or thinking clearly. At meals with the team, the athlete may play with the food or move the food on the plate to give the impression of eating, may hide the food to feign eating, or may encourage others to eat more. In later stages, athletes with anorexia, like those who have bulimia, resort to laxatives that can produce persistent abdominal pain, cause fingers to become edematous, and damage bowel muscles to further add to constipation. Severe and prolonged starvation efforts can result in dangerous electrolyte imbalance and dehydration that can become life threatening.

Primary and Secondary Signs and Symptoms of Anorexia Nervosa

Primary Signs and Symptoms

- Weight loss greater than 25% of body weight
- Behavior directed toward weight loss
- Peculiar patterns of handling food
- Intense fear of gaining weight
- Disturbances in body image
- Amenorrhea in women

Secondary Symptoms

- Constipation
- Pale and dry skin
- Dry and brittle hair
- Low blood pressure
- Electrolyte imbalances
- Dehydration
- Subnormal temperature
- Broken sleep
- Reduced pulse rate
- Brittle bones
- Slight edema around the ankles

Treatment may include hospitalization for psychological counseling, progressive and closely monitored weight gain, and an effort to establish new eating habits. Patients with anorexia are frequently reluctant to admit that they have a problem. Since they do not view themselves as underweight, changes in attitude and behavior are often difficult.

Bulimia Nervosa

Athletes who have bulimia are of normal weight but use techniques such as vomiting and ingestion of diuretics and laxatives to prevent weight gain. Patients suffering from bulimia tend to be slightly older than those with anorexia. Like those with anorexia, they have an exaggerated fear of getting fat, but they do not attempt to lose weight, only maintain it. Episodes of uncontrolled binge eating followed by vomiting are frequent. Athletes with bulimia are often outgoing perfectionists who enjoy pleasing others. Because of frequent vomiting episodes, symptoms such as enlarged salivary glands around the throat become evident, and tooth enamel is dissolved by stomach acids. Calluses on the knuckles and sores at the corners of the mouth may also be present. Irregular heart rate, muscle weakness, kidney damage, and epileptic seizures are additional symptoms that can result from frequent vomiting and electrolyte disturbances. Because outward signs are minimal and subtle, bulimia is more difficult to detect than anorexia. However, at times these conditions are found in tandem, and weight loss is evident (**bulimarexia**).

Treatment uses the same protocol as for anorexia, but it can sometimes be easier for the patients with bulimia to comply with treatment, as they often feel guilty and ashamed of their behavior, and the binge eating and vomiting is time consuming and exhausting. Admitting to the problem may be a relief, but counseling and support with a change in lifestyle and environment are necessary for successful treatment.

Obesity

Although prevalent in the general population, obesity is not normally seen in the athletic population. The number of overweight youths has more than doubled in the United States in the past 30 years, and inactivity may be the primary reason. Almost half of those ages 12 to 21 and more than one-third of high school students do not participate in regular exercise. Sumo wrestlers, football players, and heavyweight wrestlers are the athletic groups that may exhibit obesity. Body weight over 20% of the desired weight is considered in the obese range. Weight over 40 to 50% of the desired weight is considered morbidly obese and can be life threatening. Various methods of determining body fat mass relative to lean body mass are available; these are the best methods for defining desired body weight.

> For more information on determining body fat mass, refer to *Introduction to Athletic Training, Second Edition,* (Hillman 2005), chapter 4.

Nutritional counseling referral is advisable for athletes interested in lowering their body fat. A balanced diet combined with regular exercise is the most effective means of achieving weight loss, but this program should be instituted under the guidance of a nutritional counselor or physician.

SEXUALLY TRANSMITTED DISEASES AND DISEASES TRANSMITTED BY BODY FLUID

Sexually transmitted diseases are common and represent very sensitive conditions both socially and medically. These conditions can raise considerable concern and stigma among teammates, and athletes are often reluctant to report their signs and symptoms. Because of the sensitive issues surrounding sexually transmitted diseases, you must be able to deal with the athlete with professionalism and confidence. Although these conditions may involve dangers of transmission to other athletes, confidentiality and education are of utmost importance.

Human Immunodeficiency Virus (HIV) and Acquired Immunodeficiency Syndrome (AIDS)

The human immunodeficiency virus (HIV) weakens the immune system by destroying lymphocytes (T cells), impairing the body's ability to defend itself against potentially deadly infections and malignancies. Human immunodeficiency virus advances through a progression of stages, beginning with transient infections, continuing to complex diseases related to acquired immunodeficiency syndrome (AIDS), and ending in AIDS itself. Approximately 70% of those infected with HIV develop AIDS within 10 years. Acquired immunodeficiency syndrome is actually a collection of life-threatening diseases that occur as the patient's immune system becomes progressively weaker and less resistant to infection and malignancies. Normal T cell count is 800 to 1300. A patient may remain in HIV status for several years before the disease advances to AIDS; AIDS is usually defined by a drop in the T cell count below 200 as a result of HIV. At this point, the patient's health declines more rapidly.

HIV cannot be transmitted through casual contact, kissing, or touching; it is transmitted through unprotected sexual activity, intravenous drug use, breast-feeding from women infected with HIV, use of contaminated needles, and less often through transfusion of blood products. The likelihood that transfusions will cause HIV infection has decreased greatly in recent years because of improved techniques for blood screening. Although HIV can infect any age group, the greatest number of cases are seen in the most sexually active age group, ages 24 to 44. While in the late 1990s approximately 80% of HIV cases were men and 20% were women, new female cases are increasing at a faster rate than new male cases.

Although there is no cure for HIV, recent advances in medication combinations have improved the health and longevity of patients with HIV. The medical "cocktails" include an expensive combination of a relatively new class of drugs called protease inhibitors that are taken throughout the day. These medications keep HIV in check and have reduced the death rate by 50%. Athletes with HIV should notify you of the condition. Because of the persisting social stigma and often unfounded fears connected with HIV, you must respect patient confidentiality by not passing this information on. You should maintain standard sterile technique when caring for open wounds and dispose of contaminated supplies as with any other condition.

For more information on proper sterilizing techniques and contaminant disposal, refer to *Introduction to Athletic Training, Second Edition,* (Hillman 2005), chapter 8.

Hepatitis

Hepatitis is an inflammation of the liver caused by either infectious or toxic substances. It is one of the most frequently reported infectious diseases in the United States, surpassed only by gonorrhea and chicken pox. There are five known types of hepatitis: A, B, C, D, and E. They are defined by the manner of transmission and the length of time the patient can remain a carrier. Hepatitis A and E are communicated through fecal–oral transmission following food handling without proper hand washing and can evolve into epidemic situations. Hepatitis B, C, and D are transmitted through blood, semen, and other bodily fluids. Hepatitis B is hardier than HIV but is communicated in similar ways, such as sharing contaminated needles, practicing unsafe sex, and transmitting from mother to infant at birth. Hepatitis D thrives only in the presence of a hepatitis B infection. People can also contract hepatitis by eating the wrong kind of mushroom, ingesting alcohol excessively, eating raw shellfish from contaminated waters, taking too much Tylenol, and ingesting anything that causes liver inflammation.

Infectious hepatitis—hepatitis A—is most contagious before signs of jaundice appear. Hepatitis A is usually acute and without lasting effects on the liver. Hepatitis B produces more severe symptoms than either A or E, but does not carry as great a risk of causing chronic hepatitis as does hepatitis C. Although the progression is slow, occurring over 10 to 30 years, hepatitis C has the greatest chance of advancing to cirrhosis and liver failure.

Early symptoms of hepatitis include flu-like symptoms such as fever, fatigue, nausea, diarrhea, general achiness, and appetite loss. Jaundice is a hallmark. Acute viral hepatitis usually disappears within 4 to 16 weeks without any treatment beyond adequate diet and rest. Chronic hepatitis can cause periodic health disturbances and lead to cirrhosis and occasionally to liver failure.

Antibody vaccines are available for hepatitis A and B. Athletes who are sexually active, health care workers with possible exposure to hepatitis (including certified athletic trainers), and intravenous drug users are all encouraged to obtain the hepatitis B vaccine. Parents of infants should also have their babies immunized against hepatitis B. Those traveling with teams overseas should have hepatitis vaccines before leaving the country. Refer athletes suspected of having hepatitis to a physician. Care of athletes with hepatitis requires using sterile technique with open wounds and properly disposing of contaminated items.

Chlamydia

Chlamydia is the most common bacterial sexually transmitted disease in the United States. Because 75% of infected women and 50% of infected men do not show symptoms, the disease often goes untreated. Teenage girls and young women under the age of 25 have the highest incidence rate. When signs and symptoms are present, they may include painful urination (dysuria) and a pus discharge in males, or vaginal discharge, pelvic pain, and dysuria in females. Although chlamydia can be easily treated, when untreated in females it can lead to a number of severe problems including pelvic inflammatory disease, infertility, chronic pelvic pain, and tubal pregnancy with risk of death. Untreated chlamydia in males can result in urethral infection and swollen and tender testicles.

Prevention through education is the best means of treatment. Screening men and women in the high incidence age groups is also advocated. Antibiotic therapy under the guidance of a physician is the standard of care for those infected with the disease.

Genital Warts

Urethritis is an inflammation of the urethra.

Purulent means containing or consisting of pus.

Epididymitis is an inflammation of the epididymis.

Endometritis is an inflammation of the endometrium of the uterus.

Bartholin glands are small mucous glands located on each lateral inner wall of the vagina, near the vaginal opening.

Genital warts, or **condylomata acuminata**, are located in the perineum and perianal region. They are caused by the human papilloma virus (HPV), and it is estimated that 1 million new cases occur each year (Taber 1997). Genital warts are contracted through sexual contact, and the patient typically has a history of unprotected sexual contact with an infected person or with multiple partners. These viral warts begin as tiny pink swellings and may coalesce to form a fibrous overgrowth covered with thickened epithelium. They may occur singly or as colonized warts with a cauliflower-like appearance and are usually not painful. To prevent their spread, the patient should abstain from sexual contact or use a condom during intercourse until healing is complete. In women, these warts may be associated with cervical cancer; thus the patient should seek medical attention for further examination.

Gonorrhea

Gonorrhea is a bacterial infection, the infection rate of which is climbing rapidly. Females aged 15 to 19 have the highest rate of gonorrhea. Sexual intercourse is the chief means of transmission. Although symptoms are not always apparent, males can develop an acute urethritis with dysuria. Urinary frequency and urgency can also occur along with a yellow, purulent discharge. The lips of the urinary meatus can be red and swollen. Although 50% of females do not have symptoms, when symptoms are present they can include a purulent urethral discharge, a cervical discharge, or swollen Bartholin glands. In untreated cases, sterility, urethritis, prostatitis, and epididymitis may occur in males. Females may also become sterile and may develop endometritis and pelvic inflammatory disease. Either sex may develop gonococcal arthritis and conjunctivitis.

Sexual abstinence and proper condom application and consistent use are the best modes of prevention. Antibiotics are the drug of choice for treating gonorrhea.

Syphilis

Syphilis is an acute venereal bacterial condition. The syphilis bacterium is transmitted during vaginal, rectal, or oral sex; it can also be transmitted through open wounds or through direct contact with bodily fluids or blood. If symptoms occur, they are usually seen as genital or anal lesions in the form of a chancre that starts as a papule and then ulcerates. Chancres can also appear almost anywhere on the body, including the hands, eyelids, and mouth. As the chancre fades, a rash in the form of either rough, "copper penny" spots on the palms of the hands and bottom of the feet or small blotches or scales all over the body, can become visible. The rash can appear as a prickly heat rash, as slimy white patches in the mouth, or as bumps similar to chicken pox—or it may be hardly noticeable. The rash may be present for 2 to 6 weeks and spontaneously disappear. The groin lymph nodes may be enlarged. If left untreated, syphilis can progress to a secondary syphilis as the disease spreads through all tissues of the body and causes highly infectious generalized skin lesions and conjunctivitis, periostitis of the long bones, hepatitis, headaches, fatigue, weight loss, and nephritic (renal) syndrome. Late syphilis is indicated by nonspecific chronic inflammatory conditions that can affect cardiovascular and central nervous system functions.

A chancre is a sore or ulcer.

Although prevention and education are the treatment of choice, antibiotic therapy is the standard treatment for patients who have contracted syphilis. One dose of penicillin usually cures syphilis. Refer any unusual discharge, sores, or rashes, especially in the genitourinary and groin region, to a physician for diagnosis and treatment. Sterile technique is always the management technique of choice with transmissible diseases. Anyone who has been bitten or scratched by someone with syphilis should contact a physician and obtain a prescription for antibiotic therapy.

GENITOURINARY TRACT AND ORGANS

The genitourinary tract and organs include the kidneys, bladder, urinary tract, and external genitalia. Gynecological conditions are discussed separately in the next section.

Kidney Stones

Kidney stones is the common term for **urinary calculi**. Found anywhere in the urinary system, including the kidney, ureter, bladder, or urethra, kidney stones are composed of precipitated urinary salts. They occur most often in middle-aged males.

If kidney stones stay within the kidney, the patient may remain asymptomatic. If a stone moves from the kidney and obstructs the ureter, severe renal colic ensues as the smooth muscle of the ureter forcefully contracts to relieve the obstruction. The pain, which is extreme, may start in the back or flank and radiate across the abdomen into the groin, genitalia, and inner thigh. Nausea, vomiting, sweating, chills, urinary frequency or urgency, and shock may occur, as can microscopic hematuria.

Hematuria means blood in the urine.

Transport the patient to an emergency care facility for symptom relief. Renal colic is one of the most severe pains patients can experience, so morphine or another powerful analgesic is commonly administered along with antispasmodic medications. Adequate fluid intake should be encouraged. Small stones eventually pass through the ureter and are discharged. Larger stones may require surgical intervention to relieve the obstruction. This can be performed with lasers for effective yet minimally invasive results.

Urethritis

Urethritis, or inflammation of the urethra, is also known as a urinary tract infection (UTI) that is isolated to the urethra. This type of infection occurs more frequently in women than in men and is a poorly understood phenomenon. Symptoms, although not always present, may include urinary frequency and urgency, painful or burning urination, cloudy or even reddish urine if hematuria occurs, general malaise, and lower abdominal pain. Men may experience a sensation of fullness of the rectum.

Antibacterial medications usually resolve the problem within a couple of days, but antibiotics are taken for up to 2 weeks to assure a cure. Actions such as increasing fluid intake and decreasing smoking and ingestion of caffeine or alcohol may aid in reducing symptoms. Preventive steps include drinking plenty of fluids (especially water), not delaying urination, and avoiding feminine sprays and douches.

Urinary Tract Infection

As just discussed, urethritis is a form of urinary tract infection (UTI). A UTI also occurs if the bacterial infection spreads to other segments of the urinary system. In advanced cases, the infection spreads to the bladder and ureter. When kidneys are affected, symptoms of urethritis as well as other symptoms such as back pain, fever, nausea, and vomiting can be present. Although the reason for a greater incidence of UTI in women than in men is unclear, there are several conjectures. Women who use a diaphragm are more likely to develop urinary tract infections than those who use other birth control methods. Sexual intercourse can trigger an infection for some women. The female's urethra is short and close to the vagina, as well as closer to the anus than in males, so the female's bladder may be easier for bacteria to access than the male's.

Antibacterial drugs are used to treat UTIs. As with urethritis, the medication is taken for about 2 weeks even though symptoms subside after 2 days of administration. Prevention steps are the same as those listed for urethritis.

Spermatic Cord Torsion

Infarction is necrosis of a tissue or organ resulting from an obstruction of the local circulation secondary to a clot or occlusion of the vessel.

The cremaster muscle is continuous with the internal oblique and functions to draw the testicles to a more superior position in the scrotum.

The cremasteric reflex is a drawing up of the scrotal sac with ipsilateral stroking of the upper inner thigh.

Spermatic cord torsion, or testicular torsion, occurs when the testicle twists on the spermatic cord, leading to venous occlusion and engorgement followed by arterial ischemia and possible testicular infarction (figure 22.2). Torsion can also occur spontaneously in young males in the absence of trauma. Predisposing factors include anatomic abnormalities of the insertion of the tunica vaginalis or spermatic artery anomalies, a nonexistent or very long gubernaculum, a poorly placed or long epididymis, or an abnormal testicular position. Trauma to the scrotum followed by swelling or a vigorous cremaster contraction in combination with any predisposing factor can result in testicular torsion. The patient experiences a sudden or gradual onset of severe unilateral scrotal pain accompanied by scrotal swelling

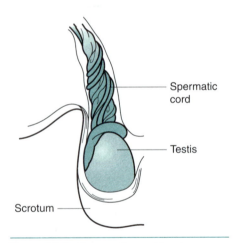

Figure 22.2 Spermatic cord torsion.

and heaviness, as well as nausea and vomiting. The involved testicle is tender and firm and is elevated in comparison to the contralateral testicle; edema is present with scrotal erythema, the cremasteric reflex is absent ipsilaterally, and scrotal elevation does not relieve the pain. This condition constitutes a medical emergency and requires immediate referral, as blood flow to the testicle is compromised.

Manual detorsion of the testicle relieves pain. If necessary, the athlete can be instructed in self-administering manual detorsion technique. Most torsions rotate inward and toward the midline, so manual detorsion must occur in the opposite direction, with a twisting outward and laterally away from the midline. This derotation may have to be repeated 2 or 3 times, depending on the athlete's pain. Manual detorsion has a 30 to 70% success rate. If the technique is successful, still refer the athlete to a physician for examination and follow-up care. If it is unsuccessful, emergency transportation to a hospital for surgical release is necessary to save the testicle.

Epididymitis

Epididymitis is an inflammation of the epididymis, one of a pair of ducts that carries sperm from the seminiferous tubule of the testicles to the vas deferens. Epididymitis can result from urinary tract infection, venereal disease, tuberculosis, mumps, or inflammation of the prostate gland or urethra. Signs and symptoms include fever, chills, inguinal pain, and swelling of the epididymis. The condition is typically treated with bed rest and antibiotics.

Hydrocele

A **hydrocele** is an accumulation of fluid around the testicle. Hydroceles are most common at birth and usually resolve without assistance by 18 months of age with the closure of the processus vaginalis. Adult hydroceles result from direct trauma, infections, or radiotherapy. Symptoms include a sensation of heaviness and mild discomfort radiating into the inguinal region and sometimes into the back. Enlargement of the scrotal sac can occur while standing and decrease while recumbent, and scrotal consistency can range from soft to tense. There is commonly no pain. Prior to treatment, a differential diagnostic examination to rule out testicular torsion must be made. It is also necessary to determine the need for surgical release of the hydrocele. Adult hydroceles often require surgical intervention; thus physician referral is necessary with any changes in the size, shape, or consistency of the testicle.

Varicocele

A varicocele is an enlargement of the internal spermatic veins that develops because of defective valves in the veins, allowing backflow into the testicle (figure 22.3). This can result in sterility. The left spermatic vein is more often affected than the right because the left vein enters the left renal vein at a right angle and can become compressed by the mesenteric artery at this site. Blood pooling with increased temperature and congestion can influence sperm production. Often the affected testicle is smaller than the other one, and when the patient is asked to bear down, blood backflow can be palpated.

Pain or a significant size difference in the testicles indicate surgical repair. Surgery is usually successful and sperm count is restored in up to 70% of patients.

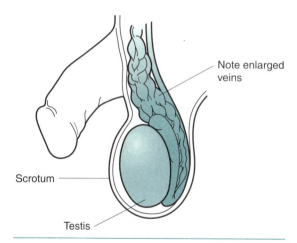

Note enlarged veins

Scrotum

Testis

Figure 22.3 Testicular varicocele.

Testicular Cancer

Testicular cancer is a highly treatable and curable cancer that occurs predominantly in males of 20 to 35 years of age. In 2003, approximately 8,000 cases were diagnosed in the United States (American Cancer Society 2003). Risk factors include family history, previous history of a testicular tumor, and cryptorchidism (an undescended testicle). While trauma is not considered a cause of testicular cancer, the tumor may be first detected during an injury examination, as a lump on the testicle is commonly the first sign. During the early stages of cancer, the athlete may be otherwise asymptomatic. In the later stages, however, symptoms such as ureteral obstruction, pulmonary symptoms, and abdominal mass may occur. Other signs and symptoms include testicle enlargement, significant decrease in the size of one testicle, feeling of heaviness in the scrotum, dull ache in the lower abdomen or groin, sudden collection of fluid in the scrotum, pain or discomfort in a testicle or in the scrotum, and enlargement or tenderness of the breasts.

Testicular Self-Examination (TSE)

As with most forms of cancer, early detection is key. While there is no research showing self-examination can reduce the number of deaths caused by testicular cancer, a monthly self-examination is recommended for those who may be at risk. The best time to perform the testicular self-exam (TSE) is during or after a bath or shower, when the scrotum skin is relaxed, making it easier to detect a lump. To perform the TSE, the American Cancer Society (2003) recommends the following steps:

1. Hold your penis out of the way and examine each testicle separately.
2. Hold your testicle between the thumbs and fingers of both hands and roll it gently between the fingers.
3. Look and feel for any hard lumps or nodules (smooth, rounded masses) or any change in the size, shape, or consistency of the testicles.
4. Become familiar with what is normal and abnormal through frequent examinations.

Palpable lumps or nodules should be differentiated from the epididymis of the normal testicles, which appears as a small bump on the upper or middle outer side of the testicle. The presence of a hydrocele (enlarged testicle due to fluid accumulation, see page 621), or varicocele (enlargement of the veins in the testicle, see page 621), may also appear as a tumor, and should be differentially diagnosed by a physician for further examination.

GYNECOLOGICAL CONDITIONS

Elite athletes frequently experience gynecological disorders, as excessive or intense exercise can cause menstrual dysfunction. Other conditions such as painful menses and vaginal infections or irritations can cause discomfort and affect athletic performance. This section also covers breast conditions.

Menstrual Dysfunction

Female athletes may complain of a variety of menstrual dysfunctions, including pain, menstrual irregularity, and loss of menses.

Amenorrhea

Amenorrhea is the absence of a menstrual cycle. There are three types of amenorrhea: primary, secondary, and irregular. Primary amenorrhea is present when menstruation has not started by age 16. There are several causative factors, including an imperforate hymen, ovarian dysfunction, and hormonal imbalance. Secondary amenorrhea occurs when menstruation stops in a woman who has previously menstruated. Factors that can produce secondary amenorrhea include pregnancy, menopause, stress, weight change, breast-feeding, anemia, excessive exercise, ovarian cysts, and medications. Irregular amenorrhea is present either when periods occur inconsistently or when only a few occur annually; causes can be related to secondary amenorrhea. Female athletes most often experience secondary or irregular amenorrhea.

Amenorrhea is often associated with disordered eating, low body weight, and excessive exercise, not all of which need be pathological. The incidence of osteoporosis (bone loss) and of stress fractures is higher in amenorrheic women than in others. Together, amenorrhea, disordered eating, and osteoporosis constitute what is termed the **female athlete triad**. Physician referral is necessary to determine the cause of amenorrhea and appropriate treatment. Hormones, hormone stimulators, thyroxin, other medications, nutrition counseling, and other measures may be indicated depending on the results of an examination and laboratory tests.

Imperforate means lacking the usual or normal opening.

Female Athlete Triad

The female athlete triad is considered a serious yet preventable syndrome composed of three interrelated conditions: disordered eating, amenorrhea, and osteoporosis. Excellent review articles (Nattiv et al. 1994; Sandborn et al. 2000) and a position stand from the American College of Sports Medicine (Otis et al. 1997) provide extensive information on this topic. While each component of the triad represents a medical problem in itself, experts agree that the combination of the three conditions can significantly affect the health of the young female athlete.

Females most susceptible to this triad meet some or all of the following criteria:

- Participating in sports where low body weight and a lean physique are considered advantageous (gymnastics, figure skating, ballet, and distance running)
- Participating in individual sports
- Participating in sports that involve judging or weight classes
- Focusing their identity around sports participation
- Excessively or suddenly increasing training
- Undergoing an adolescent growth spurt or retiring from athletics
- Experiencing amenorrhea
- Possessing a history of stress fractures
- Possessing an increased risk of fractures

Prescreening for signs and symptoms of the female athlete triad is best accomplished during the preparticipation physical examination. Medical history and physical screening should include questions regarding the following:

- Disordered eating
- Menstrual irregularities
- History of stress fractures
- Cardiac arrhythmias, bradycardia
- Life stressors, exercise habits (excessive or exercise through injury), depressive symptoms, dissatisfaction with weight or body shape, and training intensity.

Athletes identified with one component of the triad should always be screened for the other components. Also note that although these conditions are seen more often in females, males may also suffer from disordered eating and osteoporosis. There exists little research on the long-term consequences of disordered eating in males, but it has been suggested that males with delayed puberty have decreased bone mineral density and may be at increased risk for fractures (Nattiv et al. 1994).

Oligomenorrhea

Oligomenorrhea is defined as an irregular menses, characterized by infrequent or light periods or both. Causes can include rapid weight loss, anorexia or bulimia, high levels of or significant changes in exercise, and some medications and illicit drug use. Refer the athlete to a physician, who will determine the cause of the oligomenorrhea before selecting the most appropriate treatment. No treatment is required unless the cause is pathological, or unless the patient wishes to become pregnant or maintain a balance of hormone levels.

Dysmenorrhea

Prostaglandins are fatty acids that perform a variety of hormone functions.

Dysmenorrhea, also known as menstrual cramps, includes pain during menstruation that is severe enough to interfere with normal activity. Additional symptoms can include nausea, vomiting, and severe abdominal pain. Women who have dysmenorrhea have an abnormally high concentration of prostaglandins in their menstrual fluid. Release of prostaglandin into the uterus stimulates the smooth muscle to contract, limiting oxygen supply to the uterine wall by inhibiting blood supply. Once menstrual flow begins, the prostaglandin is discharged, causing symptoms to subside after the first few days of the period.

Over-the-counter analgesics and anti-inflammatories may adequately relieve pain. Hot baths and massage may also encourage muscle relaxation and increase circulation. Exercises may aid in abdominal muscle relaxation. In more severe cases, prescription prostaglandin inhibitors may be necessary to relieve symptoms. Some women also find relief with contraceptives.

Pregnancy Issues

Occasionally you may encounter and work with a physically active female who is pregnant. The following sections discuss the physiological changes that occur with pregnancy and some precautions you should be aware of with the physically active female.

Pregnancy and Exercise Considerations

Pregnancy involves the growth and development of a child in the womb and lasts approximately 40 weeks (280 days; 9 1/3 months) from the time of conception to delivery. During this time, the female experiences marked psychological and physiological changes. Physiologically, she undergoes significant cardiovascular, metabolic, and musculoskeletal changes (Wang and Apgar 1998). Cardiovascular changes include increased cardiac output, stroke volume, pulse rate, and total blood volume beginning about the sixth week of pregnancy. Metabolically, metabolic rate and body temperature increase, resulting in greater energy demands and heat production both at rest and during exercise. Body morphology also changes, with pregnant females experiencing an increase in breast size, body weight, and the weight of the fetus. These changes can shift the center of gravity anteriorly, potentially affecting balance and increasing lumbar lordosis (Wang and Apgar 1998).

Pregnancy does not preclude physically activity, but there are certain precautions pregnant athletes should follow, and they should always be closely monitored by their physician. Once you are aware that an athlete is pregnant, consult a physician before letting the athlete embark on an exercise program. Exercise levels will depend on the athlete's overall health, current physical conditioning, exercise goals, and exercise tolerance. Generally, women who have achieved a level of fitness prior to pregnancy should be able to maintain that level throughout pregnancy. However, as physiological changes occur, they may need to modify the types of activities in which they engage.

Weight-bearing exercises that increase vertical ground forces pose a concern as weight is gained; as impact forces can vary anywhere from 2 to 6 times body weight during sport activity, the impact of increased weight on the joints magnifies during these weight-bearing activities. Increased joint laxity has also been demonstrated in pregnant females secondary to dramatic changes in hormone levels (Charlton, Coslett-Charlton, and Ciccotti 2001; Dumas and Reid 1997). While some consider this increase in joint laxity to potentially contribute to strains and sprains, an increase in injury rate in pregnant females has not been documented (Wang and Apgar 1998).

Absolute and relative contraindications to exercise during pregnancy are listed in table 22.2. In the absence of these contraindications, the American College of Obstetrics and Gynecology recommends the following (ACOG Committee Opinion 2002):

- Women should be encouraged to engage in regular physical activity of moderate intensity to continue to derive the health benefits during pregnancy as they did before pregnancy.

- Epidemiological data suggests that regular exercise during pregnancy may be beneficial in the primary prevention of gestational diabetes, particularly in obese women (BMI >33).

Table 22.2
Absolute and Relative Contraindications to Aerobic Exercise During Pregnancy

Absolute
Hemodynamically significant heart disease
Restrictive lung disease
Incompetent cervix or cerclage
Multiple gestation at risk for premature labor
Persistent second- or third-trimester bleeding
Placenta previa after 26 weeks of gestation
Premature labor during the current pregnancy
Ruptured membranes
Preeclampsia or pregnancy-induced hypertension

Relative
Severe anemia
Unevaluated maternal cardiac arrhythmia
Chronic bronchitis
Poorly controlled type 1 diabetes
Extreme morbid obesity
Extreme underweight (BMI <12)
History of extremely sedentary lifestyle
Intrauterine growth restriction in current pregnancy
Poorly controlled hypertension
Orthopedic limitations
Poorly controlled seizure disorder
Poorly controlled hyperthyroidism
Heavy smoker

Reprinted, by permission, American College of Obstetrics and Gynecology Committee on Obstetric Practice. 2002. Exercise during pregnancy and the postpartum period. ACOG Committee Opinion No. 267. *Obstetrics and Gynecology* 99(1): 172.

- Due to the cardiovascular changes that occur with pregnancy, pregnant women should avoid supine and motionless standing positions during exercise as much as possible.

- In general, participation in a wide range of sport and recreational activity appears to be safe. Sport or recreational activity that has a high risk of abdominal trauma (e.g., contact sports such as ice hockey, soccer, and basketball) or falling (e.g., gymnastics, horseback riding, downhill skiing, and vigorous racket sports) should be avoided during pregnancy. Scuba diving should also be avoided throughout pregnancy.

- Exercise at altitude up to 6,000 feet appears to be safe for pregnant females. Pregnant women who engage in recreational activity at a high altitude should be made aware of signs of altitude sickness, and should stop exercise, descend to a lower altitude, and seek medical attention if noted.

- Recreational and competitive athletes without complicated pregnancies can remain active throughout their pregnancy, and should modify their activity as medically indicated. Women who engage in strenuous activities should be closely monitored by their physicians.
- While exercise during pregnancy may provide additional health benefits, women who are previously inactive or who have medical complications should be carefully examined by a physician before exercise recommendations during pregnancy are made.
- A physically active female with a history of or risk of preterm labor or fetal growth restriction should reduce her activity in the second and third trimesters.

In addition to these criteria, it is generally accepted that any exercise that results in pain, pelvic floor discomfort, excessive fatigue, or shortness of breath should be discontinued. Any pregnant female who experiences vaginal bleeding, dyspnea prior to exertion, dizziness, headache, chest pain, muscle weakness, calf pain or swelling (i.e., risk of thrombophlebitis), preterm labor, decreased fetal movement, or amniotic fluid leakage should terminate exercise and seek medical attention (ACOG Committee Opinion 2002).

Ectopic Pregnancy

An ectopic pregnancy occurs when the egg implants outside the uterine cavity, and it represents a medical emergency. The most common site of implantation outside the uterus is the fallopian tube (tubal pregnancy), but can also occur in the abdomen (abdominal pregnancy) and ovary (ovarian pregnancy), among other locations. Those who have a history of pelvic inflammatory conditions are at greater risk for ectopic pregnancies. Signs and symptoms include amenorrhea, tenderness, and pain on the affected side, which may present before the female realizes she is pregnant. With rupture of the ectopic pregnancy, signs and symptoms of shock and internal hemorrhage will also emerge and can be fatal. Treatment for ectopic pregnancy is surgical intervention soon after diagnosis is made. Any females experiencing lower abdominal pain and who might possibly be pregnant should be immediately referred to a physician for examination.

Pelvic Conditions

Pain or symptoms in the pelvic and vaginal regions are usually caused by yeast and bacterial infections. These conditions include vaginitis, candidiasis, and pelvic inflammatory disease.

Vaginitis

Vaginitis is the medical term for vaginal infections. Of the number of organisms that can cause vaginitis, the most common are bacteria, yeast, and parasites. Bacteria cause a thin, milky white or gray discharge that has an unpleasant, foul, or musty odor, and may cause discomfort or burning. Untreated conditions can lead to pelvic inflammatory disease, endometritis, cervicitis, and other obstetric complications. Treatment includes antibiotic medication. Yeast infections are discussed separately in the next section.

Trichomoniasis is a parasite that can cause a yellow-green-gray frothy or sticky discharge that sometimes has a fishy or foul odor. The condition can cause occasional itching and painful irritation. Difficulties with pregnancy can occur if the woman is infected during pregnancy. Prescription medication is necessary to treat this condition.

Vaginal infections are common among women and should be attended to when symptoms are first recognized. A correct diagnosis is crucial to effective treatment, and referral to an obstetrician for appropriate tests is necessary for an accurate diagnosis. Prevention plays a significant role in reducing the risk or spread of infection. Women can take several preventive steps. They should avoid douching since it upsets the delicate pH balance and can increase the spread of organisms; other recommendations are to avoid tight clothing and to use cotton undergarments to help keep moisture (an environment in which many organisms thrive) to a minimum. Good hygiene also prevents the spread of organisms. Scented toilet paper, feminine deodorants, and harsh soaps can further decrease the health of any irritated area. Safe sex practices help prevent sexually transmitted infections.

Candidiasis

Candidiasis, or yeast infection, is actually caused by a fungus. Small numbers of this fungus are present normally in the vagina, but when the number increases, symptoms occur. Causes include tight clothing, warm weather, stress, diabetes, pregnancy, obesity, and medications such as antibiotics, steroids, and birth control pills. Symptoms can include pain during sex, vaginal itching and burning, and a curdlike, white discharge. Candidiasis is not dangerous, and symptoms usually decrease with treatment.

Treatment includes over-the-counter antifungal medication inserted as vaginal suppositories, creams, or tablets. If the infection persists, a physician should be consulted to rule out other diseases and establish the cause. Preventive steps include wearing loose clothing and cotton underwear and avoiding douches unless instructed by a physician to use them.

Pelvic Inflammatory Disease

Pelvic inflammatory disease (PID), also called salpingitis, is a serious complication of sexually transmitted diseases. It is a bacterial infection that attacks the female reproductive system, spreading from the vagina to the womb, fallopian tubes, and ovaries. It occurs as a result of an untreated bacterial infection of the vagina. Gonorrhea is a common preceding infection. In addition to sexual transmission, females can get PID from an intrauterine device. Symptoms may not always be present but include painful stomach cramps, bleeding, fever, chills, an upset stomach, and an odorous discharge. If left untreated, the condition can lead to sterility and is in fact the major cause of sterility in young women. Women with PID have an increased risk of ectopic (tubal) pregnancy.

PID prevention includes monogamous relationships, condom use, or abstinence. Treatment includes antibiotic therapy to destroy the bacteria. Intrauterine devices should be removed before initiating therapy. The woman's sexual partner should also be examined and treated if indicated to avoid episodes of reinfection.

Breast Conditions

It is not uncommon for the breasts to feel tender before menstruation. Normal changes in the breast affect both breasts simultaneously and symmetrically. However, there may be times that an athlete comes to you out of concern, complaining of changes in the appearance or feel of the tissue in one of the breasts. In the majority of these cases the changes are benign, but they should be examined and malignancy (cancer) ruled out.

Benign Conditions

Benign (noncancerous) conditions can be caused by fibrocystic changes and fibroadenomas. Because it is often difficult to differentiate between benign and malignant changes in breast tissue without diagnostic tests, refer all patients (whether male or female) who note breast tissue changes to a physician for proper diagnosis. Two of the more common conditions are fibrocystic changes and fibroadenomas.

• **Fibrocystic Changes.** Fibrocystic changes do not represent a disease state but rather a benign development of multiple fibrous lumps or small cysts caused by an overreaction of the breast to normal hormones produced during ovulation (Tetzlaf 1998). Fibrocystic changes are common in women between 20 and 50 years of age, affecting over 50% of all women. The fibrous lumps or cysts often become larger and more tender just prior to menstruation. Coffee, tea, cola drinks, chocolate, and some diet and cold medications are thought to promote the growth of fibrocystic lumps (Tetzlaf 1998).

• **Fibroadenomas.** Fibroadenomas, benign tumors that occur most frequently in women between the ages of 18 and 35, are characterized by solid lumps of fibrous and glandular tissue. They account for nearly all breast tumors found in women under age 25 (Tetzlaf 1998). They are usually nontender, except possibly before menstruation, and are mobile when palpated.

Cancer

Breast changes such as lumps, dimpling, or puckering of the skin and thickening or swelling in the breast that do not go away may be warning signs of breast cancer, warranting immediate referral to a physician for examination. Other signs and symptoms to be concerned about include skin irritation, distortion, retraction, and scaliness and changes or tenderness in, or secretion from, the nipple. Malignant tumors not detected and treated early will continue to grow and invade adjacent, healthy tissue. As with any cancer, if left unchecked the tumor can spread to the nearby lymph nodes and travel through the lymph system and bloodstream to other parts of the body (metastasis).

Breast cancer is second only to lung cancer as a cause of cancer deaths in women. Although the risk of breast cancer increases with age and may be higher in some women, every female is at risk for breast cancer. In fact, 75% of women diagnosed with breast cancer have none of the associated risk factors other than being female or a certain age (Tetzlaf 1998). While breast cancer cannot be prevented, it can be effectively treated and cured if recognized early. Educating your athletes and encouraging breast self-examination in women 20 years and older may ultimately save a life.

Risk Factors Associated With Breast Cancer

- Age, particularly over 50
- Personal or family history of breast cancer
- Previous biopsy confirming atypical hyperplasia
- Menstruation that began at an early age
- Late-onset menopause
- Recent use of oral contraceptives or postmenopausal estrogens
- Never experiencing pregnancy or having the first child at a late age
- Higher education and socioeconomic status
- Smoking

Data from American Cancer Society, 1999, *Facts and figures.*

Breast Self-Examination

A woman who thoroughly examines her breasts each month is likely to notice any changes that might signal the onset of cancer. The few minutes it takes to perform breast self-examination (BSE) may mean the difference between detecting a cancer when it is small and still confined to the breast and detecting a cancer that is relatively large and likely to have spread beyond the breast. The purpose of BSE is for women to become familiar with how their breasts look and feel so they can readily recognize changes and report them immediately to their health care provider. Changes to watch for include a lump or thickening, dimpling or puckering of the skin, or differences in size and shape. Refer women to a physician if they have any questions concerning the following BSE steps:

1. Lie on your back with a pillow under your right shoulder. Place your right hand behind your head. Using the pads of the middle three fingers of your left hand, examine all of your right breast tissue—including tissue that extends into your armpit, up to your clavicle, and down to the bottom of your rib cage—by firmly massaging small areas in one of three patterns. Select the pattern that is most comfortable to you and use it consistently.

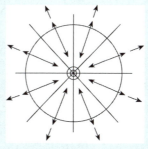

2. Examine your left breast, placing the pillow under your left shoulder, using the fingers of your right hand, and repeating the instructions for step one.

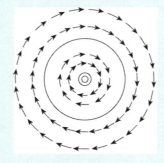

3. Repeat the examination of each breast, this time while standing with one arm behind your head. Many women find it helpful to do this part of the exam while they're in the shower because soapy hands move more easily over wet skin.

4. Stand in front of a mirror and note the texture and color of your skin as well as the shape and contour of the breast.

5. Gently squeeze the nipple of each breast and report any discharge to your health care provider at once.

6. Conduct BSE each month. If you are regularly menstruating, do it a few days after your period ends, when your breasts are less tender. Women who don't have regular periods should select a specific and consistent day of the month to perform a BSE.

SUMMARY

1. Describe and recognize the signs and symptoms of medical conditions of the endocrine system that may be encountered in the physically active.

   Pancreatic (diabetes) and thyroid dysfunction are the most common endocrine conditions you will encounter in the physically active. Diabetes mellitus is an autoimmune disorder that causes a deficiency in glucose metabolism. Signs and symptoms appear when the athlete either has too much (hypoglycemia) or too little (hyperglycemia) insulin in the body. You must be aware of the different signs and symptoms for these two conditions, since the treatments are opposite. Thyroid dysfunction results from overproduction (hyperthyroidism) or underproduction (hypothyroidism) of the thyroid hormones, which regulate the rate at which the body uses calories to expend energy. Although these dysfunctions do not prevent an athlete from participating, they may cause complications to arise during or apart from exercise. You must understand these conditions and recognize the signs of their complications in order to provide emergency assistance to the athlete when needed.

2. Describe and recognize the signs and symptoms of medical conditions of the digestive system that may be encountered in the physically active.

   Gastrointestinal complaints are among the most common medical conditions that you will encounter in physically active people. They can be caused by inflammation, viruses, bacteria, and diet. They are particularly troublesome and often restrict participation secondary to the pain and discomfort created by the accompanying symptoms. Common conditions whose associated signs and symptoms you should be aware of include appendicitis, colitis, constipation, diarrhea, esophageal reflux, gastritis, gastroenteritis, indigestion, ulcers, and irritable bowel syndrome.

3. Describe and recognize the signs and symptoms of disordered eating behaviors that may be encountered in the physically active.

Disordered eating behavior is common in the athletic population, with anorexia nervosa, bulimia, and obesity representing the more serious conditions. Anorexia is a severe psychological disorder characterized by a self-induced food aversion and extreme weight loss. Bulimia is typically characterized by an athlete of normal weight who uses techniques such as vomiting and ingestion of diuretics and laxatives to prevent weight gain. These conditions, which can be serious and life threatening, primarily affect athletes involved in activities in which body image is important and small size is advantageous, such as gymnasts, dancers, divers, jockeys, wrestlers, and crew coxswains. Obesity is less prevalent in the physically active population and is primarily restricted to heavyweight positions such as those in football and wrestling.

4. Describe and recognize the signs and symptoms of sexually transmitted diseases that may be encountered in the physically active.

Sexually transmitted diseases (HIV, AIDS, hepatitis, chlamydia, genital warts, gonorrhea, syphilis) are common and are very sensitive conditions both socially and medically. These conditions can raise considerable concern and stigma among teammates, and athletes are often reluctant to report their signs and symptoms. Because of the sensitive issues surrounding sexually transmitted diseases, you must be able to deal with the athlete with professionalism and confidence. Although these conditions may involve the danger of transmittal to others, confidentiality and education are of utmost importance.

5. Describe and recognize the signs and symptoms of genitourinary and gynecological conditions that may be encountered in the physically active.

The genitourinary tract and organs include the kidneys, bladder, urinary tract, and the external genitalia. Conditions include kidney stones, urethritis, urinary tract infections, spermatic cord torsion, epididymitis, hydrocele, varicocele, and testicular cancer. Gynecological conditions include menstrual dysfunction, pregnancy, pelvic inflammation, and breast abnormalities. In most cases, genitourinary and gynecological conditions cause sufficient pain and discomfort that the athlete will report them, but some may go undetected for some time. Screening exams and education are paramount to detection of menstrual disturbances and early detection of breast and testicular cancers.

6. Determine which medical conditions require emergency medical referral and which require physician referral for diagnosis and treatment.

Understanding the signs and symptoms and complicating factors associated with the conditions discussed in this chapter will help you recognize those that require medical follow-up or immediate referral. In particular, you must be able to differentiate those conditions that require immediate emergency care (e.g., hyperglycemia, hypoglycemia, appendicitis). Further, it is important for you to know the medical history of athletes with permanent and preexisting disease states so that you can watch for early signs of complications that may arise during sport activity.

REVIEW QUESTIONS

1. Describe the difference between a diabetic coma and insulin shock. What are the characteristic signs and symptoms of each?

2. Describe the difference between hyperthyroidism and hypothyroidism. What are the characteristic signs and symptoms of each?

3. Discuss the gastrointestinal disorders commonly seen in the physically active. What signs and symptoms would warrant physician referral?

4. Why is it difficult to examine an athlete with suspected anorexia nervosa? What signs and symptoms would cause you to suspect this condition?

5. What causes amenorrhea? What other conditions are commonly associated with amenorrhea, and what concerns might you have for an athlete with amenorrhea?

6. You learn that an athlete on the men's volleyball team has tested positive for HIV. What good judgment should govern your care for this athlete?

CRITICAL THINKING QUESTIONS

1. An athlete comes to you complaining of pain and burning with urination. What conditions might you suspect, and what questions might you ask the athlete to help determine the cause of these symptoms?

2. A thorough medical history obtained during the preparticipation physical examination at the beginning of the year can provide valuable information regarding previous medical conditions that may resurface or affect physical activity. If you were asked to design a health history questionnaire, what questions would you include after reading this chapter?

3. You learn that an athlete on your team has IDDM. What potential complications might you expect with this condition? How would you prepare for these complications, and what signs and symptoms would you look for?

4. An athlete complains of a rash in the groin area. You can tell that he is embarrassed and uncomfortable telling you this, but that he is concerned enough that he needs to talk to someone. How would you deal with this athlete, and how would your examination proceed to determine the need for medical referral?

5. You have noticed that one of your crew athletes has lost considerable weight over the past few months. You have also noted that during pregame meals she eats very little and frequently gets up to go to the bathroom before the meal is over. You also often see her running in the morning on your way into work. What conditions might you suspect, and what strategies would you use to approach this athlete with your concerns?

6. Chapter 21 discussed influenza and how some athletes with preexisting medical conditions may be at greater risk for developing serious, life-threatening complications. What conditions discussed in this chapter would you want to be aware of so you could monitor the athlete more closely should they develop influenza?

CITED REFERENCES

American Cancer Society. 2003. www.cancer.org. Accessed August 20, 2004.

American College of Obstetrics and Gynecology Committee on Obstetric Practice. 2002. Exercise during pregnancy and the postpartum period. ACOG Committee Opinion No. 267. *Obstet Gynecol* 99(1): 171-173.

Charlton, W.P.H., L.M. Coslett-Charlton, and M.G. Ciccotti. 2001. Correlation of estradiol in pregnancy and anterior cruciate ligament laxity. *Clin Orthop Rel Res* 1(387): 165-170.

Dumas, G.A., and J.G. Reid. 1997. Laxity of knee cruciate ligaments during pregnancy. *J Orthop Sports Phys Ther* 26(1): 2-6.

Nattiv, A., R. Agostini, B. Drinkwater, and K.K. Yeager. 1994. The female athlete triad: The interrelatedness of disordered eating, amenorrhea and osteoporosis. *Clin Sports Med* 13: 405-417.

Otis, C.L., D. Drinkwater, M. Johnson, A. Loucks, and J. Wilmore. 1997. American College of Sports Medicine Position Stand: The female athlete triad. *Med Sc Sports Exerc* 29(5): i-ix.

Sandborn, C.F., M. Horea, B.J. Siemers, and K.I. Dieringer. 2000. Disordered eating and the female athlete triad. *Clin Sports Med* 19: 199-213.

Taber, C.W. 1997. *Taber's cyclopedic medical dictionary*. 18th ed. Philadelphia: F.A. Davis.

Testicular Cancer. National Institute of Health Medline Plus Health Information. 2003. www.nlm.nih.gov/medlineplus/testicularcancer.html. Accessed August 20, 2004.

Testicular Cancer Resource Center. 2003. http://tcrc.acor.org/index.html. Accessed August 20, 2004.

Tetzlaf, J. 1998. *A guide to breast health care*. Chicago: Budlong Press.

Wang, T.W., and B.S. Apgar. 1998. Exercise during pregnancy. *American Family Physician April 15*. American Academy of Family Physicians. Available at www.aafp.org/afp/980415ap/wang.html. Accessed November 8, 2004.

ADDITIONAL RESOURCES

Caroline, N.L. 1995. *Emergency care in the streets*. 5th ed. Boston: Little, Brown.

Hillman, S.K. 2005. *Introduction to athletic training*. 2nd ed. Champaign, IL: Human Kinetics.

Mosby's medical, nursing, and allied health dictionary. 6th ed. 2002. St Louis: Mosby.

National Athletic Trainers' Association. 1999. *Athletic training educational competencies*. 3rd ed. Dallas: National Athletic Trainers' Association.

Putukian, M. 1998. The female athlete triad. *Clin Sports Med* 17: 675-696.

CHAPTER 23

Musculoskeletal, Nervous, and Integumentary Conditions

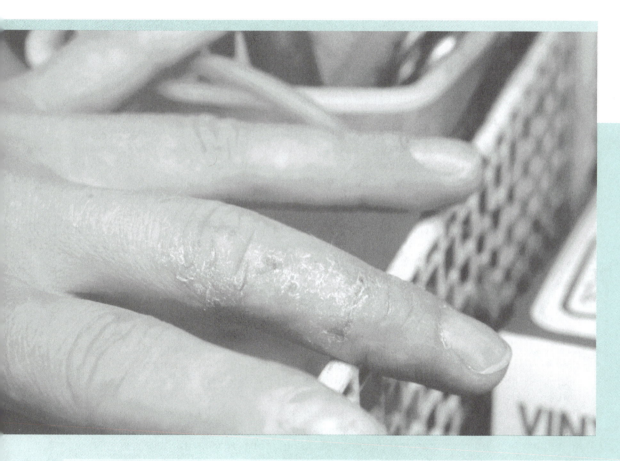

Objectives

After completing this chapter, the reader will be able to do the following:

1. Describe the signs and symptoms of skin conditions that may be encountered in the physically active

2. Describe the signs and symptoms of medical conditions affecting the musculoskeletal system that may be encountered in the physically active

3. Describe the signs and symptoms of medical conditions affecting the nervous system that may be encountered in the physically active

4. Describe the signs and symptoms of systemic diseases that may be encountered in the physically active

Doris was a 50-year-old tennis player who played at least four times a week at the local tennis club. In recent months, she began to notice increasing but intermittent pain, swelling, and stiffness in her right knee. The pain was beginning to limit her activity, so she decided to have Jason, the athletic trainer who worked at the club, look at her knee. Jason first took a history and learned that she had a history of reconstructive surgery on the right knee for a torn anterior cruciate ligament when she was 25. He also learned that she had recently increased the number of days she played tennis from 3 to 4 in an effort to lose some of the excess weight she had gained in the last year. When Jason examined her knee, he noted some mild swelling and decreased range of motion, but full strength. All special tests for ligament and meniscus injury were negative. Given her history and his examination findings, he suspected that she might be experiencing osteoarthritis and referred her to her physician for follow-up care.

This chapter addresses conditions of the integumentary (skin), musculoskeletal (muscles, bones, and joints), and nervous systems, as well as systemic diseases not previously covered. Skin conditions are common and primarily recognized by their appearance. Because of the many possible skin conditions, this chapter includes figures depicting each condition to aid your recognition. Your ability to differentiate contagious skin conditions from noncontagious conditions is particularly important when working with contact sports (e.g., wrestling) where infection can easily spread to other participants. Musculoskeletal conditions addressed in this chapter are not previously discussed in joint-specific chapters. With the exception of rhabdomyolysis, which represents an acute medical emergency, this discussion focuses on chronic inflammatory conditions of bone, joint, and muscle that are more prevalent in older adults. Systemic diseases and general medical conditions of the nervous system are rarer, but require early recognition to ensure effective and timely treatment.

THE SKIN

Skin reactions, rashes, and lesions can result from a variety of conditions and agents. Most skin conditions are not life threatening, although they can be a nuisance and linger if not treated soon after onset. Some can be treated with over-the-counter medications, but you should know your state's laws governing medication distribution and also obtain a confirmed diagnosis from a physician before administering any medication. Some dermatological conditions are contagious and others are not. You must know which are contagious so you can appropriately manage them to prevent their spreading. The best treatment for any dermatological condition is prevention. Encouraging athletes to shower, wash hands, and seek prompt medical treatment at the onset of any condition can keep most dermatological conditions to a minimum. For organizational purposes, skin conditions are classified in this chapter as infectious, inflammatory, environmental exposures, or other.

Skin Infections

Localized skin infections can result from bacterial, viral, fungal, or parasitic agents.

Bacterial Infections

Bacterial infections are typically of staphylococcal origin and are usually characterized by pustules; the hair follicle is often the site of infection.

Abscess

An abscess, which can occur in many different sites and can be either acute or chronic, is a localized infection that appears as a collection of pus (figure 23.1). Common signs and symptoms include local tissue destruction and edema. Acute abscesses usually present as a

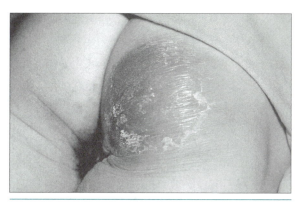

Figure 23.1 Skin abscess.
Courtesy of Kenneth E. Greer.

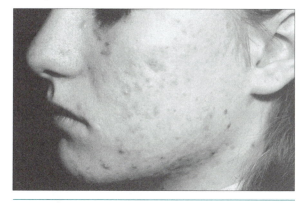

Figure 23.2 Acne vulgaris.
Courtesy of Kenneth E. Greer.

*To **debride** means to clear a wound of infectious or foreign substances in an effort to promote healing and restore healthy tissue.*

localized area of pain and increased warmth, demonstrating typical signs of inflammation. A chronic abscess is usually not as painful and is encapsulated by fibrous tissue.

Acne Vulgaris

Although acne vulgaris is commonly seen in adolescents, it can also occur as an adult-onset condition. It is the result of a heredity disorder of the hair follicles and oil glands that causes blackheads, cysts, and pustules (figure 23.2). Most cases exhibit acne lesions of varying depths on the face, neck, chest, shoulders, and back. Some people engaging in physical activity may experience a flare-up of this condition as a probable result of increased perspiration and oil production during activity. The dermatologist commonly has several options for treating acne vulgaris, including oral or topical antibacterial agents, topical antimicrobial agents, topical drying agents, and astringents to remove skin oils. Oral antibiotics are not used with preadolescents or pregnant women because of the pigmentation changes they can produce in the permanent teeth of preteens and fetuses.

Carbuncle

A carbuncle is a painful, localized staphylococcus-based infection that affects the skin and subcutaneous tissue. Commonly located on the back of the neck, carbuncles occur most frequently in men. Signs include fever, a pus-filled lesion, and local pain. At first, the skin is red and inflamed, with a hard, pus-filled core at the center (figure 23.3). Later, the skin becomes thin and disrupts, allowing pus to discharge through several openings. Refer carbuncles to a dermatologist, who can debride the area and prescribe antibiotics.

Cellulitis

Cellulitis is an inflammation of soft or connective tissue. It usually involves skin and subcutaneous tissue and has a tendency to spread. Any infecting organism can cause cellulitis, but the most frequent cause is streptococci or staphylococci bacteria that affect an area of reduced resistance following injury or other trauma. Cellulitis is characterized by a general redness of the skin, swelling, pain, and warmth that varies directly in proportion to the severity of the condition (figure 23.4). Cellulitis requires physician referral so that proper antibiotic therapy

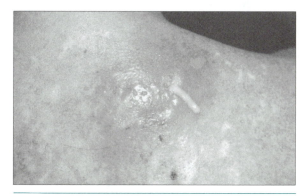

Figure 23.3 Carbuncle.
Courtesy of Kenneth E. Greer.

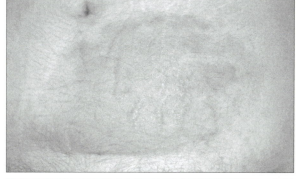

Figure 23.4 Cellulitis.
Courtesy of Kenneth E. Greer.

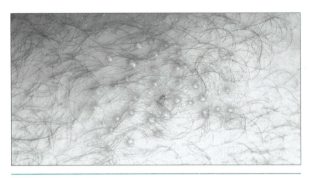

Figure 23.5 Folliculitis.
Courtesy of Kenneth E. Greer.

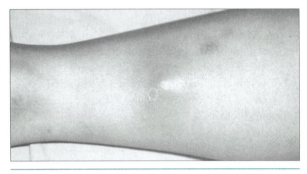

Figure 23.6 Furuncle (boil).
Courtesy of Kenneth E. Greer.

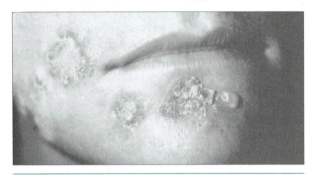

Figure 23.7 Impetigo.
Courtesy of Kenneth E. Greer.

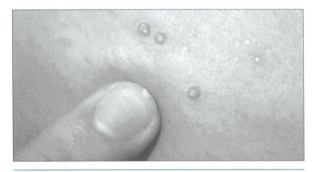

Figure 23.8 Molluscum contagiosum.
Courtesy of Kenneth E. Greer.

*A **papule** is a small raised bump on the skin that may or may not be painful.*

can be instituted. Additional treatment may include rest and heat or moist dressings as prescribed by the physician.

Folliculitis

Folliculitis, usually staphylococcal in origin, is an inflammation of the hair follicle. It frequently occurs in men with curly beards (pseudofolliculitis barbae) when the hair reenters the skin and causes a localized inflammation; however, it can occur in any hair follicle or body region. The inflammatory site becomes a pustule and displays signs of inflammation: redness, localized swelling, and tenderness (figure 23.5). The treatment is to dry the pustule with astringents or other agents used with acne vulgaris, or even oral antibiotics when the folliculitis is prominent. Scrubbing the face with an abrasive pad to prevent ingrown hair is a common method of prevention.

Furuncle and Furunculosis

The common name for a furuncle is a **boil**—a localized infection of a hair follicle (figure 23.6). The common source of infection is staphylococcus bacteria, and a boil is most often found on the neck, axillae, face, buttocks, and breasts. The local area is red, edematous, and tender. Since staphylococcal infections are highly contagious, the athlete must refrain from sport participation until the infection has healed. Should the boil rupture, the infection can spread to surrounding tissues. Treatment includes moist hot packs and 10% topical benzoyl peroxide; the physician may order oral antibiotics. Prevention includes use of soap and good hygiene in regular showering.

Impetigo

Impetigo, a contagious bacterial infection caused by either staphylococci or streptococci, is highly contagious in young children. It begins as pustules that go on to rupture and crust over (figure 23.7). These most commonly occur on the face and head but can spread to other areas. Treatment includes referral to a physician for antibiotic medication. Also advise use of soap and water for proper cleansing followed by astringents or alcohol solutions to dry the lesions.

Viral Infections

Some skin infections are viral; these include molluscum contagiosum, herpes simplex and zoster, and verruca plantaris and vulgaris.

Molluscum Contagiosum

Molluscum contagiosum, a viral contagious infection of the skin, is characterized by small, round, flesh-colored papular lesions that occur most commonly on the face, trunk, axilla, perineum, and thigh (figure 23.8). You may see many or only a few papules. Athletes in contact sports frequently transmit this disease. Physician referral is necessary for treatment with prescribed medications.

A macule is a nonraised patch of skin with altered color.

Malaise is a vague, general feeling of illness and fatigue.

Herpes Simplex

Herpes simplex infections are contagious viral infections caused by herpes virus I and II. They are characterized by an eruption of groups of vesicles (figure 23.9) and have a tendency to reactivate and reappear with stress or fever. Herpes virus I that occurs on the lips or around the nose is also called a fever blister or cold sore. Herpes virus II occurs on the genitalia. Acyclovir, an antiviral drug for herpes viruses, is available topically, orally, and by intravenous administration. Topical agents to dry the vesicles can also encourage the healing process, though prevention is the most effective means of control. Good hand-washing practices and the use of gloves when applying medication to the sore helps reduce the spread. Direct contact with the sore should be avoided.

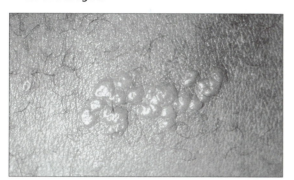

Figure 23.9   Herpes simplex I.
Courtesy of Kenneth E. Greer.

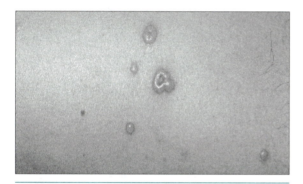

Figure 23.10   Herpes zoster (chicken pox).
Courtesy of Kenneth E. Greer.

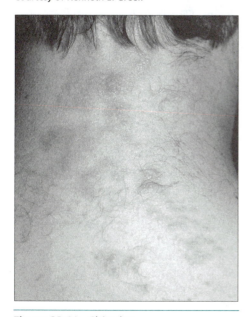

Figure 23.11   Shingles.
Courtesy of Kenneth E. Greer.

Herpes Zoster

Herpes zoster is associated with two diseases; one occurs in childhood and the other in adulthood. The childhood version is known as chicken pox (**varicella**) and the adulthood version as shingles (zoster).

- **Chicken pox** is characterized by skin lesions that begin as macules and progress to fluid-filled vesicles before they become crusty and scabbed (figure 23.10). The vesicles occur most often on the trunk, but in severe cases can spread to the face and extremities. The incubation period lasts 2 to 3 weeks. Fever and malaise can precede the appearance of macules. The older the patient, the more intense the fever and malaise symptoms. Treatment is symptomatic, aimed at reducing fever and relieving itching. The patient should avoid scratching the eruptions to prevent infection and later scarring. Encourage hand washing and bathing to minimize the risk of spreading the disease and causing an infection. The varicella vaccine that protects against severe chicken pox has been available since March 1995. Routine vaccination of children at 12 to 18 months of age is recommended. Many states require vaccination before entry into the public school system. Immunity to further episodes of chicken pox occurs with one contraction of the disease.

- **Shingles** is a viral infection that affects the posterior nerve roots and dorsal ganglion in patients usually over the age of 50. It is characterized by pain and vesicles that erupt along the inflamed nerve's cutaneous distribution on one side of the body (figure 23.11). In rare instances, vesicle eruption can be preceded for 3 to 4 days by flulike symptoms of fever, malaise, chills, and headache. The vesicles become dry and scabbed after several days and then no longer contain the virus. Pain along the nerve's pathway as a result of nerve damage from the virus—**postherpetic neuralgia**—is the most common complication; this can be severe and prolonged, lasting in some cases for months or years. Most commonly, the areas affected are the regions of trigeminal nerve and thoracic ganglia distribution. A primary complication of shingles is bacterial infections that can add to superficial tissue destruction and scarring.

Physician referral is recommended; however, there is no known treatment for herpes zoster. Acyclovir can reduce healing time, new vesicle formation, and pain duration. Symptomatic relief can occur with

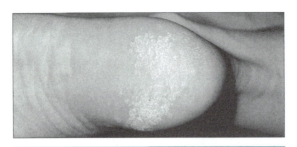

Figure 23.12 Verruca plantaris (plantar wart).
Courtesy of Kenneth E. Greer.

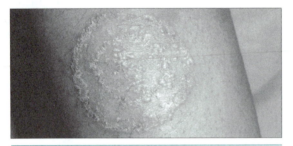

Figure 23.13 Verruca vulgaris (common wart).
Courtesy of Kenneth E. Greer.

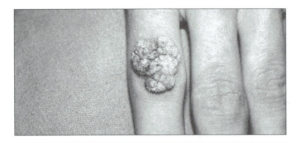

Figure 23.14 Tinea corporis (ringworm).
Courtesy of Kenneth E. Greer.

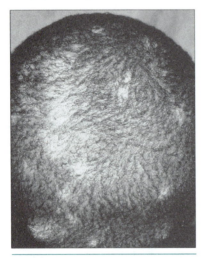

Figure 23.15 Tinea capitus (ringworm of the scalp).
Courtesy of Kenneth E. Greer.

Plaques are scaly patches.

application of topical lotions or powders. Analgesics can relieve pain.

Verruca Plantaris

Verruca plantaris is commonly referred to as a plantar wart (figure 23.12). Caused by a virus, it results in hypertrophy and thickening of the epidermis layers. It occurs on the bottom of the foot and is flattened because of the pressure of bearing weight. The thickening can cause pressure and discomfort. These warts can occur as individual lesions or can cluster in groups called **mosaic warts**. Most over-the-counter medications do not resolve plantar warts. In-season treatment includes symptomatic relief with protective or relief pads. In the off-season, referral to a physician for plantar wart removal is most effective, although there is no assurance that plantar warts will not return.

Verruca Vulgaris

Verruca vulgaris is a common wart caused by a papilloma virus (figure 23.13). These warts occur in areas of frequent trauma or infection such as the hands, elbows, knees, face, and scalp. Distinctive in appearance, they show sharp demarcation and some elevation, have either an irregular or a round border, are firm, and vary in color from light gray to near black. These warts sometimes spontaneously regress, but they can also be excised by a physician.

Fungal Infections

Fungal conditions are generally referred to as tinea or ringworm infections. Specific names reflect their location.

Ringworm

Although ringworm is one of many fungal diseases of the skin (tinea infection), the term is commonly used for a fungus that affects the scalp, trunk, and upper extremities. It is also known as **tinea corporis**. The lesion is a well-defined ringed eruption that has red or brown plaques with a raised border and may itch or burn (figure 23.14). The lesion can be dry and scaly, moist, or crusted. It spreads by direct contact with the person or animal who has the fungus or through indirect contact with items such as combs, clothing, and towels.

Topical antifungal medications, either over-the-counter or prescription, are the most common treatment. Good hand-washing technique helps reduce fungus transmission; also discourage sharing items such as combs, towels, and clothing.

Tinea Capitis

This highly contagious ringworm infection, typically seen in children, affects the scalp (figure 23.15). The lesions are scaly, grayish patches in which the hair becomes dull, broken, and thin. The affected area can include either small ringed patches or much of the scalp. You must refer to a physician for necessary topical medication, since tinea capitis does not spontaneously resolve.

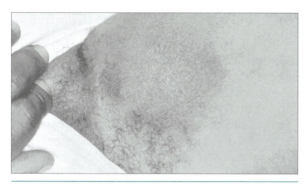

Figure 23.16 Tinea cruris (jock itch).
Courtesy of Kenneth E. Greer.

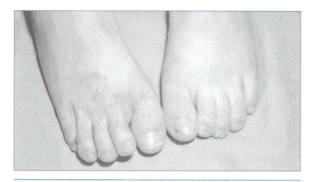

Figure 23.17 Tinea pedis (athlete's foot).
Courtesy of Kenneth E. Greer.

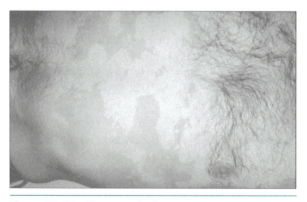

Figure 23.18 Tinea versicolor.
Courtesy of Kenneth E. Greer.

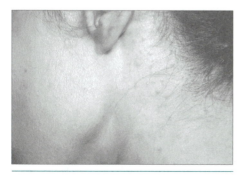

Figure 23.19 Pediculosis capitis.
Courtesy of Kenneth E. Greer.

Tinea Cruris

Tinea cruris (jock itch) is fungal infection that affects the groin (figure 23.16). It has the characteristic ringworm appearance and can cause itching, redness, scaling, and cracking. Prevention, which is the best method of treatment, includes using good showering and drying techniques, wearing clean cotton clothing, and avoiding clothes made of synthetic materials such as nylon. Antifungal medications for treating tinea cruris are available in over-the-counter and prescription doses. Not sharing towels and clothing are also good prevention habits that limit spread of the fungus.

Tinea Pedis

Tinea pedis (athlete's foot) is fungal infection that affects the feet (figure 23.17). The skin can appear red, scaly, and cracking and is often itchy. Prevention and treatment for tinea pedis is the same as for other ringworm infections. Cleansing and drying the feet properly, wearing clean socks, and avoiding walking barefoot are appropriate prevention steps.

Tinea Versicolor

Tinea versicolor is a noncontagious ringworm infection that affects the horny layers of the skin and hair follicles (figure 23.18). A yeast fungal infection, it appears first as a salmon-colored, then as a scaly, patch of skin that does not pigment. Usually found on the trunk, it appears as either a white or a brown patch of skin.

Parasitic Infestations

Parasitic infestations of lice and itch mites can infect and irritate the skin. These infections are typically found in the hair of the scalp and pubic regions.

Pediculosis

Pediculosis is an infection of the skin caused by lice (figure 23.19). The affected body region is indicated by the name: pediculosis capitis is caused by the head louse, pediculosis corporis by the body louse, and pediculosis pubis by the crab louse. Lice of this third type infest hairs of the genital region; infestation is commonly referred to as crabs. The most prevalent symptom is severe itching. Louse eggs, called nits, can be seen attached to the hair shaft close to the root as well as on clothing. Secondary bacterial infections from scratching can occur. Pediculosis is transmitted through direct contact with infected patients. Treatment includes physician referral for medication to eradicate the parasite. Thorough laundering of clothing and bed linens is also necessary.

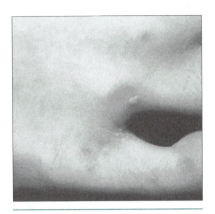

Figure 23.20 Scabies.
Courtesy of Kenneth E. Greer.

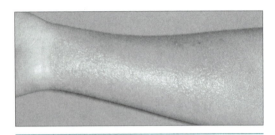

Figure 23.21 Contact dermatitis.
Courtesy of Kenneth E. Greer.

Erythema is redness of the skin.

Vesiculations are small ruptures or blistering of the skin.

Scabies

Scabies is caused by the itch mite. The impregnated female mite burrows into the skin and deposits her eggs in the tunnel. The larvae hatch and accumulate around hair follicles. The typical signs and symptoms include the appearance of elevated burrows on the skin and itching. The most common sites are the interdigital spaces of the hands and the axilla, trunk, and genital regions (figure 23.20).

Treatment includes prescribed medicated shampoo with gamma benzine hexachloride for the whole body, with repeated applications as necessary; clothing and bed linen laundering; and prophylactic treatment of team members and others in contact with the patient.

Inflammatory Conditions

General inflammatory conditions of the skin include dermatitis, eczema, and psoriasis.

Dermatitis

Dermatitis is simply defined as an inflammation of the skin. Contact dermatitis, the most common dermatitis condition, is a delayed reaction to direct contact with an allergen (figure 23.21). It is characterized by erythema, edema, itching, and vesiculations of varying degrees. The first step in treatment is to remove the offending substance. Physician referral for medications such as adrenocortical steroid ointments is recommended.

Eczema

Eczema is the generic term used to describe chronic dermatitis. It is characterized by scaling, erythematous, edematous, papular, vesicular, crusty skin and is often accompanied by itching and burning (figure 23.22). As with other forms of dermatitis, removing the irritant is key to treatment. Treatment of the lesions depends upon their stage. Moist lesions are treated with drying agents, while crusting and scaling lesions are treated with petrolatum or hydrophilic ointments.

Psoriasis

Psoriasis is a usually chronic condition of unknown etiology that exhibits characteristic eruptions on the extensor surfaces of the extremities, especially the elbows, knees, back, and scalp (figure 23.23). The eruptions are circumscribed, erythematous papules covered with silvery

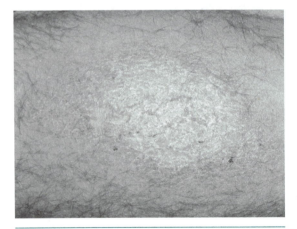

Figure 23.22 Eczema.
Courtesy of Kenneth E. Greer.

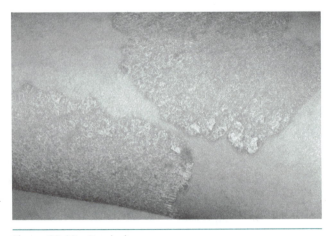

Figure 23.23 Psoriasis.
Courtesy of Kenneth E. Greer.

*A **wheal** is a reaction of the skin surface characterized by an elevated patch of skin that appears smooth and red.*

***Serum** is a watery fluid.*

***Eosinophils** are leukocytes or other granulocytes that are released secondary to an allergen or a parasitic infection.*

***Histamine** and **kinins** are chemical substances found in the body that, when released, dilate and increase permeability of blood vessels.*

scales. The frequency and duration of their recurrences and remissions vary. Refer the patient to a physician for medical care. Psoriasis is difficult to treat because it can vary considerably in type, severity, and response to treatment. Hence it requires a more individualized approach to treatment, which may include creams and ointments, oral medications, and light therapy.

Environmental Exposures

Skin lesions can be also caused by environmental conditions such as allergens and by overexposure to heat and cold. The common terms for these conditions are hives, frostbite, and sunburn.

Hives

Hives, or **urticaria,** is a dermal hypersensitivity reaction to an allergen. Common allergens include any substance that causes an abnormal reaction upon exposure, such as insect bites, foods, dust, mold, or certain medications. A wheal formation that occurs on the skin can range from small red dots to large, raised, reddened areas (figure 23.24). Wheal formation caused by exuded serum, eosinophils, and other white blood cells and local distension of blood and lymph vessels accompanies edema and erythema that result from the release of histamine and kinins.

Most people who have hypersensitivity reactions are aware of them and know the steps to take after exposure. When unprecedented reactions occur, refer the patient to the physician. Hives subside within 1 day to 2 weeks, depending on the reaction severity. Antihistamine medications and antipruritic topical agents can symptomatically relieve itching. Of course, removing the patient from the allergen is strongly recommended.

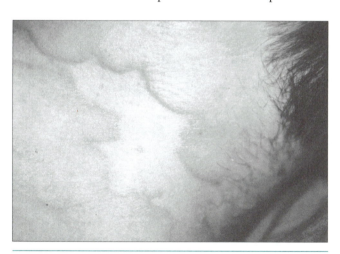

Figure 23.24   Hives in a wheal formation.
Courtesy of Kenneth E. Greer.

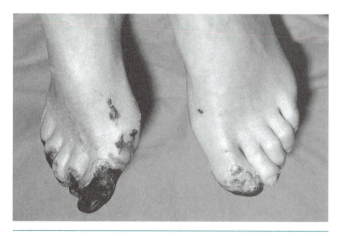

Figure 23.25   Severe frostbite.
Courtesy of Kenneth E. Greer.

Frostbite

Frostbite is a potentially serious condition of local tissue destruction consequent to exposure to cold that freezes the superficial and possibly deeper tissue layers. It can range from mild to severe. Mild cases display erythema, itching, numbness, and mild pain. If exposure to cold continues, the skin can become pale, waxy, and firm to the touch. There may be some swelling with pain, numbness, or burning that can continue for several weeks. Severe cases are characterized initially by paresthesia and painless blisters and ultimately lead to tissue destruction and gangrene (figure 23.25).

Initial treatment includes warming the tissue in warm water below 105° F (41° C). Rubbing the skin should be avoided. Immediately refer patients with signs of frostbite to a physician.

Sunburn

Sunburn, a common skin condition caused by overexposure to the sun's ultraviolet rays, is characterized by redness, pain or burning, itching, and increased skin heat. Blisters may also be present with more severe sunburns, causing the damaged skin layer to peel off a few days later. When the sunburn is severe and occurs over a large portion of the body, there may also be fever and general malaise.

Sunburn can and should be prevented with the habitual use of sunscreen, as repetitive skin damage can lead to skin cancer. Athletes with fair skin are particularly susceptible, but this is not to say that others are immune. All athletes engaged in outdoor activities, regardless of season, should protect their skin by limiting exposure when possible and by using sunscreen that blocks UVA as well as UVB rays and has a sun protection factor (SPF) of at least 15.

Other Lesions

Other lesions involving the dermis can result in tissue or fluid buildup due to mechanical friction or glandular occlusion. These conditions include blisters, calluses, and sebaceous cysts.

Blisters

A blister is a separation of the skin's dermal and epidermal layers caused by a heat buildup from friction. Fluid, either serous or blood, fills the area (figure 23.26). The preferred treatment is to protect the area with a sterile bandage. If the blister breaks, cleanse the area using sterile technique; apply an antiseptic ointment and secure with a sterile dressing. Refer large or infected blisters to a physician for lancing and debridement. Prevention is the best treatment. Athletes should wear properly fitted shoes with adequate sock protection, should break in shoes before wearing them for athletic participation, and should keep calluses well trimmed.

Calluses

Calluses are the result of excessive friction. Skin builds up in an area of high friction as a means of self-protection (figure 23.27). Calluses typically form in the feet and hands over areas of high friction, stress, and bony prominences. As the callus forms, the skin becomes thicker and less flexible and elastic, moving as an abnormally large unit and becoming more susceptible to tears. Calluses should be kept trimmed and manageable, though not completely removed so as to leave sufficient protection of more sensitive skin layers. Prevention includes wearing two pairs of socks, including a thin cotton sock next to the skin, on the feet or gloves on the hands. Use of lanolin or oils to keep the skin moist and soft can also help. If the callus should tear, treat it as any other open wound. Protection from infection is crucial. Cleanse the wound, protect it with an antiseptic or antibiotic ointment, and cover it with a sterile dressing.

Sebaceous Cysts

A sebaceous cyst is a benign cystic skin tumor that develops because of occlusion of a sebaceous gland in the dermis. It is a firm, round, movable, and nontender mass that most commonly develops on the scalp, face, back, or scrotum (figure 23.28). An infected cyst causes

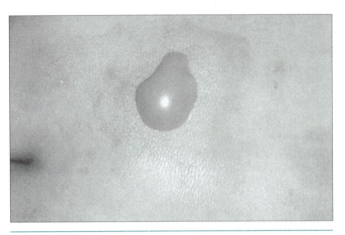

Figure 23.26   Blister.
Courtesy of Kenneth E. Greer.

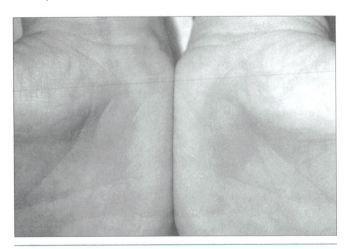

Figure 23.27   Callus.
Courtesy of Kenneth E. Greer.

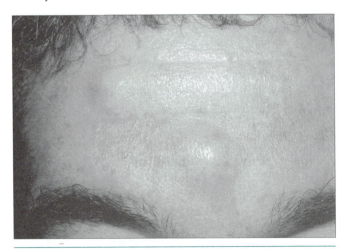

Figure 23.28   Sebaceous cyst.
Courtesy of Kenneth E. Greer.

discomfort. Treatment includes physician referral for excision of the cyst sac. If the cyst is small, the physician may puncture the cyst to drain it rather than excise it.

MUSCULOSKELETAL CONDITIONS

Muscle, bone, and joint disorders can be very disabling to the physically active. As athletic trainers increasingly care for physically active adults and mature adults, they more frequently encounter general complaints of muscle and joint pain. While joint-specific pathologies were discussed previously (see chapters 11-20), the following sections deal with more generalized muscle, bone, and joint disorders.

Bone and Joint

Chronic bone and joint conditions primarily involve arthritic conditions.

Arthritis

Arthritis is a disease characterized by pain and inflammation of one or more joints that is caused by a variety of disease processes affecting the joints, including mechanical injury, infection, autoimmune disease, and chronic, repetitive stress. Arthritis occurs when these conditions result in long-term pain, inflammation, and joint deformity. Other signs and symptoms include early morning stiffness, increased warmth around the affected joint, and reduced joint mobility. A discussion of the varieties of arthritis and their many contributing factors is beyond the scope of this chapter. Consult excellent resources such as the American College of Rheumatology (www.rheumatology.org) and U.S. National Library of Medicine (www.nlm.nih.gov/medlineplus) for more information.

Arthritis can occur in both males and females of all ages, affecting approximately 37 million people in America, or 1 out of 7. While arthritis causes athletes to limit their physical activity, inactivity can actually increase arthritis problems. According to the American College of Rheumatology (2003), research shows that arthritis patients can safely participate in appropriate, regular exercise programs; these athletes may particularly tolerate low-impact exercise, walking, swimming, and water aerobics. Exercise in the water increases buoyancy and decreases the effects of gravity, putting less weight on the joints and enabling arthritis patients to tolerate more activity. Gentle stretching, light muscular conditioning, and aerobic conditioning at moderate levels are also recommended. Athletes suffering from arthritic symptoms should consult their physician before beginning or continuing their exercise program.

Osteoarthritis

Osteoarthritis is the most common form of arthritis in the United States, most often affecting athletes over age 65 (American College of Rheumatology 2003). About 1 in 7 women over age 65 experience symptoms of knee osteoarthritis. Osteoarthritis is characterized by degeneration of the cartilagenous surface of the joint, which results in joint pain, stiffness, swelling, and decreased range of motion. Osteoarthritis can result from genetic predisposition, injury that disrupts cartilaginous surface or joint mechanics, overuse, and obesity. The joints most often affected include those in the cervical and lumbar regions, fingers, hips, knees, and great toes. Symptoms vary by location and severity. Treatment includes activity modification, anti-inflammatory medications, weight loss, and with severe degeneration, joint replacement.

Gout

Increased levels of uric acid in the blood (**uricemia**) can lead to gout, an acute arthritis marked by joint inflammation due to the disposition of urate crystals in the joints. Gout can affect any joint but is most common in the great toe, foot, and knee. Pain and swelling of the joint accompanied by chills and fever are the hallmarks of gout. You may also note hypertension and back pain. Symptoms are recurrent and more prolonged with subsequent episodes. Treatment for gout attacks typically includes nonsteroidal anti-inflammatory drugs (NSAIDs) and may include corticosteroid drugs for severe attacks. Medications that maintain uric acid levels within a normal range may prevent future attacks.

Muscular Disorders

Muscular disorders include both chronic conditions secondary to prolonged myofascial symptoms and acute trauma due to severe muscle damage.

Fibromyalgia

According to the American College of Rheumatology (2003), fibromyalgia (fibrositis) is a chronic myofascial disorder that affects approximately 2% of the United States population and is characterized by chronic musculoskeletal pain, fatigue, and localized tenderness. It occurs most often in women of childbearing age, but can affect women and men of all ages. Pain is most often experienced around the neck, shoulders, upper back, elbows, and lower back. The cause of fibromyalgia is unknown. While some patients affected by fibromyalgia have no underlying disorders, others may have conditions such as rheumatoid arthritis, irritable bowel syndrome, tension headaches, and numbness or tingling in the extremities. This disorder is often associated with sleep disturbance, psychological stress and inactivity, and altered pain sensitivity.

Fibromyalgia is diagnosed based on prolonged symptoms for 3 months or more and areas of muscle tenderness. Blood tests and X rays are used to rule out other conditions. There is no known cure for fibromyalgia at this time. Treatment usually includes medication to reduce stress and aid sleep, along with behavior modification and gentle exercise. Too much activity can exacerbate the condition.

Rhabdomyolysis

Rhabdomyolysis is an acute, sometimes fatal disease caused by severe destruction of skeletal muscle that results in injury to the kidney. Any time skeletal muscle is damaged, myoglobin is released into the bloodstream, which is ultimately filtered by the kidneys. When severe skeletal damage releases extremely large amounts of myoglobin, kidney failure may occur when the myoglobin occludes the kidney structures or breaks down, releasing metabolic by-products that can be toxic to the kidneys. Severe skeletal muscle damage may also cause fluid to shift from the bloodstream into the muscle, leading to hypovolemic shock and reduced blood flow to the kidneys.

Any disorder that damages the skeletal muscle can place a patient at risk for rhabdomyolysis, but it is more commonly associated with severe prolonged exertion, any trauma to the muscle that results in ischemia or necrosis, heatstroke, drug overdose, alcohol intoxication with accompanying tremors, and seizures and low phosphate levels (National Institutes of Health 2003). Signs and symptoms include abnormal urine color (dark, red, or cola), tenderness and weakness in the affected muscles, muscle stiffness and ache, and generalized weakness.

Rhabdomyolysis represents a medical emergency, as kidney failure can result if it is left untreated. Treatment includes early and aggressive hydration to dilute and eliminate the myoglobin from the kidneys. This may require intravenous administration of fluid until the condition stabilizes.

NEUROLOGICAL DISORDERS

Neurological disorders represent a wide range of conditions of varying etiologies that ultimately affect some aspect of the nervous system; some are acute and others are chronic. Each can result in significant complications if not recognized and properly treated.

Tetanus

Tetanus is commonly called lockjaw. Caused by the tetanus bacillus, it enters the body through an open wound that has been in contact with dirt or soil. The bacillus attaches to the local nerve, moves to the spinal cord, and becomes anchored to the motor nerves. It prevents normal synaptic inhibition so a tetanic contraction of the muscles occurs. Most commonly, it produces stiffness of the jaw and neck, with stiffness of the extremities occurring less often. Headaches, fever, and convulsions can be early symptoms. As the disease progresses, facial, back, neck, and abdominal muscles become rigid. Additional complicating factors include sphincter rigidity, dysphagia, convulsions, cyanosis, or asphyxia, and ultimately death can result. Any suspicion of tetanus infection in an athlete warrants immediate physician referral.

The best treatment is prevention with an updated tetanus toxoid immunization. Current tetanus toxoid boosters are effective for 5 to 10 years. Immediately care for wounds using proper cleansing and sterile technique. If you are uncertain of the patient's immunization status, refer the athlete to a physician so she can receive a tetanus toxoid booster as soon as possible following injury with an open wound.

Epilepsy

Epilepsy is a chronic condition characterized by recurring seizures. Seizures are a spontaneous and involuntary neurological aberration caused by unregulated and abnormal electrical brain activity; they can last from a few seconds to a few minutes. The many causes of epilepsy include head trauma, infectious diseases, metabolic disorders, tumors, congenital abnormalities, and drugs. Epilepsy can also be idiopathic in nature, without an identifiable cause, usually appearing in individuals from 5 to 20 years of age.

Possible Etiologies of Adult Seizures

The cause of seizures in adults cannot always be determined, but you should consider the following possibilities:

1. Insufficient oxygen in blood
2. Intracranial pathology
   - Head injury or space-occupying lesion (e.g., brain tumor, subdural hemorrhage)
   - Stroke
3. High fever
4. Meningitis
5. Metabolic or chemical problems
   - Low blood sugar (hypoglycemia)
   - Exposure to toxins or drug overdose
   - Withdrawal from alcohol or drugs

Although seizures are a sign of epilepsy, you should not assume that all seizures are epileptic. They can occur as single events resulting from traumatic incidents and other disorders such as extremely high fever, heatstroke, central nervous system trauma, and hyperventilation. Trauma can cause seizures at any age and may not become evident for up to 2 years following the injury. Infectious diseases such as bacterial meningitis or herpes encephalitis can also produce seizures. Other sources are premature birth or complications at the time of delivery, metabolic disorders including hypoglycemia or diabetes, drug or alcohol withdrawal, and brain tumors.

Seizures are classified as partial or focal and generalized. Focal or partial seizures affect only certain parts of the brain and usually involve only one part of the body, such as the face or arm, in a tonic–clonic activity. There is usually no loss of consciousness; other symptoms can include seeing flashes of light, pupil dilation, sweating, or tingling or jerking that can begin in one part of the body and advance to other segments. Focal seizures can progress rapidly to generalized convulsions.

Tonic refers to a sustained contraction of a muscle or muscle group.

Clonic refers to a rapid contraction and relaxation of a muscle or muscle group.

Generalized seizures are of various types, but the most common are the petit mal and grand mal seizures. Although most patients have no warning, some experience an aura or feeling that precedes an episode seconds or minutes before its onset. Precipitating factors for seizures can include stress, missed meals and medications, lack of sleep, alcohol, and fever. Petit mal seizures are brief episodes of consciousness impairment that occur in childhood and are usually outgrown by the age of 20. The patient may appear to be daydreaming or staring off into space and unaware that the episode has occurred once it is over. A grand mal seizure, also called a tonic–clonic seizure, occurs with a sudden loss of consciousness in which the person falls to the ground as the body's muscles enter a state of total tonic contractions. After about 1 minute, the body goes into the clonic phase, during which the body jerks for 2 to 3 minutes. Breathing can become shallow during the tonic phase; during the clonic phase the patient may bite the tongue or lips or experience fecal or urinary incontinence. After the seizure, the patient is very lethargic and may drift into sleep or experience additional seizures. There is usually no memory of the seizure, and the patient may have postseizure symptoms of headache, drowsiness, nausea, muscle soreness, or disorientation, sometimes lasting several days.

First aid for epileptic seizures consists of protecting the patient from nearby hazards, loosening the clothing around the neck, removing eyeglasses, and protecting the head from injury. If you know the patient has epilepsy or has a medical identification, you should turn her onto a side to allow saliva to drain and ask her if she wants to go to the hospital. If there is no history of seizure, or if she is pregnant, has diabetes, or has been injured, obtain emergency transportation to an emergency care facility.

During a seizure, there are specific actions that should be avoided. Never restrain the patient; do not place objects in his mouth, since they may obstruct breathing; and do not move him unless there is a risk of injury. Do not offer liquids until he has completely awakened.

Patients with epilepsy should carry identification indicating their condition. If the patient is an athlete, you as the athletic trainer should be informed of the situation. High risk sports such as football, skiing, and scuba diving are usually not recommended. Seizures can often be controlled with a combination of adequate rest, balanced diet, stimulant avoidance, stress minimization, and medication.

Treatment usually includes anticonvulsive medication to prevent seizures. Many drugs are available, so the specific drugs depend upon the type of seizure, the side effects of the drug, and the patient's health and age. Patients commonly try a number of drugs or combinations of drugs before finding the correct medication and dosage to bring the seizures under control. Some of the medications often used are Tegretol, Dilantin, phenobarbital, and Rivotril.

Reflex Sympathetic Dystrophy

Reflex sympathetic dystrophy (RSD) is a multisystem, multisymptom disorder. Its effect on the sympathetic nervous system results in a multitude of symptoms and problems. It usually follows an injury and most frequently affects the hand in upper-extremity injuries or the foot in lower-extremity injuries. The etiology is unknown. The primary symptom of RSD is severe, constant pain, usually a burning sensation that occurs in the involved extremity, especially distally. It is accompanied by pitting or nonpitting edema, bluish skin, coolness of the distal extremity, and reduced motor function. The color and temperature changes are thought to occur because of increased sympathetic stimulation. This abnormal sympathetic stimulation causes vasospasm of the arterioles, tissue swelling secondary to capillary release of fibrin and plasma, stiffness secondary to tissue ischemia, and eventual soft tissue fibrosis. Reflex sympathetic dystrophy can go through three stages of progression:

* **Stage I** lasts an average of 3 months and is characterized by the onset of severe, burning pain at the site of injury, accompanied by hyperesthesia, local edema, muscle spasm, limited mobility, and vasospasms that cause the skin to appear red, warm, and dry and then change to cyanotic, cold, and sweaty. In mild cases this stage may last only a few weeks and then spontaneously resolve.

Brawny edema is long-term leathery swelling of tissue.

* **Stage II,** lasting 3 to 6 months, is marked by a more severe but diffuse pain than seen in stage I. Swelling spreads and changes to a brawny edema. Spotty osteoporosis can become

Trophic refers to disordered or altered nutrition.

Ankylosed refers to joint fusion or fixation.

Dystrophy is a muscular disorder characterized by weakness and fibrosis.

Sympathectomy means removal of sympathetic nerves.

evident on X rays. Hair becomes scant and nails become brittle and grooved. Atrophy is apparent at this stage.

• **Stage III** is apparent through noticeable and irreversible trophic changes. At this stage, severe, debilitating pain may affect the entire limb and irreversible skin damage occurs. Atrophy also continues; interphalangeal joints become stiff and eventually ankylosed, and flexor tendons contract. X rays reveal more diffuse and marked osteoporosis.

If the condition continues untreated, dystrophy and then atrophy occur with less chance of recovery. The key to treatment is early recognition and intervention while the condition is still reversible. Drugs that may relieve RSD symptoms include anti-inflammatory agents, beta blockers, analgesics, tricyclics, tranquilizers, and calcium channel blockers. Nerve blocks performed as either intravenous regional blocks or sympathetic blocks are sometimes used to reduce sympathetic nerve stimulation to the area. Pain and edema control with desensitization activities and stiffness prevention are early treatments. Modalities for pain and edema control and active exercises to facilitate edema reduction and functional return are encouraged as tolerated. Extreme cases may indicate sympathectomy or the implantation of stimulators or an infusion pump.

Meningitis

Meningitis is an infection of the cerebral spinal fluid that can be either bacterial or viral. It is sometimes referred to as spinal meningitis. Bacterial meningitis is usually more severe and can result in brain damage, hearing loss, or death. Viral meningitis is rarely as serious, with recovery occurring in about 7 to 10 days. Establishing whether the cause of meningitis is bacterial or viral is crucial to effective treatment.

Symptoms are similar for all meningitis and occur over several hours to a couple of days. They include headache, stiff neck, and high fever. Nausea, vomiting, confusion, photophobia, and drowsiness can also occur. Seizures can occur secondary to meningitis.

Viral meningitis is contagious, as are some forms of bacterial meningitis. Direct contact with respiratory and throat secretions such as saliva, sputum, or nasal mucus spread this disease. Coughing, sneezing, and kissing are common means of transmitting bacterial meningitis.

Prevention is the best method to treat meningitis. Avoid contact with patients who have meningitis, and if contact occurs, use thorough hand-washing techniques. There is no vaccine against viral meningitis, but there is a vaccine against some of the bacterial meningitis strains. Treatment for bacterial meningitis includes immediate referral to a physician for appropriate antibiotics for the specific bacterial strain, prevention of dehydration, maintenance of good nutrition, and rest. There is no effective medication for viral meningitis, which usually resolves on its own, but steps to relieve symptoms, prevent dehydration, and assure proper nutrition and rest should be followed.

SYSTEMIC DISEASES

Other systemic diseases not previously covered in relation to viral, cardiovascular, musculoskeletal, joint, or neurological conditions include those that affect the blood and lymph. The following sections cover bacteremia, lymphangitis, lymphadenitis, iron-deficiency anemia, sickle cell anemia, and Lyme disease.

Bacteremia

Bacteremia (also known as bacterial sepsis or septicemia) is characterized by the presence of bacteria in the blood. It occurs when an infection overwhelms the local defenses at the original infection site (e.g., skin, respiratory, genitourinary, gastrointestinal) and enters the blood stream, initiating a systemic response that adversely affects blood flow to vital organs. Signs and symptoms include a high white cell count, increased temperature, rapid respirations, hypotension, and tachycardia. Blood cultures are used to diagnose the condition. Treatment includes an initial broad spectrum antibiotic followed by a more specific antibiotic once the location and type of the initial infection are known.

Lymphangitis

Acute streptococcal infections in the extremities can lead to lymphangitis, an inflammation of the lymphatic vessels. Signs and symptoms include red streaks extending from the infected area to the axilla or groin, fever, chills, headache, and general malaise. The area of initial infection will be red, warm, and swollen. The infection may spread to the blood stream if left untreated (see the previous section on bacteremia). Treatment includes antibiotic therapy and applying warm, moist compresses to the infected area.

Lymphadenitis

Lymphadenitis is inflammation of the lymph nodes, which can be caused by a variety of conditions resulting from bacterial infection or other inflammatory conditions that drain bacteria or toxins into the lymph. It is commonly associated with lymphangitis. Signs and symptoms include palpably hard and enlarged lymph nodes that may be warm and tender to the touch. You may also note other signs and symptoms secondary to infection such as fever, chills, and malaise. Treatment is moist heat over the affected lymph nodes and antiobiotics.

Iron-Deficiency Anemia

Anemia is characterized by a deficiency of red blood cells, hemoglobin, or total blood volume. Although there are various causes of anemia, iron-deficiency anemia occurs the most frequently. A deficiency of iron in the blood decreases the quantity of red blood cells. Since red blood cells contain hemoglobin, the oxygen carrier of the blood, anemia reduces the body's ability to deliver oxygen to cells throughout the body.

Iron deficiency occurs as a result of insufficient iron quantities in the diet, reduced iron absorption ability of the body, blood loss, or lead poisoning. Anemia is seen more frequently in women than in men because of blood loss during menstrual bleeding and because of the relatively smaller stores of iron in women.

A diet rich in iron can reduce the risk of anemia. Foods rich in iron include red meat, egg yolks, raisins, fish, legumes, and liver. Foods enriched with iron include flour, bread, and some cereals. Symptoms of iron-deficiency anemia include pale skin, fatigue, weakness, shortness of breath, low blood pressure, headache, decreased appetite, and irritability. Tests for hematocrit and hemoglobin blood levels are commonly used to identify iron-deficiency anemia.

Anemia treatment begins with identifying the cause of the condition and then taking steps to eradicate it. Iron supplements are usually provided along with a diet rich in iron. In most cases, blood levels return to normal after a 2-month treatment course. Iron supplements are best absorbed on an empty stomach, but some patients cannot tolerate the stomach upset that can occur. Since antacids and milk may interfere with iron absorption, they should not be ingested while taking iron supplements.

Sickle Cell Anemia

Sickle cell anemia is a genetic mutation of the red blood cells. Normal red blood cells are round, but sickle cells are sickle-shaped. The condition occurs most predominantly in African-Americans. About 1 in every 400 African-Americans is born with sickle cell anemia. The disease becomes apparent after the child's first year. Signs and symptoms include pain in the chest, joints, back, and abdomen that can range from mild to severe; swelling in the feet and hands; jaundice; kidney failure; repetitive infections; or gallstones or strokes at an early age.

There is currently no medication to treat sickle cell anemia. Treatment aims to prevent complications and provide symptomatic relief. Analgesics, oxygen, and fluid replacement are recommended during painful episodes. Since patients with sickle cell anemia are prone to pneumonia, vaccinations against pneumonia should be provided. Diet supplementation of folic acid can be useful. Recent attempts to cure sickle cell anemia through chemotherapy and bone marrow transplant have been successful on a limited basis.

Lyme Disease

Lyme disease first became known in 1975 when a large number of children in and around the town of Lyme, Connecticut, were diagnosed with juvenile rheumatoid arthritis. Investigations uncovered deer ticks infected with a bacterium that were responsible for the outbreak of arthritis.

Symptoms of the disease occur as a red rash in the form of a small red spot that expands over the next few days or weeks. The rash usually occurs at the site of the tick bite; it is often a red ring surrounding a clear central area and can range from the size of a dime to an area that covers the entire back. Additional symptoms can include flulike symptoms such as fever, headache, stiff neck, body aches, and fatigue. If the disease is not recognized and is left untreated, additional symptoms that can occur may include arthritis with swollen and painful joints; Bell's palsy; numbness, pain, or weakness of the limbs with poor motor coordination; an irregular heartbeat that can precipitate dizziness or shortness of breath; and less common problems such as hepatitis or severe fatigue. Early recognition is key.

The best method of preventing Lyme disease is to avoid deer ticks. Most people become infected during the summer when ticks are most prevalent and people go outside in wooded areas and grasslands where ticks are present. Walking in the center of trails and wearing long-sleeved shirts and long pants reduces tick exposure, and use of tick and insect repellents can also help. Treatment of Lyme disease includes antibiotics such as doxycycline or amoxicillin. The sooner treatment is initiated, the better and quicker the recovery.

SUMMARY

1. Describe the signs and symptoms of skin conditions that may be encountered in the physically active.

    Skin reactions, rashes, and lesions can result from a variety of conditions and agents. Bacterial infections are typically of staphylococcal origin and are characterized by pustules often located at the hair follicle. Viral skin infections include molluscum contagiosum, herpes simplex and zoster, and verruca plantaris and vulgaris. Fungal conditions are generally referred to as tinea or ringworm infections and are named based on their location. Parasitic infestations are typically found in the hair of the scalp and pubic regions and are caused by lice and itch mites that result in skin infection and irritation. Other skin conditions are caused by inflammation (dermatitis, eczema, and psoriasis); environmental exposure to allergens (hives) and excessive heat (sunburn) and cold (frostbite); and buildup of tissue or fluid due to mechanical friction (blisters, calluses) or glandular occlusion (sebaceous cysts). It is important to know which conditions are contagious in order to effectively control exposure and prevent them from spreading.

2. Describe the signs and symptoms of medical conditions affecting the musculoskeletal system that may be encountered in the physically active.

    Chronic bone and joint conditions in the physically active primarily involve arthritis, osteoarthritis, and gout, which are characterized by pain, inflammation, stiffness, and degeneration of the affected joint. Muscle conditions include fibromyalgia (fibrositis), a chronic myofascial disorder characterized by chronic musculoskeletal pain, fatigue, and localized tenderness; and rhabdomyolysis, an acute, sometimes fatal disease that is caused by severe destruction of skeletal muscle and is characterized by abnormal urine color; tenderness, weakness, and stiffness in the affected muscle; and generalized weakness. Knowing the characteristic signs and symptoms will help you differentiate these conditions from other causes of muscle and joint pain frequently encountered in the physically active.

3. Describe the signs and symptoms of medical conditions affecting the nervous system that may be encountered in the physically active.

    Neurological disorders represent a wide range of conditions of varying etiologies that ultimately affect some aspect of the nervous system; some are acute and others are chronic. Tetanus, commonly called lockjaw, is caused by tetanus bacillus, which attaches to the local nerve, moves to the spinal cord, and finally anchors to the motor nerves and causes tetanic muscle contraction. Epilepsy is a chronic condition characterized by recurring seizures that can be caused by head trauma, infectious diseases, metabolic disorders, tumors, congenital abnormalities, drugs, and otherwise unknown agents. Reflex sympathetic dystrophy (RSD) is a multisystem, multisymptom disorder that usually follows an injury and affects the sympathetic nervous system in a way that results in a multitude of symptoms and problems. Meningitis is an infection of the cerebral spinal fluid that can be either bacterial or viral. Each disorder can result in significant complications if not recognized or properly treated.

4. Describe the signs and symptoms of systemic diseases that may be encountered in the physically active.

Systemic diseases affect the blood and lymph. Bacterial conditions include bacteremia, lymphagitis, lymphadentis, and Lyme disease, which are all typically treated with antibiotics. Anemia, characterized by a deficiency of red blood cells, can be caused by a variety of factors, including iron deficiency (iron-deficiency anemia) and genetic mutation of the red blood cell (sickle cell anemia). Iron deficiency is more common in females compared to males, while sickle cell anemia is more common in African-Americans. While there is currently no medication for sickle cell anemia, iron-deficiency anemia is easily treated with diet and iron supplements.

REVIEW QUESTIONS

1. Describe the appearance and signs and symptoms of the following skin conditions:
   - Cellulitis
   - Carbuncle
   - Herpes simplex I
   - Verruca vulgaris
   - Ringworm
   - Tinea cruris
   - Pediculosis
   - Eczema

2. How do a focalized and a generalized seizure differ? What are potential causes for seizure activity?

3. An athlete reports to you with complaints of headache, stiff neck, and high fever. What medical condition should you suspect? Why would you differentiate between viral and bacterial forms of this illness?

4. A wrestler complains of itching and burning on the back of his shoulder. You examine the area and note raised, well-defined ringed eruptions that appear to be moist. What skin condition might you suspect? How would you manage this skin condition? Would you allow this athlete to return to practice? Why or why not?

5. A freshman cross-country runner comes into the athletic training room and appears quite anxious. She complains of sudden heat, itching, and burning all over her head, face, and hands. You immediately observe large welts and redness on the skin over these areas. Her history reveals no previous episodes of similar reactions. What condition might you suspect and how would you help this athlete?

6. A women's basketball player has been diagnosed with iron-deficiency anemia. The physician has asked you to counsel the athlete on proper diet to improve iron stores. What information would you share with this athlete?

CRITICAL THINKING QUESTIONS

1. As has been previously discussed, a thorough medical history obtained during the preparticipation physical examination at the beginning of the year can provide valuable information regarding previous medical conditions that may resurface or affect

physical activity. If you were asked to design a health history questionnaire, what questions would you include after reading this chapter?

2. Lymphadenitis has been defined as inflammation of the lymph nodes, which can be caused by a variety of conditions that result from bacterial infection or other inflammatory conditions that drain bacteria or toxins into the lymph. From the conditions covered in chapters 21 through 23, which conditions might you suspect could result in lymphodenitis of the cervical lymph nodes?

3. You work in an industrial clinic and a 65-year-old worker who has been physically active most of his life mentions that he has been diagnosed with arthritis. His friends have told him he had better stop exercising because it will only make his condition worse. Do you agree or disagree with their advice? How would you counsel this physically active individual regarding his condition?

CITED REFERENCES

American College of Rheumatology. 2003. www.rheumatology.org. Accessed August 20, 2004.

National Institutes of Health Medline Plus Health Information. 2003. Rhabdomyolysis. Available at www.nlm.hih.gov/medlineplus. Accessed August 20, 2004.

ADDITIONAL RESOURCES

Caroline, N.L. 1995. *Emergency care in the streets.* 5th ed. Boston: Little, Brown.

Hillman, S.K. 2005. *Introduction to athletic training.* 2nd ed. Champaign, IL: Human Kinetics.

Mosby's medical, nursing, and allied health dictionary. 6th ed. 2002. St Louis: Mosby.

Taber, C.W. 1997. *Taber's cyclopedic medical dictionary.* 18th ed. Philadelphia: F.A. Davis.

Glossary

ABCs—Airway, breathing, and circulation.

ablation—Surgical removal.

abrasion—Broad scraping or shearing off of superficial skin layers.

abscess—Localized collection of pus on any body part, caused by bacterial infection.

accessory motion—Subtle gliding movement that occurs within and between the joint's inert structures. It is usually evaluated with joint mobility tests. Also known as joint play.

acidosis—Excess accumulation of acid in the blood caused by cardiorespiratory compromise.

acromioclavicular compression test—Also known as horizontal adduction test and cross chest test.

active–assistive motion—Active motion combined with outside assistance.

active motion—Motion performed without assistance from an external source such as equipment or another individual.

active ROM—Voluntary movement of a joint through a range of motion without assistance.

acute—Of sudden onset and of short duration, typically resulting from a single event or mechanism.

adenoiditis—Inflammation of the glandular lymph tissue at the back of the pharynx.

adhesion—An undesirable attachment of two adjacent structures by fibrous connective tissue.

adhesive capsulitis—When an inflamed capsule develops adhesions and subsequent contractures causing severe limitations in range of motion.

alveolar process—The part of the maxilla or mandible that contains the tooth socket.

amenorrhea—Absence or cessation of menses.

amnesia—Loss of memory.

analgesic—Pain-reducing agent.

anaphylactic shock—Shock that occurs as a hypersensitivity reaction to an allergen.

anatomical position—The standardized position of the body on which all anatomical descriptions are based.

anatomical snuffbox—A region at the base of the thumb, formed by the extensor pollicis longus and extensor pollicis brevis tendons, in which the scaphoid bone can be palpated.

anesthesia—Absence of sensation.

angle specific torque—The torque produced at any designated point throughout the range of motion.

ankylosed—Fusion or fixation of a joint.

ankylosing spondylitis—Rheumatic disease that causes arthritis of the spine and sacroiliac joints, resulting in severe joint and back stiffness, loss of motion, and deformity as the disease progresses.

annulus fibrosis—Outer covering of the intervertebral disc that acts to withstand tension and prevent distortion of disc material.

anterior—Describes structures on or near the front of the body.

anterior distraction—Gapping test.

anterior–posterior plane—Imaginary plane that separates the body into left and right.

anterior tibial artery—The artery that courses through the anterior compartment of the lower leg, supplying the structures within the anterior compartment, then giving rise to the dorsalis pedis artery.

anterograde amnesia—Loss of an athlete's immediate memory and ability to recall events that have occurred since the injury.

anteversion—Excessive anterior angulation of the femoral head resulting in a toe-in gait.

anticholinergic—Medication to block the action of the neurotransmitter acetylcholine to relax smooth muscle.

antiemetic—Drugs that control nausea and vomiting.

antipyretic—Fever-reducing agent.

aorta—The sole vessel arising from the left ventricle that supplies blood to the primary arteries.

ape hand deformity—Deformity characterized by thumb extension and alignment in the same plane as the fingers.

Apley scratch test—Placing the hand behind the back allows simultaneous assessment of combined shoulder extension, adduction, and medial rotation. Placing the hand behind the head involves shoulder flexion, abduction, and lateral rotation.

apnea—Absence of breathing.

apophysitis—Inflammation of a bony projection or outgrowth serving as a muscle attachment.

apparent leg length discrepancy—A measurement difference when taken from the umbilicus to the left and right medial malleolus.

apprehension sign—When a patient reacts to or limits motion due to a fear or sensation of impending joint dislocation or stress.

approximation—To bring two structures near or in contact with one another.

arachnoid mater—A delicate, transparent membrane that forms the intermediate covering of the brain.

arcade of Frohse—A fibrous band located at the proximal edge of the supinator muscle near the edge of the extensor carpi radialis brevis and radial capitellar joint.

arrhythmia—Disturbance or irregularity in the rhythm of the heart.

arthrokinematics—The movement of the joint surfaces relative to one another.

articulation—A union (joint) between two bones.

assessment—A procedure through which an athletic trainer determines the severity, irritability, nature, and stage of an injury.

asymmetrical hypertrophy—Enlargement of the muscle of the ventricular septum and left ventricular walls. Also referred to as idiopathic hypertrophic subaortic stenosis.

atherosclerosis—Hardening and narrowing of coronary vessels.

athlete's foot—Tinea pedis.

atlantoaxial joint—Articulation formed between the axis and atlas.

atlantooccipital joint—Articulation formed between the skull and atlas.

atlas—First cervical vertebra.

atria—The two superior chambers of the heart that receive blood from the peripheral circulatory system (right atrium) and the lungs (left atrium).

atrophy—Wasting away or decrease in the size of a muscle or other tissue or organ.

auscultation—Listening for abdominal and thoracic sounds with a stethoscope.

autonomic nerve fibers—Nerve fibers that act on structures such as smooth muscle, glands, and blood vessels to heighten and restore body functions (e.g., blood pressure, heart rate) in response to the environment.

avascular necrosis—Tissue death resulting from a lack of blood supply.

average torque—The average amount of the tension produced by the muscle throughout its entire range of motion.

avulsion—Forceful tearing away of a part or a structure such as bone, skin, or tendon.

axis—Second cervical vertebra.

axonotmesis—Partial disruption of a nerve.

Babinski sign—Dorsiflexion of the great toe and splaying of the lesser toes with stroking of the plantar surface, indicative of a lower brain stem injury.

Baker's cyst—A popliteal cyst typically results from a herniation of the synovial cavity and accumulation of fluid in the popliteal space.

Bartholin glands—Small mucous glands located on the lateral walls of the vagina near the vaginal opening.

baseball finger—Rupture of the extensor digitorum longus tendon from the distal phalanx. Also referred to as mallet finger.

Battle's sign—Discoloration behind the ears.

benediction deformity—Wasting of the hypothenar, dorsal interossei, and fourth and fifth lumbrical muscles resulting from ulnar nerve palsy. Also known as bishop's deformity.

bicuspid (mitral) valve—The valve that blood passes through when exiting the left ventricle where it is pumped back into the periphery through the aorta.

bilateral comparison—Comparison of an injured side with an uninjured side.

bimalleolar fractures—A fracture involving both the medial and lateral malleolus.

bishop's deformity—Wasting of the hypothenar, dorsal interossei, and fourth and fifth lumbrical muscles resulting from ulnar nerve palsy. Also known as benediction deformity.

blister—Separation and accumulation of fluid or blood between superficial skin layers.

blocker's exostosis—Repetitive insult and irritation of the acromion, causing excessive bone formation and at times a palpable spur on the anteriolateral surface of the humerus. Also known as tackler's exostosis or blocker's spur.

blood pressure—Tension exerted against the arterial walls when the heart is pumping (systolic) and when at rest (diastolic).

blow-out fracture—Fracture of the orbital floor occurring as a result of a sudden increase in orbital pressure from a direct blow to the eye.

blow-out injury—An injury occurring from a hard blow to the chest while the glottis is closed, which results in rupturing of the alveoli.

boggy—Refers to a soft, spongy feel, usually the result of localized inflammation.

boil—Localized infection of skin, gland, or hair follicle. Also known as furuncle.

bolus—Rapid administration of an injectable medication.

bone spur—Bony outgrowth.

Bouchard's nodes—Nodules or bony enlargement of the proximal interphalangeal joints of the hand.

boutonniere deformity—Deformity characterized by flexion of the PIP joint and hyperextension of the DIP joint most often resulting from injury to the central slip of the extensor digitorum tendon at its insertion at the base of the middle phalanx.

boxer's fracture—A fracture specifically involving the neck of the fifth metatarsal.

brachialcephalic artery—One of the three primary arterial branches; the artery that subsequently divides into the right common carotid and right subclavian arteries.

brachial plexus—The primary neural supply to the upper extremities.

bradycardia—A heart rate that falls below the normal range.

brain stem—The stem that connects the cerebral hemispheres with the spinal cord; controls vital functions of respiration, heart rate, and blood pressure.

brawny edema—Leathery hardening or thickening of tissue due to chronic inflammation.

break test—An efficient test for strength obtained by applying isometric resistance while the joint is in a neutral midrange position.

Brudzinski test—A test used to determine nerve root irritation, meningeal irritation, or dural irritation by flexing the hip.

bulimarexia—Eating disorder characterized by both anorexic and bulimic behaviors.

burners—Nerve injury (usually brachial plexus) with classical symptoms of immediate sharp, burning pain radiating down the distal extremity.

bursa—Synovial-filled membrane that lies between adjacent structures to limit friction and ease movement.

bursitis—Inflammation or swelling of a bursa.

burst fracture—Fracture of the C1 vertebra. Also known as a Jefferson fracture.

café au lait spots—Darkened patches of skin.

calcaneal exostosis—A condition characterized by excess calcium formation resulting in increased prominence of the posterior calcaneus, commonly referred to as pump bump.

capsular pattern—A pattern of limited joint motion that is unique to each joint, resulting from restriction in the joint capsule.

capsular restriction—A restriction in joint range of motion due to capsular adhesions or scarring.

capsulitis—Inflammation of the joint capsule.

cardiac tamponade—Hemorrhage within the enclosed and inelastic pericardial cavity.

cardinal sign or symptom—A classic sign or symptom highly indicative of that condition.

cardiogenic shock—A condition characterized by inadequate blood flow and cardiovascular system collapse due to inadequate cardiac output.

carpal tunnel syndrome—A condition of the wrist and hand characterized by compression of the median nerve as it passes through the carpal tunnel.

cauda equina—The terminal portion of the spinal cord.

cauda equina syndrome—Compression of the terminal portion of the spinal cord usually caused by a central disc herniation resulting in bowel and bladder dysfunction.

caudal—Away from the head.

central nervous system—The brain and spinal cord.

cephalad—Toward the head.

cerebellum—Portion of the brain that controls motor functions that regulate posture, muscle tone, and coordination.

cervical plexus—The primary sensory supply to the neck and scalp and the primary motor supply to the neck musculature and the diaphragm.

cervical radiculitis—Pain referred down the arm from cervical nerve root compression.

cervical whiplash—Sudden forced extension of the neck followed by forced flexion.

chalazia—A sebaceous cystlike tumor on the eyelid.

chancre—A sore or ulcer.

Cheyne-Stokes respiration—Breathing pattern characterized by a rhythmic fluctuation between hyperpnea and apnea.

chronic—A condition of gradual onset and of prolonged duration usually resulting from an accumulation of minor insults or repetitive stress.

chronic instability—Abnormal joint laxity due to permanent slackening of a joint ligament or capsule.

chuck grip—A grip that measures the force exerted between the thumb and index digit pads.

clonic—A rapid contraction and relaxation of a muscle or muscle group.

clonus—A very brisk and exaggerated reflex response.

clonus test—A test that determines whether the central nervous system is functioning properly by rapidly stretching a muscle.

closed chain—A segment where the distal end is fixed or in contact with the ground.

closed kinetic chain—Movement of the body with the distal segment working against a fixed or immovable object.

closed wound—An injury that does not disrupt the skin surface.

clubbed—Large and convex.

clunk test—A test for glenoid labrum integrity.

comminuted—To break into pieces or multiple fragments.

comparable sign—A positive response indicating either a reproduction or an alteration of the athlete's symptoms.

compartment syndrome—A significant rise in intracompartmental pressure caused by severe bleeding within a muscular compartment that can compromise neurovascular structures.

compound dislocation—An injury in which a displaced joint penetrates the skin surface so that the bone is exposed.

compound fracture—An injury in which a displaced fracture penetrates the skin surface so that the bone is exposed.

compression—To squeeze or press together.

compression force—Placing direct pressure on a surface or soft tissue.

concussion—A transient alteration in brain function without structural damage caused by an agitation or shaking of the brain.

condylomata acuminata—Genital warts.

conjunctivitis—An irritation and inflammation of the outer surface of the eye or inner eyelid, more commonly known as pinkeye.

contrecoup-type injury—An injury occurring when the moving head makes contact with an immovable or more slowly moving object. Also referred to as a deceleration injury.

contusion—The compression of soft tissue by a direct blow or impact sufficient to disrupt or damage the small capillaries in the tissue, commonly referred to as a bruise.

coronal plane—Imaginary plane that separates the body into front and back.

cortical sensation—Identifying a particular structure or texture by feeling the object with the eyes closed.

costochondritis—Inflammation of the costochondral junction.

costoclavicular syndrome test—Also referred to as the military brace position test.

coup-type injury—An injury in which the brain is traumatized at the location of impact when the head is stationary and is struck by a moving object.

coxa valga—Femoral neck angulation >135°.

coxa vara—Femoral neck angulation <120°.

Cram test—Another name for the bowstring test; identifies compression on the sciatic nerve.

crank test—A test that assesses anterior shoulder dislocation.

cremaster muscle—A muscle that is continuous with the internal oblique and functions to draw the testicles to a more superior position in the scrotum.

cremasteric reflex—A drawing up of the scrotal sac with ipsilateral stroking of the upper inner thigh.

crepitus—A crackling, grating, or grinding sensation caused by abnormal movement between two structures.

cretinism—Hypothyroidism in the very young, resulting in stunted growth, sparse hair growth, improperly developed reproductive organs, and mental retardation.

cross chest test—Also known as the horizontal adduction test.

cubital tunnel syndrome—A term that collectively describes ulnar neuropathy and compression at the elbow.

cubital valgus—Excessive valgus angulation of the extended elbow.

cubital varus—A decreased valgus angulation or actual varus angulation of the extended elbow. Also referred to as gunstock deformity.

cyanosis—A bluish or purplish discoloration of the skin due to deficient oxygenation of the blood.

De Quervain's disease—Tenosynovitis of the abductor pollicis longus and extensor pollicis brevis tendons and their sheaths on the radial side of the thumb.

debride—To clean a wound of infectious or foreign substances in an effort to promote healing and restore healthy tissue.

decerebrate posturing—A rigid extension of all four extremities with the arms internally rotated and pronated, which is a sign of upper brain stem injury.

decorticate posturing—A rigid extension of the legs and flexion of the arms, wrist, and hands toward the chest, indicative of injury above the brain stem.

deep fascia—A thick, fibrous, continuous structure that envelops and separates muscles.

deep fibular nerve—Innervates the muscles in the anterior compartment of the leg and provides sensation for the skin between the first and second digits of the foot.

deep tendon reflex—An involuntary muscle contraction in response to a tendon tap.

deep vein thrombophlebitis—The inflammation of a deep vein.

degenerative—Chronic deterioration of a joint or tissue structure over time.

degree of freedom—The number of directions a segment is free to move.

dental caries—Cavities.

dermatome—An area of skin innervated by a single spinal nerve root.

detailed history—A comprehensive investigation of the patient's chief complaint, mechanism of injury or nature of illness, associated signs and symptoms, and any preexisting factors that may contribute to the current complaint.

diabetes—An autoimmune disorder that causes a deficiency in glucose metabolism.

diabetic coma—Unconsciousness due to a lack of insulin. Also referred to as hyperglycemic shock.

diastolic pressure—Measures the pressure exerted against the artery walls when the heart rests (i.e., left ventricle relaxed).

differential diagnosis—An evaluation to rule out the involvement of other joints or regions as the cause for the symptoms.

diplopia—Double vision.

dislocation—Complete disassociation or displacement of one joint surface on another.

distraction—An assessment or mobilization technique where longitudinal force is applied to a joint to separate opposing joint structures.

dorsalis pedis artery—The artery that supplies the foot.

drawer test—A manual test that glides one joint surface on another to examine for instability.

drop arm test—A test that assesses the integrity of the rotator cuff.

dura mater—The outermost covering of the brain consisting of a tough fibrous tissue that serves as the inner lining of the skull and provides protection to the brain.

dyspepsia—Either improper digestion or deficient absorption of food in the digestive tract.

dysphasia—Pain with swallowing.

dyspnea—Difficulty in breathing.

dysrhythmia—A disturbance in the normal heart rhythm, such as a premature or late beat.

dyssynchrony—A misfiring or mistiming of a muscle contraction.

dystrophy—Muscular disorder characterized by weakness and fibrosis.

ecchymosis—Discoloration of tissue.

edema—Swelling resulting from fluid accumulation in the interstitial tissues.

effusion—When fluid escapes and collects in the surrounding tissues.

embolism—Obstruction of a blood vessel by a blood clot.

end feel—The quality of the feel or sensation felt by the evaluator when applying pressure to the joint at the end of the range of motion.

endometritis—An inflammation of the endometrium of the uterus.

endurance—The muscle's capacity to produce force over a series of consecutive contractions or its ability to maintain a sustained contraction over a period of time.

eosinophils—Leukocytes or other granulocytes that are released secondary to an allergen or a parasitic infection.

epicondylitis—An overuse injury to the tendinous attachments of the flexor–pronator group at the medial epicondyle or the extensor–supinator group at the lateral epicondyle. Also referred to as "tennis elbow."

epididymitis—An inflammation of the epididymis.

epidural hematoma—A tear in the middle meningeal artery resulting in a rapidly expanding hematoma in the epidural space.

epidural space—The space between the skull and dura mater.

epilepsy—A chronic condition characterized by recurring seizures.

epiphysis—A secondary ossification center or growth plate.

epistaxis—Nosebleed.

Epstein-Barr virus (EBV)—A member of the herpes group of viruses, which is the source of most cases of infectious mononucleosis, or "mono."

erythema—Redness of the skin.

essential history—History that influences immediate examination and care.

evaluation—The systematic process that allows the clinician to make a clinical judgment.

eversion—The outward movement of the sole of the foot away from the midline of the body.

examination—To inspect closely; to test the condition of an injury or illness.

exercise-induced asthma (EIA)—Asthma that occurs during exercise.

exostosis—Excess calcium formation resulting in increased prominence of a bone surface.

expectorant—A drug used to increase flow and decrease the viscosity of mucus in the respiratory passageway.

extension—Movement that decreases the angle of a joint.

extensor lag—Inability to fully extend the knee during active motion, but full passive motion is present.

extracranial—Outside the skull.

extrinsic—Originating, or coming from, outside.

extrusion—Avulsion or disassociation of a tooth from the tooth socket.

Faber (flexion, abduction, external rotation) test—Also known as the Patrick test or Jansen's test; used to identify limited mobility of the hips.

fascia—A fibrous membrane that supports, separates, and envelops muscle.

fasciculation—Involuntary contraction of muscle fibers innervated by a single motor unit.

fatigue—A reduced capacity to do work.

faun's beard—A hairy patch overlying the lumbar spine, indicative of spina bifida occulta.

female athlete triad—A combination of amenorrhea, disordered eating, and osteoporosis.

femoral hernia—A condition occurring when the abdominal viscera protrude through the femoral ring and into the femoral canal just inferior to the inguinal ligament.

femoral nerve—Innervates the iliopsoas and knee extensor muscles.

fibular—Another name for peroneal, referring to the fibula.

fibular (peroneal) artery—An artery that descends obliquely from its origin toward the fibula and courses along the posterior lateral aspect of the leg to supply the popliteus muscle and muscles of the posterior and lateral compartments of the lower leg.

fibular (peroneal) nerve—The lateral or posterior division of the sciatic nerve, supplying the hip extensors, abductors of the thigh, and extensor/dorsiflexor muscles of the foot and ankle.

fibularis muscle—Another name for peroneus muscle, referring to the muscles attaching to the fibula.

first degree—An injury classification characterized by mild tissue disruption and disability.

five-object recall—A test that examines for anterograde amnesia through the verbal presentation of five unrelated objects.

flail chest injury—An injury characterized by multiple fractures of three or more adjacent ribs.

flatfoot—A condition caused by hypermobility resulting from increased ligament laxity and muscle weakness on the plantar surface of the foot. Also known as pes planus.

flexibility—The degree of pliability or adaptability of a muscle, tendon, or joint.

flexion—Movement that increases the angle of the joint.

focused history—An investigation of the patient's chief complaint and any problems that are readily apparent or that need attention before transporting the patient off-site.

forearm splints—Periostitis occurring in the forearm.

forefoot—Composed of the tarsometatarsal, intermetatarsal, metatarsophalangeal, and interphalangeal joints.

Fowler test—The relocation test used to assess anterior instability. Also known as the Jobe relocation test.

fracture—Disruption or break in the continuity of a bone.

frontal plane—Imaginary plane that separates the body into front and back. Also referred to as the coronal plane.

fulcrum test—A test that assesses the possibility of a femoral stress fracture.

functional deformity—Deformity that does not involve permanent structural changes and typically results from mechanical dysfunction.

furuncle—An infection of the hair follicle. Also known as a boil.

gamekeeper's thumb—Ulnar collateral ligament rupture of the first metacarpophalangeal joint. Also known as "skier's thumb."

ganglion—A cyst that is characterized by herniation of synovial fluid through the joint capsule or synovial sheath of a tendon. Also known as a synovial cyst.

gapping test—Stress test for the anterior sacroiliac ligaments.

genicular branches—Nerve branches that supply the knee joint.

genu recurvatum—Excessive knee hyperextension.

genu valgus—Lateral angulation of the tibia relative to the femur.

genu varum—Medial angulation of the tibia relative to the femur.

gingivitis—Inflammation of the gums that results from the presence of bacteria typically caused by food deposits and inadequate brushing or flossing.

glenoid labrum—A ring of fibrocartilage that deepens the glenoid fossa to increase glenohumeral stability.

glide—Movement that occurs when a point on one surface contacts new points on the opposing surface. Also known as a slide.

glide force—A force applied to the joint where the distal surface is moved in a straight (transverse) plane on the proximal joint surface.

glucocorticoid—An adrenal cortical hormone primarily used to protect against stress and to affect protein and carbohydrate metabolism.

gluteus medius lurch—A drop of the non-weight-bearing pelvis and hip during its swing-through phase. Also known as Trendelenburg gait.

goiter—Enlargement of the thyroid gland.

golfer's elbow—Also known as medial epicondylitis.

goniometer—The tool used for measuring joints.

goniometry—The measurement of joint angles.

guarding—A protective, voluntary muscle spasm in an effort to protect an injured area.

gunstock deformity—A carrying angle less than the normal 5° or 15° valgus angulation. Also known as cubital varus.

hangman's fracture—A fracture of the pedicle or pars of the C2 vertebra.

Hawkins test—A test that compresses the supraspinatus tendon against the coracoacromial ligament to test impingement of the supraspinatus tendon.

heart—The muscle that pumps blood through the lungs and the peripheral circulatory system.

heartburn—A condition in which the acid from the stomach enters the esophagus.

Heberden's nodes—Nodules or bony enlargement of the distal interphalangeal joints of the hand.

heel spur—A bony outgrowth on the anterior inferior surface of the calcaneus due to tractioning of the plantar fascia.

hematocele—Rapid blood accumulation within the membrane surrounding the testicle.

hematoma—A localized mass or "blood [hema] tumor [toma]" caused by an accumulation of blood in a confined area of a tissue or space.

hematuria—Blood in the urine.

hemipelvis—A condition in which one side of the pelvis is smaller than the other.

hemophilia—A genetic condition in which the blood does not clot.

herniation—Development of a protruding structure (e.g., vertebral disc) or organ (e.g., intestine) through its outer wall or cavity where it is contained.

Hibbs' test—A test of the posterior sacroiliac ligaments. Also known as the posterior distraction test.

high blood pressure—A condition involving an elevated systolic (>140 mmHg) or diastolic (>90 mmHg) blood pressure associated with generalized arteriolar vasoconstriction. Also known as hypertension.

hindfoot—Composed of the distal tibiofibular (syndesmosis), talocrural (tibia, fibula, and talus), and subtalar (talus, calcaneus, navicular) joints.

hip anteversion—Excessive anterior angulation of the femoral neck that results in a toe-in gait.

hip pointer—A contusion to the iliac crest.

hip retroversion—Decreased anterior angulation of the femoral neck producing a toe-out gait.

histamine—Chemical substance found in the blood that, when released, causes dilatation and increased permeability of blood vessels.

history—A carefully taken record of past and current events that aid in diagnosis of an injury or illness.

Hopkins Verbal Learning Test—Examines verbal memory and learning.

horizontal adduction test—Cross chest test.

humoral—A bodily fluid or semifluid such as a hormone.

hydrocele—Fluid accumulation within the membrane surrounding the testicle.

hyperemia—Redness of the eye.

hyperesthesia—Heightened or increased sensitivity to sensory stimuli.

hyperglycemic—A condition that occurs if there is too little insulin and glucose levels are elevated above normal levels. Also known as high blood sugar.

hyperglycemic shock—Shock induced by a lack of insulin (abnormally high blood sugar). Also referred to as diabetic coma.

hyperkinesis—Abnormal increase in movement or purposeless muscle movement.

hypermobility—Excessive motions in one or more planes.

hyperpnea—Rapid, deep breathing.

hypertension—Elevated blood pressure, usually considered when pressure is greater than 140/90 mmHg.

hypertonia—Excessive muscle tone.

hypertrophy—An increase in the size of a muscle or other tissue or organ.

hyphema—An accumulation of blood in the anterior chamber of the eye.

hypoesthesia—Diminished sensation.

hypoglycemic—Low blood sugar.

hypotonia—Flaccid muscle tone.

hypovolemic shock—A condition that occurs as the result of decreased blood volume in the circulatory system. Also referred to as hemorrhagic shock.

hypoxia—Lack of oxygen.

imperforate—Lacking the usual or normal opening.

impingement syndrome—Encroachment in the subacromial space that decreases the area through which the supraspinatus and subacromial bursa pass underneath the subacromial arch.

incision—A cut through the full thickness of the skin usually caused by a sharp object or instrument and resulting in smooth, even wound edges.

infarction—Necrosis of tissue or organ from obstruction of local blood flow.

inferior vena cava—The vein that brings deoxygenated blood from the lower body into the heart.

inguinal hernia—Protrusion of the small intestine through the inguinal canal or abdominal wall.

instability—Abnormal or excessive joint laxity or excursion.

insulin—A peptide hormone responsible for glucose utilization.

insulin shock—Shock resulting from a severe hypoglycemic reaction resulting from an overdose of insulin.

intervertebral foramen—The opening between two adjacent vertebrae that allows passage of the paired spinal nerves.

intra-articular—Within the joint capsule.

intracranial—Within the skull or cranium.

intrathecal—Within the spinal canal.

intrathecal pressure—Pressure within the spinal canal.

intrinsic—Originating, or coming from, inside a body segment.

intrusion—A condition in which the tooth is driven into the socket.

ischemia—Tissue anemia caused by a lack of blood flow to an area.

isometric—Muscle contraction at a fixed joint position where there is no shortening or lengthening of the muscle fibers.

isotonic strength—Strength required to lift a fixed amount of weight through a range of motion.

J sign—Abduction or lateral rotation of the leg that indicates tightness of the IT band.

Jansen's test—A test used to identify limited mobility of the hip, also known as the Patrick test or Faber (flexion, abduction, external rotation) test.

Jendrassik's maneuver—A technique that increases the nervous system's sensitivity to improve deep tendon reflex response.

jersey finger—Rupture of the flexor digitorum longus tendon from the distal phalanx of the finger.

Jobe relocation test—Test used to assess anterior instability. Also known as the Fowler test.

jock itch—A fungal infection in the groin region. Also known as tinea cruris.

joint mice—Loose fragments within the joint.

joint mobilization—A passive evaluation of joint movement to assess the capsular structures of the joint.

joint play—Accessory motion.

Jones' fracture—A fracture of the base of the fifth metatarsal usually caused by tractioning of the peroneus brevis tendon.

Kehr's sign—A sign characterized by pain radiating into the left shoulder and partially down the arm, usually indicative of a spleen injury.

Kernig test—A test in which the neck is flexed to determine nerve root irritation, meningeal irritation, or dural irritation.

ketoacidosis—Increased acidity in the blood due to excess of ketone bodies.

kinins—Chemical substances found in the body that, when released, dilate and increase permeability of blood vessels.

kyphosis—Excess posterior convexity of the thoracic spine.

labored breathing—When the patient experiences difficulty speaking or exerts unusual effort to inhale.

laceration—Tearing of the skin resulting in jagged, uneven wound edges.

Lachman-Trillat test—Another name for the Lachman test. Also known as the Ritchie test or the Trillat test. Examines the integrity of the anterior cruciate ligament.

Lasegue's test—Another name for the straight leg raise test.

lateral pinch grip—Grip that measures grasping strength by placing the dynamometer between the pad of the thumb and the medial aspect of the index finger.

lateral plantar nerve—Innervates the muscles of the foot.

laxity—Hypermobility or increased joint movement.

length–tension relationship—Describes the force a muscle can generate when it has contracted or extended to any specific length.

Lisfranc's fracture—A dislocated fracture of the midfoot characterized by one or more displaced proximal metatarsals.

Little League elbow—A valgus traction force injury of the medial elbow that may start out as an inflammatory response or apophysitis and progress to an avulsion of the apophysis if the repetitive stress continues.

Little Leaguer's shoulder—Epiphyseal fracture of the proximal humeral growth plate.

load and shift test—Test for anterior and posterior instability of the glenohumeral joint.

long latency reflex—A reflex that receives input from higher brain centers and may involve one or more interneurons that mediate the reflex response.

long loop reflex—A reflex that receives input from higher brain centers and may involve one or more interneurons that mediate the reflex response.

loose-packed position—Positioning of the joint where the ligaments are at their resting length and under the least amount of tension.

lordosis—Excessive anterior convexity of the cervical and lumbar spine.

lower motor neuron—Peripheral motor nerves that originate in the spinal cord and innervate skeletal muscle.

lower motor neuron lesion—Injury to nerve structures in the anterior horn of the spinal cord and in the spinal and peripheral nerves.

lumbar plexus—A network of nerves arising from the ventral rami of the first four levels of the lumbar spine, L1 through L4.

lumbarization—The S1 vertebral segment remains mobile and separate from the sacrum, appearing as a sixth lumbar vertebra on X ray.

lumbosacral trunk—A large nerve that joins the sacral plexus and is considered separate from the lumbar plexus.

Lundington's test—Examination for tear of the tendon of the long head of the biceps.

lung collapse—A reduction in lung volume. Also know as a pneumothorax.

luxation—Complete disassociation of two joint surfaces. Also referred to as dislocation.

lymphocytes—Cells in the blood and lymphatic tissue that provide immunity from invading organisms.

MacIntosh test—Also known as the lateral pivot shift maneuver.

macrophages—The major phagocytic (destroyer) cells of the immune system.

macule—A nonraised patch of skin with altered color.

malaise—A vague, general feeling of illness or fatigue.

malingering—Pretending to be injured.

mallet finger—Avulsion of the extensor digitorum longus from the distal phalanx. Also known as baseball finger.

mallet finger test—A common name for the extensor tendon avulsion test.

malocclusion—An inability to approximate the upper and lower jaw or teeth in a normal bite.

manual muscle test (MMT)—A graded strength test performed by applying manual resistance to a segment to evaluate a particular muscle or muscle group.

manual strength test—Any strength evaluation where the examiner applies the resistance.

medial plantar nerve—Innervates the muscles of the foot.

medial sural cutaneous nerve—The nerve that supplies sensation to the lateral aspect of the ankle and foot.

mediastinum—Cavity that houses the heart, thoracic parts of the great vessels, the trachea, the left and right bronchi, and related structures.

meninges—The three layers that cover the brain and spinal cord.

metabolic acidosis—Increased acidity in the tissues due to build up of anaerobic byproducts and increased permeability of the capillary walls.

metabolic alkalosis—Increase in the plasma concentration of carbon dioxide.

metabolic shock—Cardiovascular collapse secondary to a loss of body fluid as a consequence of illness that causes diarrhea, excessive urination, or vomiting.

metastasis—The spread of malignant cells through the lymphatic system from one body part to another.

metatarsalgia—A general term used to describe metatarsal pain. Also used as a term for Morton's neuroma.

midfoot—Composed of the talocalcaneonavicular, cuneonavicular, intercuneiform, and calcaneo-cuboid joints.

miserable malalignment syndrome—Another name for patellofemoral pain syndrome.

monosynaptic reflex arc—When one afferent neuron is stimulated by its sensory receptor and directly synapses with an alpha motor neuron, resulting in muscular excitation or inhibition.

mosaic warts—Warts clustered in groups.

motor tests—Tests used to assess neuromuscular integrity and muscle strength.

muscle fasciculations—Involuntary muscle contractions that occur secondary to injury or pain, involving only a few muscle fibers innervated by one motor unit.

muscle spasm—Involuntary muscle contraction involving the entire muscle, which occurs secondary to injury, fatigue, or pain.

muscle spindles—Specialized muscle fibers arranged parallel to the contractile muscle fibers. They sense changes in muscle tension and length and control muscle tone.

muscle tremors—Involuntary muscle contractions involving several motor units, which occur secondary to injury or pain.

myocardial—Muscle of the heart.

myositis—Inflammation of a muscle or its connective tissue.

myositis ossificans—A condition that occurs when the body's inflammatory response during absorption of a hematoma causes calcification or bony deposits to form in the muscle.

myotendinous unit—A unit composed of both contractile (muscle) and noncontractile (tendon and fascia) connective tissues that work together to move one body segment on another.

myotome—A muscle or muscle group that is innervated by a single nerve root.

myxedema—A condition that occurs secondary to chronic hypothyroidism marked by drowsiness, cold body temperature, and possible coma.

Neer impingement test—Test for rotator cuff impingement.

Nelaton's line—A line from the ischial tuberosity to the ipsilateral ASIS used to determine congenital hip dislocations.

nerve plexus—Multiple spinal nerves interconnecting through a series of uniting, dividing, reuniting branches that ultimately result in mix peripheral nerves that emerge from the plexus as terminal branches.

neuralgia—Ache or pain along the distribution of a nerve.

neurocognitive testing—Determines cognitive function for immediate memory, delayed memory, and concentration.

neurogenic—Originating in or controlled by the nervous system.

neurogenic shock—A condition that occurs when there is damage to the spinal cord and the nerves that innervate smooth muscle, resulting in loss of vascular tone.

neuroma—Thickening of a nerve, or "nerve tumor," secondary to chronic irritation and inflammation.

neuropathy—A general term to describe any pathological condition of the nerve.

neuropraxia—Transient or temporary loss in nerve function.

neurotmesis—Complete severance of a nerve.

neurovascular bundle—Major arteries, veins, and nerves running together in a thin fascial sheath.

nociceptor—Pain receptor.

nursemaid's elbow—Subluxation or dislocation of the radioulnar joint, where the radial head is pulled down into and becomes caught in the annular ligament.

nystagmus—Involuntary lateral oscillatory movement of the eyes.

objective—A sign or symptom that is perceptible to other persons or is measurable.

observation—A visual recording or assessment.

obturator nerve—Innervates the adductor muscles of the thigh.

open chain—A segment where the distal end is not fixed or in contact with the ground.

open wound—An injury that disrupts the continuity of the skin.

ophthalmoscope—An instrument used in a routine eye exam to detect injury or disease in the interior structures of the eye.

orthostatic hypotension—A condition in which the blood pressure drops when a person suddenly moves to a standing position.

osteochondral—Referring to bone (osteo) and cartilage (chondral).

osteochondritis dissecans—Avascular necrosis of a joint's articular surface.

osteochondrosis—Alterations and degenerative changes of the subchondral bone. Precursor to osteochondritis dissecans.

osteokinematics—The movement of the long bones that produces motion.

osteophyte—A bone spur or bony outgrowth.

otorrhea—Fluid draining from the ears.

otoscope—A light source combined with a magnifying lens and specula used to examine the inner ear.

overpressure—An application of pressure at the end of a joint's physiological motion to assess end feel and ligamentous integrity.

overuse injury—An injury due to repetitive microtrauma that often follows periods of inadequate rest or recovery, overactivity, or repetitive overloading of a structure.

pallor—Loss of skin coloration due to decreased blood flow.

palpable—Detectable by touching or feeling.

palpation—A skilled evaluation using the sense of touch to identify soft tissue or bony abnormalities.

palsy—Partial or complete paralysis resulting from pressure on a nerve.

papule—A small raised bump on the skin that may or may not be painful.

paresthesia—Impaired or altered sensation such as a tingling, burning, or numbing.

parietal pleura—The outer wall of the pleural sac that adheres to the external wall of the pleural cavity.

pars interarticularis—The region of bone between the superior and inferior articular facets.

passive motion—Motion performed without the assistance of the patient.

passive ROM—Movement of a joint through a range of motion by someone other than the person being assessed.

patella alta—A patella that sits abnormally high in the femoral groove.

patellofemoral pain syndrome (PFPS)—Vague term describing the general term anterior knee pain. Also known as miserable malalignment syndrome and patellofemoral stress syndrome (PFSS).

patellofemoral stress syndrome (PFSS)—Patellofemoral pain syndrome.

pathological reflexes—Abnormal reflexes specific to particular diseases.

peak torque—The greatest torque produced at any point in the range of motion.

pediculosis capitis—A parasitic infection of the hair on the head, caused by the head louse.

pediculosis corporis—A parasitic infection of the body, caused by the body louse.

pediculosis pubis—A parasitic infection in the pubic region, caused by the crab louse.

periodontitis—Loss of alveolar bone and recession of the gum line due to bacteria. Also known as pyorrhea.

periosteum—The fibrous membrane covering the bone.

periostitis—Inflammation of the outer lining of the bone (periosteum).

peripheral circulatory system—Includes arteries, arterioles, capillaries, venules, and veins that communicate with the various tissues of the body.

peripheral nervous system—All the neural structures except the brain and spine, including the cranial nerves arising from the brain and the cervical, thoracic, and lumbosacral spinal nerve roots arising from the spinal cord.

pes cavus—An abnormally high or excessive arch.

pes planus—An abnormally low or absent arch. Also known as flatfoot.

photophobia—Sensitivity to light.

phrenic nerve—A crucial nerve that arises from C3 through C5 that is the only motor nerve supplying the diaphragm.

physiological motion—The active motion of the joint that occurs in the planes of motion. Flexion, extension, adduction, abduction, and rotation are examples of physiological motions.

pia mater—The inner meningeal membrane of the brain.

pitting edema—Soft tissue swelling that results in skin depression after pressure is released.

plantar arch—Artery formed by the dorsalis pedis and lateral and medial plantar arteries that gives off digital branches to the toes.

plantar flexion—The movement of the sole of the foot in an inferior direction, as occurs with pointing the toes.

plaques—Scaly patches.

plica—A fold in the synovial membrane on the anterior aspect of the knee.

popliteal pressure test—Another name for the bowstring test.

posterior—Describes structures on or near the back of the body.

posterior tibial artery—The artery that passes deep in the posterior compartment of the lower leg after giving rise to the peroneal artery near the distal border of the popliteus muscle.

postherpetic neuralgia—Pain along a nerve pathway as a result of a virus.

Pott's fracture—Avulsion fracture of the medial malleolus and shear fracture of the lateral malleolus.

power—The time required to perform work.

primary survey—The initial evaluation that examines for immediate life-threatening conditions.

prolapse—A bulge or weakening of a structure (e.g., disc bulge).

prominence—Outgrowth.

pronation—To rotate downward. In the foot, this represents a composite of three motions occurring at the joint—eversion, dorsiflexion, and abduction in the open chain; in the closed chain, eversion, plantar flexion, and abduction. In the forearm, this represents rotating the hand downward or posteriorly.

pronator teres syndrome—Compression of the median nerve at the elbow.

proprioception—Awareness of position or movement of the body or a body segment.

prostaglandins—Fatty acids that perform a variety of hormone functions.

protrusion—A condition of being thrust forward or projecting outward.

psychogenic shock—A transient condition of shock that results in fainting due to fear, anxiety, or emotional stress that causes a sudden involuntary nervous system reaction, vasodilation, and pooling of blood in the peripheral blood vessels.

pudendal nerve—Arises from separate branches of S2 through S4 to supply the muscles of the perineum and provide sensation to the external genitalia.

pulmonary arteries—The arteries that deliver deoxygenated blood to the lungs.

pulmonary embolism—Obstruction of the pulmonary artery usually due to a thrombus (blood clot) in the lower extremity breaking loose.

pulse—A palpable and rhythmic throbbing or wave in the arteries caused by contractions of the heart.

pulse rate—The rate at which the heart is beating, usually expressed in beats per minute (bpm).

pump bump—Increased prominence of the posterior calcaneal tuberosity. Also known as a calcaneal exostosis.

puncture—A small hole or wound caused by a sharp, penetrating object.

Purkinje fibers—Extend from the bundle branches (originating from the AV node) to the myocardium in the ventricle to complete the cardiac conduction system.

purulent—Containing or consisting of pus.

pyorrhea—Loss of alveolar bone and recession of the gum line as a result of bacteria. Also known as periodontitis.

quadrant position—Placement of a spinal segment in lateral flexion, extension, and rotation to the same side as the symptoms.

quadriceps angle (Q-angle)—The angle created by a line from the anterior superior iliac spine through the midpoint of the patella and a line from the tibial tubercle through the midpoint of the patella.

raccoon eyes—Discoloration around the eyes caused by skull fracture.

radial nerve palsy—Injury to the radial nerve.

radicular—Pain referred into the extremity.

radiculitis—Referred pain secondary to nerve root compression.

rales—A crackling, popping, or bubbling sound heard with auscultation of the lungs.

range of motion (ROM)—The arc of motion through which a body segment moves in a specific cardinal plane of motion.

Reagan's test—A test to assess lunate instability. Also known as the lunatotriquetral ballottement test.

rebound tenderness—Pain with stretch of the peritoneum when the abdominal wall is depressed and then released.

referred symptoms—Symptoms experienced away from the site of injury.

reflex—An involuntary muscle contraction in response to a stimulus (e.g., tendon tap).

renal colic—Extreme pain that starts in the flank or back and radiates across the abdomen into the groin, genitalia, and inner thigh.

respirations—Rhythmic breathing or air exchange in and out of the lungs.

respiratory alkalosis—A deficiency of carbonic acid in the blood caused by excessive elimination of CO_2.

resting position—The position where the joint capsule is loosest and the bone ends are the least congruent with one another.

retinacula—Thickenings in the deep fascia that hold a tendon in place when a muscle contracts.

retrograde amnesia—Loss of memory and inability to recall events before the traumatic event.

retroversion—Decreased anterior angulation of the femoral neck resulting in a toe-out gait.

Reye's syndrome—A rare, often fatal childhood disease that can damage the brain and other vital organs. Reye's syndrome has been linked to using aspirin in children.

rhinorrhea—Fluid draining from the nose.

rhinovirus—Viral infection of the upper respiratory system.

rhonchi—A loud whooshing sound heard with auscultation of the lungs, indicating mucus in the bronchi.

rigidity—A boardlike feeling that does not decrease when the muscles are relaxed that indicates internal bleeding.

Ritchie test—Another name for the Lachman test. Also known as the Lachman-Trillat test or the Trillat test.

roll—Movement that occurs when a point on one surface aligns with a point on its opposing surface.

rotation—Turning a segment on its axis.

rubeola—A highly contagious viral infection. Also known as measles.

Ryder method—Test used to identify retroversion and anteversion of the hip. Also known as Craig's test.

sacralization—A congenital fusion of the L5 and S1 vertebrae. On X ray there appears to be only four lumbar vertebrae.

sacral plexus—The lumbosacral trunk and the ventral rami of the S1 through S4 sacral spine nerves.

sacroiliac rotation—When the ilium rotates on the sacrum unilaterally.

sagittal plane—Imaginary plane that separates the body into right and left. Also referred to as the anterior–posterior plane.

salpingitis—A serious complication of sexually transmitted diseases in which a bacterial infection attacks the female reproductive system, spreading from the vagina to the womb, fallopian tubes, and ovaries. More commonly known as pelvic inflammatory disease (PID).

Salter-Harris classification system—The most widely accepted classification system for epiphyseal injury.

scaption—A position of shoulder abduction to 90° in a scapular plane, which is 30° anterior to the frontal plane.

scapular winging—A protrusion of the vertebral border of the scapula away from the posterior chest wall as a result of serratus anterior muscle weakness.

Scheuermann's disease—Juvenile kyphosis, or a growth disorder characterized by inflammation and osteochondritis of the thoracic vertebrae.

sciatica—Referred pain down the lower extremity along the sciatic nerve distribution.

sciatic nerve—The main branch of the sacral plexus. It is formed by spinal nerves L4 to S3.

scoliosis—A lateral or S curvature of the spinal column.

screw home mechanism—The biomechanical movement of the femur on the tibia as the knee extends and flexes.

second degree—An injury classification used to describe moderate tissue disruption and disability.

second-impact syndrome—An autoregulatory dysfunction of the brain that causes rapid and fatal brain swelling, usually a result of a secondary brain insult that is often minor.

sensory discrimination—Differentiating stimuli between two or more distinct points.

sensory nerves—Receive information from the peripheral environment and within the body and forward this information to the central nervous system in order to regulate the body's functions.

septic shock—A condition that results in severe dilation of the blood vessels and cardiovascular system collapse in response to bacterial infection.

sequelae—The progressive course of a pathological condition.

sequestration—Separation. Describes an advanced stage of disc herniation where the inner disc material becomes separated from the annulus fibrosis.

serous fluid—Watery fluid that moistens surface membranes.

serum—A watery fluid.

shear force—A force that is directed parallel to a joint or soft tissue surface.

shin splints—A general term used to describe pain and inflammation of the musculotendinous unit or periosteum along the anteromedial border of the tibia. Also known as medial tibial stress syndrome.

shock—A condition of inadequate peripheral blood flow, secondary to trauma, that results in cardiovascular collapse.

shoulder abduction test—Nerve root compression relief test.

sign—Evidence of injury that is observed or can be objectively measured.

silver fork deformity—Dorsal displacement of the distal fragments of the radius and ulna in relation to their proximal shafts; characteristic deformity of a Colles' fracture.

SINS—Stage, Irritability, Nature, and Severity of an injury.

sinus dysrhythmia—A common occurrence in which pulse rate varies with the respiratory cycle, naturally slowing with expiration and increasing with inspiration.

SI units (Système International d'Unités)—The international standard for reporting measurements.

skier's thumb—Ulnar collateral ligament rupture of the first metacarpophalangeal joint. Also known as "gamekeeper's thumb."

skin—The organ that covers the entire surface of the body.

snowball crepitus—A form of crepitus that sounds and feels as if you are compressing or rubbing the surface of a snowball with your fingers.

SOAP notes—Documentation of **s**ubjective findings, **o**bjective findings, overall **a**ssessment, and subsequent **p**lan for the athlete based on an assessment.

spasm—Involuntary muscle contraction.

Speed's test—A test used to examine the integrity of the biceps tendon.

spin—Movement that occurs when one surface rotates on a stationary axis like a spinning top.

spina bifida occulta—A congenital malformation of the lumbar spine characterized by incomplete closure of the posterior lamina at birth.

spinal stenosis—A developmental or congenital narrowing of the spinal canal.

spondylitis—An inflammation of the facet joint and its surrounding capsule.

spondylolisthesis—A secondary condition to bilateral spondylolysis, characterized by a forward subluxation of the involved vertebrae in relation to the vertebrae directly below.

spondylolysis—A fracture of pars interarticularis located between the inferior and superior facets.

spondylosis—Degenerative changes of the vertebrae and disc.

spoon-shaped nails—Severely concave nails that may indicate fungal infections.

sprain—Stretching or tearing of a ligament or capsular structure.

Sprengel's deformity—A deformity characterized by an underdeveloped scapula that sits high on the posterior chest wall, caused by a failure of the scapula to descend properly.

Spurling's test—Cervical compression with the neck in extension and rotation to the involved side.

stability—Maintenance of equilibrium or relationship of joint structures with an imposed force.

Standardized Assessment of Concussion (SAC)—Examines the immediate and prolonged effects of mild head injury on mental status, and it tracks symptom resolution over time to assist with informed decisions on return to play.

stener lesion—A complication of ulnar collateral ligament injury of the thumb in which the adductor aponeurosis gets caught between the ruptured ends of the ligament and prevents healing.

stenosis—A stricture of any canal.

stenotic—Marked or characterized by narrowing of a tunnel or canal.

stiff neck—Torticollis.

stingers—Common name for brachial plexus injuries with the classical symptoms of immediate sharp, burning pain radiating down into the arm.

stone bruise—Heel contusion.

strain—Stretching or tearing of a muscle or tendon.

stress test—A method of applying force to a structure to evaluate its integrity.

stridor—A high-pitched crowing that indicates an airway obstruction.

stroke test—Another name for a sweep test.

structural deformity—Deformity characterized by permanent structural changes in the bone or joint, which are usually congenital.

sty—An infection or obstruction of a ciliary gland of the eyelid.

subacute—Interim between acute and chronic, usually referring to later stages of the inflammatory process.

subarachnoid space—Space between the arachnoid mater and the pia mater that contains cerebral spinal fluid.

subdural hematoma—Bleeding in the subdural space.

subdural space—Space between the arachnoid mater and the dura mater.

subjective—Information gained from impression or perception; not readily observed.

subluxation—An incomplete disassociation of two joint surfaces.

substitution—Using other muscles to aid or replace the function of the intended muscle.

sulcus sign—A depression in the skin below the acromion with distraction of the glenohumeral joint.

superficial fascia—Fascia that lies just beneath the skin and covers the entire body.

superficial fibular nerve—Innervates the fibular muscles in the lateral compartment of the leg and provides sensation for the skin over the distal anterior aspect of the leg and the dorsum and digits of the foot.

superficial reflexes—Cutaneous reflexes elicited by stimulating the skin over areas where the central nervous system mediates movement.

superior gluteal nerve—Arises from the sacral plexus (L4-S1) to supply the gluteus medius and minimus and the tensor fascia latae.

superior vena cava—The vein that brings deoxygenated blood from the upper body into the heart.

supination—To rotate upward. In the foot, this represents a composite of three motions occurring at the joint—inversion, plantar flexion, and adduction of the foot in the open chain; inversion, dorsiflexion, and adduction in the closed chain. In the forearm, the motion represents rotating the hand upward or anteriorly.

supine—Lying on the back.

supracondylar fracture—Transverse fracture of the humerus just superior to the condyles.

supraspinatus strength test—A test that assesses the integrity of the supraspinatus. Also called the empty can test.

swan-neck deformity—A deformity caused by hyperextension at the PIP joint and hyperflexion at the DIP joint due to disruption of the volar plate and tensioning of the flexor tendons.

sympathectomy—Removal of sympathetic nerves.

sympathomimetic—A group of medications that mimic the actions of the sympathetic nervous system to cause vasoconstriction and open respiratory passageways.

symptom—A subjective complaint or an abnormal sensation described by the patient that cannot be directly observed.

syncope—Fainting or temporary loss of consciousness caused by inadequate blood flow to the brain.

syndesmosis—An articulation formed between two bones by a ligament.

synergists—Muscles that work with the prime mover to assist joint motion. Their contribution to joint motion varies depending on joint orientation and position.

synovial fluid—Fluid secreted by the synovial membrane to provide joint lubrication.

systolic pressure—Measures the pressure against the artery walls when the heart pumps (i.e., left ventricle contracting).

tachycardia—Rapid pulse.

tachypnea—Presence of rapid respirations.

talotibial exostosis—Excess bone growth on the anterior dome of the talus or distal tibia.

tendinitis (tendonitis)—Inflammation of a tendon.

tennis elbow—An overuse injury to the tendinous attachments of the flexor–pronator group at the medial epicondyle or the extensor–supinator group at the lateral epicondyle. Also known as epicondylitis.

tenosynovitis—Inflammation of the synovial sheath covering a tendon.

tensile force—Traction or pulling away of a structure.

tension pneumothorax—A condition in which lung collapse and increasing pressure in the pleural cavity causes the mediastinum to shift away from the injured side, compressing the heart and healthy lung and compromising their function.

theater sign—Anterior knee pain that is exacerbated by ambulation after prolonged sitting.

third degree—Injury classification used to describe severe, complete tissue disruption and disability.

thoracic outlet syndrome (TOS)—A clinical term that describes compression of the neurovascular structures as they exit through the thoracic outlet at the base of the neck.

thrombus—Blood clot.

tibial branch—Nerve branch that supplies the gastrocnemius, soleus, plantaris, and popliteus muscles.

tibial varum—Medial angulation or bowing of the tibia.

tinea corporis—A fungus that affects the scalp, trunk, and upper extremities. Also known as ringworm.

Tinel's sign—Pain or radiation of symptoms reproduced with percussion or "tapping" over a nerve.

tinnitus—Ringing in the ears.

tip grip—Grip that determines opposition strength by measuring the force exerted between the tip of the thumb and the tip of the other digits.

tonic—Refers to a sustained contraction of muscle.

torque—The force exerted by a muscle about a joint's axis of rotation.

torticollis—A deformity characterized by a lateral curvature of the cervical spine. Also known as wryneck and stiff neck.

traction—Applying a longitudinal force to a joint to separate the proximal from the distal portion.

transient neuropraxia—Temporary sensory changes such as burning, tingling, or numbness, or motor changes (weakness to temporary paralysis) in both the upper and lower extremities as a result of spinal cord compression.

transverse—Horizontal orientation or at a right angle to the long axis of a structure of the body.

transverse plane—Imaginary plane that separates the body into top and bottom.

tremor—Involuntary contractions of multiple motor units.

Trendelenburg gait—A drop of the non-weight-bearing pelvis and hip during its swing-through phase. Also known as a gluteus medius lurch.

trichomoniasis—Parasitic infestation of the genus Trichomonas.

tricuspid (AV) valve—The valve through which blood passes from the right atrium to the right ventricle.

trigger finger—Tenosynovitis of the flexor tendon sheath, most commonly seen in the third and fourth digits, resulting from thickening or nodules in the synovial sheath.

trigger point—A focal, hyperirritable area in the muscle or fascia that results in referred symptoms of pain, particularly when pressure is applied.

Trillat test—Another name for the Lachman test. Also known as the Lachman-Trillat test or the Ritchie test.

trophic—Disordered or altered nutrition.

true leg length discrepancy—A measurement difference in left and right leg length when measured between the ASIS and the medial or the lateral malleolus.

Tunnel of Guyon—A space between the pisiform and hamate bones through which the ulnar nerve passes.

turf toe—Sprain of the first metatarsophalangeal joint. Also known as great toe sprain.

twist force—A rotational force.

uncinate processes—The bony lip on the lateral aspect of the cervical vertebral body.

unhappy triad—Combined injury to the anterior cruciate ligament, medial collateral ligament, and medial meniscus.

upper motor neuron—Motor nerves originating in the cerebral cortex that send stimuli from the brain to the motor nuclei of the spinal cord.

upslip—When one ilium rides higher on the sacrum than the other ilium.

urethritis—Inflammation of the urethra.

uricemia—Excess uric acid in the blood.

urinary calculi—Kidney stones.

urticaria—Dermal hypersensitivity reaction to an allergen. More commonly known as hives.

vaginitis—Inflammation or infection of the vagina caused by microorganisms.

valgus—A medially directed force or angulation of the joint.

valgus stress—A medially directed force applied to the lateral aspect of a joint to cause gapping of the medial joint and test the integrity of the medial joint structures.

Valsalva maneuver—A test in which the athlete holds her breath and bears down or similarly blows into a closed fist to increase intrathecal pressure. A positive sign indicates a herniated disc or other space-occupying lesion within the spinal canal.

varicella—The childhood version of herpes zoster. Also known as chickenpox.

varus—A laterally directed force or angulation of the joint.

varus stress—A laterally directed force applied to the medial aspect of a joint to cause gapping of the lateral joint and test the integrity of the lateral joint structures.

vasomotor—Smooth muscle control of blood vessel size.

vasovagal—Reflex dilation of blood vessels.

venipuncture—Puncturing a vein with a needle or similar device to draw blood, deliver fluids intravenously, deliver medications, and so on.

ventricles—The two inferior chambers of the heart that pump blood into the lungs for oxygenation (right ventricle) or into the peripheral circulatory system to deliver the newly oxygenated blood to the body (left ventricle).

vertebral canal—The space formed by the anterior body and posterior arch of each vertebrae that houses and protects the spinal cord.

vertigo—Dizziness.

vesiculations—Small ruptures or blistering of the skin.

vibration test—Another name for a percussion test.

viral myocarditis—Inflammation of the heart muscle caused by a viral infection.

visceral pleura—The inner layer of the pleural sac that adheres to the surface of the lung.

volar—Palmar aspect of the wrist and hand.

Volkmann's ischemic contracture—Contracture deformity of the wrist and hand resulting from ischemic necrosis of the forearm muscles.

wheal—A reaction of the skin surface characterized by an elevation of a patch of skin that is smooth and red in appearance.

wheezing—A high-pitched whistling sound heard with auscultation, commonly noted with bronchial restriction in association with asthma.

winging of the scapula—Protrusion of the vertebral border of the scapula away from the posterior chest wall as a result of serratus anterior weakness.

wipe test—Another name for sweep test.

work—The total force applied over the length of a contraction and displayed as the area under the strength curve.

wryneck—Torticollis.

Yergason's test—A test for assessing bicipital tendinitis.

Index

About the Authors

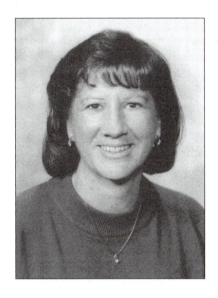

Sandra J. Shultz, PhD, ATC, CSCS, is associate professor and co-director of the Applied Neuromechanics Research Laboratory at the University of North Carolina at Greensboro. As a certified athletic trainer since 1984, she has a broad clinical perspective with experience at the collegiate, high school, and clinical settings, as well as at the Olympic and international levels.

Before coming to the University of North Carolina at Greensboro, Dr. Shultz taught and conducted clinical research in the sports medicine and athletic training program at the University of Virginia. She also served as associate director of athletic training and rehabilitative services at the University of California at Los Angeles where two of her primary responsibilities were the direct health care of student-athletes and the education of student athletic trainers.

Dr. Shultz is a member of the National Athletic Trainers' Association (NATA), the American College of Sports Medicine (ACSM), and the National Strength and Conditioning Association (NSCA). She currently serves as chair of the NATA Convention Program Committee. Previously she served on the NATA's Entry-Level Education Committee, Pronouncements Committee, and Appropriate Medical Coverage for Intercollegiate Athletics Task Force. She is actively involved in research related to injury risk of the anterior cruciate ligament in female athletes and has received grant funding from the National Federation of State High School Associations, the NATA Research and Education Foundation, and the National Institutes of Health. She is the primary author of the National Federation of State High School Athletics Association's *Sports Medicine Handbook* and the NATA's *Appropriate Medical Care for Intercollegiate Athletics.* She is also an editorial board member for the *Journal of Athletic Training.*

Dr. Shultz received her PhD from the University of Virginia and her master's degree from the University of Arizona. She received the Freddie H. Fu, MD, New Investigator Award from the NATA Foundation in 2003.

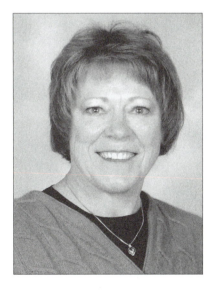

Peggy A. Houglum, PhD, ATC, PT, is an assistant professor at Duquesne University in Pittsburgh. She has more than 30 years of experience in rehabilitation providing patient and athlete care. Her extensive background as a certified athletic trainer and physical therapist has provided her with a unique perspective regarding rehabilitation programs that make therapeutic exercise techniques appropriate and effective for treatment of athletic injuries.

Dr. Houglum has clinical experience in a variety of settings, including acute care and rehabilitation hospitals, sports medicine clinics, and athletic training facilities. She has also served as an athletic trainer with the United States Olympic Sports Festivals, Olympic Games, and World University Games.

A member of the American Physical Therapy Association's Sports Medicine Section and National Athletic Trainers' Association (NATA), she is currently chair of the NATA Continuing Education Committee. Houglum also created the NATA's first formal continuing education programming in 1991. She was named to the NATA Hall of Fame, the association's highest award, in 2002, and received NATA's Most Distinguished Athletic Trainer Award in 1996. Dr. Houglum is also clinical applications editor of the *Journal of Athletic Training.* She received her PhD in sports medicine from the University of Virginia, and she received her master's degree in athletic training from Indiana State University.

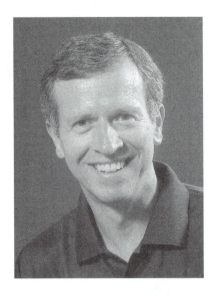

David H. Perrin, PhD, ATC, is dean of the School of Health and Human Performance and a professor at the University of North Carolina at Greensboro.

For 13 years, Dr. Perrin served as a member of the NATA Professional Education Committee, helping to write the guidelines for accreditation of both undergraduate and graduate athletic training education programs. For 15 years, he directed the graduate programs in athletic training and sports medicine in the Curry School of Education at the University of Virginia. He was editor in chief of the *Journal of Athletic Training* from 1996 to 2004 and was the founding editor of the *Journal of Sport Rehabilitation*. He is author of *Isokinetic Exercise and Assessment* and *Athletic Taping and Bracing*, editor of *The Injured Athlete, Third Edition*, and coauthor of *Research Methods in Athletic Training*.

Dr. Perrin's research interests include injury risk factors of the anterior cruciate ligament in female athletes. His awards from the National Athletic Trainers' Association include the Sayers "Bud" Miller Distinguished Educator Award, the Most Distinguished Athletic Trainer Award, the William G. Clancy, Jr., MD, Medal for Distinguished Athletic Training Research, and induction into the NATA Hall of Fame. He is a fellow of the American College of Sports Medicine and a fellow of the American Academy of Kinesiology and Physical Education.

Dr. Perrin received his master's degree from Indiana State University and his PhD from the University of Pittsburgh. In his free time, he enjoys traveling, exercising, and vacationing at his lake cottage in Vermont.

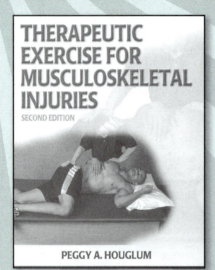
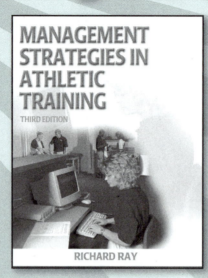
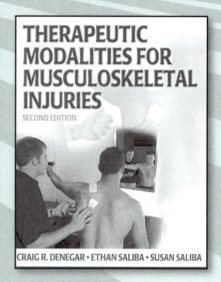
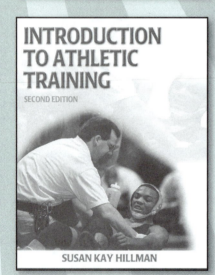
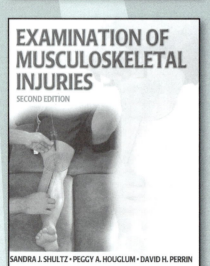